100 DRUGS
THAT WORK

100 DRUGS
THAT WORK

A Guide to the Best
Prescription and Non-prescription Drugs

Mike Oppenheim, M.D.

Lowell House
Los Angeles

Contemporary Books
Chicago

This book is not intended to encourage treatment of illness, disease, or other medical problems by the layman. Any application of the recommendations set forth in the following pages is at the reader's discretion and sole risk. If you are under a physician's care for any condition, he or she can advise you about information described in this book.

Library of Congress Cataloging-in-Publication Data

Oppenheim, Michael, 1940-
    100 drugs that work: a guide to the best prescription and non-prescription drugs / Mike Oppenheim.
        p. cm.
    Includes index.
    ISBN 1-56565-115-4
    1. Drugs—Popular works. I. Title. II. Title: One hundred drugs that work.
RM300.O67 1994
615'.1—dc20   93-23654
                                                               CIP

Some material reprinted in slightly different form from June 29, 1993, issue of *Family Circle,* © 1993, Family Circle, Inc.

Other material in somewhat different form appeared originally in *Better Homes & Gardens.*

The chapter "Ten Overused Drugs" used by permission of Meredith Corporation. All rights reserved.

Request for such permissions should be addressed to:
Lowell House
2029 Century Park East, Suite 3290
Los Angeles, CA 90067
Publisher: Jack Artenstein
Director of Publishing Services: Mary D. Aarons
Project editor: Peter L. Hoffman
Text design: Mary Ballachino/Merrimac Design

Manufactured in the United States of America
10 9 8 7 6 5 4 3 2

Contents

Part III: Drugs for digestive disorders, 119

**Part IV: Drugs for neurological and psychological
        disorders, 147**

Part V: Drugs for pain, 183

Part VI: Hormones and drugs for metabolic disorders, 211

How to Read This Book

A few weeks ago, a patient rushed in, her face so puffy that she could barely speak. I gave her an injection, and within five minutes she recovered. She was enormously relieved and I felt pleased with myself, too.

Drugs produce marvels like that, and doctors enjoy the results as much as patients. In this case, my pleasure was tempered by the knowledge that I had cured a reaction to another injection given an hour earlier. Drugs have their inconvenient side, but they *can* work wonders.

For the sheer thrill of a dramatic cure, family doctors must rely on drugs (surgeons experience this thrill more often: every appendectomy is a lifesaving cure—the most surgery I can do is remove a sliver or some earwax, but even that gets me intense gratitude; doctors love gratitude).

If a patient arrives in agonizing pain, I can make it vanish in minutes. I can calm a violent allergy, clear up asthma, and relieve vomiting. I can cure "blood poisoning" in a week and tuberculosis in a few months—genuine miracles by our grandparents' standards.

Drugs cure bacterial infections and normalize most high blood pressure. If acid burns your stomach, a drug will stop acid production; if you'd rather not get pregnant, I can provide a fairly safe means.

The drugs in this book encompass almost every one a family doctor uses. You've all taken half a dozen of them, probably from the sections on hormones or drugs for pain, infection, or digestive or respiratory problems. If other sections leave you cold, be patient. Sooner or later you'll discover an intense interest in a drug you or someone close to you must take every day, such as a blood pressure or arthritis pill.

Expect your doctor to give you some information when handing over the prescription, but not as much as you'll find here. Every medical student learns to discuss every treatment, but after a few thousand penicillin prescriptions, most doctors' penicillin lectures grow shorter. Besides, doctors genuinely believe you're not interested; polls always find we underestimate our patients' desire for information.

Even so, we give more than you hear. I'm constantly disturbed when patients insist I never gave them the information I give everyone. Doctors forget that being in the office is routine for us but stressful for patients who miss half what we say, a truth confirmed by researchers who quiz patients as they are leaving doctors' waiting rooms.

Doctors are creatures of habit. Some stick to familiar drugs (usually the best policy), but delay too long changing to those that are clearly superior. Others embrace the newest with the same eagerness many laymen show toward the latest car or computer. Although both new and old drugs usually work, they may not be the "treatment of choice." You'll learn the best treatment here.

■■■

Besides working, the hundred drugs in this book are the best, but don't despair if you're taking one I haven't included. Look at the end of the chapter where I list members of the same family. For example, dozens of diuretics resemble hydrochlorothiazide (Hydrodiuril, Esidrix, Oretic) except for a few differences trumpeted in advertisements that are not terribly important. Others have disadvantages that may or may not matter. Perhaps they cost more, produce more side effects, or have appeared too recently for nastier side effects to come to light, but most work fine. If chlorothiazide (Diuril) or polythiazide (Renese) happens to be your doctor's favorite, you're getting a good drug.

Many of the best have been around a while. The newest antibiotic in this book appeared in the early 1980s, and I don't see major changes on the horizon despite a half dozen new antibiotic approvals every year. All are stunningly expensive; most duplicate existing drugs, a few improve our treatment of obscure infections, but I wouldn't be surprised if my antibiotic section held up for the rest of the century. Dramatic advances in most fields are not terribly common—perhaps one or two per decade (AIDS and anticancer drugs are an exception; that's why I don't include them). New drugs often provide unpleasant surprises after a few million patients have tried them (FDA approval comes after tests on a few thousand).

Drugs also have a frustrating habit of losing efficacy. A reliable rule of pharmacology states that early studies, especially those carried out by the discoverer, provide the best results. Many drugs that seem terrific when released gradually fade from sight. One wise doctor told a class of medical students: "Always use a new drug when it's first released—while it still works." Sensible doctors stick to a familiar drug until a new one proves to be clearly superior.

Reading the Headings Within Each Chapter

Pay attention to "treatment of choice," another way of saying "best." Penicillin is the choice for strep throat. If you're allergic to penicillin, then erythromycin is best. You should not receive any other drug for strep throat without a good reason. One might be that the best choice upsets your stomach. Alternate drugs may work, but they never work better—and if they work equally well, they may have other disadvantages such as higher cost. You'll read more about alternates under the following heading on "good" drugs. So don't think badly of a drug that isn't a first choice. Many disorders have several equally good treatments and not a single treatment of choice.

"How it works" explains how a drug acts both to help you and to bother you with possible side effects. Doctors are taught that patients should know about these, but they rarely spend much time on drug action, partly because they've forgotten.

"How dispensed" lists forms (tablets, liquid, powder) as well as treatments for common disorders. If you receive a different dose or length of therapy, make sure you know why. For example, your doctor may prescribe a smaller dose because you are a small person (a good reason) or because he believes a small dose works as well as the usual one (he might be right, but ask for an explanation).

"Translating the label" lists drug names and that can be bewildering because almost every drug has two or more names (notice "hydrochlorothiazide" above). One is "generic," simply the name of the chemical the drug is made from (such as acetaminophen). Sometimes the company holding the patent and others that hope to carve out a market share sell the drug under a snappier brand name (*Tylenol, Datril, Panadol, Anacin-3*), hoping their advertisements will drive the generic name from your mind or (in the case of a prescription drug) the doctor's.

This confusion is inevitable as long as manufacturing drugs remains a competitive business, but I don't strongly disapprove. People who favor selling drugs by generic name eat Jello and blow their noses on Kleenex without guilt, and when they need a quick duplicate, they don't call their copying machine a "Ricoh" or a "Canon," but by another manufacturer's name. If you want the cheapest drug and are too shy to ask your doctor, ask the pharmacist for a generic when you hand over the prescription. Even if the doctor has written the brand name, it's legal almost everywhere to substitute.

All medical journals and some popular publications use generic names, adding the brand name as an afterthought: ". . . treatment of Flanagan's disease is phenylethylpropazolidine hydrate (Zappo). . . ." If that confuses you, it confuses doctors no less. Some writers omit brand names entirely, often forcing me to consult the Physician's Desk Reference ("the PDR") to find out what the author is talking about. In this book I highlight the most popular name. If everyone knows the generic (penicillin, codeine) that's what I use. Rival pharmaceutical companies may gnash their teeth, but if one brand name is clearly the most popular, I prescribe it. I never tell a patient I'm prescribing diphenoxylate-atropine or diphenhydramine. I say "Lomotil" or "Benadryl" even if I'm prescribing a generic.

This section also includes a list of other drugs in the same class. Unless I say otherwise, consider them acceptable alternatives.

■■■

Read what I write under "side effects," "interactions," and "allergies," but understand that the only drugs with *no* bad effects are those with no effects at all. When doctors prescribe, they've balanced the benefits with the risks and decided the benefits win.

I mention fewer than a half dozen drugs that cause reactions with blood thinners (see drug 38). Blood thinners are so tricky that a host of medications can cause some hazardous problems when combined with them, so your doctor must know all the drugs you're taking before prescribing one. If you don't know, go to your medicine cabinet and memorize them. If your memory isn't reliable, carry a list. Don't expect them to be "in the chart."

If a drug turns your teeth yellow, and you discover I didn't mention that, understand that I include *common* side effects: those most patients complain about. But I also include some rare ones I learned in medical school and read about in journals, but have never seen in twenty years of practice. I couldn't possibly list all reported, rumored, and hypothetical reactions.

If you're interested, you'll find all of the side effects in the Physician's Desk Reference. Like most doctors, I get a free copy every year and give the old one to nonmedical friends. They're always eager to receive what they believe is a doctor's secret book, but you can buy a PDR in bookstores. I advise against it, but if you want to know every bad thing a drug can do, the PDR tells you. I consult it every day, mostly to refresh my memory on dosages and length of therapy, but I also run my eyes over the innumerable "warnings," "precautions," "adverse reactions," and "contraindications," that fill the pages. Now and then I decide a drug is too risky for a particular patient, but mostly I go ahead despite a frightening list of side effects.

Laymen who consult the PDR about a drug I've prescribed are invariably unnerved.

"It says this causes liver damage."

"No, it doesn't. The warning says it occasionally makes liver tests abnormal. You don't need to worry about that, but I probably wouldn't give it to someone with severe liver disease."

"It says this drug may cause blindness . . . ."

"That's what it says, but no one has ever seen a case; I think a related drug did that, so the FDA insisted the manufacturer include the warning . . . ."

"It says this drug can cause a rash . . . ."

"Any drug can do that, but it doesn't happen very often . . . ."

"But I'm susceptible to rashes . . . ."

If you do buy a PDR, have a doctor on hand to calm your fears. Never rely on any book (including this one) as a guide to whether you need a particular drug.

■■■

Under "interactions," I describe how each drug might act combined with food, alcohol, other drugs, pregnancy, and nursing.

Sometimes I include its effect on sex. If advice under "pregnancy" and "nursing" seems wishy-washy, you must understand both the limitations of science and the average American doctor's fear of lawsuits.

As far as science goes, we obviously can't test new drugs on pregnant women to determine if they cause birth defects. We performed such tests in the past, although not deliberately. Doctors didn't worry about birth defects until the 1950s. Pregnant women in past generations received so many older drugs so often that we're pretty sure several of those drugs are safe. Penicillin and Tylenol are examples. However, not even the best study can "prove the negative." If bananas cause birth defects, sooner or later we'll prove it if we test enough women. But we can never say with certainty that they *don't* cause defects because, maybe, with a larger number of subjects . . . . Animal tests help, but they're not 100 percent applicable to humans.

Of course, we can *say* a risk is extremely small. Doctors train for long periods and worry a great deal about subjecting you to small but catastrophic risks in exchange for fairly certain benefits. One person in 50,000 who takes penicillin drops dead, but when a patient needs penicillin, I prescribe it. Mostly, our decisions are right. When they're wrong, we're often sued.

One effect of these suits is that doctors would rather not give any drug to a pregnant woman. Theoretically, that is correct practice because we can never prove a drug does not cause birth defects. But when confronted by a desperately miserable woman with a splitting headache, a fiery vaginal infection, or a month of vomiting, doctors don't enjoy delivering pious lectures on the virtue of a drug-free pregnancy.

In the past I consulted the PDR, but drug companies are as frightened as doctors so they confine themselves to unhelpful mush like "physicians should exercise caution in prescribing to pregnant women." Many doctors will prescribe if relieving suffering seems essential, and the woman decides, after listening to our warning of the risk, that she wants the drug.

The patient's decision does not relieve us of our responsibility, but medicine is a noble calling, and I believe doctors must accept greater risks than other professions in exchange for the privilege of practicing—whether it's the risk of catching AIDS or being sued.

Although I'll take risks for my own patients, I'm not willing to shoulder the burden for the rest of the world, so this book doesn't give anyone permission to take any drug during pregnancy or while nursing or at any other time. That's *your* doctor's responsibility.

What You Should
Know About Costs

Browsing magazines at my neighborhood drug store, I was startled to hear a woman burst into tears. Standing at the pharmacist's window, she had just learned the price of her prescription: $90 for a ten-day supply of an antibiotic. She didn't have that much with her, she explained. Couldn't he give her something less expensive?

"A pharmacist can't do that," he explained. "And there's no generic Ceclor."

Ah, Ceclor! I thought to myself. *A source of so many brutal surprises.* Cefaclor (Ceclor) is the most popular member of the cephalosporin class of antibiotic. Pediatricians commonly prescribe it for middle-ear infections for which it is a fine treatment—equal to the best. For reasons never clear to me, doctors also prescribe it to adults either as a placebo (for "bronchitis," or colds or flu) or for infections that it cures. Yet Ceclor *is not the treatment of choice for any adult infection.*

Most doctors have only a vague idea how much drugs cost, but I'm an exception because I buy them for one of my sidelines: I'm the doctor for most Los Angeles hotels. Like you, I hate buying expensive things (cars, computers, medical services) for which the quoted price means nothing because it's always inflated by "extras" that are essential: like radios in cars or keyboards for computers. So, my fee for a hotel visit includes the cost of any drugs I carry in my bag and hand out at the time of my visit.

When hotel guests ask if there is an extra charge for medication, they are always pleased when I say no. Whether it's a ten-day course of antibiotics or a hefty injection, my cost is rarely more than a few dollars—and I never give less than the best.

I *never* buy Ceclor, but if I did, I'd pay $2.15 for a single 250-mg capsule in 1993. At three times a day for ten days, that comes to $64.50—and I buy wholesale! At $90 retail, that woman was getting a bargain!

Overhearing more, I learned the woman had a skin infection for which ordinary penicillin (six cents a pill!) seemed fine. Suggesting that would have been wildly unethical, so I continued to read my magazine and was pleased to hear the pharmacist offer to phone and ask for a different prescription.

"No," she responded firmly. "This must be the best; otherwise he wouldn't prescribe it."

That was so wrong I had to speak up. Identifying myself as an M.D., I assured her that many fine antibiotics would work as well and a call from the pharmacist would not offend the doctor. After reaching the office and explaining the problem, he turned and told her the doctor felt Ceclor was exactly what she needed.

"Tell him the price!" I whispered. He nodded.

This story ends happily, but it's a true story, so the happiness isn't perfect. Stunned no less than his patient by the cost, the doctor decided Ceclor wasn't absolutely necessary.

However, like many doctors, he was in love with cephalosporins and reluctant to switch. In that case, suggested the pharmacist, the doctor might consider cephalexin (Keflex), the oldest member of the family and therefore the cheapest. Relieved, the lady left with $30 worth of pills—still three times the price of a course of penicillin, but I couldn't tell her that.

Critics of medical costs denounce pharmacies for varying wildly in their charges, and it's true you can pay double or triple for the same prescription if you pick the wrong store. Critics also denounce doctors for not prescribing generics routinely. But these are feeble obstacles to someone who wants to save money. A few phone calls will find a pharmacy with the lowest price. Anyone who wants a generic should simply ask the pharmacist. Unless the doctor has taken the trouble to write "DNS" (do not substitute) on the prescription, that's what you'll get.

Phoning from the pharmacy is not likely to catch on, so the time to prevent drug shock is before the doctor writes the prescription. You'll find plenty of help here, and once you've read this book you'll know more about drug prices than your doctor. If he or she wants to give you Noroxin at $2.50 a pill (wholesale!) for your bladder infection, you can politely ask what the objections are to sulfa at six cents.

Make a mental adjustment when you read "wholesale costs." Retail prices vary so much I couldn't guess what they'd be, but most pharmacies pay the same wholesale. Don't expect to pay less than double wholesale at the biggest discount pharmacy; triple or quadruple is more likely. You should also know that, besides its markup, the pharmacy adds several dollars for the labor of counting the pills and typing the label, so don't be surprised if you pay $5 for pills that cost fifty cents wholesale.

Finally, the cost you'll see here is the lowest I pay, so it will be for a generic even if the chapter title is a brand name. A 25-mg Benadryl capsule costs 20 cents wholesale, but I pay 1.6 cents for 25 mg of generic diphenhydramine.

Huge medical organizations insist on special treatment, so they may pay half my costs. Kaiser-Permanente is huge, so members should expect to benefit. Anyone over 50 can join the American Association of Retired Persons and buy cheaper than retail. AARP's address is 1909 K Street NW, Washington, DC 20049.

PART I
Antibiotics and Other Drugs for Infections

Antibiotics kill germs but not viruses. In fact, when researchers studying viruses in the laboratory pour antibiotics over a culture to prevent bacterial contamination, the viruses grow quite happily.

Germs turn out to be easy prey because they are complex living creatures that move, breathe, eat, and reproduce much the same as higher animals. Finding chemicals that interfere with these processes (i.e., antibiotics) is not too difficult. Viruses are *much* harder to kill. Far tinier than a germ, a virus outside a living cell resembles a crystal. It also behaves like one; it's inert. No drug can block a virus's essential function because none exists. Boiling water or a strong antiseptic can destroy a virus, but that is not practical when treating patients. Experts debate whether any virus can actually be called "alive."

A virus remains inert until it enters a living cell. Once inside it begins to reproduce, but unfortunately, it does that by taking over your cell's reproductive apparatus so the cell (not the virus) manufactures more viruses. Now that the virus is doing something, we can interfere, but since your own cells are doing the work, fighting a viral infection can wreak havoc; many antiviral drugs are very poisonous. Researchers are gradually growing more clever, so newer antivirals like Zovirax (16.) are surprisingly safe. Even better ones are coming, but the twenty-first century will be with us before drugs to attack viral infections work as well as antibiotics do against germs.

▌
Penicillin

Arranging flowers one morning sometime before 1945, a woman pricked herself on a rose thorn. Late that day her fingertip became sore. The next day it grew painful enough to bring her to the doctor, who prescribed a salve and hot compresses. Three days later, sweating with fever, her hand inflamed and swollen, she entered the hospital, where nurses wrapped the arm in hot towels. Weeks passed as the infection climbed higher. When her fingers became black and gangrenous, the doctor considered amputating the arm. Sometimes it helped, but in this case the infection had spread too far. Pus oozed from sores that sprang up from head to feet; a convulsion revealed that an abscess had formed in her brain. As the gangrene advanced and her fever rose, she mercifully sank into a coma and died.

That was "blood poisoning," a term so terrifying 50 years ago that we still remember it. As frightening as "cancer," it called up images of an agonizing, drawn-out illness that killed men and women in their prime of life. Today, the woman would take her sore finger to a doctor, receive a few dollars' worth of penicillin, and be well in a few days. When I perform a similar miracle every week or two, my patients never give it a thought.

You may have heard of Alexander Fleming's discovery of penicillin. Returning to his London laboratory on a Monday in 1928, he noticed that several culture dishes had been left out without lids, so mold had settled out of the air and grown over the bacteria. Instead of discarding the contaminated plates, Fleming made the observation that won him his Nobel prize. Although most dishes contained mold overgrowing bacteria, one revealed a circle of dead bacteria surrounding a single mold colony. Fleming realized the colony was secreting something that killed bacteria.

Twenty years later, when Fleming became a medical superstar, popular writers invented the usual nonsense required for someone who makes a great discovery. They portrayed him as a visionary who foresaw the millions of lives to be saved and who worked tirelessly against great odds to bring his discovery to fruition. The truth is that after a few years' research, Fleming lost interest in penicillin. He published no papers on it after 1932. That year he had the honor of making the Presidential address at the Royal Society of Medicine. He could choose his own subject—and he didn't choose penicillin.

The story of penicillin—and of antibiotics in general—begins with Louis Pasteur in the nineteenth century. It's wonderful to read about not only because the stories are fascinating but because it ends happily with one of the great positive accomplishments of human ingenuity. The best book on the subject is *In Search of Penicillin*, by David Wilson (Knopf, 1976). It's out of print, but your library can locate a copy.

You probably don't recognize the names Howard Florey and Ernst Chain, who shared Fleming's Nobel prize. They converted penicillin from an obscure substance known only to bacteriologists (its status in 1938) into the most miraculous drug of the century.

Researchers at Oxford, Florey and Chain wanted to investigate natural substances that killed bacteria. To choose which to study they did what any sensible scientist does: went to the library and read through scientific journals. They found three candidates; one was penicillin.

The first bacterial inhibitor candidate turned out to be toxic, so Florey and Chain turned to penicillin. That was not as easy as it sounds. All they had to go on was an interesting mold juice full of a thousand impurities and impossible to test even on animals. When Fleming and others had tried to purify the juice, the penicillin disappeared. After months of tiresome trial-and-error the Oxford researchers developed a laughably (to our eyes) cumbersome process that required a refrigerated room in which technicians ("penicillin girls") wearing overcoats and mufflers mixed and shook gallon bottles of ether with mold juice to isolate tiny quantities of precious powder.

No journalistic invention can overdramatize the first penicillin treatment in 1941. The patient was Albert Alexander, a policeman who had scratched his cheek while gardening. Blood poisoning developed, and after two months Alexander was near death with draining abscesses covering his body, one eye lost, and his lungs filling with infection. One day after the first dose of penicillin his fever dropped and the abscesses stopped draining. By the fourth day the policeman was eating and feeling well, but the supply of penicillin was running out despite desperate efforts to extract penicillin from his urine to give a second round. After five days there was no more, and he died.

Penicillin is treatment of choice for:

1. *Cellulitis.* This is "blood poisoning" except it no longer gets to that point. A skin infection caused by the streptococcus, it begins after a minor injury, in many cases too minor to be noticed. The victim notices somewhere on the body a painful, red area that quickly spreads. Only the most stoic patient can stay away from the doctor more than a few days. I prescribe 500 mg of penicillin four times a day for ten days and expect improvement in a few days.

2. *Strep throat.* Mostly a disease of children, this streptococcal infection produces a sore throat, fever, swollen neck glands, and *no cough or cold symptoms.* Most adult sore throats are viral infections, although your doctor will probably give you an antibiotic anyway.

   Penicillin V 250 mg four times a day works fine, *but you must take it for ten days.* Even without treatment, strep goes away in four or five days, but several weeks later a small percentage of victims develop rheumatic fever, a mysterious illness that inflames the heart and often produces permanent valve damage. Before heart attacks took over in the 1940s, rheumatic heart disease was the leading cardiac killer—and it's still not rare.

   Mothers often ask for a "shot of penicillin" to make their child well more quickly. Despite popular belief, penicillin shots don't work significantly faster than pills.

3. *Pneumococcal pneumonia.* Forty years ago, this section would have been titled simply "pneumonia." At that time when someone came down with a severe cough and fever, and a chest x-ray showed pneumonia, the pneumococcus was probably responsible (that's how the germ got its name).

   Life is more complicated today. Obscure microorganisms like legionella (remember the Legionnaire's disease panic in the mid-1970s?; it turned out to be a fairly common pneumonia) and mycoplasma have risen to prominence. Although pneumococcal pneumonia remains common, mycoplasma causes more lung infections in otherwise healthy people, and penicillin can't kill mycoplasma. Unless your doctor can isolate the pneumococcus (not easy unless he sticks a needle into your lung, and we do that only on someone seriously ill), erythromycin (5.) is the treatment of choice for pneumonia.

4. *Syphilis.* Still a common sexually transmitted disease. Treatment of early syphilis is with an injection of a long-acting penicillin. Pills never work. Advanced syphilis requires several weekly injections.

DOCTOR OPPENHEIM ON INJECTIONS. I treat strep by injection for one reason: when I don't trust the patient to take the full course. Taking all ten days of penicillin is so critical for preventing rheumatic fever that research projects have tried to make it simpler. They've discovered that 500 mg twice a day works as well as 250 mg four times. *Do not stop.*

MEDICAL SECRET. If your doctor prescribes less than ten days of antibiotic, he doesn't believe you have strep. Except for diphtheria, strep is the only bacterial throat infection experts recognize. If you have a virus, your doctor is giving you antibiotics so you won't think you've wasted your time coming to the office. Experience has taught us that patients with a miserable sore throat yearn for "strong" medicine and are disappointed when we prescribe throat lozenges and aspirin.

But if you're an exception, let the doctor know quickly. Say something like "I just want to know why I'm sick and what to do. I don't want an antibiotic unless it'll really help." Don't wait until he announces you need one because he probably won't reverse himself. If you're still not sure you need an antibiotic, *take it.* Patients who decide on their own to ignore a doctor's instructions get into terrible trouble. Either speak up or follow orders.

5. *Meningitis.* Provided it's caused by the meningococcus or pneumococcus, usually the case in adults and older children.
6. *Human and animal bites.* Giving an antibiotic to prevent infection seems reasonable, but it doesn't work well, and we do it only in a few circumstances. Human bites are one; they lead to nasty infections so frequently that everyone should be treated immediately. An animal bite is not as dangerous, so we may simply clean it and leave it alone, but if an infection develops, penicillin is the treatment: 500 mg four times a day for a week or two.
7. *Lyme disease.* But *only* in pregnant women and young children. Adults take 500 mg four times a day for three weeks. One of the tetracyclines is best for other adults; I discuss Lyme disease in the tetracycline chapter.
8. *Less common (but not rare) infections* like trench mouth, anthrax, listeriosis, gas gangrene, lung abscess, yaws, and actinomycosis.

Penicillin is good for :

Gonorrhea, in those areas of the world where penicillin-resistant bacteria cause only a few cases. Nowadays this excludes most parts of the world, so the traditional, punishing, double-penicillin shot is passing into history.

How it works

Penicillin poisons bacteria by weakening their cell walls so they crumple and the germ falls apart. You should appreciate this precise action; it means penicillin can't poison *you* because human cells don't have walls, only thin rubbery membranes. Other antibiotics are more or less toxic to *all* living cells, so doctors can give only a limited dose, but we pour in titanic amounts of penicillin for deadly infections like meningitis—20 times more than we'd use for a routine illness.

How dispensed

Pills of 250 and 500 mg and liquids of 125 and 250 mg per teaspoon. Unlike more convenient drugs, you must take penicillin three or four times a day, although twice a day works for strep throat. You must also *always* empty the bottle. Doctors prescribe antibiotics in exactly the amount needed to cure your infection. If any remains when you stop, you've done something wrong.

Injectable versions come in many forms: long-acting (benzathine penicillin, L-A Bicillin) for syphilis and strep throat, short-acting (procaine penicillin, Wycillin, Pfizerpen) for gonorrhea, and a mixture of both (C-R Bicillin) sometimes used for strep throat in children because the injection is less painful.

Translating the label

Other names are Penicillin V, phenoxymethyl penicillin, Betapen, Pen-Vee K, and Veetids.

Side effects

Penicillin rates high here. As usual, the PDR lists horrifying reactions, but in practice they rarely occur. Penicillin doesn't routinely upset the stomach or cause drowsiness—two side effects that worry my patients most.

Interactions

Food. No problem; you can take penicillin before or after eating.

Alcohol. No problem.

Drugs. Don't take other antibiotics at the same time; some seem to cancel penicillin's action. Experts warn that penicillin and other antibiotics lessen the activity of birth control pills and can result in spotting and even pregnancy. I don't know any doctor who has encountered that, but we do worry about it.

Pregnancy. No evidence it causes birth defects. As an old drug, penicillin reaps the benefit of a massive experiment that couldn't be done today (we didn't realize it was an experiment at the time). During the 1940s and 1950s when doctors worried less about birth defects, pregnant women received plenty of penicillin. It did not cause harm—which was not the case with a few other antibiotics such as sulfa and tetracycline.

Nursing. Penicillin is excreted into milk. Sensitization to drugs and foods occurs most often during the first year of life, so I'm more reluctant to give penicillin to women who are nursing than when they were pregnant.

Allergies

Fatal allergic reactions are more common with penicillin than other antibiotics, although most follow injections, not pills. Less serious reactions (itching, rashes, fever) are not rare but are less common than everyone believes. Not all rashes signal an allergy, and an upset stomach (rare with penicillin but common with other drugs) is almost always simple irritation, not an allergy.

If you're genuinely allergic to penicillin, erythromycin works fine for cellulitis as well as streptococcal and pneumococcal infections, although it's three times more expensive and has more annoying side effects. Many doctors prescribe one of the cephalosporins (Keflex, Velosef, Ceclor). Although these work as well, they're 5 to 50 times more expensive! Tetracycline is the alternative for syphilis.

Wholesale cost:

Penicillin is cheap. In 1993, I paid three cents per 250-mg pill, six cents for 500 mg. A one-shot injection for strep throat cost $11.

2 Amoxicillin • 3 Augmentin

Soon after penicillin appeared, scientists began tinkering with the molecule. The first "semisynthetic" penicillin had identical action, but was more reliable when taken orally because it resisted acid breakdown. This was penicillin V, discussed in the previous section.

During the 1950s, more tinkering produced ampicillin, which kills the same germs as penicillin plus several more. Ten years later, amoxicillin appeared. Effective against the same germs as ampicillin, it's absorbed better from the GI tract and produces a higher blood level so the dose is three times a day instead of four. For years after its release, amoxicillin cost more than ampicillin, and its advantages weren't great enough to overcome that. Now that costs are the same, there's no reason to use ampicillin.

The most popular prescription drug in the world, amoxicillin is also the leading seller in the U.S., making up 5 percent of *all* prescriptions. Although a valuable antibiotic, amoxicillin owes much of its popularity to wide use as a placebo. Doctors prescribe it extensively for colds and other viral infections.

Amoxicillin is treatment of choice for:

Middle ear infection. Mainly a disease of children, it typically begins during an upper respiratory infection and causes an earache. Occasionally, a child too young to talk will be feverish and fussy, and the doctor discovers the infection by looking in the ear. I can't remember seeing an infection in an older child who didn't also have pain.

Overdiagnosing middle ear infections in a young child is wise because infections can damage the developing ear. For older children and adults, this is another convenient diagnosis (like "strep" and "bronchitis") that enables the doctor to prescribe an antibiotic for a viral infection. Here are clues that make a middle ear infection unlikely:

- Pain in both ears. The left ear is entirely separate from the right, so germs rarely invade both simultaneously, but the generalized congestion of a cold routinely does this. Treatment is decongestants.

· Pain during rapid pressure changes: flying, swimming, driving through mountains. The middle ear contains air as well as a passage (the eustachian tube) opening into the back of the nose. During pressure changes, air moves in and out through the eustachian tube. When the tube is blocked by congestion from a cold or allergy, air is trapped in the ear. Changes in pressure force the eardrum to balloon in and out, and that hurts. Treatment is decongestants and nasal spray.

· Pain after cleaning your ear with a cotton swab, being careful (as you assure your doctor) not to shove it in too far and puncture the drum. You have damaged the delicate lining of the canal and caused an infection—an *external* ear infection, not the one amoxicillin cures. Suspect an external infection if it hurts to pull your earlobe. Treatment is usually antibiotic ear drops.

These are good but not infallible clues. Call your doctor if your ear hurts, and go to the office if you can't reach him.

Amoxicillin is good for:

1. *Urinary tract infections*
2. *Sinus infections*
3. *Exacerbations of chronic bronchitis*
4. *Gonorrhea*

Amoxicillin and ampicillin, essentially identical, work for everything penicillin does, but they should never be prescribed instead of penicillin because they are *not* superior and cost three times more. Gonorrhea is the exception. For someone terrified of injections, a large oral dose of amoxicillin is a substitute for a shot of penicillin in those cases where penicillin still works (penicillin pills *never* work for gonorrhea).

How they work

Exactly the same as penicillin, but they kill a few more species of germs. When it first appeared, ampicillin cured serious intestinal infections including those caused by Salmonella (typhoid is one) and Shigella. But in poor countries, anyone can buy antibiotics over the counter like aspirin, and everyone takes them like aspirin, so these germs became resistant.

Closer to home, Hemophilus, one bacteria that causes middle ear infections, is showing signs of resistance, so by the mid-1990s the best treatment will probably be Augmentin, a combination of amoxicillin with a chemical called clavulanate that neutralizes this resistance. An excellent antibiotic, it's still under patent and very expensive.

How dispensed

Amoxicillin: capsules of 250 and 500 mg, chewable tablets of 125 and 250 mg, and liquids of 125 and 250 mg per teaspoon. For small children there are drops containing 50 mg per ml. The adult dose is 250 to 500 mg three times a day.

Augmentin: tablets of 250 and 500 mg of amoxicillin plus 125 mg of clavulanate; chewable tablets containing 125 mg of amoxicillin and 31.25 mg of clavulanate and another chewable tablets with twice this dose. Finally, there is an oral suspension of 125 mg of amoxicillin and 31.25 mg of clavulanate and another with double this concentration. The dose is identical to amoxicillin.

Ampicillin: capsules of 250 and 500 mg, a liquid of 125, 250, and 500 mg per teaspoon, and drops with 100 mg per ml. Four times a day is the proper schedule.

Translating the label

Amoxicillin: Amoxil, Polymox, Trimox, Wymox. With clavulanate there is only Augmentin.

Ampicillin: Omnipen, Polycillin, Principen.

Side effects

Diarrhea is fairly common, especially in children, because these drugs kill more colon bacteria than plain penicillin. Augmentin is the worse offender. This is not an allergic reaction nor does it mean the drug isn't working. Unless it's intolerable, keep taking it.

Interactions

Food. No problem; you can take them before or after eating.
Alcohol. No problem.

Drugs. The same as penicillin.

Pregnancy. Probably as safe as penicillin although no one knows for sure. Being newer, they weren't casually given to pregnant women, but no one seems alarmed.

Nursing. Like penicillin, mothers excrete these into their milk, so they shouldn't be prescribed without a good reason.

Allergies

If you're allergic to penicillin, you're allergic to amoxicillin, ampicillin, and Augmentin.

The ampicillin rash is not an allergy, but you must know about it because your doctor might not.

Ten percent of everyone given ampicillin or amoxicillin erupts with small pink spots three or four days later. For an unknown reason this happens to over 90 percent of patients with infectious mononucleosis ("mono"—a viral infection for which antibiotics are useless). The rash is sometimes itchy, but never intensely so. Stopping the antibiotic isn't necessary, and the spots fade after a few days.

As mentioned in the previous section, alternative antibiotics are never superior, always more expensive, and often have more unpleasant side effects, so you don't want "allergic to penicillin" in large red letters on your chart unless it's true. If you think you have an ampicillin rash, suggest this. But if the doctor maintains it's an allergy, believe him unless you can find another who disagrees. Remember, the doctor on the spot takes priority over this book.

Wholesale cost

I pay 7 cents for a 250-mg amoxicillin capsule, 6 cents for ampicillin; 500 mg costs slightly less than twice as much. Augmentin is steeper: $1.60 for 250 mg, $2.50 for 500 mg.

4
Dicloxacillin

Like amoxicillin, a form of penicillin, but unlike amoxicillin doesn't kill a greater variety of germs than penicillin. It's actually weaker against most, but superior at killing staph, a particularly common and virulent germ.

Dicloxacillin is the best treatment for:

Staphylococcal skin infections. You've probably suffered them at some time during your life. Common ones:

Impetigo. Small blisters appear on the face and quickly burst, leaving itchy, crusty patches. Affects other areas of the body less often. Although mostly a disease of children, impetigo is not rare in adults.

Folliculitis, an infection of hair follicles that produces many small, painful pimples, which I see most often in the beard area, armpits, and buttocks.

Boils (furuncles, carbuncles). Another hair follicle infection, these are larger, painful lumps. A boil is a mass of pus: a thick paste of living and dead staphylococci plus the cells fighting them. Antibiotics can't penetrate to the center of the pus, so they never cure it. A boil must be drained; if you wait long enough that happens spontaneously, but relief is quicker when a doctor does it. We often give antibiotics to prevent the infection's spreading, but they probably aren't necessary once draining begins.

Mastitis, breast infection that produces painful, red, swollen area around nipple, usually during nursing.

Dicloxacillin is good for:

Cellulitis and strep throat: the first two listings in the penicillin section. Doctors give dicloxacillin if they're worried about staph. Once they're certain staph isn't involved, they should switch to regular penicillin.

How it works

When Fleming noticed something killing germs on his culture plate, the dead germs were staphylococci. Until well into the 1940s penicillin killed staph nicely. Then some infections persisted despite huge doses, and doctors were introduced to antibiotic resistance—a problem that still plagues us.

Researchers discovered that some staph secreted a chemical that destroyed penicillin. Called penicillinase, it worked by breaking the penicillin molecule at one spot. Once broken, the antibiotic became powerless. Today most staphylococci make penicillinase.

Then scientists produced one of the great triumphs of science. Having learned how penicillinase works, researchers studied how to frustrate it. Since it attacks a single spot on the penicillin structure, why not attach a bulky molecule nearby to prevent penicillinase from coming near? So they did, and it worked. Soon a family of "penicillinase-resistant penicillins" sprung up, each with a different molecule shielding the vulnerable spot. Some (methicillin, nafcillin, oxacillin) are given intravenously for severe staph infections. Dicloxacillin is the most popular oral form, although cloxacillin (Tegopen) works as well.

How dispensed

Capsules of 125, 250, and 500 mg and a suspension containing 62.5 mg per teaspoon. The usual adult dose is 250 to 500 mg four times a day.

Translating the label

Dicloxacillin brand names are Dynapen and Pathocil.

Side effects

Same as penicillin.

Interactions

Food. Best taken on an empty stomach.
Alcohol. No problem.
Drugs. Same as penicillin.

Pregnancy. No one is certain if it's safe.

Nursing. Like penicillin, mothers excrete it into their milk.

Allergies

Penicillin allergy includes dicloxacillin.

Wholesale cost

27 cents for 250-mg capsule; 47 cents for 500 mg.

5
Erythromycin

Secreted by a fungus discovered in Philippine soil in 1952, erythromycin rivals amoxicillin as the most popular antibiotic for people who don't need an antibiotic. If you have a cold, sore throat, viral respiratory infection, flu, or "bronchitis," and your doctor suspects you won't be satisfied with aspirin and cough medicines, you'll probably receive erythromycin. After a few days you'll recover and give the antibiotic credit. When that happens a few times, you'll assume your particular infection requires erythromycin.

Despite extensive use as a placebo, erythromycin remains one of the most valuable antibiotics for treating common bacterial infections.

Erythromycin is treatment of choice for:

1. *Pneumonia* in otherwise healthy people. Pneumonia means "lung infection," so there are as many pneumonias as there are microorganisms—hundreds. You're always better off if a doctor knows which one caused your infection, but that is difficult with pneumonia. Many organisms produce similar symptoms (cough, fever, and feeling ill), the same physical exam (the doctor hears crackles as the air you breathe bubbles through pus in the lung),

and a typical chest x-ray (patches of fluid where there should be clear lung).

In the most common lab test, you cough into a cup and the lab cultures the sputum to identify whatever germs grow. Although easy to perform, the test is unreliable, because germs that normally live in the throat fly out with the sputum, and that's usually what the lab finds.

Despite our clever machines and tests, we still identify a disease best by examining a piece of it. We can get a piece of pneumonia by sticking a needle through your chest into a lung, sucking out some pneumonia fluid, and sending it to the lab. Although far superior to a sputum culture, it's slightly risky, so we reserve it for patients sick enough to be hospitalized. When a patient isn't that sick, we assume it's one of the common germs (viruses don't often cause pneumonia).

When I see a healthy adult with pneumonia, I prescribe erythromycin for two weeks, then see the patient in a month to make sure the x-ray has returned to normal. I want to be called if there's no improvement in a few days, but that rarely happens because erythromycin cures the most common "community-acquired" pneumonia caused by a microorganism called mycoplasma. It also cures the second most common: pneumococcal pneumonia. Penicillin only cures the second, so you shouldn't get it without a definite diagnosis. As a bonus, erythromycin is also the best treatment for—

2. *Legionnaire's disease.* You may remember the hysteria in the mid-1970s when hundreds of American Legion conventioneers fell ill and dozens died. Rumors of food poisoning or a toxin in the air conditioning ruined the hotel that hosted the convention, but the cause proved to be an obscure but surprisingly common bacteria. Although preferring to attack smokers and people with chronic illness, Legionnaire's may be a fairly common pneumonia in the general population.

3. *Cellulitis and strep throat.* Provided you're allergic to penicillin. Other antibiotics that work are more expensive but probably not superior.

Erythromycin is good for:

1. *Chlamydial infections.* These are a large family including the most common sexually transmitted bacterial infection. Tetracyclines are treatment of choice, so you'll find out more in that section.

2. *Pertussis (whooping cough)*. Given early, it shortens the illness, but it's useless once severe coughing begins.
3. *Staphylococcal skin infections.*
4. *Acne.*

How it works

Although mostly a substitute for penicillin, erythromycin works differently by attaching to structures inside the bacteria that manufacture proteins, blocking their action. Since living things are mostly protein, a bacteria that can't make protein can't grow or multiply, but it doesn't die.

You might think an antibiotic that kills germs works better than one that doesn't. Some doctors think so, too, but they're wrong. If an antibiotic restrains germs causing an infection, the body's defenses quickly get the upper hand and wipe them out. If the body's defenses are weak, antibiotics are not so helpful. If defenses are absent, no antibiotic can keep an infection at bay.

How dispensed

Tablets of 250, 333, 400, and 500 mg and a suspension containing 100, 125, 200, and 400 mg per teaspoon. One gram a day (1,000 mg) is minimum for an adult, two grams for pneumonia and more serious infections.

Translating the label

Erythromycin comes under a torrent of names but most begin with "E" or "I": ERYC, Erythrocin, EryPed, E-mycin, Ery-Tab, E.E.S., Ilotycin, and Ilosone. Wyamycin and PCE are the exceptions.

Side effects

Erythromycin produces fewer serious side effects but more complaints than any antibiotic. A solid minority of patients have stomach pain; others suffer nausea and vomiting, a sign of stomach irritation, not allergy, and it's not dangerous. If you can stand the discomfort, there's no reason to stop, but if it's too unpleasant, ask your doctor to switch to something else. Doctors routinely advise taking erythromycin with food, but I'm not sure that helps.

Now that I've told you erythromycin might upset your stomach, don't refuse it unless you've already experienced this. The odds are better than 50/50 it won't, and you should try to take the best antibiotic for the job.

Interactions

Food. Absorption is better on an empty stomach although some coated and delayed-release capsules are supposed to overcome this.

Alcohol. Erythromycin is excreted through the liver and is also slightly irritating to that organ, so experts discourage drinking at the same time. Although healthy people shouldn't worry, they should obey this warning.

Drugs. Erythromycin can increase the blood level of theophylline (Theo-dur, Theo-bid), a common antiasthma drug, and carbamazepine (Tegretol), an epilepsy drug, as well as digitalis, so you're more likely to suffer side effects from these drugs. Tell the doctor if you're taking them; don't assume he or she knows. Older patients on the blood thinner coumadin (Warfarin, Panwarfin) must be watched closely because the combination can make their blood even thinner.

Pregnancy. As one of the oldest antibiotics, many pregnant women took erythromycin before we realized that might be risky, and no one noticed birth defects. Today erythromycin is treatment of choice for pregnant women with syphilis who are allergic to penicillin because alternatives aren't safe; we are more reluctant to give erythromycin for less severe infections.

Nursing. Excreted into milk but probably safe.

Allergies

Very rare. Almost everyone who insists he or she is allergic has suffered only a stomach upset.

Wholesale cost

Eight cents for 250 mg, 18 cents for 500 mg.

The Cephalosporins:
Keflex, Ceclor, Rocephin

A cephalosporin spelling bee might be an annual event at the AMA convention, won by the doctor with the best memory for trivia. Dozens are available; more appear every year; all the names sound alike: cephalothin, cefazolin, cephalexin, cefaclor, cefamandole, cefotaxime, ceftriaxone . . . . Three have proven useful for my office and hotel patients, and my knowledge of the rest remains sketchy. But they are a scientific triumph. Once the news of penicillin spread, researchers ransacked the dank basements, swamps, and garbage dumps of the world, searching for lifesaving molds. The search continues, and millions of samples have produced dozens of important drugs, not all antibiotics. Among the most precious was Cephalosporium fungus isolated in 1948 from a sewage outlet off the Sardinian coast. Like penicillin, it killed staphylococci. Unlike penicillin, it still does.

Unpatented penicillin is cheap, so drug companies don't advertise it much. Cephalosporins are patentable and expensive, and companies have publicized their virtues with great success. They are vastly overprescribed.

The molecule resembles penicillin, and the first cephalosporins weren't a significant improvement. Tinkering with the molecule quickly produced a flood of similar cephalosporins. At first they were nearly identical to the original, but by the 1970s some killed new varieties of bacteria, so they received a separate title as "second-generation cephalosporins." In the 1980s, newcomers killed different germs, so they became the third generation. Further generations are in the works.

Don't make the mistake of many patients and a few doctors by assuming that new or "broad spectrum" antibiotics are superior. They are merely different. Third-generation cephalosporins work best against bacteria that attack hospitalized or seriously ill patients. They tend to be weaker than the old first generation in fighting staph, strep, and similar germs that cause infections that I see in the office.

Here are three of the best:

6
Cephalexin (Keflex): A First-Generation Cephalosporin

Cephalexin is treatment of choice for:

Nothing. Specialists use first-generation cephalosporins for certain serious infections, but they are not the treatment of choice for anything I see in the office.

Cephalexin is good for:

1. *Cellulitis*
2. *Strep throat*
3. *Some pneumonias*
4. *Staphylococcal skin infections*
5. *Urinary tract infections.*

In other words, it substitutes for one of the penicillins. For the first four above, erythromycin is cheaper, but if a patient has had a bad experience I'll use cephalexin. I also use it for an uncomplicated urinary tract infection when a patient is allergic to both penicillin and sulfas.

How it works

Like penicillin, cephalosporins interfere with construction of the bacterial cell wall.

How dispensed

Tablets and capsules of 250 mg and 500 mg and a suspension containing 125 and 250 mg per teaspoon. Usual dose is 250 mg four times a day, 500 mg for severe infections and pneumonia. 500 mg twice a day works as well for strep throat.

Translating the label

Cefalexin is also known as Keflex, Keftab, Biocef, Cefanex, and Zartan.
Although it's the most popular of the first generation, you may encounter:
· Cefadroxil (Duricef)
: Cephradine (Velosef)
· Cefazolin (Ancef, Kefzol)

Side effects

The great popularity of cephalosporins is not entirely the result of fashion and publicity. Doctors appreciate the low incidence of side effects and so do patients. Allergic reactions happen less often than with penicillins and upset stomachs less often than with erythromycin.

Interactions

Food. Absorption is quicker on an empty stomach, but all will be absorbed eventually, so taking it after meals is all right.

Alcohol. No problem.

Drugs. Same as penicillin.

Pregnancy. Probably safe; given to rats, huge doses don't cause birth defects. Since animal tests aren't always applicable to humans, that doesn't prove cephalosporins are harmless, so doctors are reluctant to prescribe them unless there's no choice.

Nursing. Excreted into milk but no one has noticed any problems.

Allergies

Since cephalosporins resemble penicillin, you might think their allergies overlap. Experts certainly worry and constantly warn doctors about prescribing them to patients allergic to penicillin. Doctors tend to do it anyway, and I've never had a problem, but I wouldn't give a cephalosporin to anyone who's had a serious reaction to penicillin.

Wholesale cost

Cost is 15 cents for 250 mg capsule; twice that for 500 mg.

7
Cefaclor (Ceclor): A Second-Generation Cephalosporin

Cefaclor is treatment of choice for:

Nothing.

Cefaclor is good for:

1. *Cellulitis*
2. *Strep throat*
3. *Some pneumonias*
4. *Staphylococcal skin infections*
5. *Middle ear infections* (for those in children many consider cefaclor the treatment of choice)
6. *Urinary tract infections*
7. *Sinus infections*
8. *Exacerbations of chronic bronchitis*

This list may explain cefaclor's amazing popularity. Like laypeople, doctors often believe the more germs an antibiotic kills, the better it is. The truth is the exact opposite. If a doctor is smart enough to discover the exact germ causing an infection, the best drug kills it and no other. This is one reason why penicillin is such a good antibiotic. It has a "narrow" spectrum.

How it works

Second-generation cephalosporins kill a modestly larger number of bacteria than the first generation. That increases their utility for children with ear infections and older smokers with chronic bronchitis, but cheaper antibiotics work as well.

How dispensed

Capsules of 250 and 500 mg and suspension containing 125, 187, 250, and

---

THE DOWNSIDE OF BROAD-SPECTRUM ANTIBIOTICS.
Without a diagnosis, killing as many different germs as possible is a messy, inferior tactic. The drug might miss the responsible germ, kill its rivals, and make things worse. It will certainly create havoc among the scores of germs that live peacefully on your skin and in your mouth, digestive tract, and genitals. Havoc includes digestive upsets, itchy fungal infections, and "superinfections" from obscure germs that resist most antibiotics.

---

375 mg per teaspoon. Adult dose is 250 mg three times a day, 500 mg for severe infections.

Translating the label

Cefaclor is still under patent, so you'll only see it as Ceclor.
Other second generations include:
- Cefuroxime (Ceftin, Zinacef, Kefurox)
- Cefamandole (Mandol)
- Cefoxitin (Mefoxin)
- Cefonicid (Monocid)
- Cefmatazole (Zefazone)
- Cefprozil (Cefzil)

Side effects

As uncommon as first generation.

Interactions

No different from first generation—except that several occasionally produce flushing and headaches when taken with alcohol. Cefaclor is not one of those.

Allergies

The same.

Wholesale cost

$2.10 for 250-mg capsule; $4.20 for 500 mg. That's wholesale.

8
Ceftriaxone (Rocephin): A Third-Generation Cephalosporin

Ceftriaxone is treatment of choice for:

Gonorrhea. Increasing penicillin resistance of the gonococcus boosted ceftriaxone into the top category in most areas of the country by the 1980s.

Ceftriaxone is good for:

Early syphilis, severe bone, joint, and abdominal infections; meningitis and pneumonia as well as most infections treated by second generation. Except for gonorrhea and early syphilis (one of the few infections best treated by a single shot), you shouldn't encounter third generation cephalosporins unless you're sick enough to be in the hospital.

How it works

Same as the others. Thirty years of practice have turned biochemists into virtuosos at rearranging the cephalosporin molecule. New varieties of third generation are pouring onto the shelves in such quantities that any list will be out of date by the time you read this. Many are valuable in killing obscure and difficult germs that attack victims of cancer, immune deficiency, or serious chronic illness. By the time you need one, you'll have little interest in discussing their pros and cons.

How dispensed

Ceftriaxone can't be taken orally; it comes in a powder which the doctor or pharmacist prepares just before injection; 250 mg of ceftriaxone treats gonorrhea. Oral third-generation cephalosporins exist but offer no great advantage.

Translating the label

Ceftriaxone is also Rocephin.

Side effects

To some people, the injection is not particularly painful, and the short duration of therapy means other side effects are even less likely than with longer courses.

Interactions

None with a single shot of ceftriaxone. High-dose, long-term therapy with third generation is a different matter, and many cause a bleeding tendency or interact with alcohol.

Allergies

As uncommon as with earlier cephalosporins.

Wholesale cost

Cost is $12 for 250 mg of ceftriaxone. Seriously ill patients in the hospital may require ten times that dose every day.

9
Sulfas

A guaranteed winner in any trivia contest: Who won the first Nobel prize for discovering an antibiotic? It wasn't Alexander Fleming for penicillin, but Gerhard Domagk in 1938. He discovered the sulfas in 1932.

Domagk worked at the Bayer Company in Germany (named after the inventor of aspirin), subsidiary of giant I.G. Farben chemical company. I.G. Farben was developing new fabric dyes, and Domagk discovered that injecting one of these dyes into mice protected them against bacterial infections. Other researchers criticized him for using animals—not because they were tender hearted but because animal tests are messy and complicated and many researchers believed animal experiments were inaccurate compared to testing against bacteria in a test tube. Luckily, Domagk ignored them because his dye didn't kill germs in a test tube. It must be taken internally and broken down; one breakdown product is an antibiotic.

That was Prontosil, a name that still brings a thrill to some very old doctors. Unlike penicillin, which failed early tests because it was in such short supply, Prontosil was a simple, cheap chemical that produced dramatic results from the very beginning. Besides curing serious infections, Prontosil turned patients bright yellow in the process (it was, after all, a dye). Fortunately, that effect wasn't too desirable, so researchers removed the dye portion of the molecule and were left with sulfanilamide.

We find it hard to appreciate what a revolution this drug produced in the minds of doctors. They had been searching for drugs to cure infections for a century—and had found plenty. But doctors are as logical as anyone else, and logic is a bad basis for science. Logic says that to kill bacteria you must poison them, so medical researchers investigated poisons and developed drugs containing arsenic, mercury, bismuth, and other very unpleasant chemicals. Until as late as the 1940s, victims of syphilis received weekly injections of very nasty arsenic or bismuth compounds. Treatment might last a year, but doctors believed it worked (modern historians are doubtful).

As late as the 1930s, many good scientists insisted that searching for drugs to cure infections was a waste of time. Anything that worked would be too poisonous, they believed. That attitude may have influenced Fleming to give up on penicillin.

The great contribution of the sulfas had nothing to do with their ability to kill germs. They're not very powerful, and germs often develop resistance (poor Albert Alexander, who was almost saved by penicillin, had received sulfas unsuccessfully). Sulfas taught doctors that drugs could kill germs without poisoning the patient. As soon as they realized that, they rushed to find them, and within ten years discovered most of the antibiotics still in use.

Sulfas are treatment of choice for:

Nocardiosis. This is a rare infection by a fungus that usually causes pneumonia and occasionally abscesses in the brain or elsewhere. Nocardiosis is one of the few remaining infections on which sulfas work best. This is a far cry from the 1940s when sulfas were best for strep, staph, meningitis, gonorrhea, and many intestinal infections.

Sulfas are good for:

Urinary tract infections. Sulfas are so cheap they verge on the treatment of choice for uncomplicated bladder infections (but not for kidney infections that produce high fever and make you ill). Bladder infections only cause symptoms of an irritated bladder—the urge to run to the bathroom too often, difficulty getting the urine out, burning.

How it works

Sulfas block manufacture of the folic acid vitamin. Without it, bacteria stop growing. Sulfas don't interfere with human folic acid because our cells can't manufacture it. We get it whole in our diet.

How dispensed

Common sulfas appear in 250 and 500 mg tablets and suspension of 250 mg per teaspoon.

One gram three or four times a day for five days is a reasonable treatment. Twenty years ago the treatment lasted two weeks, but that isn't necessary, and doctors who still do it are behind the times. If you think you have an especially difficult problem, longer treatment isn't helpful because sulfas are only good for *uncomplicated* bladder infections. If your symptoms are persistent or recurrent you should (a) find out why and (b) not take sulfas.

Two-thirds of all patients (mine included) don't take drugs as directed. Good studies prove this again and again, so experts exhort us to explain the importance of following instructions. When we explain carefully, studies show that two-thirds still don't follow instructions. This is a big problem with bladder infections because symptoms disappear a few days into treatment, so patients tend to stop too soon and risk a recurrence. In an effort to make things simpler, experts have explored shorter courses. Ten years ago, there was a rage for single-dose treatment. Two grams of sulfa taken at once cures most bladder infections, but a minority of patients soon relapse, so the treatment fell out of fashion. Three days' treatment is becoming popular, and may work as well as five days.

Translating the label

Dozens of sulfas have been developed, but you're likely to encounter the following:
- Sulfisoxazole (Gantrisin)
- Sulfamethoxazole (Gantanol)
- Sulfamethizole (Thiosulfil Forte, Urobiotic)

Side effects

As antibiotics go, sulfas have more than their share of side effects, but most patients never experience them.

"Drug fever" is a common side effect of any drug and not rare with a sulfa. Let your doctor know if a new fever develops after several days of treatment. An upset stomach occurs as often as a fever—about 3 percent of the time.

Black readers receiving a sulfa should mention "glucose-6-phosphate-dehydrogenase deficiency" or simply "G-six-P-D deficiency." Like sickle cell anemia, it's a hereditary blood disorder limited mostly to blacks: about 10 percent of men and a much smaller number of women. Most victims feel fine unless they take certain drugs that quickly destroy their defective red cells, causing severe anemia. That doesn't happen all the time, and some reactions are so mild the patient doesn't complain. As a result, many doctors (who learn about G6PD in medical school) forget they should prescribe something else to black patients. This side effect also applies to several other drugs.

Interactions

Food. None.

Alcohol. None.

Drugs. Antidiabetes pills (Diabinese, Micronase, Glucotrol) are distantly related to the sulfas. When taken together the sulfas can increase the antidiabetic action and lower blood sugar too much. That usually doesn't happen, but your doctor should be aware.

Sulfas may also increase the bleeding tendency of those taking blood thinner, but so many drugs bear this warning I'm not sure how useful it is.

Pregnancy. Doctors didn't notice birth defects when they prescribed sulfas indiscriminately from the 1930s to the 1950s so they may be safe in early pregnancy. Sulfas are definitely dangerous during the last few months because they can wreak havoc in the fetus's immature blood stream and cause permanent brain damage.

Nursing. Forbidden for the same reason.

Allergies

Serious allergic reactions and rashes are fairly common—but that means about 2 percent of the time.

Wholesale cost

About 6 cents for a 500-mg tablet.

10
Trimethoprim-Sulfamethoxazole (TMP/SMX)

A distant relative of the sulfas, trimethoprim is popular in Europe but never caught on in the U.S. However, during the 1960s it breathed new life into the fading sulfas when it was discovered that, taken together, they make a more powerful drug. Both inhibit folic acid, but since they do it in different ways, bacteria can't easily develop resistance. Germs tend to become resistant to one antibiotic at a time, so when two are present, one will still kill. TMP/SMX works against the same bacteria as the original sulfas discovered in the 1930s; unlike them, it still works.

Two antibiotics are not necessarily better than one. Many combinations interfere with each other, and side effects are always greater. We often give several antibiotics to hospitalized patients with life-threatening infections, but TMP/SMX is one of the few useful combinations for outpatients.

Trimethoprim-Sulfamethoxazole is treatment of choice for:

1. *Mild kidney infections.* Generally affecting young women, these cause fever and chills with some midback pain, often with nausea and vomiting. Women with a bladder infection and low back pain often believe they have a kidney infection, but that isn't so. A kidney infection should make you feverish and ill; bladder infections don't. I hospitalize everyone with a kidney infection who looks fairly sick, but oral antibiotics will treat a mild infection.
2. *Pneumonia in someone with AIDS or a positive HIV test.* This is probably Pneumocystis carini, not a germ but a one-celled protozoan that practically never infects anyone with a normal immune system.
3. *Montezuma's revenge.* Intestinal infection that produces cramps, diarrhea, and occasionally vomiting and affects about 1/3 of everyone who travels to poor parts of the world. Experts warn you to avoid uncooked food and un-

treated water, but good studies show that people who obey get sick just as often.

Trimethoprim-Sulfamethoxazole is good for:

1. *Acute prostate infections.* Women suffer most urinary infections in the bladder, men in the prostate, a gland just outside the bladder that produces ejaculatory fluid. Solitary bladder infections are rare in men, but an infected prostate tends to affect the bladder, so men suffer the same symptoms as women in addition to fever and pain in the prostate area.
2. *Sinus infections.*
3. *Exacerbation of chronic bronchitis.*
4. *Urinary tract infections.* Unlike sulfas, TMP/SMX is also good for difficult and recurrent infections.
5. *Middle ear infections.*

How it works

Like sulfas, trimethoprim interferes with a germ's ability to make folic acid, but it interferes at a different stage, so the combination does a better job.

How dispensed

Tablets containing 80 mg of trimethoprim and 400 mg of sulfamethoxazole and double-strength tablets containing twice as much of each. There is also a suspension with 40 mg of trimethoprim and 200 mg of sulfamethoxazole per teaspoon. One double-strength tablet twice a day is the usual adult dose.

Translating the label

A popular antibiotic, you'll find it as Septra, Bactrim, and Trimeth/ Sulfa.

Side effects

Same as with sulfas, but more frequent. Perhaps 10 percent of patients will have some sort of unpleasant reaction, mostly rashes, headaches, and upset stomachs.

Interactions:

Food. None.

Alcohol. None.

Drugs. Same as with sulfas.

Pregnancy. As with sulfas, dangerous in late pregnancy.

Nursing. Forbidden.

Allergies

About 6 percent of patients have allergic reactions, mostly an itchy or painful rash.

Wholesale cost

Nine cents for single-strength tablet, 11 cents for double.

II Tetracycline • I2 Doxycycline

One of the first prizes from the great mold-screening rush of the 1940s was tetracyclines, a family of antibiotics, all of which attack the same bacteria (unlike the various penicillins and cephalosporins which chemists have altered to kill more varieties). Although one type of tetracycline, doxycycline, has some advantages, a broader spectrum isn't one of them.

But the spectrum is broad enough: dozens of common bacteria, and more dozens of rare ones as well as several classes of microorganisms too small and primitive to be germs but not small enough to be viruses—rickettsiae, mycoplasma, and chlamydia. Tetracyclines even attack a few protozoa such as amebas and malaria parasites. Only during the past decade have new and wildly expensive antibiotics approached the spectrum of the tetracyclines, and they're not useful enough to mention here. I prescribe tetracyclines every day.

Tetracyclines are treatment of choice for:

1. *Chlamydial infections.* These tiny microorganisms, barely visible through a microscope, are sometimes considered bacteria and sometimes placed in a separate category. Chlamydia cause "nongonococcal urethritis," the most common sexually transmitted disease. In men this produces an annoying discharge from the penis, but woman may suffer severe pelvic pain and sterility. Other chlamydial diseases are rare and exotic in the U.S., but not necessarily elsewhere: trachoma (the leading cause of blindness in poor parts of the world), psittacosis (parrot fever), and lymphogranuloma venerum, a classic old venereal disease long superseded by aggressive new-comers like herpes and AIDS.

2. *Rickettsial infections.* Another tiny microorganism causing uncommon but frightening diseases that you've probably heard of: Rocky Mountain spotted fever, typhus, Q-fever.

3. *Cholera.* Spread through contaminated water, epidemics still occur in parts of the world and even occasionally in the U.S. Symptoms are fever and violent diarrhea. Untreated, patients die of fluid loss from the diarrhea.

4. *Lyme disease.* Spread by ticks, it's become a minor media disease and can be unpleasant if not caught early.

   Days to weeks after the bite, the infection reveals itself as a red dot that expands to a red blotch, often with a clearing center like a bull's-eye. It's painless and fades in a few weeks but is often accompanied by flu symptoms. Unlucky patients don't notice the rash and dismiss the illness as a virus.

   Months afterward, about 20 percent of victims develop neurological symptoms such as severe headache, numbness, burning pains, or temporary paralysis of certain nerves such as those of one side of the face. Sometimes the disease affects the heart, causing irregular beats, palpitations, and dizziness. Once again, these last a few weeks.

   About half of untreated patients eventually develop arthritis in the larger joints, most often the knees. Although this usually disappears, a few victims continue to have recurrences.

5. *Acne.* Excellent for suppressing pimples, we often give low doses for long periods. Most likely, tetracycline works by inhibiting a germ that lives in your pores. Although effective, tetracycline isn't the best for all acne. Topical creams are safer and work fine for mild pimples. Blackheads and white-

heads require Retin-A (90.). For overwhelming pimples and disfiguring cysts, you need isotretinoin (Accutane, 92.).

Tetracyclines are good for:

1. *Gonorrhea.* In someone allergic to penicillin and on whom the doctor doesn't want to risk even a cephalosporin.
2. *Prostate infections.*
3. *Syphilis.* In someone allergic to penicillin.
4. *Exacerbations of chronic bronchitis.*
5. *Mycoplasma pneumonia.* The most common pneumonia in healthy young adults.
6. *Montezuma's revenge.*
7. *Bubonic plague.*

How it works

All tetracyclines block a cell's ability to make proteins. Animal cells don't make proteins the same way as bacteria, so tetracyclines don't interfere with human metabolism.

How dispensed

Most short-acting tetracyclines come in 250- and 500-mg capsules and a suspension containing 125 mg per teaspoon. Long-acting tetracyclines such as doxycycline come in 50-mg and 100-mg tablets and a suspension of 25 mg per teaspoon. For the short-acters, 250 mg four times a day is a reasonable starting dose for acne and mild infections, but I use 500 mg for other infections. The usual dose of doxycycline is 100 mg twice a day.

Translating the label

The most popular short-acting tetracycline is plain tetracycline. Plenty of others exist (chlortetracycline, oxytetracycline, methacycline, demeclocycline), but none has any advantage. Brand names for tetracycline are Achromycin, Tetracyn, and Sumycin.

Doxycycline (Vibramycin, Monodox, Vibra-Tabs, Doryx) is the leading long-acting tetracycline. You'll occasionally see minocycline (Minocin), which may be slightly better for acne but otherwise has no advantages and more side effects.

Side effects

Considering how often I use it (mostly for acne and V.D.), I hear few complaints. Except for an occasional bout of diarrhea, it doesn't upset the stomach. Now and then a woman complains of an itchy vaginal discharge after a week of treatment. That happens because tetracyclines eliminate so many germs normally present in the vagina that yeast (also normally present) multiply enough to make her aware of them.

Experts warned that tetracyclines cause photosensitivity: an exaggerated sunburn after exposure to the sun. Many pharmacists routinely attach a sticker to the vial, warning the patient to stay out of the sun. This reaction doesn't occur often, so some doctors forget to mention it.

Never take outdated tetracyclines. Like outdated film, most outdated drugs are probably O.K. or perhaps weaker, but *outdated tetracyclines become poisonous.*

You should know that tetracyclines have an avid attraction for calcium. Given to young children, they combine with calcium in developing teeth, so adult teeth grow in permanently stained. A week or so of treatment probably won't do that, but no child under age eight should receive tetracycline.

Interactions

Food. Besides calcium, tetracyclines combine avidly with other metals including iron, aluminum, magnesium, and zinc. This means that if you take them with dairy products (rich in calcium), antacids (which may contain aluminum, magnesium, or calcium), iron pills, or mineral supplements, they will attach and travel through the GI tract without being absorbed. Don't take a tetracycline within two hours of these foods.

Food reduces absorption of plain tetracycline, so take it on an empty stomach. Doxycycline and minocycline don't have this drawback. Dairy products also don't interfere with doxycycline, but the other metal interactions still apply.

CATTLE RANCHERS ALSO USE TETRACYCLINES DAILY. The meat you buy in the supermarket contains tetracyclines because commercial animal feed contains it. Ranchers and other growers are convinced that feeding animals antibiotics prevents disease and makes them grow faster. The Department of Agriculture maintains that only tiny amounts remain in the meat you buy—too little to cause problems. I have no reason to doubt them, but I don't want to eat even tiny amounts of tetracycline, so I buy only meat guaranteed not to contain antibiotics. It doesn't taste better, costs about 50 percent more, and is mostly available in health food stores.

Alcohol. No problem.

Drugs. The usual warnings about blood thinners apply. Like erythromycin, tetracycline occasionally increases the blood level of digitalis and carbamazepine (Tegretol). If your doctor is treating your high cholesterol with agents that bind cholesterol in the digestive tract such as cholestyramine (Questran) or colestipol (Colestid), he should know that these also bind tetracyclines. Tetracycline interferes with the action of penicillin, so a doctor should never prescribe them together.

Pregnancy. Besides tooth staining, tetracyclines can lead to dental defects and even bone defects if taken during pregnancy.

Nursing. Excreted into milk, so nursing mothers shouldn't take it.

Allergies

True allergies are rare.

Wholesale cost:

Tetracycline: 2.5 cents for 250 mg, 5 cents for 500 mg.

Doxycycline: 11 cents for 100 mg.

Since 100 mg twice a day of doxycycline costs almost the same as 500 mg four times a day of tetracycline, I prefer doxycycline except when using low doses for acne.

13
Macrodantin

In many ways an ideal antibiotic, Macrodantin (generic name is nitrofurantoin) concentrates in the bladder where it's needed, but nowhere else, so it's useless for infections outside the urinary tract. Doctors underuse Macrodantin—partly because it's old and out of fashion, but also because new drugs have fewer side effects.

Macrodantin is good for:

Bladder infections. It's also excellent for prevention. Recurrent episodes of cystitis plague many young women. If they can pinpoint the cause—usually sex— one pill taken afterward usually prevents the infection. Macrodantin is probably safer for this purpose than other antibiotics because it doesn't affect bacteria in other parts of the body such as the colon.

How it works

Once absorbed, nitrofurantoin binds so tightly to proteins in the blood that very little diffuses into tissues as blood flows through the body. In fact, blood containing this drug won't kill bacteria, but the kidneys detach the antibiotic from the protein, so it reaches a very high concentration in urine. Researchers aren't certain how that works except it interferes with some essential bacterial function.

How dispensed

Tablets of 25, 50, and 100 mg; 50 mg four times a day for a week probably cures average infections, but many doctors give 100 mg.

Translating the label

Macrodantin and long-acting form, Macrobid, are the only brand of nitrofurantoin.

Side effects

Macrodantin's lack of popularity owes much to its effect on the stomach: 25 to 50 percent of users suffer nausea or vomiting. Other side effects are rare over the usual week of therapy.

Check the sulfa chapter for my warning about blacks and glucose-6-phosphate-dehydrogenase deficiency. This is another drug those afflicted must avoid unless their doctor approves.

Interactions

Food. Taking Macrodantin with food increases absorption and may or may not diminish stomach irritation.

Alcohol. No effect.

Drugs. Nothing important.

Pregnancy. Forbidden around term because it can provoke anemia in the fetus. No evidence exists for birth defects if taken earlier.

Nursing. Tiny amounts appear in milk, so it may be safe.

Allergies

One percent suffer allergic skin rash. Fewer suffer a violent pulmonary hypersensitivity reaction with fever, chills, cough, shortness of breath, and a chest x-ray that looks like pneumonia. Once the drug is stopped, symptoms disappear quickly. Long-term users can suffer a more severe lung reaction, but there's no reason to take nitrofurantoin daily for long periods.

Wholesale cost

Cost is 25 cents for 50 mg, 50 cents for 100 mg.

14
Metronidazole (Flagyl)

Women who tell me they have a "yeast infection" are usually wrong. Fungi (yeast) cause 20 to 40 percent of annoying vaginal discharges. Nearly all the rest are from a single-celled protozoan (trichomonas) or from bacteria. Unlike yeast treatment, a simple pill takes care of both.

Available since the 1960s, Flagyl's value has grown with the years despite being useless against all common bacteria such as staph or strep. Not only is it one of the safest drugs against protozoa and amoeba, it kills most anaerobic bacteria (germs that only live where no oxygen exists). These cause serious infections deep inside the body such as brain abscesses, peritonitis, and other intestinal infections. If you need Flagyl for these, you'll probably be hospitalized.

Flagyl is treatment of choice for:

1. *Trichomonas.* Causing 10 to 30 percent of vaginal infections, it produces an unpleasant discharge usually accompanied by itching. Yeast infections tend to itch more, but doctors who diagnose a vaginal infection by symptoms are as inaccurate as their patients. A glance at your discharge under the microscope takes only a minute.
2. *Bacterial vaginosis.* A collection of anaerobic bacteria with names like Gardnerella or Hemophilus, these cause half of all vaginal infections. The average victim has a bad smelling discharge with little itching.
3. *"Amebic dysentery."* Don't blame this for ruining your Mexican vacation; that illness is probably the one I discussed in the Sulfa chapter. Despite the impressive name, amebic infections are usually less violent, producing gas, cramps, and foul smelling, loose bowel movements that come and go. Only rarely does this appear as typical "dysentery"—violent bloody diarrhea, high fever, and severe cramps.
4. *Giardiasis.* Another one-celled creature distantly related to trichomonads, it lives in the small bowel, producing bloating, cramps, belching, and flatulence. Spread by contaminated water, giardia are the most common cause

of waterborne diarrhea in the U.S. Experts find them in about 4 percent of stool sent for evaluation. Not rare, giardiasis doesn't produce a violent illness, so victims may suffer for months before a doctor thinks of it.

Flagyl is good for:

1. *Severe infections by many anaerobic bacteria.*
2. *Several skin disorders.* It relieves acne rosacea, a common affliction that produces pimples and redness over the cheeks and nose, mostly in middle-aged women. Smelly leg ulcers and bedsores often respond promptly to metronidazole (infections from anaerobic bacteria tend to smell bad). Finally, many dermatologists try metronidazole for several stubborn, chronic disorders including hives, psoriasis, and gum inflammations. A subtle bacterial infection may lie behind these, but no one is certain.
3. *Inflammatory bowel disease.* With names like ulcerative colitis and Crohn's disease, these difficult ailments produce chronic bowel inflammation with diarrhea and abdominal pain. One miserable complication of Crohn's disease is persistent draining abscesses around the anus. Metronidazole in high doses heals these better than any other medication and also helps suppress the pain and diarrhea of Crohn's disease.

How it works

Flagyl seems to damage DNA, the genetic material that controls heredity and cell reproduction.

How dispensed

In 250- and 500-mg tablets and a vaginal gel.

250 mg three times a day for a week works fine for trichomonas and bacterial vaginosis. In their perpetual effort to persuade you to take all your pills, researchers found that two grams taken in one dose works almost as well for trichomonas, and that's what I use. That doesn't work for bacterial vaginosis, but someone who doesn't want to take a pill can use a vaginal cream (Metrogel-Vaginal) for vaginosis. Giardiasis also responds to 250 mg three times a day, but amebas, skin disorders, and inflammatory bowel disease require much higher doses.

Translating the label

Flagyl is the most popular brand of metronidazole. Others are Protostat and Metric.

Side effects

Twelve percent of patients report upset stomach, mostly nausea but occasionally vomiting, abdominal pain, or diarrhea. Eighty-eight percent don't, so give the drug a chance. Alternative drugs are worse. Occasionally, patients get a harmless metallic taste in the mouth.

Interactions

Food. No problem.

Alcohol. "Can I drink while I take this?" may be the most common question patients ask when I hand over a prescription. Many are convinced that large numbers of drugs, usually antibiotics, react violently with alcohol. In fact, few drugs do, and patients are surprised and sometimes skeptical when I tell them drinking is O.K. I don't tell them that with Flagyl. *Don't touch alcohol* while taking it and for 48 hours afterward because there's a small chance of a "disulfiram reaction."

Disulfiram (Antabuse) is occasionally given to alcoholics in an effort to stop them drinking. When a person with Antabuse in the blood drinks alcohol, he suffers flushing, vomiting, cramps, and a splitting headache. This sounds like a terrific way to cure alcoholism, but it plays only a minor role in treatment programs. I discuss it in a later chapter.

Only a small minority ever have that reaction, and I've never seen a case, but I hear the warning so often I must repeat it.

Drugs. Naturally, no one taking Antabuse should take Flagyl. It may also increase the effect of blood thinners; then again it may not. So many drugs can cause problems with blood thinners that I won't mention this again unless it's a major risk.

Pregnancy. Although there's no evidence that it causes birth defects, any drug that damages DNA is worrisome, so it's forbidden during the first three months of pregnancy. We are not anxious to prescribe it during the last six months either, but we may give in if a patient can't stand her trichomonas infection. No good alternative exists.

Nursing. Metronidazole causes cancer in rats. Although no evidence exists
for this in humans, this is enough to make it off limits during nursing because
we are always more careful with infants.

Allergies

Pure allergies and rashes are rare.

Wholesale cost

Four cents for 250 mg, eight cents for 500 mg. The much newer vaginal gel
costs $22, and a skin cream goes for $19 per ounce.

15
Vermox

Americans consider worms helpful in the garden and undesirable in the family
pet, but they rarely feel a personal involvement. My patients associate worms
in humans with inhabitants of tropical nations with low incomes and careless
personal hygiene. News of their own worms comes as a shock.

Nature abhors a vacuum; you and your digestive tract are a rich source of
food not only for you and your native bacteria, but dozens of parasites that can't
survive elsewhere. Keeping worm-free requires more handwashing and proper
food handling than even Americans have patience for, so many of us accommodate a modest number of intestinal parasites. Only a minority harbor enough to
produce symptoms but it's not a small minority—perhaps 30 million. I mentioned protozoal parasites in the Flagyl chapter. Here are some worms.

Vermox is good for:

1. *Pinworms.* Thirty percent of North Americans have them, mostly young children and their parents. Tiny, threadlike worms that live harmlessly in your colon, they make themselves known at night when the female wiggles out the anus to lay eggs. This tickles, so nighttime anal itching is a clue although doctors should think of pinworms for anyone with anal itching at any hour of the day.

   You catch pinworms by swallowing the eggs which are, obviously, associated with feces. You might think it's easy to avoid swallowing feces, but it turns out to be almost impossible if children live in the house and difficult even if they don't.

   We make the diagnosis by seeing the female worm, which is about half an inch long (the much smaller male remains inside). Traditionally doctors hand out Scotch tape with instructions to apply the sticky side to the anus at night, then bring it in for microscopic exam. If no worms turn up, we treat anyway because Vermox is safe and cheap. Everyone in the house must take it.

2. *Ascariasis.* Unlike the tiny pinworm, an ascarid is a robust creature the size of an earthworm that lives off the contents of your small intestine. Eggs pass out in feces and remain alive for years in dry soil. Like pinworms, you must swallow them to acquire worms.

   Heavy infections occur where children are allowed to defecate in the soil around the house, and in these areas 100 percent of children and most adults are infected. Experts estimate that ascarids live in one quarter of the world's population, but U.S. inhabitants make up only four million. Heavy infections cause abdominal pain, malnutrition, and occasionally a surgical emergency when a mass of worms obstructs the bowel or a single worm crawls up a narrow duct and gets stuck.

   Complications are rare in the U.S. where most victims harbor too few to produce symptoms. Americans discover their ascarids in the toilet when one accidentally slips out. Nothing brings a healthy person to the doctor faster than excreting a worm; always put it in a bottle and bring it along. Not only will this educate the doctor who has probably never seen one, but it assures you of treatment. If you merely announce that you've passed a worm the doctor will nod sympathetically (patients often see things in their stool that aren't there) and order a "stool for ova and parasites," an expensive test that will be negative if you have only a few worms.

3. *Hookworms.* Unlike ascarids, which eat your food, hookworms eat your blood by biting into the wall of your small intestine. Worldwide, they drink nine million quarts daily from 900 million victims, making up the leading cause of iron deficiency anemia in poor countries. Hookworms were a serious U.S. public health problem until well into the twentieth century when shoes became fashionable even among the poor, but they still live in the soil of the south from Texas to Virginia.

Like other worms, their eggs pass out in the feces, but a hookworm returns by a more direct route. When a bare foot steps on a larva, it penetrates the skin and migrates to the intestine. Just as healthy humans can give blood every few weeks, they can support several thousand hookworms without severe symptoms, but it's not a good idea. Walking barefoot over most of the world puts you at risk.

How it works

Vermox directly poisons worm cells, making it impossible for them to take up or use glucose. Higher animals handle glucose in a different manner, so Vermox has no affect on them.

How dispensed

Chewable tablet of 100 mg.

For pinworms, one tablet treats everyone over age two. Sometime we prescribe a second after two weeks.

Treating ascariasis and hookworm requires one tablet twice a day for three days.

Translating the label

Vermox is the only brand of mebendazole.

Equally effective is another drug, pyrantel pamoate (Antiminth), although dosage varies with age.

Side effects

Uncommon because so little is absorbed. Abdominal pain and diarrhea occasionally occur when masses of worms are killed and expelled.

Interactions

Food. None.
Alcohol. None.
Drugs. None.
Pregnancy. No problems in humans but it causes birth defects in rats. We don't give it during the first three months and only later if essential.
Nursing. There's no information; probably inadvisable.

Allergies

Almost none at normal doses. Rare reports of rashes and hair loss at high doses for severe infections.

Wholesale cost

Cost is $4.50 per tablet.

16
Zovirax

The first important, nonpoisonous treatment for a viral disease, Zovirax marked a major medical triumph of the 1980s—mostly as a harbinger of better things to come. It was not as major a triumph as antibiotics during the 1930s because they cured common infections. Zovirax cures a few uncommon infections and suppresses common ones, still a big advance.

We have mastered the art of inventing drugs that kill bacteria without killing you at the same time. Looking back, this was easy. Germs are complicated creatures. Because they carry out many functions (breathing, reproducing) in different ways than higher animals, we can interfere with them without harming you. For example, antibiotics such as tetracycline and erythromycin prevent certain germs from manufacturing proteins without bothering your cells because they make proteins through a different process.

A thousand times smaller than germs, a virus is basically a small collection of genes like those in each of your cells plus a simple protein coating. Under the electron microscope, it resembles a pretty crystal with symmetrical borders. Since it doesn't breathe, eat, move, or divide, scientists debate whether a virus can be called "alive."

Outside a cell, a virus is inert. You can destroy it by boiling or dousing it with strong disinfectant, but this is impractical inside your body. Once a virus enters the body, antibodies can attack it, and that's why good immunizations exist for many viral diseases (polio, smallpox, hepatitis, measles, rubella, yellow fever). An immunization is simply a weak dose of the virus that your defenses can easily overcome. Once your immune system has been exposed, it attacks future infections of the same virus so rapidly you're not aware.

When a virus attaches itself to a cell, a small hole appears in the cell membrane, and the viral gene enters; the protein coat stays outside. Once inside, the virus migrates to the cell nucleus, inserts itself into the cell's genes, and disappears. Some viruses remain silent for years or even forever, but for most diseases the interval is days or weeks during which the virus takes control of the cell. Then the cell stops its normal activities and begins manufacturing viruses. Eventually the cell fills up with viruses, dies, and falls apart, releasing viruses to infect other cells.

You can see the problem. Even when a virus is multiplying, the host cell does all the work. Drugs that attack viral infections block that activity, but blocking the activity of your own cells causes difficulties, and early antiviral drugs were poisonous. They were similar—and sometimes identical—to anticancer drugs. As scientists learn precisely what a virus does inside a cell, they will design drugs that don't cripple a normal cell's activity.

Acyclovir (Zovirax) is the first. Although not very toxic, it works against only two members of a single virus family.

Zovirax is treatment of choice for:

1. *Herpes simplex skin infections.* A huge media splash erupted during the early 1980s when genital herpes was described as America's most devastating plague and our punishment for enjoying the sexual revolution. As always, the media spread fear and nonsense until 1983, when it decided that AIDS, not herpes, was America's most devastating plague, etc. There is always a media disease.

   During a herpes attack, the virus kills a small patch of skin, producing one or several sores that heal in a week or two. Although they can be excruciatingly painful, this is not necessarily so. Many are only itchy or mildly annoying. Herpes can affect any area of the body. Most people think first of the genitals, but herpes often attacks the lip (fever blister), inside the mouth (canker sore), on the fingertips (whitlow) or anyplace else. Perhaps the most aggravating feature is its tendency to recur, often every few months, but this doesn't happen forever. After a few years, recurrences grow less frequent and eventually stop.

2. *Herpes simplex encephalitis (brain infection) and herpes in the newborn.* Both are fairly uncommon but devastating, usually fatal without treatment, leaving most survivors with brain damage. Zovirax works miracles here.

3. *Chicken pox and herpes zoster (shingles).* Everyone knows chicken pox—a mild childhood illness caused by another virus of the herpes family. You can't catch chicken pox twice because antibodies from the first infection snap up any virus that gets into the blood, but the virus remains dormant in nerves at the base of your spine.

   Now and then the chicken pox virus reactivates, travels down the nerves of that particular segment of spine and inflames a patch of skin on one side of the body, producing painful blisters that heal in a few weeks. These are shingles. Shingles only affects a strip of skin on one side because a different spinal nerve serves the other.

   Shingles and even chicken pox are dangerous and sometimes fatal in someone with an immune system weakened by diseases such as AIDS or leukemia. Acyclovir shortens an attack of ordinary shingles and chicken pox and saves lives in a widespread infection. However, the chicken pox virus is only one tenth as sensitive to acyclovir as herpes simplex, requiring a much higher dose. I only use it for severe attacks.

Zovirax inhibits the rest of the herpes family including the Epstein-Barr virus that causes infectious mononucleosis. Unfortunately, Epstein-Barr is even less sensitive to acyclovir so the dose is too high to be practical, but future drugs will do better. Just as the 1930s marked the dawn of the antibiotic era, the 1990s will see the beginning of an explosion of good antivirals.

How it works

When a cell reproduces, it first duplicates its own genes which are composed of deoxyribonucleic acid (DNA). A cell accomplishes this by using a large protein called an enzyme that plucks small molecules from the surrounding fluid and attaches them one after another to make an exact DNA copy. One of these small molecules is called thymidine. Zovirax resembles thymidine but is not identical. If an enzyme mistakes Zovirax for thymidine and attaches it to the growing DNA, that ruins the copy because it's impossible to attach the next molecule to the other end of the Zovirax. Fortunately your normal enzyme isn't very sensitive to Zovirax, mostly ignoring it and picking out genuine thymidine.

Taking over the cell, herpes simplex forces it to make a slightly different copying enzyme which seems to prefer Zovirax to genuine thymidine, so every effort to make new viral DNA stops short. When herpes zoster takes over, its copying enzyme is less sensitive to Zovirax, so much more of the drug is necessary to interfere with its reproduction.

How dispensed

Tablets of 200 mg and an ointment.

I never use the ointment unless patients request it after I've explained it doesn't work. I discuss the ointment in the drugs-that-don't-work chapter.

Dosage: 200 mg of tablets five times a day for ten days treats a first attack of herpes simplex; five days treats a recurrence. Begun soon after symptoms appear, this cuts down the number of blisters and speeds healing of those already present. Zovirax doesn't stop recurrences and isn't necessary if the attack isn't bothersome. This is hard to get across to some patients who feel that such an ugly infection demands treatment.

Chicken pox and shingles require four times this dose.

Translating the label

Zovirax is the only available brand of acyclovir.

Side effects

One good feature of newer drugs is better information. The FDA has been demanding better statistics on the bad effects as well as the good, so I can be specific about Zovirax.

—About 3 percent of patients suffer nausea and vomiting.

—Less than 1 percent suffer headache.

Other side effects such as diarrhea, dizziness, and loss of appetite are even less common. Zovirax is a remarkably benign drug.

The above statistics are for short courses. As with all drugs, the longer you take it, the more problems appear. Doctors occasionally give Zovirax for long periods to suppress recurrences; that works only as long as you take it, so I don't try to prevent recurrences unless the patient is truly miserable. Given Zovirax for up to six months, 13 percent of patients suffer diarrhea, 9 percent nausea and vomiting, 8 percent dizziness, and 4 percent joint pains.

Interactions

Food. Food doesn't delay absorption.

Alcohol. None.

Drugs. No significant problems.

Pregnancy. Although there's no evidence it causes birth defects, no doctor wants to give a pregnant woman a drug that interferes with DNA synthesis, even if it only works in viruses. A developing baby is churning out DNA.

Nursing. Forbidden for same reason.

Sex. No problems reported.

Allergies

Very rare.

Wholesale cost

One dollar for 200-mg capsule. $36 for 15-gram tube of ointment.

17
Amantadine

The first nonpoisonous antiviral has been around for 30 years and remains the only drug that shortens an influenza attack. Unfortunately, it seems a dead end. A peculiar molecule with a structure unrelated to other drugs, amantadine has frustrated attempts to create similar treatments for other viral illnesses. The future of antiviral drugs probably lies with those that interfere with viral reproduction (like Zovirax) or boost the immune response (like interferons).

Amantadine is the treatment of choice for:

Influenza A. This is the epidemic flu that occurs most winters, attacking 20 percent of the population during an average "flu season," but up to half in a bad year. Typical flu arrives suddenly with fever, chills, headache, body aches, and intense misery; it lasts about a week. Cough and sore throat occur, but they are not the major complaint. Given within two days of onset, amantadine shortens the illness by several days.

Amantadine is good for:

1. *Preventing influenza A.* Given daily during an epidemic, it provides over 70 percent protection—similar to the flu vaccine, which is preferable.
2. *Treating Parkinsonism.* Influenza can devastate a nursing home, so amantadine is passed out generously during an epidemic. Soon after its release, patients with Parkinsonism mentioned that their tremor had improved, so doctors discovered this new application. Later I'll mention that antihistamines such as Benadryl (see 82.) also help mild Parkinsonism. Amantadine works slightly better.

How it works

No one knows its action on the influenza virus. Some experts believe it discourages injection of the infectious viral nucleus into the cell after the virus attaches to the outside. Amantadine helps Parkinsonism by increasing secretion of neurotransmitters from nerves harmed by the disease.

How dispensed

As 100-mg tablets and a syrup containing 50 mg per teaspoon; 100 mg twice a day is usual dose although we usually reduce that by half in patients over 65.

Translating the label

Symmetrel is the only brand of amantadine.

A relative, rimantadine (Flumadine) works as well with fewer side effects. Developed in 1980, it's widely used in Europe, and in August 1993 was approved for use in the U.S.

Side effects

Five to 10 percent of patients complain of dizziness, insomnia, nausea, or difficulty concentrating. A few become depressed or confused.

Interactions

Food. None noted.

Alcohol. None.

Drugs. No distinct interactions, but the elderly are sensitive to drugs that act on the brain, particularly when taking more than one such as amantadine plus a tranquilizer or antidepressant. On the other hand, amantadine doesn't interfere with flu vaccine, so a good tactic during an epidemic is to be immunized, then take amantadine for two weeks until the vaccine takes hold.

Pregnancy. Causes birth defects in rats, so we discourage its use.

Nursing. Heavily excreted in milk and considered unsafe.

Sex. None noted.

Allergies

Not common—fewer than 1 percent suffer.

Wholesale cost

20 cents for 100-mg tablet.

18
Griseofulvin

My patients spend a great deal of time rubbing creams between their toes, between their legs, over their skin, and even on their nails and scalp in an effort to cure a fungal infection or "ringworm." They usually fail because—

1. It's not a fungus. In adults, most itchy rashes on the body or scalp are something else. Rashes on the face are hardly ever ringworm. Only between the legs and toes are the odds in their favor.
2. They reinfect themselves. Most itchy rashes between the toes are genuine fungal infections, and a few weeks of antifungal cream gets rid of it. But a fungus growing between your toes certainly grows over your feet, too, and within a few weeks it spreads back.
3. Creams don't work. That is, they don't work where skin is too thick to penetrate: over the palms, soles, and heels. They also won't penetrate far into nails or hair follicles.

No permanent harm results from treating yourself for a superficial fungal infection until frustration drives you to the doctor's office. Even then you might come away with another cream no better than you've been using because doctors don't like giving drugs for such a minor problem. Unfortunately, nothing else works.

An old antibiotic used in animals since the 1940s and humans since the 1960s, griseofulvin only kills funguses that live on skin, hair, and nails. It has no affect on bacteria or even a "yeast," a class of fungus that infects the vagina and occasionally skin.

Griseofulvin is treatment of choice for:

1. *Fungal infections of the scalp and hair.* Although more common in children,

these are not rare in adults and produce a host of symptoms from itching and scaling to patchy (not generalized!) hair loss to painful sores and oozing. The diagnosis is not easy; the doctor shouldn't make it without a microscopic examination of the hair.

Fungi grow slower than bacteria; they also die slower, so we treat for much longer. Curing a scalp fungus takes at least a month.

2. *Fungal infections of the nails.* Rubbing a cream onto an infected but dead nail is futile. To eliminate the fungus you must swallow griseofulvin, which enters your bloodstream and soaks into new, living nail deep under the skin. As this nail dies and grows forward, the antibiotic remains, so fungus in the diseased nail can't grow backward. Eventually healthy nail grows out completely, the last of the infected nail is clipped off, and you're cured.

This takes time: six months for fingernails, at least a year for toes. And there's no guarantee. Sometimes it doesn't work; sometimes the fungus reappears after successful treatment. But if you hate the sight of your nails, griseofulvin may help, although you may have to persuade your doctor. It's an underused therapy.

3. *Fungal infections of the feet.* You can stop the miserable itching between your toes by applying a cream, but an extensive eruption over the soles and heels requires griseofulvin for a few months.

My feet never bothered me, but they always appeared dry and scaly. I assumed this was how feet were supposed to look until I began taking griseofulvin for my toenails. After a month, my feet became pink and smooth, and they've remained so.

Griseofulvin is good for:

Ringworm and similar fungal infections of the skin. Creams do fine for fungi over the arms, legs, and body, but they aren't practical for a very extensive infection.

How it works

Griseofulvin prevents fungi from reproducing by preventing DNA and protein production. It works so well for superficial infections because almost all of the drug concentrates in skin, hair, and nails. Researchers find only tiny amounts elsewhere in the body.

How dispensed

Tablets of 125, 165, 250, 330, and 500 mg plus a suspension containing 125 mg per teaspoon.

Different brands are not comparable, and the label on the bottle gives no clue, so your doctor should know which is which. This occurs because griseofulvin is extremely hard to absorb, so makers grind it into a very fine powder. Some is "microsized" and some "ultramicrosized," i.e., smaller than microsized. Neither is superior but ultramicrosized requires a smaller dose because more is absorbed. One gram per day of microsized treats nail infections as well as two thirds of a gram of ultramicrosized. Skin infections require half as much of either.

Translating the label

Microsized griseofulvin comes as Grifulvin, Grivate, and Grisactin. Fulvicin P/G, Grisactin ultra, and Gris-PEG are ultramicrosized.

Side effects

Treating my own toenails, I noticed an annoying headache for the first week of my treatment, but it disappeared. Headaches affect 15 percent of users. It's also one of the few drugs to cause photosensitivity. This probably occurs even less often than with the tetracyclines, but since treatment takes so long it's something to think about.

Liver, blood, and kidney abnormalities occur rarely. Your doctor may test your blood and urine if you're on a long course, but don't be upset if he doesn't. It's not essential unless you already have a liver, blood, or kidney problem—in which case I doubt if any doctor will give griseofulvin.

Interactions

Food. Griseofulvin is one drug that you should take on a full stomach—not to prevent irritation but because absorption is quicker. In fact, since it's much more soluble in fat than water, I've read recommendations to take it after "a fatty meal." This isn't essential.

Alcohol. It may aggravate the effect of alcohol, producing flushing and palpitations. This is not the same violent "disulfiram" reaction I mentioned with metronidazole, but be careful.

Drugs. Reviewing griseofulvin's interactions, I came upon a statement in the PDR that the drug's effect on the liver may increase the breakdown of estrogens, including the estrogens in birth control pills, thus decreasing their contraceptive action.

That's the first time I've heard this about griseofulvin, but the rumor that women on the pill can get pregnant if they take antibiotics has been drifting around for a decade. I don't know what to make of it; no patient of a doctor in my circle has gotten pregnant because of this, and few doctors mention the possibility.

Pregnancy. Two cases of Siamese twins have occurred since 1977 in women taking griseofulvin. No one has seen other defects, but animal tests reveal some, so it's forbidden in pregnancy or even in someone thinking of getting pregnant.

Nursing. Griseofulvin concentrates in the skin, so very little comes out in milk, but it's probably not a good idea to nurse if you're on long-term therapy.

Allergies

Hives and other allergic rashes happen rarely.

Wholesale cost

Microsized: 60 cents for 250 mg, $1 for 500 mg.
Ultramicrosized: 35 cents for 165 mg, 60 cents for 330 mg.
At retail, a year of therapy runs into money.

19
Miconazole

Most itchy rashes are not the result of ringworm or a fungal infection, although the chances are better if you itch in a warm, damp place: between the legs, between the toes, under the breasts, less often under the arms.

Repeating what I said in the last section, intensely itchy rashes on dry areas (arms, legs, trunk) are almost certainly something else—most likely a local irritation or allergy. Funguses on dry areas don't itch very much.

Ringworm, of course, is not a worm, but the description of a typical fungal rash—a pink area surrounded by circular, scaly raised border that slowly enlarges. Don't expect this in very damp areas; you may see only a generalized itchy redness.

Fungi are plants that, unlike green plants, can't make their own food, so they live off dead matter. Your hair and skin surface are dead, so fungi live quietly on your body just as many germs do. When something happens to favor one or another organism, it multiplies, takes over, and causes trouble. Since fungi grow best where it's warm and wet, you'll understand where they're likely to appear.

Once you've diagnosed a fungal infection, it's all right to treat yourself. Even if you're wrong, no great harm results. Although half a dozen relatives of miconazole are marketed by other drug companies, most require a prescription. When first released in the 1970s miconazole was a prescription item, but the FDA changed this around 1987. Don't assume that this was because miconazole isn't as "strong." The FDA doesn't consider strength in its decisions, only safety. Over the past 15 years the FDA has been slowly reviewing all prescription drugs and releasing those deemed safe enough for over-the-counter sale in its effort to lower medical costs. You should appreciate this. Miconazole's rivals are equally safe, but their makers may believe that keeping them as prescription drugs is more profitable. Clotrimazole, a competitor, is now available over-the-counter. Approval came at the same time as miconazole, but its manufacturer waited several years before making the change.

Miconazole is treatment of choice for:

1. *Fungal infections between the legs, between the toes, under the arms and breast.*
2. *Mild fungal infections of the rest of the skin.*
3. *"Yeast" vaginal infections.* These typically cause intense itching and a vaginal discharge resembling cottage cheese.
4. *Thrush.* A yeast infection of the mouth and throat, it produces white patches that may or may not be painful. Fairly common in young children, it mostly affects adults who are chronically ill, immune suppressed, or malnourished, but (like a vaginal yeast infection) it can appear after antibiotic therapy.

Miconazole is good for:

Tinea versicolor. Although another common skin fungus, tinea versicolor ("fungus that changes color") is worth a separate discussion. It's so common I see several cases every week—usually in someone who comes in for another problem. Preparing to listen to the heart or chest with my stethoscope, I notice a few dozen pink- or salmon-colored spots. When I point them out, patients tell me the spots have been around for years, waxing and waning, becoming more vivid during the summer.

Tinea versicolor doesn't itch and only affects the chest, shoulders, and upper back, so patients are slow to wonder about it. The rash flares during summer because the fungus blocks sunlight, so the skin underneath doesn't tan. When the tan fades, the rash fades.

Treatment isn't necessary if it doesn't bother you. Any antifungal works, but rubbing a cream onto the chest and back is awkward, so I prefer a lotion containing selenium sulfide (Selsun, Exsel). Apply it after a shower, wait ten minutes, then wash it off. Do this daily for two weeks. Recurrences are almost guaranteed. To prevent this, use the lotion once a week forever.

How it works

Miconazole damages the membrane of the cell, making it difficult to take in nutrients and divide.

How dispensed

Over-the-counter miconazole comes as a cream, powder, spray, vaginal cream, and vaginal suppository.

To treat skin infections, apply a thin film twice a day. Itching should disappear in a week, but if you don't continue for at least a month, you'll soon have your infection again. Remember that fungi die slowly. For yeast infections, use the cream or suppository daily for a week.

Equally effective, prescription imidazoles (the family that includes miconazole) come as all of the above plus "troches"—tablets that dissolve in the mouth. Larger suppositories are available for a three-day course, and a very large suppository for a single dose. More convenient, they may work slightly less well than a week's treatment. For thrush, suck on a troche five times a day for two weeks.

Translating the label

Miconazole's OTC brand name is Micatin, but the name is Monistat if you receive it by prescription. Monistat is also the name of the vaginal cream and suppository. Other popular antifungals:

Clotrimazole is sold as Lotrimin, Mycelex, and Gyne-Lotrimin.

You can buy it over-the-counter. Those listed below remain available only by prescription as of 1993:

- Butoconazole is Femstat.
- Terconazole is Terazol.
- Econazole is Spectazole.
- Oxiconazole is Oxistat.
- Sulconazole is Exelderm.
- Tioconazole is Vagistat.
- Ketoconazole is Nizoral.
- Ciclopirox is Loprox.
- Naftifine is Naftin.
- Itraconazole is Sporana.

Side effects

Applied to skin, a rare patient notices some burning. The vagina is rather more sensitive. Used for a week, a few percent of women feel discomfort, but less than 1 percent stop treatment. Suppositories seem less irritating with about 1 percent of women complaining.

Interactions

Food. Treating thrush, it's unwise to eat while sucking the troche.

Alcohol. Don't drink while sucking a troche.

Drugs. None known.

Pregnancy. Large oral doses caused birth defects in rats, but intravaginal doses didn't.

Since a small amount is absorbed thorough the vagina and more through the digestive tract, it shouldn't be used during the first three months of pregnancy unless absolutely necessary. Troches shouldn't be used during any part of pregnancy.

Little drug penetrates beyond the skin, so using the cream or lotion is all right.

Nursing. No one knows if miconazole appears in breast milk, so the PDR advises doctors to "exercise caution" in prescribing it to nursing women. I honestly don't know how to do that except by not prescribing it. Perhaps your doctor knows better.

Allergies

If the cream burns, that's probably a local reaction, not an allergy. Unless it hurts too much there's no harm in continuing.

Wholesale cost

One ounce of generic miconazole is $2. A week of vaginal cream or suppositories is $10. Two weeks of clotrimazole troches (miconazole troches aren't available) cost $53.

20
Pyridium

Although a pain reliever, phenazopyridine (Pyridium) is almost always prescribed together with an antibiotic for a urinary tract infection, so I include it in this section. An ingenious drug, it does only one thing but does that well.

Pyridium is treatment of choice for:

Burning on urination; also for urgency, excessive frequency, and other symptoms that signal irritation of the bladder and urethra—usually from an infection but also from injuries or procedures such as passing a catheter.

How it works

As a local anesthetic. Useless at killing bacteria, it won't cure an infection, but it also won't interfere with a urinalysis or urine culture, so feel free to take one to relieve the discomfort before seeing a doctor. I prescribe enough so a patient has some left over, and I encourage her to save them for her next infection. Never take an antibiotic under these circumstances. It won't relieve symptoms quickly but often makes the urinalysis deceptively normal.

How dispensed

In 100 and 200-mg tablets; 200 mg every eight hours is usual dose. Two days is a good treatment period because the antibiotic will be working by then, and any minor injury will have healed.

Some doctors prefer an antibiotic combined with phenazopyridine (Azo-Gantrisin, Azo-Gantanol, Urobiotic), but this is unnecessary. After two days you won't need the phenazopyridine, so you'll be taking a useless drug.

Translating the label

Phenazopyridine is sold under the brand names Pyridium or Pyridiate.

Side effects

Although experts report a 10 percent incidence of stomach upset, my patients who take it for a few days don't complain. One hundred percent of patients can expect their urine to turn bright orange.

Black women with G-6-P-D deficiency shouldn't take phenazopyridine, but (remember my discussion in the sulfa chapter) women inherit this disorder much less often than men.

Interactions

Food. Take after eating.
Alcohol. None.
Drugs. None.
Pregnancy. Although probably all right, it's rarely essential.
Nursing. Probably all right.

Allergies

Less than 1 percent.

Wholesale cost

Three cents for 100 mg, 5 cents for 200 mg.

PART II
Drugs for
Cardiovascular Problems

During the nineteenth century, "heart disease" meant rheumatic heart disease, a vivid ailment doctors could follow using the primitive techniques of the day: observation and the stethoscope. Both remain equally useful today despite proliferation of complex testing methods.

Rheumatic heart disease followed rheumatic fever, a common childhood illness that occasionally occurred after a strep throat infection (we still aren't sure why). Children suffered fever, joint pains, rashes, and inflammation of the heart that was often fatal. Although much less common in wealthy countries today, rheumatic fever is still around, but it's become less serious in the twentieth century. Deaths are rare, and rheumatic heart disease occurs less often.

Nineteenth-century rheumatic fever lasted months and left some victims with a damaged heart. Others recovered but began showing signs of heart valve leakage during their 20s or 30s. Rheumatic heart disease doesn't cause chest pain, but heart failure. A heart with a leaky valve can't pump efficiently so a victim first notices fatigue after exertion. Then normal activities become difficult. Because the heart pumps too weakly, blood piles up outside, waiting to pass through. Outside the heart are the lungs, so in "congestive heart failure," lung vessels swell with blood, interfering with breathing. Patients cough and wheeze; colds and minor lung infections make them much sicker. As the heart weakens still more, fluid oozes out of the engorged vessels into the lung itself; a doctor can hear the noise of air bubbling through fluid; the patient gasps for breath. Nowadays, we can eliminate this water and strengthen the heart, but the nineteenth-century doctor could mostly observe and sympathize. He also prescribed drugs and believed they worked, but they didn't. Even those doctors still use today (such as digitalis) don't work well with rheumatic heart disease.

Although heart attacks occurred before this century, they were less common, and doctors were only vaguely aware of them. One reason: rheumatic heart disease produces interesting murmurs audible by stethoscope; a heart suffering a heart attack often sounds normal. Until well into the twentieth century, medicine recognized a disorder called "acute indigestion" that was often fatal. President Harding died suddenly in 1923 with this diagnosis. Soon after, the electrocardiogram came into use; a heart attack produces very specific ECG abnormalities, so doctors had something to get their teeth into, but it wasn't until the 1940s that coronary artery disease passed rheumatic heart disease as the leading cause of cardiac mortality.

Doctors knew about high blood pressure in the nineteenth century, but they considered it a "vital sign" like temperature and pulse—something that you watched when a patient was sick, but not a disease in itself, an attitude that lasted until around 1930. Anyway, no good method existed to lower blood pressure. That didn't really change until after World War II. President Franklin Roosevelt had very high blood pressure for the last years of his life. By 1945, he was probably sick enough to affect his performance in office; the stroke that killed him was the end result.

Progress in treating high blood pressure has been pleasant to follow because there's been so much. During the 1940s and 1950s, we controlled blood pressure with rice and fruit diets, sympathectomy (an operation that cut nerves controlling blood pressure, which didn't work very well), and several drugs that invariably made patients sleepy, dizzy, impotent, and constipated.

By the 1960s patients with modest high blood pressure led a fairly normal life provided they could tolerate the foul-tasting potassium required by high-dose diuretics. More severe pressures still demanded unpleasant drugs, although beta blockers were a vast improvement. By the 1970s, calcium channel blockers allowed most hypertensives to lead normal lives, and the appearance of angiotensin-converting enzyme inhibitors during the 1980s have increased that to almost 100 percent. Today, no one should die of high blood pressure or even suffer mild inconvenience.

We haven't done as well with coronary artery disease. By the time cholesterol buildup in the coronary arteries reduces blood supply to the muscle as a whole (causing heart failure), or nearly blocks one blood vessel (causing chest pain or angina), or completely blocks that vessel (causing a heart attack), medical science can't give you back a normal heart. In contrast, as long as treatment keeps a hypertensive's blood pressure normal, he or she literally doesn't have the disease.

We can carry blood around a coronary blockage with bypass surgery, blow up a balloon inside a narrowed artery to stretch it (angioplasty), or even vaporize the obstruction with a laser. As time passes, we will get better at these very expensive and complex techniques, but they will never substitute for a heart without plaques.

Prevention accomplishes that—keeping your cholesterol low, staying thin, not smoking, leading an active life. This is less impractical than it sounds because Americans have been doing pretty well: Over the past 30 years, heart attack deaths have dropped 40 percent.

We have fairly good drugs that strengthen the heart, reduce its workload, increase blood supply, and suppress irregular beats generated by diseased muscle, but these are temporary expedients. Dissolving the buildup would restore the heart to normal, but this is not as easy as it sounds. Cholesterol plaques are rock-hard. Some evidence exists that drastically (not modestly) lowering your cholesterol gradually reduces the buildup; I encourage that.

Diuretics

21 Hydrochlorothiazide • 22 Dyazide • 23 Lasix

Most patients who ask me for antibiotics don't need them. The situation is clearer for diuretics; almost everyone who asks doesn't need them. These are young women who tell me they are "retaining water" and feeling bloated, or patients of any age with swollen ankles at the end of the day. Except to some women who genuinely swell before their period, doctors do not enjoy giving diuretics for these problems. Bloating is a symptom of intestinal muscle spasm, not excess "water" (and not, if you've read my other books, gas).

Swollen ankles after standing occur when your leg veins leak under the weight of all the blood above, and fluid oozes out. Veins grow more porous with age, so readers with no problem now may eventually notice it. Doctors call this a "cosmetic problem," because it looks bad but isn't dangerous. To alleviate the condition, doctors tend to urge you to eliminate salt from your diet, wear tight stockings, and put your legs up. Although that works, drugs work better. In my youth I delivered lectures on the unwisdom of poisoning your kidneys to eliminate harmless water. Patients mostly nodded politely, but looked discouraged. Nowadays if a patient still yearns for a diuretic after I've done my best, I'll prescribe a small dose.

Patients who receive a diuretic are getting one of the great triumphs of medicine. Modern diuretics have saved more lives than antibiotics with less publicity. Most lives have been saved treating high blood pressure, and despite an onslaught of good new drugs, diuretics remain among the best. They also help victims of heart failure and improve the quality of life in several other ailments.

Diuretics are treatment of choice for:

1. *High blood pressure.* With so many families of antihypertensives available, it's inevitable that many doctors find one or another preferable for various subclasses of patient, and you'll read about them in drugs 31 to 38. But for the average, healthy person with a diagnosis of high blood pressure, diuretics remain at the top. They are also the cheapest by far. At the mention of "cheap," patients are quick to let me know that money is no object; they want what's best for them. Then I have to defend myself, and it's surprisingly hard to convince a patient that a pill costing a penny works as well as one costing a dollar.

2. *Heart failure.* Rheumatic valvular disease caused most nineteenth-century heart failure. Most of today's failures occur when progressive coronary artery narrowing either kills a segment of heart or leaves the entire organ too little blood to support normal activities. You'll remember the symptoms from the previous section.

Health writers love to praise the miraculous healing properties of the human body. Although there is much truth in this, I read too much worshipful gush; it drives me to think of ways in which our body behaves stupidly and makes a bad disease worse. Heart failure is one.

As a heart beats more weakly, circulation to the kidney drops. Sensing "too little blood coming through," the kidneys retain salt and water to increase blood volume. Normally, the kidneys are very helpful in adjusting the body's fluid balance. If you're bleeding or dehydrated, they hold back salt and water that would normally pass out in the urine. Your life may depend on it. But in heart failure this is exactly the wrong thing to do. The poor heart can't handle the usual volume of blood; the last thing it needs is more.

Diuretics force the kidney to do what a sensible kidney should have done all along. The effect is dramatic in an emergency room where a patient struggling to breath through "pulmonary edema" recovers in half an hour after an injection of Lasix.

Diuretics are good for:

1. *Edema caused by severe kidney and liver disease.*
2. *Many rare diseases with names like diabetes insipidus, renal tubular acidosis, and hypoparathyroidism where the body's mineral or fluid balance is out of kilter.*
3. *Some kidney stones.* Hydrochlorothiazide and its relatives reduce calcium excretion. After a person has passed a calcium kidney stone (not all are calcium; always save your stone!), taking a diuretic daily prevents future stones.
4. *Osteoporosis.* Women who take diuretics in the hydrochlorothiazide family after menopause suffer fewer fractures, probably because they lose less calcium in the urine. This news is only a few years old, so doctors don't yet prescribe them for this purpose, but that may change.

How they work

They work on the kidneys. Popular writers like to explain that kidneys filter the blood, but that's so simplified it's wrong, although they do extract a great deal of fluid from blood passing through: a quart every eight minutes, which works out to 180 quarts a day. If you urinated everything the kidney filtered, you'd shrivel like a prune and die in half an hour.

Fortunately 179 quarts return to the bloodstream; only about one quart leaves the body as urine. As filtered fluid travels down thousands of kidney tubules, the cells lining those tubules are fiercely active, not only reabsorbing fluids and minerals but excreting and exchanging others.

Many body wastes aren't filtered at all—they're excreted by cells in the tubules, which also take back many salts and minerals and exchange them for others. The kidneys filter over two pounds of ordinary salt, sodium chloride, every day. The tubules reabsorb 99 percent. If you're on a low-salt diet, that becomes 100 percent. None appears in the urine, so a doctor can confirm that you're not cheating. Besides getting rid of wastes, the kidneys carefully regulate the amount of fluid, salts, and minerals in your body.

Diuretics have no effect on filtration; they block salt reabsorption. As salt spills out of the kidney into the bladder it carries the water that dissolves it.

Thiazides such as hydrochlorothiazide work on the far end of the tubule, and at that point 90 percent of the salt has already been reabsorbed, so thiazides don't produce a violent diuresis. They also work for a long period—half a day to a day.

Lasix (furosemide) and its relatives are called "loop" diuretics because they act on a middle area of the tubule that makes a 180-degree turn. Most salt is absorbed here, so these drugs produce a larger volume of urine, but act only for a few hours.

Dyazide and *Maxzide* are a combination of hydrochlorothiazide and another drug, triamterene. Triamterene is a poor diuretic, but we use it for another purpose.

Diuretics force the kidney to excrete potassium along with sodium, and this has always worried doctors, sometimes with good reason. Lack of potassium makes the heart more irritable and prone to abnormal rhythms. This is not of much consequence in a healthy heart, but something to think about if you have heart disease, and worrisome if you're taking digitalis (see drug 24.), a drug that also makes the heart more irritable.

In the past, everyone given diuretics received a large bottle of potassium chloride and a lecture on the evils of a low potassium. A wise doctor made the lecture memorable, anticipating the patient's first taste from the bottle. You might assume that potassium chloride tastes like its close relative, sodium chloride, but it tastes far worse. I suspect patients weren't reliable about taking potassium, and sympathetic doctors prescribed too little: several teaspoons instead of tablespoons per day. Potassium tablets have no taste, but they're more expensive and often damaging to the stomach.

Triamterene solved this problem in a way very satisfying to scientific doctors who like a drug that does one single thing. Triamterene blocks the ability of kidney cells to excrete potassium. When released during the 1960s, it was too expensive to compete, but now that the price has dropped there's less reason to prescribe plain potassium. I haven't done so in years, but I also don't give triamterene except to patients on a diuretic plus digitalis and to a few hypertensives with cardiac rhythm disorders. Healthy people taking diuretics do indeed have a lower potassium, but, except for checking the level every year, I don't treat it, and most doctors do the same.

How dispensed

Hydrochlorothiazide is available in 25- and 50-mg tablets. Fifty mg twice a day is the usual dose for heart failure and other disorders causing edema. Larger doses don't produce more diuresis. In the past this was also the starting dose for high blood pressure, but we've discovered that lower doses often work as well. Today, I begin with 25 mg a day, and sometimes 12.5 mg a day is enough.

Hydrochlorothiazide-triamterene combinations contain 25/37.5 mg, 25/50 mg, or 50/75 mg. Since triamterene is included only to prevent potassium loss, the amount of hydrochlorothiazide determines the dose.

Lasix comes as 20-mg, 40-mg, and 80-mg tablets, an oral solution containing 10 mg per milliliter, and an injectable solution of the same concentration.

Forty mg twice a day treats most edema. Unlike thiazides, loop diuretics produce more effect as the dose increases, so we occasionally give titanic doses for stubborn edema or recalcitrant heart failure—up to 600 mg per day.

Although loop diuretics lower blood pressure, they're too strong to use routinely, and thiazides work less violently. Only when thiazides fail should a doctor consider switching, and this happens most often in high blood pressure

---

Patients with edema worry about their fluid intake. After all, isn't edema water? In fact, water flows freely out the kidney. If you drink too much water, it turns quickly into urine. If you eat salt, however, the kidney must find water to dissolve it, so it reabsorbs more. To reduce your blood volume and eliminate edema you must get rid of salt; that's why patients with high blood pressure and heart failure must avoid salt. They can drink as much water as they want (unless, of course, they have kidney disease).

combined with kidney failure. Loop diuretics continue to work during kidney failure, but thiazides lose their effectiveness.

Translating the label

Hydrochlorothiazide may come as Hydrodiuril, Esidrix, Oretic, or Hydrochlor. Too many other thiazides exist to list here; none works better or costs less. Their generic names end with -thiazide (chlorothiazide, polythiazide, bendroflumethiazide, etc.). Hydrochlorothiazide-triamterene is known as Dyazide and Maxzide. Hydrochlorothiazide dominates the market so completely that no company combines triamterene with another thiazide although this would work as well.

Lasix dominates the market for furosimide, although many generics exist.

Other loop diuretics are ethacrynic acid (Edecrin), which has been around as long as Lasix but isn't used much because of a few more unpleasant side effects, and bumetanide (Bumex): new, heavily promoted, not superior, and (like all new drugs) much more expensive.

Side effects

Any drug that blocks kidney function can produce a dazzling variety of fluid and mineral abnormalities. Checking for them provides a major source of income for clinical laboratories. During exam time, medical students' calculators work busily, searching for solutions to complex electrolyte problems. Mathematically inclined doctors become kidney specialists.

Daily diuretic use can elevate the uric acid, glucose, calcium (loop diuretics lower calcium), and cholesterol but lower sodium, potassium, chloride, and magnesium. Then again they may not, or the change may have no importance.

As noted, a low potassium level marks the most significant abnormality, important to avoid in someone with severe medical problems. It's less important in healthy people with high blood pressure and won't happen if you only take a diuretic now and then. I check blood potassium once a year in my hypertensives, and urge them to avoid salt because sodium and potassium excretion rises and falls together.

I pay less attention to potassium than my patients who read ominous warnings in women's magazines and self-help books. Mostly healthy, they don't worry about dangerous cardiac rhythms; what catches their eye are other symptoms of potassium deficit: "weakness, lethargy, and muscle fatigue . . . ."

Chronic fatigue is a common complaint among healthy patients. Entire books cover the subject, but this isn't one because I have no brilliant solution. If my patients aren't currently tired, they worry about it, especially if they are taking a drug that may cause it. Some patients accept my reassurance that fatigue from low potassium is rare, but others don't, so I find myself prescribing Dyazide or Maxzide to patients who don't need them. In fact, that's the most common reason I prescribe them.

Treating gouty patients, I remember that diuretics raise the uric acid level and provoke an attack of gout, but I've never witnessed this. I worry a little about raising blood sugar. Theoretically this can unmask diabetes in someone who's on the verge, but it doesn't happen often. I also haven't found that it creates difficulties controlling my diabetics' blood sugar, although that's another possibility.

Despite the many metabolic derangements diuretics can produce in theory, they are remarkably benign. They don't produce the four effects patients hate the most: upset stomachs, drowsiness, impotence, or constipation.

Interactions

Food. No significant problems.

Alcohol. Beer drinkers should take care. As a resident, I hospitalized a middle-aged man who had lapsed into a semicoma while socializing with friends. He was on a diuretic, and his potassium was slightly low, but the sodium was the lowest I'd ever seen. My colleagues wondered how he'd lost so much salt, but I pointed out that losing that much is unlikely; his low sodium showed that the man was waterlogged—his blood was dilute. I had the advantage of remembering an amusing article in a British medical journal describing comatose beer drinkers who were also taking diuretics.

Remember that diuretics force the kidneys to excrete salt, not water. In fact, a kidney under the influence of a diuretic is reluctant to excrete water unless it contains salt. Beer is a very low sodium drink, so it's mostly water, and drinking a dozen bottles in an hour can put you in the hospital because the kidney holds onto the water, waiting for salt to appear. If beer were saltier, the kidneys could handle it better.

Drugs. Antidiabetes pills (Diabinese, Micronase, Glucotrol) are distantly related to diuretics, so one occasionally finds a conflict; usually it's only necessary to change the dose of the diabetes drug. A big conflict exists between diuretics and lithium, used to treat mania and depression. Although chemically related to sodium, lithium is much more toxic, and you shouldn't take a diuretic if you're on lithium.

Diuretics potentiate the action of other blood pressure pills, but we consider this a useful side effect.

Never take potassium if you're on Dyazide or Maxzide, and that includes many salt substitutes (check the label) and low-sodium milk (often high in potassium). never take one class of drug that tends to raise the potassium: the angiotensin-converting enzyme inhibitors that I'll discuss a few chapters further on.

Pregnancy. No diuretic except Lasix causes birth defects in animals. All diuretics are probably safe in humans, but there's also little reason to give them during pregnancy.

Nursing. Diuretics seem safe; too little information exists on Dyazide/ Maxzide.

Allergies

I never see them, but they can occur. Hives and sun sensitivity are probably the most common.

Wholesale cost

Hydrochlorothiazide is a bargain. I pay about $5.60 for a thousand 25 mg, $6.50 for 50 mg.

One generic 40 mg Lasix goes for about a penny.

You pay a premium for triamterene plus hydrochlorothiazide; one combination pill costs 16 cents.

24
Digitalis

Digitalis strengthens the heart, an action anyone can understand. It also slows the heartbeat. Both actions have been known for thousands of years, so those who believe that ancient and primitive cultures have much to teach us about medicine use the digitalis family of drugs as an example.

I have as much respect for folk medicine as folk dentistry. Those healers were clever, but it's safer to get sick in the twentieth century. If you believe natural medicine is superior, you can obtain digitalis from plant extracts among western herbalists or dried toad skin in the Orient, but don't try it. Natural digoxin can kill you. African tribes used it as arrow poison.

The Romans used it as rat poison. Physicians in many cultures prescribed it as an emetic (to cause vomiting) and a diuretic. Digitalis isn't a diuretic, but prescientific physicians didn't understand heart disease. However, they knew edema when they saw it, and occasionally they hit the jackpot.

During the final stage of heart failure, blood stagnates because the feeble heart can't pump fast enough, so fluid oozes into the tissues, and the poor victim swells enormously. Today we treat congestive heart failure before this happens, but in the past "dropsy" was not rare. Giving digitalis strengthened the heart; when blood flowed normally, tissue fluid returned to the circulation, edema disappeared, and the patient felt much better. Miracle cures thrill doctors as much as patients, so healers around the world used digitalis whenever they saw a patient with edema. Not being a diuretic, it usually didn't work, but as long as it worked now and then, doctors were happy to continue.

During the eighteenth century, English physicians made the first scientific observations on digitalis. This was the conclusion of the best doctors:

1. Make sure the patient has dropsy.
2. Give foxglove (the plant containing the drug).
3. If the patient doesn't vomit, give more.
4. If the patient doesn't vomit, give more.
5. (more of the same...)
6. When the patient starts to vomit, stop.

They concluded (correctly) that vomiting meant digitalis was working. We would conclude (also correctly) that vomiting was a sign of digitalis poisoning. Digitalis toxicity is still too common—among the drug's leading side effects—but we do our best to avoid it.

Fortunately, we don't have to give the herb that contains hundreds of chemicals and an unpredictable amount of digitalis. We have the unnatural, but pure drug, so we can calculate how much you need, give the right amount, and then wait, confident that it will work. The best doctor in the eighteenth century had no way of knowing how much digitalis he was giving, and he couldn't allow his desperately ill patient to wait days while he carefully gave increasing amounts. So he stuffed foxglove into his patient until he saw the first evidence of an effect: vomiting.

Digitalis is good for:

1. *Heart failure.* A diuretic is usually the first treatment and may relieve mild failure by itself, but when the heart needs added strength only digitalis provides it.
2. *Excessively fast heart rates*—provided they originate in the atrium, the small chamber where blood arrives first. These have names like atrial fibrillation, atrial flutter, and paroxysmal atrial tachycardia. We never use it to treat rhythms beginning in the ventricles below the atriums. I explain why below.

How it works

Heart muscle contracts in response to an electrical impulse. Each heart cell gradually accumulates a quantity of electrically charged calcium. When the charge reaches a certain level, special proteins in the cell suddenly contract. Then the charge builds up again. Digitalis allows the calcium to build to a higher level, so the eventual contraction is more forceful.

Many drugs like adrenalin make the heart pump more blood, but they also force it to work harder, consuming more oxygen and energy. This is like whipping a sick horse; we don't want to make an injured heart work harder. Under the influence of digitalis the heart becomes more efficient—it pumps more blood without working harder.

To understand how digitalis slows the pulse, you must understand how the heart is built. From high school science, you'll remember that the heart is really two separate pumps with four chambers: two small ones (atriums) on top that empty into two larger chambers (ventricles) on the bottom. Blood from the body empties into the right atrium, which pumps it down to the right ventricle, which pumps it to the lungs to absorb oxygen. Blood returning from the lungs pours into the left atrium, which pumps it down to the left ventricle, which pumps it back out to the body.

Obviously, the entire heart can't contract at the same time. The atriums must contract first, so the electrical signal for a heartbeat begins in the atrium. It spreads across both atriums, but a barrier exists between the atrium and ventricle, and electricity can cross only through a small area called the atrioventricular node. The node slows the current for an instant to allow the atriums to contract, then passes it to the ventricles.

Atriums are not essential. If they stop pumping, blood pours through into the ventricles, which do almost all the work. The heart becomes slightly less efficient, but most patients don't notice. Unfortunately, atriums usually fail because they are contracting too fast to do any good. In atrial fibrillation they quiver without contracting at all. In atrial flutter, contractions are so fast—perhaps 300 times a second—that no pumping takes place.

Although you can live normally with atrial fibrillation, a few minutes of ventricular fibrillation kills you. Luckily, each atrial signal still pauses at the atrioventricular node, so the ventricle doesn't mimic the atrium's fibrillation or flutter or even "tachycardia" (meaning fast heartbeat). But the pause isn't very long; the node can pass enough to make the ventricle race dangerously fast—perhaps 150 to 200 beats a minute (a normal heart beats 60 to 80 times). This is not a healthy speed.

Digitalis is a big help here because it makes the atrioventricular node even slower at passing an electrical signal. When the ventricle is racing because the atriums are beating too fast, digitalis will slow it to a normal rate. It won't slow a normal heart, and it's positively dangerous if the rapid rate originates in the ventricles (see side effects below).

How dispensed

Tablets of .125, .25, and .50 mg, an injectable solution, an elixir of .25 mg per teaspoon, and capsules containing .05 and .10 mg.

Digitalis must saturate your tissues to provide the maximum benefit, so a doctor may give five times the usual amount on the first day, a "loading dose." We do this if a patient needs to feel better quickly. But if there's no hurry, it's safer to give the usual dose, .25 mg per day for an average adult, and wait. Used this way, ten days may pass before a patient is properly "digitalized."

Translating the label

"Digitalis" is a family of similar chemicals. Twenty years ago half a dozen were available, but nowadays almost the only one prescribed is digoxin, also known as Lanoxin or Lanoxicaps. A rare doctor may use a longer-acting relative, digitoxin (Crystodigin), and the above doses don't apply.

Side effects

Writing a prescription for an antibiotic or pain medication, I take a quick look at the patient. Someone very large or small might cause me to make a minor dose adjustment, but prescribing the right amount of digoxin requires more careful calculation. I want to know a patient's weight plus the "lean body weight" as well as the kidney function. I must also know about other medical problems as well as medications he or she is taking. Digoxin is tricky, probably the most dangerous drug a family doctor commonly uses. In surveys of serious side effects, it's always near the top. Five to 20 percent of everyone on digoxin is affected sooner or later; about 20 percent of reactions are life threatening. We divide them into:

1. *Cardiac—about half of all side effects.* You must take the good with the bad, and when digitalis strengthens the heart it makes it more irritable: prone to extra beats and certain irregular rhythms. Patients are often unaware, but doctors want to know, so anyone taking digoxin has frequent electrocardiograms.

A low potassium combined with digitalis makes the heart still more irritable, so anyone on diuretics and digoxin must take extra potassium or triamterene.

Another good-with-the-bad: since it slows the heart, it sometimes slows it too much. If digoxin works so well on the atrioventricular node that no current passes, a patient has "complete heart block." You might assume that the heart stops and the patient drops dead, but this rarely happens—at least not immediately—because the ventricles beat spontaneously (although slowly) even without a signal. But complete heart block is not healthy.

2. *Gastrointestinal—one quarter.* Before vomiting occurs, victims of digitalis toxicity lose their appetite and feel queasy. This is so common that diet pills once contained large amounts of digitalis. This is still true in some parts of the world, but unlikely in the U.S.

3. *Nervous system and other—one quarter.* Although not very common, yellow vision is a unique effect of digitalis toxicity. Blurry vision, weakness, headache, and psychotic reactions happen now and then.

Despite all these unpleasant possibilities, most people taking digoxin feel fine—and a good deal better than before they began.

Interactions

Food. None.

Alcohol. None.

Drugs. Innumerable. Diuretics don't really "interact," but they lower potassium; so does oral cortisone. Among other drugs mentioned in this book:

— Beta blockers (Drugs 32. and 33.), and calcium channel blockers (Drugs 34. and 35.) also suppress the atrioventricular node and encourage heart block.

— Antibiotics may kill intestinal bacteria that inactivate digoxin, so more will be absorbed. I don't know of a doctor who pays attention to this, and a week or two of antibiotics is probably safe.

— Opiates (Part IV) may increase absorption by slowing transport through the intestines.

— Antacids (Part III) may interfere with absorption.

— Quinidine (Drug 25.) and verapamil (Drug 34.) increase blood levels for unclear reasons.

— Thyroid (Drug 71.) is safe if you're taking it to replace a real deficiency. Make sure this is the case; excess thyroid makes the heart more irritable.

Pregnancy. There's no evidence of birth defects, but only women with serious heart disease should get it.

Nursing. Some appears in breast milk, but much less than the usual dose for an infant.

Sex. Rumor has it that digitalis can cause impotence and diminished sexual drive, but this must be rare.

Allergies

Despite the mass of side effects, genuine allergy is almost unheard of. In one huge study of drug reactions, 9,399 patients who took digitalis suffered none.

Wholesale cost

About 4 cents per .25-mg tablet.

25
Quinidine

Quinidine is a form of quinine, an ancient drug used to treat malaria and dozens of other diseases. It didn't work for the "other diseases," but since it worked so well for malaria our ancestors loved using it.

Two hundred years ago, an occasional patient treated for malaria noticed that his irregular pulse became regular, so quinine was the first antiarrhythmic drug. In the middle of the nineteenth century, quinidine was isolated and given its name by, of all people, Louis Pasteur. You may remember Pasteur as the famous bacteriologist, but he began life as a chemist and made important discoveries. He discovered stereoisomers, and quinidine is one of two stereoisomers of quinine.

Many chemicals exist as stereoisomers, identical in structure except they are mirror images. Your left and right hands are mirror images. They're identical, but when faced in the same direction you can't superimpose them. One chemical stereoisomer has slightly different properties from the other, and it turns out that quinidine affects the heart more strongly than natural quinine, a mixture of both stereoisomers.

Quinidine is treatment of choice for:

Preventing atrial fibrillation and atrial flutter. In the past, doctors gave quinidine to "convert" the heart back to a regular rhythm, but it took high doses and only worked a third of the time. A low-voltage shock from a cardioverter (also used for cardiac arrest) works better with fewer side effects. Once the rate is regular, doctors give quinidine hoping to keep the heart from reverting. Sometimes that isn't possible, but persistent atrial fibrillation or flutter is not dangerous unless the rate is too fast. If so, treatment is digoxin.

Quinidine is good for:

1. *Preventing life-threatening cardiac rhythms.* Mostly this means ventricular fibrillation, the common cause of cardiac arrest. Once revived, a victim will probably receive quinidine to lessen the chance of a recurrence. Not quite as life-threatening is ventricular tachycardia (tachycardia means "fast heart") in which the ventricle overrides the usual signal from the atrium and beats too rapidly on its own.
2. *Suppressing extra beats.* "Premature contractions" on an electrocardiogram look larger and uglier than normal beats. This makes many doctors nervous, and they can't resist the urge to make them disappear. Although a few types are ominous, there's no evidence that the average extra beat leads to more serious rhythms and requires treatment—especially with a drug as risky as quinidine. If your family doctor treats your extra beats, make sure you hear an explanation of why your beats are particularly dangerous. It wouldn't hurt to consult a cardiologist.
3. *Treating malaria.* It works fine when quinine isn't available.

How it works

Quinidine slows electrical conduction through the heart and even through an individual heart cell, so it decreases irritability and "automaticity." Automaticity means the heart can beat even when there is no electrical signal—a useful quality when something blocks the usual signal, but risky in an irritable heart.

How dispensed

Tablets of 200, 275, and 300 mg and long-acting tablets of 300 and 324 mg. Dosage varies according to how well the rhythm is controlled, but it's usually one or two regular tablets four times a day, or one or two of the long-acting two or three times.

Translating the label

Look for "quin": Quinaglute, Quinidex, and Cardioquin.

Side effects

Remember I said digitalis is the most dangerous drug a family doctor commonly prescribes. Quinidine is more dangerous, but family doctors don't use it much. When I see a patient on the drug, a cardiologist has usually prescribed it.

Cardiac side effects are opposite from those of digitalis: quinidine weakens the heart and makes it less irritable. The weakening is usually not significant, but we don't like to prescribe it to someone already in heart failure. Making an irritable heart less irritable is helpful, but treating someone whose electrical conduction is already slow can stop the heart entirely. When a patient suffering "heart block" requires quinidine, a cardiologist may put in a pacemaker first.

An upset stomach is the leading noncardiac side effect. Switching to different formulations may or may not help.

Before chemists isolated the drug, patients got their quinine by eating the bark of the cinchona tree. This named the side effect called "cinchonism": ringing in the ears, temporary loss of hearing, dizziness, blurred vision, and nausea. It still occurs in sensitive individuals.

Side effects are so troublesome that almost one third of patients can't tolerate them. Fortunately, most occur so quickly that experts advise giving the first dose in the office. A patient with no problems after a week will probably do fine.

If you're black and you don't remember my paragraph about G-6-P-D deficiency in the sulfa chapter, take a look. Quinidine is another drug that causes anemia in those with G-6-P-D.

Interactions

Food. None.
Alcohol. None.

Drugs. Blood level of digoxin doubles on the usual dose of quinidine. Diuretics, Tagamet, and verapamil increase the blood level of quinidine; the epilepsy drugs, Dilantin and phenobarbital, decrease it. Antacids delay absorption. Doctors can safely give quinidine with these drugs provided they adjust the dose.

Pregnancy. No clear evidence of birth defects, but it shouldn't be given unless essential.

Nursing. Probably O.K.

Sex. None.

Allergies

Hives, itching, flushing, and asthma are not common and usually occur during the first few weeks.

Wholesale cost

Twenty-five cents for a 324-mg timed-release tablet, seven cents for a plain 200-mg tablet.

26
Nitroglycerin—Short-Acting

The man who synthesized nitroglycerin in 1846 did what many scientists did in that freewheeling century: he tasted it. And got a headache.

Nineteenth-century doctors loved drugs with quick and interesting action, so nitroglycerin was a hit. Placed under the tongue, a large dose produced giddiness and a throbbing headache that began in less than a minute and rarely lasted more than half an hour. Patients knew they were getting something powerful. For 30 years, doctors prescribed nitroglycerin enthusiastically for a host of ailments before concluding it worked only for one.

Nitroglycerin is treatment of choice for:

1. *Relieving acute angina.* Angina is chest pain caused by lack of oxygen to part of the heart. Patients begin noticing it after several decades of cholesterol buildup when their coronary arteries are partly filled by cholesterol "plaque." The buildup doesn't completely block an artery (killing the muscle and causing a heart attack), but it allows only enough blood through to supply oxygen during normal activity. During hard work (climbing stairs, mowing the lawn, digesting a heavy meal, losing your temper) the heart requires more blood, but no more can pass the obstruction. Deprived of oxygen, the muscle hurts. Feeling intense chest heaviness or ache, an angina victim usually stops whatever he or she is doing. After a few minutes, the heart slows and requires less oxygen.

   The inadequate blood supply becomes adequate again, and pain stops. Doctors define angina as "chest pain provoked by exertion and relieved by rest."

   Nitroglycerin relieves acute angina within minutes. If it doesn't, you probably don't have angina. By middle age, chest pains are a common affliction, and most aren't angina. Family doctors overprescribe nitroglycerin because it's safe and because proving that chest pain is angina is not easy (an ordinary electrocardiogram won't do it).

2. *Preventing acute angina.* Veteran angina sufferers use nitroglycerin five minutes before an activity that brings on an attack: taking out the trash, washing windows, having sex.

Nitroglycerin is good for:

Smooth muscle spasm. "Smooth" muscle is any muscle you don't use for moving around ("skeletal" muscle). Smooth muscle lines your blood vessels, digestive tract, glands, ducts, and organs. Some very severe chest pains are not angina but muscle spasm of the esophagus. Many people have spasm of the arteries in their fingers, causing pain and even gangrene and ulcerations. Nitroglycerin is worth a try.

How it works

Since narrowed coronary arteries lead to angina, experts assumed nitroglycerin worked by dilating those arteries. Like many reasonable assumptions in medicine, that turns out to be wrong. Nitroglycerin works mostly by relaxing arteries and veins outside the heart. By relaxing arteries, blood pressure drops, so the heart ejects blood with less effort. Veins return blood to the heart; when relaxed, they hold more blood, so less pours into the heart. With less to pump, the heart needs less oxygen.

This truth about nitroglycerin is slightly discouraging. It doesn't allow the heart to work harder, but only lowers the workload.

How dispensed

Sublingual nitroglycerin is the common form. You'll find it as .15-, .30-, .40-, and .60-mg tablets. They dissolve under the tongue in a few minutes.

One can spray nitroglycerin from a can—also under the tongue. Use up to three doses of the sublingual form or spray over 15 minutes. If pain persists, see a doctor quickly.

Translating the label

Although usually generic, the sublingual tablet also comes as Nitrostat.

The spray is Nitrolingual.

Side effects

The major discomforts are not "side" effects but the proper action of the drug. You should expect them. The drop in blood pressure causes dizziness. Everyone should sit down after taking a tablet. Users aren't guaranteed a headache, but they should experience at least a vague throbbing. Flushing often occurs because skin blood vessels are dilated. When no symptoms occur, tablets may be outdated.

Interactions

Food. None, but you should avoid eating while using it.

Alcohol. Combined with nitroglycerin it can drop blood pressure drastically and produce intense dizziness.

Drugs. Very few with short-acting nitroglycerin.

Pregnancy. Although it's an old drug, few pregnant women need nitroglycerin, so nothing is known, and I can't even find records of animal tests.

Nursing. The short-acting form disappears from the blood quickly, so it's probably O.K.

Sex. Although an erection occurs when blood pressure drops in the penile arteries and blood flow increases, nitroglycerin apparently doesn't help or hinder.

Allergies

Rashes and severe reactions are extremely rare.

Wholesale cost

Four cents for sublingual tablet, $23 for can of spray.

27
Long-Acting Nitrates: Isosorbide Dinitrate (Isordil, Sorbitrate)

Nitroglycerin prevents angina nicely, but the effect wears off in half an hour, so drug companies worked hard to keep nitrates in the blood for long periods and eventually succeeded. Defeating the liver was their major problem.

Dissolving nitroglycerin under the tongue works because veins in the mouth carry blood directly to the heart, which pumps it out to the body. Swallowed nitroglycerin also gets into the blood, but veins from the digestive tract first flow through the liver, a huge, complex organ that processes nutrients and almost everything else you swallow. Very little nitroglycerin that enters the liver emerges from the other end.

Oral nitrates appeared after World War II. Doctors prescribed them; patients took them more or less as prescribed. When asked, patients agreed they were having less angina. But they weren't, researchers found on closer study. Pain is one symptom easily influenced by a placebo (unlike, say, vomiting or fever). Almost any drug given by an enthusiastic doctor diminishes pain for a while.

Researchers tried larger and larger oral doses and various chemical relatives, finally developing genuinely useful long-acting nitrates. Isosorbide dinitrate works fine.

Isosorbide dinitrate is good for:

1. *Relieving acute angina.* Sublingual Isordil or chewable Sorbitrate works although not as quickly as plain nitroglycerin—perhaps in three minutes instead of two—so we only use it when a patient can't tolerate nitroglycerin.
2. *Preventing angina.*

How it works

All nitrates work alike, but "toleration" becomes a problem with long-acting forms. After a week, they stop working (that's why, although nitrates lower blood pressure, they're not a practical treatment). The bright side is that toleration disappears in less than a day when they're not used. So we try to prescribe long-acting nitrates for most of the day, but not all. If you need continuous protection, calcium or beta blockers work better.

How dispensed

Isosorbide dinitrate comes as:
   — a sublingual tablet of 2.5, 5 and 10 mg.
   — a chewable tablet of 5 and 10 mg.
   — a tablet to swallow containing 5, 10, 20, 30, and 40 mg (notice larger dose).
   — a slow-release tablet or capsule containing 40 mg.

We treat acute angina with a 2.5- or 5-mg sublingual tablet or twice this amount of chewable tablet. Preventing angina requires double this dose; it works for two to three hours. The swallowed tablets are supposed to work for six hours, the slow-release for eight to twelve hours. One begins with the lowest dose and builds until relief appears.

Translating the label

Isordil and Sorbitrate are brands that have been around for 30 years, but plenty of generics are available, plus less common brand names: Dilatrate and Iso-bid.

Many other long-acting nitrates are on the market including:

— Pentaerythritol tetranitrate tablets: Peritrate.

— Plain nitroglycerin in slow-release tablets: Nitroglyn, Nitrong.

— Isosorbide mononitrate (Ismo), slow-release tablet.

— A "buccal" tablet held between cheek and gum; dissolves over several hours: Nitro-gard.

— Nitroglycerin ointment absorbed through skin: Nitro-bid.

— Patches stuck to skin that slowly release nitroglycerin: Deponit, Mini-tran, Nitrodisc, Transderm-Nitro.

Patches have become the rage because they are so convenient, but they're not superior, and the smaller patches may not work at all. As I've mentioned, keeping a constant blood level of a nitrate leads to tolerance, and many patients who faithfully change their disks every day receive only a placebo effect. I like to prescribe a four-times-a-day pill three times a day.

Side effects

Similar to short-acting nitrates.

Wholesale cost

For sublingual tablets, 3 cents apiece.

Less than a penny apiece for 5- and 10-mg oral tablets. Slightly more for large sizes.

The 40-mg timed-release tablet would cost me about six cents.

Twenty cents for a 5-mg chewable.

Technology doesn't come cheap; I'd pay over a dollar for a patch.

Cholesterol-Lowering Drugs: Niacin, Questran, Lopid

Next to quitting smoking, lowering cholesterol is the healthiest action the average person can take. Nowadays, only a minority can benefit from not smoking, but almost everyone should work on cholesterol. The lower your level, the better off you are. If you can push it down to 150 mg per 100 cc, cholesterol will not settle onto your arterial walls and build up into rock-hard, obstructive plaques. Your risk of hardening of the arteries (atherosclerosis), which leads to heart attacks and strokes, will drop to near zero.

The Nature of the Problem

When I entered practice 20 years ago, a lab slip for a blood cholesterol looked like all lab slips. Printed near the space for the result were normal values: 180 to 300. When a patient's level rose above 250, we grumbled that he was on thin ice and should start trimming fat from his beef. But, after all, anything under 300 was normal. Today the slip contains an essay on the meaning of different levels plus a table of normal values for subcategories of cholesterol (HDL, LDL, etc.). It's an improvement in some ways, but not all.

Do you know what a "normal" test is? You're in good company if you don't because many doctors are unsure. To illustrate, let's say scientists develop a new test: a blood porcelain. Part of their task is to draw blood from a few hundred average people and measure the porcelain level. Perhaps everyone's result lies between 7 and 45. The researchers calculate where 95 percent lie (say between 11 and 35), and like magic that becomes the normal range. So "normal" is only a statistical term; it means 95 percent of the population fits inside.

Finding a normal value by measuring general population works fine if almost everyone is healthy. But what if that isn't so? If you measure body weights during a famine, how useful are 95 percent of the results? ("You weigh 82 pounds, Mr. Jones, but that's . . . let me check . . . that's within normal . . . ").

In the same way, American cholesterol values are wildly distorted because so many of us are diseased. You know heart attacks and so forth are our leading cause of death, but you probably don't know humans shouldn't have atherosclerosis (this isn't true for all diseases; for example, even a perfectly healthy person has a certain cancer risk). In cultures where normal values of cholesterol are *really* normal—say between 80 and 150—no one's arteries harden and fill up with cholesterol.

Early in my career, experts were growing skeptical of our cholesterol statistics. At first they told us to treat everyone with a level above 260. Within a few years, they lowered this to 240, then 220, and by the late 1980s I was reading instructions to take action at the 200 level. That includes most of my patients! Experts also found subtypes of cholesterol: low density lipoprotein cholesterol (LDL, a bad one that we should lower) and high density lipoprotein cholesterol (HDL, good cholesterol; the higher the better). Many of my patients worry about their subtypes, but I don't. These are useful for borderline situations, but getting your total cholesterol under 200 remains the goal. Drugs help, but they're only essential in rare inherited defects in cholesterol metabolism. Everyone else can accomplish this by diet.

Diet Before Drugs

If this were a book on lowering your cholesterol, you wouldn't be reading it because no publisher would publish it. No market exists for a book that makes statements like: Most of you won't follow a diet that lowers your cholesterol a great deal. Modestly changing your diet won't do it. That will modestly lower your cholesterol. To reach a level where your risk of atherosclerosis is near zero involves a radical change: an extremely low-fat, high-fiber, nearly vegetarian diet. The Pritikin diet is an example (Pritikin got rich, and his book sells well, but most people give up on it).

Although eccentric, the healthiest diet isn't necessarily unpalatable. I follow it, and I love eating, although friends have long since stopped inviting me to dinner because I refuse to eat many common foods. So it takes a compulsive character that most people don't have. Try, but remember that life is short, and food one of its great pleasures.

When We Think About Drugs

Today, doctors reduce blood pressure to normal nearly 100 percent of the time with almost no side effects. We reduce cholesterol somewhat with a high incidence of side effects, but we've been treating blood pressure aggressively for 40 years, cholesterol about 20. Eventually we'll do better.

We try diet first. If you can't bring your level below 240 in six months, we try drugs. In the future, we'll bring everyone below 200 even if it requires drugs, but today we're not sure the risk outweighs the benefits for levels below 240. So if your cholesterol is 220, and your doctor says you don't need drugs, he's probably right. But that's still too high.

Knowledge that a hundred million Americans would happily pay to eat steak and eggs without guilt has not escaped the drug companies, and they are working hard to tap into this bonanza.

Although no breakthroughs are in sight, I expect steady improvements. Three drugs that work today are:

1. Niacin—the cheapest.
2. Questran—the safest.
3. Mevacor—the most pleasant.

28
Niacin

Also known as nicotinic acid, this is a vitamin, but don't think of it as a nutrient. Niacin deficiency doesn't raise cholesterol and taking an adequate amount doesn't lower it. To lower cholesterol we use niacin as a drug—giving at least a hundred times the body's requirement.

How it works

In massive doses, it diminishes production of LDL and, as a side benefit, increases HDL. After a month, total cholesterol should drop 10 to 15 percent.

How dispensed

Tablets of 50, 100, 250, and 500 mg and sustained-release capsules of 125, 250, 400, 500, and 750 mg.

Twenty-five milligrams satisfies your nutritional needs, but this won't touch an elevated cholesterol. That requires 3,000 to 6,000 mg.

Translating the label

Look for "Ni..." Brands include Niacor, Nicobid, Nicolar, and Slo-Niacin.

Side effects

Anyone who thinks megavitamins make you feel better should try a few grams of niacin. Almost everyone feels an intense flushing; their skin turns red, feels hot, and sometimes itches. We try to minimize that by beginning with a low dose and advising taking it on a full stomach. We also assure patients that flushing diminishes after a few weeks, and we may be right. Taking an aspirin half an hour before helps. Finally, we can prescribe the slow-release capsules, but that weakens the major advantage of niacin: cheapness. Also, a few (not many) patients on the sustained release form have suffered liver inflammation that returns to normal after changing to the regular form. Until doctors decide if this is significant, stick to the regular tablets.

Massive niacin upsets 10 to 20 percent of the stomachs it encounters; we don't give it to ulcer patients. It also raises uric acid (which can precipitate gout) and makes the blood sugar of diabetics harder to control.

Interactions

Food. Take it with food.

Alcohol. The combination makes flushing worse.

Drugs. Since flushing results from relaxed, dilated blood vessels, and since hypertension pills also relax blood vessels, you might expect a conflict, and this sometimes happens.

Pregnancy. No reported problems, but it's a bad idea for pregnant women to take large doses of anything essential for normal body function. The developing fetus should have everything it needs but not too much.

Nursing. Avoid it. Too much of a good thing might not be good for an infant.

Sex. No reported problem.

Allergies

Rare. Itching and flushing aren't allergies.

Wholesale cost

Cost is 1.5 cents for a 500-mg tablet. That comes to 9 to 18 cents per day. Compare this to the two following drugs.

Seven cents for a 500-mg sustained-release capsule.

29
Questran

My 1968 pharmacology text states that cholestyramine (Questran) "may lower plasma cholesterol, but it is not used for that purpose." In a short section (part of the chapter on vitamins) the book mentions without enthusiasm other cholesterol-lowering drugs. Except for niacin, all are little used today or have been withdrawn because of toxicity. In 1968, we knew that a high cholesterol was bad, but no studies showed that lowering it saved lives, so we didn't pay much attention unless the level was sky-high.

Demonstrating that lowering cholesterol prevents heart attacks proved maddeningly elusive. Although expensive, the studies themselves were easy. Scientists recruited a few hundred or (better) a few thousand adults, then divided them up into a control and a treatment group. The treatment group promised to take their medicine faithfully and follow a low-cholesterol diet. Then researchers waited five or ten years to see what happened. Invariably they discovered that the subjects didn't take their medicine faithfully or stick as closely to the diet as they promised. As a result, their cholesterol fell only slightly compared to controls. If their heart attack rate dropped, it dropped so little experts quarreled nastily over whether that proved anything.

Deep in their hearts, cholesterol researchers yearn to study smoking. One has only to watch a few hundred smokers and nonsmokers for a few years to discover the smokers are dropping like flies. No one can produce such impressive results with cholesterol, but things are improving. By the late 1980s some studies managed to push cholesterol down a modest amount so that the modest drop in heart disease convinced the majority of doctors. I'm convinced. The best study used Questran.

Questran is treatment of choice for:

Intense itching from liver disease. The liver produces bile that flows into your small intestine to help digest fats. When disease obstructs bile flow, it backs up into the blood. Bile in the blood causes itching, which can make the patient more miserable than more ominous symptoms of the disease itself. As you'll learn below, Questran increases excretion of bile (if outflow from the liver is completely blocked, it doesn't work). We also try Questran for intense itching when the liver isn't diseased and we can't find the cause. Sometimes it helps.

How it works

Using cholesterol as a major ingredient, the liver makes about a pint of bile a day. After helping with digestion, 95 percent is reabsorbed at the far end of the small intestine, returned to the liver, and used again.

Questran binds strongly to bile in the small intestine. Reabsorption can't occur, so the bile plus the Questran passes out in your stool. Faced with a lack of recycled cholesterol, the liver looks elsewhere for a supply and extracts it from the blood. The drop in cholesterol is similar to that produced by niacin— 10 to 15 percent.

How dispensed

Cartons containing 60 9- or 5-gram packets. Both contain the same amount of Questran—4 grams. You can also buy it in large cans.

Two to six packets a day is usual dose. The consistency of sand but less tasty, Questran must be mixed with water or juice.

Translating the label

The 9-gram packets are original Questran. To reduce the volume of each dose, the manufacturer managed to pack the same amount into 5 grams: Questran Light.

Colestipol (Colestid), a competitor, is a related drug that probably works as well.

Side effects

Neither bile nor Questran absorbs water, so a large, dry mass enters the colon after each dose. Almost everyone complains of constipation, so we urge patients to take plenty of bran and fluids. Bloating, belching, nausea, and flatulence also occur as colon bacteria react to this new source of food.

Along with uninspiring taste, these side effects are tiresome, and many patients give up after a few weeks or months. But all this unpleasantness occurs inside the digestive tract. Unlike all other cholesterol-lowering drugs, Questran and Colestid aren't absorbed into the blood, so they're the safest.

Interactions

Food. Bile dissolves fat, so fat-soluble vitamins (A, D, E, K, and folic acid) leave the body along with it. Rarely a problem for anyone on a nutritious diet, but some doctors give supplements.

Alcohol. No problems.

Drugs. Questran not only binds bile, but a long list of drugs, but that should not cause trouble if you take your drugs one hour before or four hours after Questran.

Pregnancy. Although not absorbed, Questran may lower the fat-soluble vitamin level enough to make it risky, even with supplements.

Nursing. Risky for the same reason.

Sex. An occasional report of increased sexual drive.

Allergies

Hives and asthma occur rarely.

Wholesale cost

Cost is $80 for 60 packets, $35 for can of 42 doses, about $1.60 to $5.40 per day if you buy the can.

30
Mevacor

Megavitamins and intestinal binders are crude and unpleasant. Progress means real drugs with fewer annoying side effects (but an occasional serious one). When doctors began to take cholesterol seriously in the 1960s, drug companies perked up. By the 1970s, Japanese investigators found an excellent possibility in the familiar Penicillium mold, and other companies rushed to screen their molds to find a similar compound, but not so similar that they couldn't patent it. Merck Sharp & Dohme won the race in the U.S. and Mevacor appeared in 1987.

How it works

Mevacor belongs to a class of drugs called hydroxy-methylglutaryl coenzyme A (HMG CoA) reductase inhibitors. HMG is the most important enzyme your liver uses to manufacture cholesterol from simpler molecules; blocking its action reduces the level 20 to 40 percent. Consuming cholesterol partly nullifies that, so patients can't relax on their diet.

How dispensed

Tablets of 20 and 40 mg.

Treatment begins with 20 to 40 mg per day, which may work, but higher doses work better. Increase monthly to a safe maximum of 80 mg.

Translating the label

Mevacor is the brand name of lovastatin. After years of Mevacor's dominance, competitors began appearing in 1992. Although not superior, they may bring down the price.

Pravachol is the brand name of pravastatin.

Zocor is the brand name of simvastatin.

Side effects

Patients on niacin and Questran rarely forget what they're taking, but almost everyone on Mevacor feels fine. A few suffer headaches, constipation, or bloating.

A few percent also suffer liver and muscle abnormalities, so doctors should order a periodic blood test.

Interactions

Food. Take after meals.

Alcohol. None noted, but Mevacor shouldn't be used in the presence of liver disease.

Drugs. Severe muscle damage, often with kidney failure, has occurred when Mevacor is used with niacin as well as another cholesterol-lowering drug, gemfibrozil (Lopid), and an immune-suppressant cyclosporine (Sandimmune).

Pregnancy. Forbidden; titanic doses cause birth defects in rats, but not in mice. Remember Mevacor interferes with an important human enzyme, so there's no telling how that might affect a developing fetus.

Nursing. Forbidden.

Sex. No reported problems.

Allergies

Fairly common. Five percent of users experience rashes and itching and smaller numbers photosensitivity, fever, joint pains, and shortness of breath.

Wholesale cost

Two dollars for a 20-mg tablet, $3.60 for 40 mg. Daily cost is similar to Questran. Knowing anticholesterol therapy is probably a lifetime regimen should encourage you to work on managing by diet alone.

31
Clonidine (Catapres)

A relic of earlier days of hypertension treatment (i.e., the 1970s), clonidine was revived with the development of a skin patch. Swallowed, cheapness is its only advantage in blood pressure therapy, but tantalizing evidence exists that Catapres is useful for preventing migraines and quitting smoking.

Clonidine is treatment of choice for:

Nothing, but the patch is probably equal to the best for high blood pressure.

Clonidine is good for:

1. *High blood pressure.* When I was in training in 1975, Catapres had just been released, and I remember lectures from our hypertension experts extolling its virtues and lack of side effects. They urged us to substitute it for the current leading antihypertensive, Aldomet (still available, but fading). We obeyed, but patients were not impressed. Many complained it made them drowsy—which was their complaint about Aldomet, too. Following instructions, we assured them that might disappear in a few weeks if they persisted. I'm not certain this was accurate. I never liked either Aldomet or Catapres; at that time, beta blockers (next section) were still not approved for high blood pressure, but many of us prescribed them anyway. The Catapres patch does produce less drowsiness. Patients prefer a weekly patch to daily pills, so that would be near the treatment of choice if it weren't so expensive.

2. *Preventing migraine.* Anyone with more than a few migraines a month should take a drug daily to reduce their frequency. Dozens exist, including beta blockers, antidepressants, antihistamines, calcium blockers—and clonidine. A sufferer who hasn't tried them all is having more headaches than necessary. Rarely used in the U.S., clonidine is among the top migraine drugs in Europe. Remind your doctor if he hasn't thought of it.

3. *Quitting smoking; quitting narcotics.* At least once a year a medical journal publishes a study showing clonidine suppresses symptoms of either narcotic or cigarette withdrawal. Although the researchers are reputable, clonidine hasn't made a big splash among those who treat these problems.

How it works

Clonidine partly blocks the sympathetic nerves of your autonomic nervous system.

No one knows what causes common hypertension, but as soon as scientists learned how the body regulates blood pressure, they found ways to lower it by interfering with this regulation. Since early in the century we've known the body has more than one nervous system. The "voluntary nervous system" consists of much of your brain and spinal cord plus nerves that supply your muscles. It's called voluntary because you control it.

But you also have an "autonomic nervous system" made up of parts of the brain, spinal cord, and other nerves that supply organs, glands, blood vessels, heart, digestive tract, and other support systems. This system handles the body's routine housekeeping without conscious control (other writers claim you can exert control by techniques such as biofeedback; there is some truth in this, but it's oversold).

The earliest antihypertensives developed 50 years ago blocked the entire autonomic nervous system. Although this system goes about its business silently, anything that depresses its activity brings it vividly to your attention. Those early drugs lowered more than blood pressure. Patients stopped sweating, their saliva dried up, their eyes stopped focusing, their bowels and bladder fell silent, their mental processes slowed, and they slept a great deal. They were not happy people.

But scientists kept working and learned to separate the autonomic system into a "sympathetic" and "parasympathetic" division. Despite some overlap, the sympathetic system monopolizes control of blood pressure, so drugs that avoid parasympathetic blocking produce fewer unpleasant side effects. Clonidine does that.

Later researchers have subdivided the sympathetic system still further and developed drugs with even fewer side effects. The latest drugs avoid bothering the autonomic system entirely.

How dispensed

Tablets of 0.1, 0.2, and 0.3 mg and three patches programmed to deliver same amount daily over a week's time. Starting dose for high blood pressure is 0.1 mg twice a day. If necessary the dose is increased every month to a maximum of 0.3 mg twice a day. Begin treating migraine with 0.1 mg at bedtime and increase by 0.1 mg monthly to the same maximum.

Translating the label

Never a big seller, Catapres remains the only brand of clonidine.

Side effects

About 40 percent of those taking the tablet complain of a dry mouth. One third feel drowsy. Sixteen percent feel dizzy. Ten percent suffer constipation. Catapres is not hard on the stomach; only 5 percent of patients have nausea or vomiting.

The patch does better. One quarter of users have dry mouth, and 12 percent feel drowsy. Although the rate of stomach upset is the same, dizziness and constipation are rare.

Interactions

Food. None.

Alcohol. Clonidine may increase the sedative effect of alcohol, but that is true of any drug that causes drowsiness.

Drugs. Because they stimulate the sympathetic nervous system, antidepressants may interfere with clonidine's action and require an increased dose.

Pregnancy. No reported problems in humans but a few in animal tests.

Nursing. Probably safe.

Sex. Studies show a 3 percent incidence of loss of sexual desire or impotence. This is the risk when a patient isn't told. In my experience, the rate skyrockets when I announce I'm about to prescribe a drug that very rarely causes sexual problems. References also mention that delayed ejaculation occurs and women sometimes complain of inhibited orgasms.

Allergies

Less than 1 percent for the tablets. The patch often produces local skin irritation, and about 20 percent of users can't tolerate it. The risk is over twice as great for whites as blacks.

Wholesale cost

Two cents for a .2-mg tablet. Other doses differ by only a fraction of a cent.

The smallest patch costs about $7.

Beta Blockers

32 Inderal • 33 Lopressor

"Finally a high blood pressure drug with no side effects," boasted a medical journal advertisement introducing propanolol (Inderal) in the mid-1970s. Until its appearance, powerful antihypertensives (diuretics weren't in that class) made so many patients sleepy, constipated, or impotent that doctors struggled to keep them taking their pills. Now I could assure patients that wouldn't happen.

Today no one praises beta blockers for lack of side effects, but that shows how much progress we've made. Everyone treated for high blood pressure in the 90s expects to feel fine. That wasn't so in the old days.

I've introduced Inderal as a high blood pressure treatment because that's mostly why family doctors prescribe it, but beta blockers have other useful actions.

Beta blockers are treatment of choice for:

1. *Preventing a second heart attack.* Once someone has survived the first, taking Inderal daily lowers the risk of another. Don't confuse that with preventing your first heart attack. Only aspirin does that.
2. *Essential tremor.* A tiresome hereditary disorder in which hands tremble during active movements but not at rest. It's not as disabling as the other common movement disorder, Parkinson's disease, which beta blockers don't help.
3. *Stage fright.* Don't get your hopes up. Beta blockers don't reduce fear, but they block the physical effects of adrenaline, a hormone released when you're frightened. You know adrenaline is working when your muscles tense and you sweat, tremble, and feel your heart pound. These uncontrollable symptoms make it difficult for musicians and public speakers to perform, so they benefit from a beta blocker.

Beta blockers are good for:

1. *High blood pressure.* Being old, they're cheap and still very useful.
2. *Angina.*
3. *Aggressive, impulsive behavior in the presence of brain damage.* Especially useful in hyperactive and uncontrollable patients with mental retardation, they lack the dangerous side effects of antipsychotic drugs such as Thorazine.
4. *Cardiac rhythm disorders, especially excessively fast heart rates.*
5. *Idiopathic hypertrophic subaortic stenosis.* When you read of a young athlete suddenly dropping dead, this might be the reason. IHSS is a congenital heart abnormality whose cause we don't know (so it's "idiopathic"). Part of the heart below the aorta ("subaortic") becomes overgrown and thick ("hypertrophic"). Usually that causes no problem at rest, but when the heart beats fast during exercise this thick area gets in the way, blocking exit of blood into the major artery, the aorta (stenosis means narrowing). In other words, the faster the heart beats, the less blood it ejects. As I explain below,

beta blockers prevent the heart from speeding up.

6. *Preventing migraine.* Although we don't understand why, many antihypertensives reduce frequency of migraine. Sufferers should try them.

How it works

You'll remember from the clonidine section how blocking the entire autonomic nervous system lowers blood pressure and produces miserable side effects. When researchers discovered that the autonomic system had a sympathetic and parasympathetic division, other researchers produced drugs like clonidine that blocked only the sympathetic. Patients suffered less, but they still suffered.

Working hard, researchers found that organs stimulated by the sympathetic nervous system had two sorts of receptors: alpha and beta. Alpha receptors concentrated in blood vessels, eyes, and skin, beta receptors in the heart and lungs. When only alpha receptors were stimulated, a subject became alert, blood pressure rose, pupils dilated, and sweat flowed. Stimulating beta receptors increased heart rate and relaxed the bronchioles (we treat asthma by stimulating beta receptors with Adrenalin and similar drugs; patients breathe easier but their hearts pound). Strangely enough, blocking either alpha or beta receptors lowers blood pressure.

By preventing the heart from beating rapidly, beta blockers reduce its oxygen requirements and prevent angina. They also make the heart beat more weakly, not a problem in an otherwise healthy heart, but we don't prescribe them to someone whose heart is already failing.

Having discovered alpha and beta receptors, researchers looked further and found beta receptors came in two forms: B1 and B2. The heart contains mostly B1; B2 predominates in the lungs and muscles. Propanolol blocks both, fine for most patients but troublesome in asthmatics and chronic bronchitics who have hypersensitive bronchiole muscles. Blocking B2 receptors can constrict them and aggravate wheezing.

Lopressor, the first selective B1 blocker, has less effect on the lungs, but so far all B1 blockers have some B2 activity, especially at high doses. With so many other good drugs available, doctors should avoid beta blockers in anyone with these lung disorders.

With so many systems and receptors to play with, researchers are having a field day inventing drugs that block, stimulate, or bypass them. Doctors can now prescribe a beta blocker that also stimulates the sympathetic nervous system. Although that sounds like a contradiction, these drugs do everything propanolol does without slowing the heart. Not slowing the heart is rarely important.

It turns out there are A1 and A2 receptors as well as drugs that block them along with beta receptors; some also stimulate the sympathetic system as a bonus. Although your chance of needing them is slight, doctors love new drugs, and companies promote them heavily, so you may get one when Inderal would do just as well.

How dispensed

Inderal comes as a 10-, 20-, 40-, 60-, and 80-mg tablet plus a long-acting capsule of 60, 80, 120, and 160 mg. There is an injectable form containing 1 mg per milliliter.

Plain metoprolol (Lopressor) comes as 50 and 100 mg tablets and an injectable of 1 mg per milliliter. A long-acting metoprolol (Toprol) comes as 50-, 100-, and 200-mg tablets.

Dosages. For high blood pressure: begin with 40 mg of Inderal twice a day. Allow a week to see if it works; double the dose if it doesn't. One can give a maximum of 640 mg per day. Occasionally a three times a day schedule is needed if pressure rises before the end of 12 hours. Patient takes a long-acting capsule once a day. Begin Lopressor at 50 mg twice a day to a maximum of 400 mg a day. Toprol's usual dose is 100 mg once a day to a maximum of 400 mg.

Angina. Same as high blood pressure.

Rhythm disorders. Ten to 30 mg of Inderal three or four times a day. Metoprolol isn't FDA approved for these disorders, but similar low doses probably work as well.

IHSS. Twenty to 40 mg of Inderal three times a day or 50 mg of Lopressor twice a day.

Preventing migraine. Begin with 40 mg twice a day of Inderal and gradually increase until it helps or you reach 120 mg twice a day. That may take months. Start Lopressor at 50 mg twice a day and work up to 100 mg twice a day. Inderal works better than Lopressor, but don't give up until you've tried several beta blockers.

Tremor. Same as for migraine.

Stage fright. Use small doses, 20 mg of Inderal, an hour before a performance.

Translating the label

Propanolol's brand name is Inderal.

Metoprolol is known as Lopressor. Toprol-EX is a long-acting form.

Other beta blockers are newer and not superior, but plenty of doctors use them. Here's what's available; a few more will appear by the time you read this.

A. Nonselective beta blockers (similar to Inderal)
   - nadolol (Cogard)
   - timolol (Blocadren)
   - penbutolol (Levatol)
B. B1 blockers (similar to Lopressor)
   - atenolol (Tenormin)
   - betaxolol (Kerlone)
C. Beta blockers that stimulate sympathetic system
   - carteolol (Cartrol)
   - acebutolol (Sectral)
   - pindolol (Visken)
D. Beta blocker that also blocks alpha
   - labetalol (Normodyne, Trandate)

Side effects

Twenty years ago, welcoming Inderal for its lack of side effects, I stressed the big three listed in the first paragraph. Drowsiness, constipation, and impotence remain uncommon, but other complaints occur more often. Most common is a vague fatigue that 90 percent of users do not experience (10 percent do; sometimes we should look on the bright side). Perhaps 5 percent feel depressed. Insomnia and vivid dreams are the most peculiar side effect and not uncommon at highest doses. Unfortunately, most of the dreams are nightmares.

Although not really a side effect, beta blockers slow the heart, usually to less than 60 beats per minute. This is so predictable that when I don't find a slow pulse, I suspect my patient isn't taking the drug I prescribed. With the action of adrenaline blocked, the heart doesn't accelerate in response to stress, most likely the explanation for the fatigue some patients feel.

As mentioned, nonselective beta blockers may aggravate breathing difficulty in asthmatics and chronic bronchitics; B2 blockers do the same at higher doses.

Theoretically, beta blockers weaken the heart, which isn't noticeable in a reasonably normal heart, but patients with heart failure should receive a different drug. Since they slow electrical conduction, we don't like to give a beta blocker to anyone with a defect in electrical conduction ("heart block") or a disorder producing a slow pulse.

Interactions

Food. Take the drug with or after meals.

Alcohol. Slows rate of absorption, but problems are rare.

Drugs. Many. Sometimes doctors seem as eager to block beta receptors as they once were to remove tonsils. Like tonsils, receptors are useful so you should keep them in working order if possible. Many surgeons insist that a patient stop a beta blocker before a major operation. Anesthetics and blood loss lower blood pressure; mostly this causes no problems, but a surgeon or anesthesiologist who wants to give a drug to raise blood pressure or stimulate the heart, doesn't want to fight through the effects of a beta blocker.

Insulin and other antidiabetes drugs. Beta blockers are risky with diabetics. During an insulin reaction, a patient experiences sweating, a pounding heart, headache, and trembling. Diabetics learn these are signs of low blood sugar, but they're really the effects of excess adrenalin released during hypoglycemia. Beta blockers can eliminate those early warnings, so we try not to prescribe them for diabetics.

Tagamet and Thorazine increase blood levels of beta blockers so your doctor may reduce your dose (or increase the other drugs).

These drugs decrease blood levels: two antiseizure drugs, Dilantin and phenobarbital, as well as Rifampin (an antibiotic, mostly used for tuberculosis), and aluminum hydroxide, an ingredient in antacids.

It's considered hazardous to combine a beta blocker with a calcium channel blocker (next section) because both slow the heart and depress conduction. Sometimes a cardiologist will take that chance.

Pregnancy. Toxic to animal fetuses in very high doses. No evidence of harm in humans, but we avoid it.

Nursing. Probably safe.

Sex. The parasympathetic nervous system encourages erections, and alpha receptors stimulate ejaculation. Since few beta receptors exist in the penis, impotence shouldn't be a problem, but now and then I hear about it. Rarely, someone of either sex complains of lowered sexual drive.

Allergies

Rare.

Wholesale cost

Propanolol: 1.5 cents for 10-mg tablet to 3.5 cents for 80 mg. Convenience has a price: long-acting capsules range from 40 cents for 60 mg to 75 cents for 160 mg.

Metoprolol remains under patent for a few more years, so you'll buy only Lopressor at 50 cents for a 50-mg tablet, 75 cents for 100 mg. Toprol sells for 45 and 70 cents and $1.30. The other beta blockers are at least as expensive.

Two Calcium Blockers

Although still excellent drugs, beta blockers turned out to produce more side effects than we realized. Around 1980, when our enthusiasm for beta blockers began to wane, a new class of drugs appeared that treated the same disorders in a different way and caused different and probably fewer side effects. Although a significant advance, calcium blockers were heavily promoted and overprescribed, and soon they multiplied to the same confusing excess as beta blockers. But they're good drugs—and the differences between them are greater than among individual beta blockers.

Calcium blockers are good for:

1. *High blood pressure.*
2. *Angina.*
3. *Rhythm disorders, especially those producing a fast heart rate.*

4. *Preventing migraine.*
5. *Relaxing muscles.* Thereby preventing asthma, treating premature labor and premature ejaculation, menstrual cramps, and spasm of the esophagus and other areas of the digestive tract. None enjoys FDA approval for these indications, and I've never felt the urge to try them, but no law forbids it.

How they work

Most patients and even a few doctors take the name literally and worry about interaction with calcium supplements and osteoporosis, but "blocking" has nothing to do with calcium in the diet, digestive tract, blood stream, or bones. These drugs only obstruct the tiny amounts that flow in and out of cells in the heart and arteries, regulating electrical conduction and muscle contraction. When this calcium flow is blocked, conduction slows and muscles relax. Since these drugs don't interfere with the autonomic nervous system, they lack the tiresome side effects of earlier cardiovascular drugs, but do introduce a few of their own.

Calcium blockers not discussed here

Like beta blockers, they are flooding the market. None is clearly superior for common disorders, but subtle differences in their action on the heart or blood vessels may persuade your doctor to prefer one. Most are heavily promoted, so you may receive:
  · diltiazem (Cardizem, Dilacor)
  · nicardipine (Cardene)
  · nimodipine (Nimotop)
  · isradipine (Dynacirc)
  · felodipine (Plendil)
  · amlodipine (Norvasc)
  · bepridil (Vascor)
  · nitrendipine (Baypress) and nisoldipine—two not yet FDA-approved but that may have changed by the time you read this.

34
Verapamil

The first successful calcium blocker, it was approved for treating angina in 1982, but not for high blood pressure until 1987. Even so, doctors often prescribed it before 1987 (once a drug is FDA-approved for one problem, doctors are free to use it for anything).

Among calcium blockers, verapamil is treatment of choice for:

1. *High blood pressure.* It's the cheapest and has fewer annoying side effects than other blockers. Verapamil is best for high blood pressure in someone without serious heart disease. It slows electrical conduction more than most blockers, so we avoid it in anyone whose conduction is already depressed. We also use another blocker for hypertensives with heart failure because verapamil slightly reduces the force of contraction.
2. *Cardiac rhythm disorders.* If digitalis won't slow the rate in someone with atrial fibrillation or flutter, adding verapamil helps. It also prevents and treats episodes of "paroxysmal supraventricular tachycardia," an alarming disorder that occasionally produces a racing heart in otherwise healthy people.
3. *Preventing migraine.* Europeans use calcium blockers more liberally for migraine, and several still unapproved in the U.S. work even better, so keep your eyes open.

How dispensed

In 40-, 80-, and 120-mg tablets plus long-acting capsules containing 120, 180 or 240 mg and an intravenous solution of 2.5 mg per milliliter.

Usual dose is 80 mg three times a day or one long-acting capsule daily. We can go as high as 120 mg three times a day of the regular tablet or one long-acting capsule twice a day.

Translating the label

Brand names are Calan, Verelan, and Isoptin. Some long-acting brands have -SR (sustained release) after the name.

Side effects

Constipation is leader with 7 percent complaining. A few users experience dizziness, fatigue, headache, or ankle swelling.

Interactions

Food. None, but take the -SR brands with food; one long-acting form, Verelan, can be taken with or without food.

Alcohol. None known.

Drugs. Verapamil increases blood level of digitalis; when the two are used together, digitalis dose must be reduced. With similar actions, beta and calcium blockers can depress the heart too much when used in combination, but occasionally it's worth the risk. Verapamil counteracts the effect of quinidine (drug 25.) and lowers the blood level of lithium.

Pregnancy. Toxic to rat embryos.

Nursing. Excreted in milk, so not advisable during breast feeding.

Sex. Although rare, I've seen an occasional report of impotence.

Allergies

About 1 percent.

Wholesale cost

Seven and 10 cents for 80- and 120-mg tablets. One dollar for 240-mg long-acting tablet.

35
Nifedipine

Among current calcium blockers, nifedipine stands opposite to verapamil in actions and side effects. Although we use it for the same problems, it has distinct advantages and drawbacks that you should know.

Among calcium blockers, nifedipine is treatment of choice for:

1. *Angina.*
2. *High blood pressure in patients with significant heart disease.* Nifedipine relaxes narrow coronary arteries more vigorously than verapamil, but interferes less with electrical conduction and strength of contraction. On the other hand, it produces more unpleasant side effects.

How dispensed and how to take it

Ten- and 20-mg capsules plus long acting capsules containing 30-, 60-, and 90-mg.

The starting dose is 10 mg three times a day and the maximum 30 mg three times a day. One can take the entire dose once a day in the long-acting form.

Translating the label

Brand names are Procardia and Adalat. After careful consideration, the Pfizer Company rejected -SR as the extension indicating sustained-release Procardia. Its choice was -XL (extra long).

Side effects

Most are related to its vigor in relaxing blood vessels: flushing, light-headedness, and a mild throbbing headache in about 10 percent of patients. Four percent notice swollen ankles, 2 percent palpitations. Only rarely are these bad enough to force the doctor to change drugs. These reactions occur far more often than with verapamil; to compensate, nifedipine almost never causes constipation.

Interactions

Similar to verapamil except for surprisingly different drug interactions.

Beta blockers. The combination of a calcium and beta blocker lowers blood pressure and calms the heart much better than either one alone—but at the price of too much calming and lowering. Here, nifedipine has the advantage over other calcium blockers. Because of its minimal effect on electrical conduction and strength of contraction, it's the safest calcium blocker to use with a beta blocker. For the same reason, it's less likely to conflict with other drugs that treat rhythm disorders such as quinidine.

Digitalis. Again nifedipine performs better; although it may raise digitalis levels, this is rarely significant.

Allergies

No different from verapamil.

Wholesale cost

Thirty cents and 50 cents for the 10- and 20-mg capsule, $1.10, $2, and $2.30 for the long-acting forms.

Alpha Blockers

36
Hytrin

A modest advance over clonidine, alpha blockers appeared in the late 1970s several years after a more substantial advance, beta blockers. Overshadowed, they never caught on, and I can't recall prescribing them, but other doctors do now and then.

Hytrin is good for:

1. *High blood pressure.* I suspect that alpha blockers have as many miscellaneous uses as calcium and beta blockers, but lack of popularity is a big disadvantage because some new treatments turn up unexpectedly. For example, doctors learned that beta blockers prevent migraines when patients treated for angina or high blood pressure began mentioning it.

2. *Prostatic hypertrophy.* An organ the size of a small walnut resting just under the bladder in men, the prostate manufactures half the ejaculatory fluid which it secretes into the urethra running conveniently down the middle of the prostate. For unclear reasons, every man's prostate swells beginning around age 45. By the 60s a substantial fraction of men notice difficulty urinating as the growing prostate presses on the urethra, and about 10 percent require surgery to cut away the obstruction. When obstruction is less serious, drugs can shrink the prostate enough to make symptoms less unpleasant. It turns out that the smooth muscle in the prostate contains alpha receptors and alpha blockers relax this muscle.

How it works

Drugs blocking all alpha receptors exist, but they make the heart too irritable. Drugs in this chapter block only alpha-1 receptors, so they lower blood pressure with little effect on other organs except the prostate.

How dispensed

As 1-, 2-, 5-, and 10-mg tablets.

Treatment starts with 1 mg at bedtime and may be increased every few weeks. Most high blood pressure and urinary difficulty responds to less than 5 mg per day, but a doctor can go as high as 20.

Translating the label

Hytrin is the brand name of terazosin.

The first alpha blocker was prazosin (Minipress); it works as well as Hytrin but must be taken twice a day. The newest is doxazosin (Cardura), released in

1991. Chemists can generate as many alpha blockers as other classes of antihypertensive, but fewer have reached the market—again because they aren't terribly popular.

Side effects

One percent of patients faint within an hour of taking the first dose because blood pressure falls so rapidly. That doesn't happen if the person is lying flat, so always take the first few doses in bed at night.

For the others, Hytrin improves on clonidine, but doesn't measure up to the newer antihypertensives. About 20 percent of users experience dizziness, 10 percent fatigue, 5 percent one of the following: nausea, drowsiness, palpitations, nasal congestion, and ankle swelling.

Interactions

Food. None.

Alcohol. None.

Drugs. Surprisingly, no significant interactions.

Pregnancy. No birth defects in animal studies and no reports in humans, but we prefer not to prescribe it.

Nursing. Small amounts appear in milk, so it's rarely necessary to discontinue nursing.

Sex. No significant problems reported.

Allergies

Rashes appear in 1 to 2 percent.

Wholesale cost

About a dollar a tablet for all doses. Generics will appear soon, dropping the price, but for now the cheapest alpha blocker is generic prazosin at six cents for 1 and 2 mg, twelve cents for 5 mg.

Angiotensin-Converting Enzyme Inhibitors

37
Lisinopril (Zestril, Prinvil)

Progress in high blood pressure treatment is satisfying to contemplate—more satisfying than, say, progress in arthritis or headaches, which has been steady but modest. From sympathetic blockers in the 1950s to beta blockers in the 1960s and calcium blockers in the 1970s, we have done even better in the 1980s by developing angiotensin-converting enzyme (ACE) inhibitors. Although no better at lowering blood pressure (easy with even the earliest drugs) they have reduced the old antihypertensive side effects to the vanishing point. They have a few new side effects, but remain among the most benign blood pressure drugs.

Lisinopril is the oldest of the once-a-day ACE inhibitors and among the cheaper of this expensive family of antihypertensives.

Lisinopril is good for:

1. *High blood pressure.*
2. *Heart failure.* Cardiologists use ACE inhibitors for difficult cases because it lowers blood pressure without affecting the heart, so cardiac workload declines.

How it works

ACE inhibitors block the enzyme that converts angiotensin I (which has no effect on blood pressure) into angiotensin II, a natural substance that powerfully constricts the arteries. Angiotensin II probably serves a useful function, and an excess probably doesn't cause hypertension, but lowering its level relaxes arteries and reduces blood pressure.

How dispensed

As 5-, 10-, 20-, and 40-mg tablets.

Usual starting dose is 10 mg a day. May be increased every two to four weeks to 40 mg. If that doesn't control pressure, we often add a small dose of diuretic such as 12.5 mg of hydrochlorothiazide.

Translating the label

Lisinopril is sold as Zestril or Prinvil.
- Rival ACE inhibitors:
- Captopril is sold as Capoten.
- Enalapril is Vasotec.
- Fosinopil is Monopril.
- Benazepril is Lotensin.
- Ramipril is Altace.
- Quinapril is Accupril.

Side effects

Angiotensin II has no influence on the heart, so lisinopril doesn't speed, slow, or weaken it or interfere with electrical conduction. Lisinopril doesn't affect the autonomic nervous system, so users shouldn't experience impotence, dizziness, drowsiness, or bowel problems.

Unlike diuretics, ACE inhibitors don't cause potassium loss; in fact the opposite occurs, so a diuretic combined with an ACE inhibitor is excellent treatment for stubborn high blood pressure. ACE inhibitors also have no effect on blood sugar, cholesterol, or uric acid.

Despite fewer traditional side effects than any major antihypertensive, lisinopril has several of its own. Two percent of users show kidney abnormalities; this doubles or triples if the patient takes diuretics or already has kidney disease. A doctor should test the blood for kidney function a few weeks after beginning therapy.

Blood pressure drops so quickly in 1 percent of patients that they become intensely dizzy; one in a thousand faints. Be careful during the first few doses.

A unique side effect of ACE inhibitors, an annoying dry cough, appears 2–3 percent of the time.

Finally, all the side effects in the first paragraph that aren't supposed to occur, occur. But not very often.

Interactions

Food. None. Users shouldn't take salt substitutes that contain potassium.

Alcohol. None.

Drugs. Avoid any drug that might elevate blood potassium such as Dyazide or Maxzide—diuretics that contain an additional drug to inhibit potassium loss. Because ACE inhibitors also inhibit potassium loss, taking potassium supplements is forbidden, but it's not necessary to avoid high potassium foods.

Ibuprofen (Motrin, Advil, Nuprin) and other nonsteroidal anti-inflammatory drugs (drugs 61. and 62.) can also lead to elevated potassium.

An ACE inhibitor can raise blood lithium to a toxic level (potassium and lithium are chemically related). If a patient is taking both, the doctor should test blood for lithium more often than usual.

Pregnancy. In general, women who need blood pressure drugs should continue them if they become pregnant, but NOT ACE inhibitors. Increased fetal deaths have occurred in women taking them.

Nursing. Tiny amounts are excreted in milk, so it may be safe.

Sex. Rare reports of impotence and decreased sexual desire.

Allergies

Rare but unpleasant. About one patient in a thousand suffers a violent reaction called angioedema in which the face, lips, tongue, and hands swell suddenly. Rashes, often with itching and fever, affect 1 to 2 percent.

Wholesale cost

Lisinopril is a bargain if you can't tolerate other antihypertensives, but not otherwise; 5-, 10-, and 20-mg tablets cost about 80 cents; I'd pay over $1.25 for the 40-mg.

38
Warfarin (Coumadin)

During the early years of this century, cattle in the midwest occasionally bled to death for no apparent reason. In 1924, a veterinarian found the cause: spoiled sweet clover that farmers often substituted for corn as winter cattle feed. Over the next decades, researchers isolated the responsible agent and developed a useful relative: warfarin. Experts agreed a chemical that prevents blood clotting could be useful, and this proved correct. A superb rat poison, warfarin remains popular around the world.

In 1951, a man swallowed rat poison in a suicide attempt, but survived. Peculiar events often stimulate medical progress, and this was one. Doctors who observed this case wondered if warfarin might prevent clots safely in humans, and within three years a large trial sponsored by the American Heart Association seemed to show a benefit in patients suffering a heart attack.

That was important news. Besides causing heart attacks and most strokes, blood clots in the circulatory system and lungs are a major source of disability and death. Before warfarin, doctors had no effective treatment, so they plunged ahead with so much enthusiasm the drug soon acquired a bad reputation. Blood thinners are dangerous and probably cause more catastrophic bleeding than benefit to someone suffering a heart attack or stroke. Despite this, 30 years of experience and research have shown they're genuinely helpful in many conditions.

How it works

Warfarin blocks the action of vitamin K, a vitamin that stimulates the liver to manufacture several proteins that participate in the complex process of clotting. The liver secretes these proteins into the blood where they circulate until needed. Injured tissue releases substances that trigger coagulation, so when blood reaches a damaged area the clotting proteins undergo a chemical change, forming a sticky clot that covers the damage.

This result is useful when a blood vessel is torn during an injury. Unfortunately, sometimes the "damage" is a thick, rough cholesterol plaque that accumulates after 40 or 50 years on the American diet. A clot may mistakenly form on this plaque and completely block a blood vessel (in the heart this defines a heart attack). Sometimes clots form on a plaque, then break off and get stuck in a narrower vessel— perhaps the lung or brain. Clots also form when blood stops flowing—especially when it stagnates in the large leg veins of someone who lies quietly in bed for several days. Warfarin is useful for all these conditions. Although it won't dissolve clots already in place, it prevents them from growing and discourages new ones from forming.

Vitamin K is not one of the fashionable vitamins, so no one takes it to feel better. An excess doesn't make your blood more likely to clot, and deficiency is almost unheard of because it's present in many foods and manufactured by bacteria in your colon. Newborns, however, have no colon bacteria and only a marginal amount of the vitamin in their body, so they routinely receive a shot of vitamin K.

Warfarin is good for:

1. *Preventing blood clots in veins.* Clots form in the large veins of people who are immobile (for example, after surgery), or who have diseases such as cancer that make the blood more clottable, or heart failure where blood flows sluggishly. Sometimes clots form for no obvious reason. Warfarin isn't helpful for short-term prevention after surgery because it takes too long to work; doctors use an injectable drug called heparin that I don't discuss because it's only used in hospitals.

2. *Preventing emboli* (i.e., clots that break off and lodge somewhere else) in (A) Someone who has already had one. Clots occasionally grow large enough to obstruct a vein, but far more damage occurs when a piece breaks off and obstructs a more essential organ—especially a lung or the brain. A patient who has suffered one pulmonary or cerebral embolus will take warfarin until the risk of more emboli passes—anywhere from several months to years. (B) Someone at high risk who has never had an embolus. Anyone with an artificial heart valve requires anticoagulation. Doctors think about warfarin in patients with long-term atrial fibrillation (see digitalis), heart failure, and rheumatic heart disease (see cardiovascular drug introduction).

3. *Preventing a second heart attack.* In a recent study, patients who received

warfarin after a heart attack suffered 34 percent fewer recurrences. Although this is an improvement over aspirin (about a 20 percent reduction), the study is too new, and more researchers must get the same results, before it becomes standard therapy. Beta blockers and aspirin are much safer.

4. *Preventing strokes in someone who has had a heart attack.* The study above showed a dramatic 55 percent reduction, but the same caution applies.

How dispensed

Tablets of 1-, 2-, 2.5-, 5-, 7.5-, and 10-mg.

Once you take warfarin, several days pass before the level of clotting protein in the blood drops, so doctors sometimes start with a "loading dose" of about 10 mg for two to four days before dropping to a "maintenance dose" of 2 to 10 mg. The doctor will check how fast the blood clots with a test called a partial thromboplastin time (PTT), and he will do this every day until the time is right, then every one to four weeks as long as you are under treatment. Despite testing, sometimes blood becomes too thin and bleeding occurs, but that is less common than in the past. Twenty years ago doctors routinely kept the PTT at twice normal (for example, 20 seconds instead of 10). Today we prefer one and a half times or less, a safer level but still effective.

Translating the label

Coumadin is the only significant brand of warfarin.

Side effects

We give warfarin to interfere with coagulation, so bleeding is not really a "side" effect—it's an unwanted consequence of the effect we want. About 10 percent of patients treated for a year suffer a significant hemorrhage—into the digestive tract, a joint, the urinary tract, or the brain. About .5 to 1 percent die. In a recent study in which patients were kept on a fairly low dose (PTT less than one-and-a-half times normal), only 4 percent bled. Bleeding is often a serious complication, but you shouldn't forget we give this drug to avoid even worse consequences.

Interactions

Food. Although food slows absorption, all is absorbed eventually. Patients should avoid large amounts of green leafy vegetables because they contain vitamin K; modest amounts are all right.

Alcohol. Reports exist of alcohol both increasing and decreasing warfarin's effect.

Drugs. So many drugs conflict it's safest to assume that all are forbidden unless your doctor says otherwise. He or she should certainly give you a long, long list or simply forbid any drugs without prior approval. That includes aspirin and vitamin supplements. Naturally, vitamin K is forbidden because it cancels the anticoagulant effect. Vitamin C can do the same.

Pregnancy. Absolutely forbidden. It causes both birth defects and hemorrhage in the fetus.

Nursing. Only an inactive form appears in the milk, so it's probably all right except in premature infants. Your doctor should have the last word.

Sex. A rare report of priapism (painful, long-lasting erection) turns up, but no one knows if warfarin is responsible.

Allergies

Rashes, hives, and fevers occur, but rarely.

Wholesale cost

About five cents for the 1-, 2-, 2.5-, and 5-mg tablets, eight cents for 7.5-mg and 10-mg.

PART III
Drugs for Digestive Disorders

39
Tagamet

It's fun to read about great accidental discoveries like penicillin, but medical progress depends on finding things we *know* must exist. Among the most satisfying examples is cimetidine (Tagamet), the first of a family of antiulcer drugs called histamine-2 blockers.

As late as the 1960s when I was a medical student, doctors injected histamine into patients to measure gastric acid production. Histamine causes a normal stomach to pour out more acid, and the stomach of an ulcer patient should pour out even more. This was not a pleasant experience. A patient sat for hours with a tube down the nose while the doctor had the tedious job of sucking out acid every 15 minutes. The test was also inaccurate; patients with ulcers sometimes produced more acid than normal, but sometimes they didn't. Doctors knew that but were reluctant to give it up because the test was so logical. Ulcers are caused by stomach acid, so we should measure it.

The histamine that provokes acid secretion is the same chemical that the body produces during an attack of hay fever. Antihistamines suppress hay fever, but not acid secretion. Experts theorized (correctly, it turned out) that the human body has two histamine "receptors," which they called H1 and H2. Common antihistamines blocked H1 receptors in the skin, nose, and lungs that produced the itching, runny nose, and wheezing of hay fever, but had no effect on stomach receptors. H2 blockers had to exist, so researchers began searching.

By the late 1960s the first H2 blocker reached the market in Europe and was quickly withdrawn after several patients died. Europeans are more adventurous, so new drugs are usually available several years before they appear in the U.S. Our FDA wants more evidence of safety than its European counterparts, so drugs released here have fewer nasty surprises. Don't assume this method is superior; holding back an important drug for several years can also cause needless suffering.

Tagamet appeared in the early 1970s in Europe (we didn't get it until 1977), and quickly shot to the top of the drug best-seller list, surpassing even Valium. An excellent and safe acid suppressor, competitors eager to share the market haven't improved on Tagamet although at least one (Zantac) outsells it.

Tagamet is treatment of choice for:

Nothing. Although H2 blockers are fine drugs, other drugs work equally well.

Tagamet is good for:

1. *Stomach and duodenal ulcers ("peptic ulcers").* An ulcer is a hole. Peptic ulcers happen when acid damages the surface of the upper digestive tract. Although they can occur without symptoms, the traditional complaint is gnawing pain on an empty stomach relieved by food or antacid. Pain is usually centered just below the rib cage.

   Pay attention to that description because most stomach pain isn't ulcers, and H2 blockers are probably the most overprescribed nonantibiotic. Thus, pain on a full stomach is not typical of an ulcer because food should neutralize acid.

   Diagnosing an ulcer isn't easy. I'm reassured when patients have typical complaints, but fewer than half turn up with an ulcer when tested—and these tests aren't cheap: about $500 for endoscopy, the most accurate. The majority have vague ailments we call "gastritis" or "dyspepsia," tiresome but not serious.

   Although finding an ulcer is expensive, treatment is cheap, so good doctors often go ahead with a trial of therapy if the patient isn't very sick and is suffering the first attack. Therapy is *always* six weeks of Tagamet or other H2 blocker taken every day. I see many patients who take a Tagamet now and then when their stomach acts up. That doesn't work.

2. *Preventing a peptic ulcer from recurring.* "Once an ulcer, always an ulcer," is a medical cliche with a good deal of truth. Even without treatment most ulcers heal in a few months, but many return. Taking half the usual Tagmat dose daily greatly reduces recurrences, but only as long as treatment contin-

ues. Most doctors wait to treat the ulcer when it returns unless recurrences are particularly frequent or severe.

3. *Reflux esophagitis with heartburn,* which occurs when gastric contents back up into the esophagus ("reflux" means flowing backward). Unlike the lining of the stomach, the esophagus isn't built to withstand acid, so reflux causes a burning sensation in the chest. Everyone suffers this now and then, but if it occurs regularly—especially when you go to bed at night— see a doctor. At first you'll probably get antacids plus advice on keeping acid where it belongs: not eating for several hours before bedtime, raising the head of your bed, and avoiding cigarettes, alcohol, chocolate, and coffee, which encourage backup. If that doesn't help, most doctors move on to H2 blockers or Reglan (drug 43.). A new drug (Prilosec—40.) is becoming the choice.

4. *Zollinger-Ellison syndrome, systemic mastocytosis, and multiple endocrine adenomatosis.* These are rare diseases accompanied by massive oversecretion of gastric acid. You don't have to know about them. H2 blockers were the treatment of choice until the early 1990s when Prilosec, drug 40, took over.

How it works

"No acid, no ulcers," is another medical cliche; stomachs that can't make acid almost never get an ulcer. H2 blockers don't eliminate acid entirely. You'll do better with omeprazole (Prilosec), but doctors use it for only the most stubborn cases. A little acid is a good thing. Although not essential for digestion, it helps. More important, acid kills organisms swallowed with food. People with less stomach acid (and even those on H2 blockers) are more susceptible to intestinal infections. Those with zero acid can't absorb vitamin B12 (they require injections) and are susceptible to stomach cancer, but you shouldn't worry about this with the usual month or two of H2 blocker therapy.

Taken at bedtime, 800 mg of Tagamet cuts acid by 85 percent over the next eight hours but hardly at all after that. This works fine.

How dispensed

Tablets of 200, 300, 400, and 800 mg, a liquid containing 300 mg per teaspoon, and an injectable form with 300 mg in 2 cc.

In the past, patients took Tagamet four times a day or twice a day, but a large evening dose works equally well, so 800 mg at bedtime is the best treatment for an active ulcer, 400 mg for preventing a recurrence.

Translating the label

Cimetidine comes only as Tagamet, but the patent expires in 1994, so readers will have access then to generics.

Other H2 blockers approved in the U.S.:
- Ranitidine (Zantac)
- Famotidine (Pepcid)
- Nizatidine (Axid)

Side effects

About 1 percent of users notice dizziness, drowsiness, or diarrhea, but these are usually mild. Less often, he or she develops confusion and hallucinations within a few days after beginning; this disappears soon after stopping.

All of Tagamet's rivals advertise that they offer fewer side effects and drug interactions, and they may be right. They're worth a try if you have a bad reaction, but side effects are not common, and I prefer drugs that have been around the longest unless a good reason exists to switch. Lower price is a reason, but the newer H2 blockers are slightly more expensive; generic cimetidine, of course, is far cheaper.

Interactions

Food. None.

Alcohol. Both Tagamet and Zantac increase blood levels, perhaps by increasing absorption and slowing its breakdown. Other H2 blockers don't seem to do this.

Drugs. Taking an antacid within a couple of hours interferes with absorption. Tagamet has a tendency to interfere with breakdown of certain drugs and increase their blood level. Those usually mentioned are blood thinners, beta blockers, Dilantin, and tranquilizers. Although bad effects are not common, your doctor should know all the drugs you're taking.

Pregnancy. No reports of problems in either animals or humans.

Nursing. Considered unsafe because it's heavily secreted into milk.

Sex. Impotence has appeared in men receiving very high doses for the rare diseases mentioned above, but not in the doses used for ulcers. Men have reported swollen or tender breasts, but that is rare at the usual doses.

Allergies

Rashes and drug fever occur rarely.

Wholesale cost

Cost is 80 cents for 200- and 300-mg tablet, $1.40 for 400 mg, $2.50 for 800 mg. Tagamet costs about 15 percent less than its major rival, Zantac.

40
Prilosec

Drug development moves fast. When I began this book, I decided not to include Prilosec, which was approved in 1990, as a different and stronger inhibitor of stomach acid than the Tagamet family. Gastroenterologists warned us not to be too eager to use this highly promoted new drug. It's not necessary to wipe out all acid to cure gastric disorders, they explained. A modest decrease usually works. Furthermore, a stomach with zero acid makes doctors uncomfortable. I worry about this factor in the Tagamet section, which was written before I changed my mind about Prilosec.

During the year that followed, I watched experts change their minds. Human studies showed it didn't produce the rare tumor researchers noticed in rats. The FDA approved it for treatment of ordinary ulcers; experts decided more acid suppression is indeed better, especially for several rare diseases as well as reflux.

Prilosec is treatment of choice for:

1. *Zollinger-Ellison syndrome, systemic mastocytosis, and multiple endocrine adenomatosis.*
2. *Reflux esophagitis with heartburn.* It provides quicker symptom relief and healing than H2 blockers, but some experts encourage doctors to begin with the familiar older drugs.

Prilosec is good for:

Stomach and duodenal ulcers. Despite higher healing rates and quicker pain relief, H2 blockers work pretty well, so doctors tend to prefer them. But I suspect that may change.

How it works

Not a histamine blocker, Prilosec binds directly to acid-secreting cells in the stomach and shuts them down. Twenty mg a day, the usual ulcer treatment, cuts secretion by more than 90 percent. Higher doses do better, but until we have more experience we won't use them except for the rare disorders in category 1 above.

How dispensed

As 20-mg capsules; 20 mg a day treats ulcers and reflux. The diseases in category 1 require at least three times more.

Translating the label

Prilosec is omeprazole.

Side effects

Although usually tolerated, Prilosec makes more patients uncomfortable than H2 blockers. Three to 5 percent suffer either headache, nausea, diarrhea, or abdominal pains.

Interactions

Food. Take on an empty stomach. A delayed-release capsule, it's only absorbed after reaching the intestine.

Alcohol. None noted.

Drugs. May increase blood level of Valium, Dilantin, blood thinners, and Tagamet.

Pregnancy. Some defects in animal studies; none noticed in humans, but it's a good rule to avoid new drugs.

Nursing. No information; probably worth avoiding.

Sex. None reported so far.

Allergies

Rashes in 1.5 percent.

Wholesale cost

$3.50 for a 20-mg capsule.

41
Sucralfate

In the early 1980s, a drug appeared that healed ulcers as well as H2 blockers with fewer side effects. Even better, this drug isn't absorbed into the body, but works locally on the ulcer. Despite wide use, sucralfate has never caught on. Certainly, it lacks the wild popularity of H2 blockers, and doctors don't use it as a placebo for garden-variety indigestion, but I believe it's a slightly superior ulcer treatment.

Sucralfate is good for:

1. *Stomach and duodenal ulcers.* My treatment of choice. Doesn't affect acid flow, so it's not useful for the rare diseases mentioned earlier (Zollinger-Ellison, etc.).
2. *Preventing an ulcer from recurring.*

How it works

For decades, ads for digestive aids have boasted they "coat" the stomach. Your mother gave you milk or another soothing liquid for the same purpose. They didn't work. Your digestive lining oozes fluid and is covered with a layer of slimy mucus; nothing much can stick to it. All foods and medicines obey the law of gravity, collecting in a puddle at the lowest point in your stomach.

Until sucralfate, that is. It reacts with gastric acid to form a glue-like gel that sticks to the ulcer surface. Sucralfate sticks to healthy tissue, too, but less firmly. Food and antacids don't wash it off, and the coating from one dose lasts about six hours. Most likely, that protects the ulcer from further acid injury.

How dispensed

In 1-gram tablets. The original dose was one tablet an hour before meals and at bedtime, but it turns out that two tablets twice a day work as well. We use half this dose to prevent a recurrence. The ulcer usually heals in six weeks.

Translating the label

Sucralfate is Carafate, and no other company seems interested in marketing a competitor.

Side effects

Very little enters the bloodstream, so side effects are almost unknown. About 2 percent of users have constipation.

Interactions

Food. Take on empty stomach.

Alcohol. None.

Drugs. Since it works by being sticky, sucralfate also binds drugs. Give it two hours to settle into the ulcer before taking another medication.

Pregnancy. Probably safe.

Nursing. You'd think no sucralfate would appear in breast milk, and you might be right, but no one has studied the matter, so we don't know. It's probably safe.

Allergies

Reported, but extremely rare.

Wholesale cost

Cost is 70 cents a tablet.

42
Antacids

Advertising has convinced everyone that man fights a continual battle against stomach acidity, so laymen consume huge quantities of antacid. Although they may take Maalox or Mylanta to relieve discomfort coming on after a big meal, that accomplishes nothing because food itself neutralizes stomach acid. Fortunately, antacids are largely harmless.

In the past, doctors also gave antacids for vague digestive upsets; nowadays we prefer to overprescribe Tagamet or Zantac, so if you get an antacid you probably need it.

Antacids are good for:

1. *Gastric and duodenal ulcers.* I treat ulcers with Tagamet for convenience, not because it's superior. The cure rate with antacids equals that of H2 blockers.
2. *Reflux esophagitis with heartburn.*

How they work

Any alkali neutralizes acid. Sodium bicarbonate has been popular since Roman times and remains particularly satisfying because bicarbonate plus acid liberates carbon dioxide, and the large belch that follows is audible proof something good is happening. Bicarbonate works quickly, but provides such a huge dose of sodium that even healthy people should take it only now and then.

Commercial antacids are barely absorbed into the blood, and they don't produce gas as they neutralize acid. One ingredient, aluminum hydroxide, works much slower than baking soda and is constipating. A few products contain this alone. A second ingredient, magnesium hydroxide, works fast and causes diarrhea (milk of magnesia is pure magnesium hydroxide). Most commercial antacids combine aluminum and magnesium in the hope of providing quick but long-acting acid control plus no bowel upsets. Sometimes that succeeds, but you may have to switch a few times to find one that suits you.

Many antacid manufacturers add simethicone and boast that this relieves gas and bloating. I discuss simethicone in the "drugs that don't work" section.

A few antacids contain calcium carbonate, a better acid neutralizer, but also (in the case of calcium) a stimulator of stomach acid secretion, so experts frown on them. These are probably safe for occasional use, but I don't discuss them here.

How dispensed

As tablets and liquid. Use liquid. The tablets must dissolve completely in the stomach, and no one knows if that happens.

Pay attention to your doctor's instructions because the label undoubtedly recommends far too little—usually a few teaspoons. An effective treatment is two tablespoons one and three hours after meals (to prolong the action by mixing with food) plus two tablespoons at bedtime. That's 14 tablespoons per day, so a good antacid course is not much cheaper than Tagamet.

Translating the label

I don't have a favorite antacid. You should choose on the basis of flavor, cost, and the effect on your bowels. Don't worry about those labeled "extra strength." That just affects the dose. Don't pay attention to extras like simethicone. Do notice the sodium content if you're on a low-salt diet.

A few that follow substitute other aluminum or magnesium compounds for the hydroxide, but that makes no difference.

- Maalox
- Mylanta
- Gelusil
- Di-Gel
- Riopan
- Aludrox
- WinGel
- Marblen
- Gaviscon
- Antacids containing only aluminum hydroxide: Amphojel, Alternagel

Side effects

Very few if you obey the label and take tiny amounts.

A genuine ulcer-curing course will probably loosen or tighten your bowels. If that becomes too unpleasant, switch brands. If diarrhea is persistent, try pure aluminum hydroxide. In my experience, no one becomes constipated enough to require pure milk of magnesia, but it's a possibility.

Interactions

Food. None.

Alcohol. None.

Drugs. Antacids interfere badly with the absorption of iron and the tetracyclines. Use another antibiotic. If you're taking iron as a general tonic, taking antacids is all right because they don't interfere with placebo affect.

Pregnancy. Probably O.K.

Nursing. Probably O.K.

Sex. No problems.

Allergies

Never heard of anyone allergic to antacids, but anything is possible.

Wholesale cost

About $2.20 for 12 ounces of generic liquid. Serious users should buy in quantity. Fourteen tablespoons per day equals a quart every five days.

43
Reglan

A few years ago I made a hotel call on an Australian family whose child was vomiting. I'm often shocked at drugs prescribed in foreign countries, and that was my reaction when the mother showed me the metoclopramide syrup she had given her seven-year-old. Our FDA approves metoclopramide (Reglan) for several serious gastrointestinal disorders, but not for the usual upset stomach.

"That's a powerful drug," I cautioned her. "You shouldn't give it to a child." She looked puzzled. Later, I wondered if I overreacted. Australia is a civilized country, and the bottle contained instructions for a child's dose, so it was probably safer than I thought. Reglan's PDR entry teems with ominous warnings, but they aren't any more ominous than those under drugs American doctors prescribe for vomiting. Like foreign food and fashion, foreign taste in drugs may seem strange, but it's not necessarily inferior.

Reglan is good for:

1. *Reflux esophagitis with heartburn.*
2. *Nausea and vomiting.*

The FDA has approved it only for limited and serious indications: before cancer chemotherapy, to prevent postoperative vomiting, or to treat a form of stomach paralysis that affects diabetics. This is another case where doctors are free to use an approved drug any way they choose, but Reglan has never caught their attention. Current drugs work fine, but Reglan is useful when they don't.

How it works

By increasing muscle contraction of the upper digestive tract, Reglan tightens the end of the esophagus and speeds progress of food out of the stomach. Food moving forward is less likely to back up.

How dispensed

Five- and 10-mg tablets plus a syrup and injectable containing 5 mg per milliliter.

Ten mg before meals and at bedtime is a starting dose for reflux and vomiting.

Translating the label

Although an old drug, Reglan is the only current brand name of metoclopramide.

Side effects

Fairly common with continuous therapy. Oddly, both drowsiness and agitation occur 10 percent of the time. Less than 1 percent of users have more alarming reactions such as tremor, depression, muscle twitches, and uncontrollable movements. That makes Reglan sound risky, but similar reactions occur with the "phenothiazines," America's choice for nausea and vomiting.

Interactions.

Food. Take before meals.

Alcohol. Increases drowsiness side effect.

Drugs. Sedatives, sleeping pills, tranquilizers, and narcotics also increase drowsiness. Because it increases stomach emptying, Reglan may reduce absorption of drugs that require time in the stomach (such as digitalis) but speed absorption of drugs that require the small intestine (antibiotics, acetaminophen). Narcotics such as codeine and Percodan reverse metoclopramide's action.

Pregnancy. No problems in animal tests, but the usual warnings apply.

Nursing. Metoclopramide appears in breast milk, so once again the PDR urges doctors to "exercise caution." That probably means you should avoid it.

Allergies

Hives and wheezing occur rarely, mostly in patients with asthma.

Wholesale cost

Cost is 2.5 cents for 5 mg, 3 cents for 10 mg.

44
Lomotil

A derivative of opium, a natural substance known since the dawn of civilization, large doses made people sleepy and relieved pain, but smoking opium for pleasure didn't become popular in the Orient until the eighteenth century. It spread to Europe and led to a modest amount of addiction but never caught on. Opium was not outlawed until well into the twentieth century. Western societies prefer alcohol.

Despite opium's evil reputation, people through the ages mostly took it to relieve diarrhea. In areas with poor sanitation (everywhere before the twentieth century and in most of the third world today) intestinal infections, parasites, and diarrhea from spoiled food were universal. A bottle of tincture of opium was a mainstay of even the poorest family. Mothers fed it to their babies and still do in many countries. Tincture of opium remains available here; you may know it as paregoric (see label below).

Codeine and other opium derivatives given for pain work equally well for diarrhea, but doctors prefer drugs targeted for one ailment, and Lomotil is by far the most popular.

Lomotil is good for:

Diarrhea. Lomotil combines an opium derivative, diphenoxylate, with atropine. In huge doses (and without the atropine!) diphenoxylate causes euphoria and might lead to dependence, but this doesn't happen in ordinary use. Almost insoluble in water, diphenoxylate can't be injected.

How it works

All opiates decrease the propulsive action of muscles in the digestive tract. Food remains in the stomach and takes longer to move through the small intestine and colon. As a result, more water is absorbed and intestinal contents become thicker.

The atropine in Lomotil has no useful action because it's present in such small amounts. The manufacturer added it with the commendable aim of preventing abuse. Atropine blocks the action of parasympathetic nerves (see the clonidine section), so anyone taking a few dozen pills will feel ill, not euphoric.

How dispensed

Tablets and liquid. Usual adult dose is two pills or two teaspoons every six hours.

Translating the label

Lomotil is brand name. Motifen is a competitor that replaces diphenoxylate with a closely related opiate, difenoxin. Other good opiate antidiarrheals include:
- Lopermide (Imodium)
- Paregoric (Donnagel, Parapectolin)

A nonopiate, bismuth subsalicylate (Pepto-Bismol–drug 45), also works.

Side effects

Constipation leads the list, so stop taking Lomotil once diarrhea diminishes. Continual use of opiates produces tolerance to their more pleasant effects but not to constipation. Addicts are chronically constipated. Other side effects are rare at the usual doses—mostly nausea or drowsiness.

Interactions

Food. None.

Alcohol. May increase drowsiness.

Drugs. Lomotil may make sedatives and tranquilizers more sedating.

Pregnancy. No birth defects, but a decrease in maternal weight gain during animal studies. We avoid it unless it's essential.

Nursing. Probably O.K. if used occasionally.

Sex. No problems.

Allergies

Although genuine allergies are rare, identical rashes are not because opiates provoke the release of histamine. Sensitive patients react with generalized itching, flushing, or hives.

Wholesale cost

Cheap. One cent for a generic pill.

45
Pepto-Bismol
(bismuth subsalicylate)

An old but useful drug with new uses popping up now and then, generic competitors are surprisingly hard to find, but they're available.

Pepto-Bismol is good for:

1. *Diarrhea.* As good as Lomotil or Imodium.
2. *Preventing traveler's diarrhea (Montezuma's revenge).* It's difficult to convince

many patients because they have heard that taking antibiotics daily prevents traveler's diarrhea, so they assume a pink medicine sold without a prescription must be inferior. In fact, both work equally well, reducing the risk by about two thirds.

Pepto-Bismol is not very good for:

Treating ulcers. But it's not entirely useless and is occasionally prescribed. Bismuth subcitrate (long available in Europe but not in the U.S.) heals ulcers as well as Tagamet, and other bismuth compounds are under active investigation. Keep your eyes open for FDA approval; these drugs are cheap and safe.

How it works

In treating diarrhea the salicylate in bismuth subsalicylate probably works locally in the intestine to suppress inflammation—an action similar to aspirin, also a salicylate but one absorbed too quickly to work.

Pepto-Bismol probably prevents traveler's diarrhea by suppressing bacterial growth. That may also explain its action in treating ulcers, which rarely occur in the absence of certain stomach bacteria. In fact, evidence is growing that bismuth compounds plus certain antibiotics heal ulcers and keep them healed better than acid blockers. I predict that this will be the ulcer treatment of choice before the end of the century.

How dispensed

Tablets as well as bottles of 4, 8, 12, and 16 ounces.

To treat diarrhea with regular-strength Pepto-Bismol, take two tablets or two tablespoons every half hour to a maximum of eight doses. The dose for the maximum-strength liquid is also two tablespoons, repeated every hour to a maximum of four doses.

Preventing traveler's diarrhea requires two tablets or two tablespoons of the regular strength four times a day for the duration of the trip.

Translating the label

Pepto-Bismol is bismuth subsalicylate. Maximum-strength Pepto-Bismol contains somewhat less than twice the concentration.

Side effects

Often blackens both the tongue and stool; harmless.

Manufacturer warns of the possibility of "salicylism" that I discuss in the aspirin section. Although reasonable because bismuth subsalicylate distantly resembles other salicylates, it must be rare.

Interactions

Food. None.

Alcohol. None.

Drugs. Aspirin's warnings apply, but probably for safety's sake rather than actual experience. Bismuth subsalicylate doesn't irritate the stomach like aspirin and has little effect on blood clotting.

Pregnancy. Salicylates are not a good idea, and we don't like giving heavy metals like bismuth either.

Nursing. Probably O.K.

Sex. No problems.

Allergies

If you're allergic to aspirin or other salicylates, you might be allergic to bismuth subsalicylate.

Wholesale cost

Two dollars for an 8-ounce bottle of the regular strength or 30 chewable tablets.

46
Activated Charcoal

As a child I bought cans of black lumpy material to pack into my aquarium filter. Water from my tropical fish tank first flowed through a clump of fiberglass to remove large particles, then through the charcoal, which extracted waste gases and impurities. Medical science didn't have much other use for activated charcoal at the time, but that has changed.

Activated charcoal is good for:

1. *Removing poisons from the digestive tract.* All emergency rooms stock a supply. You should keep a bottle in the house, especially if you have young children.

2. *Flatulence.* The average person passes rectal gas up to 20 times per day. Vegetarians pass more. Everyone believes they pass too much.

   Bacteria living in your colon generate gas by feeding on carbohydrates that have arrived undigested from the small intestine. Despite the general opinion that fat is hard to handle, your small intestine digests fats (and proteins) very well, so only a tiny fibrous residue enters the colon. This is of no interest to the germs; they thrive on the much larger volume of plant remains containing carbohydrates too complicated for human digestive enzymes but not for theirs.

   Although my patients are skeptical, no disease produces excess gas in an otherwise healthy person. In fact, a nutritious high-roughage diet is very gassy. Once produced, gas moves in the same direction as the rest of your colon contents. It doesn't reverse itself and cause belching; that's swallowed air. It's not absorbed into the blood. Drugs like simethicone that are supposed to break up bubbles are clearly nonsensical because the gas is still there.

   Only activated charcoal makes gas disappear. In studies where volunteers ate a gassy meal, those who took activated charcoal expelled less gas than those given a placebo. In real life, many of my patients are convinced it helps, others are not impressed. It's possible huge doses work better, but no one has studied this.

3. *Diarrhea.* That's what the advertisements claim, but put it well down on my

list. Most diarrhea results from a hyperactive colon or excess fluid in the stool. Charcoal doesn't influence those.

How it works

No relation to burned toast, this is purified charcoal that's been heated and exposed to steam to make its surface extremely absorbent. A surprising number of toxins and gases simply stick firmly to the charcoal.

How dispensed

Tablets containing from 250 to 600 mg. For home treatment of poisoning buy a bottle that combines activated charcoal with water or sorbitol, an indigestible sugar that causes diarrhea. Sorbitol is supposed to make the liquid palatable and speed expulsion of the poison.

The dose for gas is 500 to 1000 mg to a maximum of 4000 mg per day. A poison victim should drink the entire bottle, but try to speak to a doctor or poison control center before proceeding.

Translating the label

Activated charcoal is sold over-the-counter, so learn to look for labels and avoid products with additional ingredients. Plain activated charcoal is extremely safe even in large doses, but all bets are off if you get a mixture.

For poisoning, names include Charcoaid and Actidose.

Side effects

Essentially none although it can turn stool black.

Interactions

Food. None.

Alcohol. None.

Drugs. Needless to say, it absorbs good as well as bad chemicals. Don't take another drug within two hours of a dose of charcoal.

Pregnancy. No known problems.

Nursing. O.K.

Allergies

None known.

Wholesale cost

Three dollars for 100 tablets of 240 mg.

47
Ipecac

Although its recent popularity owes much to the epidemic of eating disorders such as bulimia, syrup of ipecac remains a valuable drug that every parent should keep on hand. Despite being riskier than giving activated charcoal to a child who has swallowed something he shouldn't, inducing vomiting with ipecac is more reliable.

Ipecac is good for:

Making someone vomit. Notwithstanding its vigorous action, syrup of ipecac is safe and sold without a prescription.

How it works

By stimulating an area in the brain that causes vomiting, most likely ipecac also irritates the digestive tract because it works in the presence of drugs such as Compazine or Thorazine that suppress the same brain area.

How dispensed

In bottles of one half and one ounce.

Give one teaspoon for a child under age one, one half ounce (one tablespoon) to children over age one and adults. Vomiting occurs less often if the stomach is empty, so give a glass of water afterward. The dose can be repeated if no vomiting occurs within 20 minutes. Ipecac takes at least 15 minutes to work, but pumping the stomach is no faster. Always try to talk to a doctor or poison control center before taking action.

Don't give ipecac to anyone unconscious or drowsy or to expel a corrosive such as strong acid, alkali, or lye or a petroleum product such as kerosene, gasoline, paint thinner, or cleaning fluid.

Translating the label

You want syrup of ipecac, never ipecac fluid extract 14 times more concentrated. Read the label.

Side effects

None with occasional use, but we don't like to leave it in the digestive tract. If vomiting doesn't occur, the doctor will pump the stomach to remove it. Ipecac contains emetine, a drug useful for parasitic infections, but toxic to the heart. This causes no problem in a single dose and only rarely when treating parasites, but bulimics who take ipecac daily can suffer permanent damage.

Interactions

Food. None.

Alcohol. None.

Drugs. Activated charcoal absorbs ipecac, so don't give it at the same time. Naturally, you should avoid antivomiting drugs.

Pregnancy. No problem in a single dose.

Nursing. No problems.

Allergies

None reported.

Wholesale cost

Cost is $1.65 an ounce.

48
Scopolamine

An ancient remedy, scopolamine occurs widely in nature in plants of the belladonna family such as henbane. Belladonna is Italian for "beautiful woman." Centuries ago men considered widely dilated pupils sexy, belladonna eyedrops accomplished that.

Belladonna dilates pupils by blocking nerves that are part of the autonomic nervous system (see Catapres section). Scopolamine blocks autonomic nerves throughout the body and was once used extensively for these properties. Because it inhibits salivary and lung secretions, doctors gave it before anesthesia. Scopolamine's blocking action affects the brain, causing drowsiness and (after the drug wears off) amnesia. Because large doses caused hallucinations and wild behavior, anesthesiologists quickly switched when more predictable preop drugs appeared.

Obstetricians took longer and were using it during my medical school obstetrics rotation in a Brooklyn hospital in 1970. At that time, doctors already knew giving narcotics and general anesthesia to a mother depressed the newborn too much, but natural childbirth wasn't fashionable and clever local anesthetic techniques weren't available. Neither a painkiller nor an anesthetic, scopolamine was safer, but its hallucinations combined with labor pains drove women crazy. They had to be tied down and shrieked continually, so the delivery room was a nerve-racking place, but after the drug wore off they remembered nothing. Only the medical students remembered, and no one fell in love with obstetrics.

Scopolamine is treatment of choice for:

Motion sickness. Although this leads to nausea and vomiting, once you're sick no drug works well. You must take scopolamine *before* you need it. Some antihistamines work, but scopolamine works better. You can only find it as a skin patch because the oral form produces too many side effects.

How it works

Scopolamine blocks many autonomic nerves, and you'll discover which ones if you're sensitive to the patch. It prevents motion sickness by blocking nerves leading from the balance organs in your ear and to the nausea center in the brain. Once the center goes into action, blocking its nerves isn't terribly helpful, but scopolamine is mildly effective as an antinauseant.

It also blocks nerves that govern secretion by the salivary and sweat glands as well as respiratory and digestive tract. You can still find it in digestive remedies (Donnatol, Donnagel), but in doses too small to work. Larger doses would be unpleasant—see below.

How dispensed

A one-inch-square disc. Four hours before you depart, stick it to a clean, hairless area behind an ear and change it every three days.

Translating the label

Transderm-Scop is the only patch available.

Side effects

Expect a dry mouth—two thirds of users notice it. Drowsiness affects one in six. In the past, over-the-counter sleeping pills contained scopolamine, but antihistamines have taken its place.

The belladonna effect on pupils is no longer fashionable, but it occurs almost as often as drowsiness, accompanied by difficulty focusing and blurred vision. More vivid side effects are rare: confusion, memory disturbances, hallucinations.

Interactions

Food. None.

Alcohol. Avoid; alcohol increases drowsiness and all the mental side effects.

Drugs. Avoid drugs that block the same autonomic paths: antihistamines, antidepressants, and other belladonna drugs.

Pregnancy. No reported problems, but we don't recommend it.

Nursing. Not recommended; infants are sensitive to belladonna.

Sex. None reported.

Allergies

Only a rare rash.

Wholesale cost

Cost is $44.00 for packet of 12.

49
Compazine

When my phone rings at 2 A.M., the likely caller is a hotel guest in the throes of vomiting—the most frequent reason for a wee-hour call. If my beeper sounds while I'm jogging at 6:30, it's probably also a vomiter, but one too polite to wake me earlier.

I owe much of my success as a hotel doctor to vomiters; since I practice part-time and write part-time, I can usually get away. Although I have several rivals in the city, all have busy practices. Most sick guests will wait a few hours. Now and then, however, a busy executive, arms wrapped around the toilet, puts enormous pressure on hotel staff to produce a doctor immediately. Nothing delights me more than switching off my computer and rushing off to a new hotel.

Vomiting makes for a gratifying visit because patients are desperately ill, and I can usually help. Even if I can't, the illness rarely lasts long, so I get the credit when it passes. Almost invariably I give an injection of Thorazine, a powerful antivomiting drug. That puts me in a distinct minority because almost every American doctor prefers Compazine, a close relative. No logical reason exists why Compazine is their choice for severe vomiting just as there's no reason for our religious avoidance of metoclopramide. All work well and have similar side effects. I'll explain my preference for Thorazine in the next section.

Compazine is good for:

1. *Severe psychotic disorders such as schizophrenia.* You probably associate Thorazine with mental illness, but Compazine works as well. Both are members of the phenothiazine family, also known as major tranquilizers. Just as doctors rarely prescribe Thorazine for vomiting, psychiatrists rarely use Compazine for schizophrenia.
2. *Nausea and vomiting.*
3. *Hiccups.* I cure hiccups by rubbing the midline of the soft palate with a tongue depressor. Before I learned this from another doctor, I also gave drugs. The tongue depressor technique works better.
4. *Anxiety.* Although helpful, Compazine and other phenothiazines have too many side effects for long-term use. "Minor" tranquilizers like Valium and BuSpar are safer.

How dispensed

Tablets of 5 and 10 mg, long-acting capsules of 10, 15, and 30 mg, and a syrup of 5 mg per teaspoon. Also available are suppositories of 2.5, 5, and 25 mg plus injectable solution containing 5 mg per cc.

Usual adult dose is 10 mg every four hours or one 25 mg suppository or long-acting capsule twice a day.

Translating the label

Generic name is prochlorperazine. Most phenothiazines have long chemical names ending in -azine. Doctors can't tell them apart, so you'll hear the brand name. Here are others used for nausea and vomiting:

  · Thorazine (chlorpromazine)
  · Phenergan (promethazine)
  · Trilafon (perfenazine)
  · Temaril (trimeprazine)

These are not phenothiazines but we use them interchangeably:

· Vistaril (hydroxyzine)
· Tigan (trimethobenzamide)

How it works

Compazine and most phenothiazines have no action in the digestive tract itself but suppress an area in the brain that controls nausea and vomiting. Fortunately, that's the site of action of most drugs and illnesses that cause nausea.

Compazine doesn't affect the balance organs in your inner ear, so there's no point in taking it for motion sickness. Since it doesn't act in the GI tract, it won't protect against the local irritation of drugs like erythromycin or aspirin.

Side effects

Long-term use produces some alarming symptoms I'll mention in the chapter on Thorazine, but these are unlikely after a single injection or a short course of pills. The most common minor reactions are dizziness, drowsiness, dry mouth, and constipation, but I can't remember anyone complaining. Patients prefer almost any symptom to nausea.

Every few decades a doctor gets a major surprise, as I did from the patient described in the introduction of this book. Having received a Compazine injection an hour before, she had suffered a rare "dystonic reaction." If I hadn't remembered a similar case from medical school 25 years ago, I might not have made such a clever diagnosis. Long ago, a patient arrived in our emergency room looking to the left, insisting he couldn't straighten his head. Everyone suspected faking until one doctor remembered. Although very uncommon, a single dose of a phenothiazine may produce a striking muscle spasm, usually of the neck, back, or tongue. These are a pleasure to treat because a single shot of the antihistamine, Benadryl, produces a dramatic cure.

Interactions

Food. None.
Alcohol. Phenothiazines enhance the effect.
Drugs. Phenothiazines increase actions of strong narcotics such as morphine or Demerol. We avoid the combination when some actions (sedation, de-

pression of respiration) would be dangerous. But since phenothiazines also increase their painkilling action, we may deliberately combine them for this purpose.

Since phenothiazines work on the brain, they interfere with many drugs that treat neurological conditions such as Parkinsonism. They sometimes interfere with high blood pressure medication.

Pregnancy. Although not recommended, obstetricians occasionally use it for severe vomiting.

Nursing. Probably O.K. in low doses and for short periods.

Sex. No problems for short courses.

Allergies

Fairly common although they usually take at least a week to appear. Most consist of hives or other itchy eruptions, and they occur in 5 percent of users.

Wholesale cost

Fifteen cents for a 5-mg tablet, 30 cents for 10 mg. One 25-mg suppository costs over $2.50, and a 10-mg injection about $1.50.

PART IV
Drugs for Neurological and Psychological Disorders

50
Thorazine

Synthesized in France in 1950, chlorpromazine (Thorazine) was the first of the major tranquilizers that revolutionized treatment of mental illness. A deceptive phrase, "major tranquilizer" does not mean "heavily sedating." Although Thorazine makes patients drowsy, other antipsychotic drugs aren't sedating at all. "Major" stands for major psychiatric illnesses. Thorazine and its relatives don't cure them, just as Inderal doesn't cure high blood pressure, but patients are better off.

Your family doctor probably doesn't provide primary care to many severe psychiatric illnesses. Nor does he or she think of Thorazine when a patient is vomiting, although it works as well as its relative, Compazine. But I like it, so it's included here.

Thorazine is good for:

1. *Severe psychosis.* Major tranquilizers eliminate wildly disorganized thinking: hallucinations, delusions, fears, and the disruptive behavior that accompany severe psychoses such as schizophrenia. Despite portrayals in the movies and on TV, the mentally ill are not carefree eccentrics or victims of unhappy childhoods, but genuinely sick and suffering. Once a schizophrenic stops hearing terrifying voices, his or her behavior grows calmer. Some recover completely and don't require drugs, but relapses occur, and many become chronically ill.

Talking to patients with chronic schizophrenia, on or off drugs, is disturbing. They are not the colorful characters in "One Flew Over the Cuckoos Nest." Something is missing. But at least you can talk to them when they're taking their medication. This change was so dramatic that psychiatrists concluded many institutionalized mentally ill could live in the community provided they took medication and received ongoing care. Delighted at the chance to save tax money, state governments jumped at the chance to close mental hospitals. Hundreds of thousands of the mentally ill received (1) a prescription for Thorazine, (2) an appointment to a local mental health clinic, and (3) directions to the exit. Mental hospitals were torn down and replaced by condominiums.

It turns out that good community care for severely ill schizophrenics costs more than keeping them in a mental hospital. Communities didn't want to spend the money, so these sick people make up the largest and most permanent segment of the homeless.

2. *Nausea and vomiting.* I once gave Compazine injections like most American doctors, but I've switched. Ten milligrams of Compazine takes up 2 cc. The equivalent of Thorazine, 25 mg, is only 1 cc, a less painful injection. In addition, Thorazine seems more sedating than Compazine, and patients appreciate the rest after a night of vomiting. Finally, although I don't charge for drugs, I buy them, and Thorazine injectable is two-thirds less expensive.

3. *Anxiety.* As with Compazine, we don't use Thorazine much for ordinary neuroses because of side effects. Also, the "tranquility" of the major tranquilizers isn't as pleasant as Valium and its relatives, so patients don't grow to prefer them.

4. *Hiccups.* As good as Compazine. Not as good as rubbing the throat with a tongue depressor.

How it works

No one knows. Experts have described dozens of actions on the brain, but no one really knows which are useful and which merely explain side effects. I suspect the theory that mental illness is caused by stress and an unhappy childhood has been a drag on progress. If that theory is correct, drugs are only modestly helpful, and proper treatment is kindness and understanding. In fact, kindness and understanding work pretty well for milder emotional disorders (milder illnesses respond to almost anything), but drugs work better for serious, crippling mental illness.

There is a good parallel with tuberculosis, the leading killer of the nineteenth century. During the last century, everyone agreed T.B. was caused by stress, poor diet, overwork, and the burdens of modern living in polluted cities. Governments responded by building sanitariums where patients received rest, good food, and country air. It was a poor treatment. No one was cured. Once we found out what really caused T.B. (germs) we could look for a treatment that worked (something to kill germs). Once we succeeded in the 1950s, sanitariums closed, patients with T.B. continued their usual stressful, poorly nourished lives, but their disease vanished if they took their drugs faithfully.

Although the stress theory still has advocates, more psychiatrists are wondering if mental illness isn't a real brain disease. Major tranquilizers didn't weaken the stress theory because they were far from a cure. Yet they did amazing things and stimulated a rush of brain research that moved into high gear in the 1970s. In a decade or two, we'll have better drugs.

How dispensed

Tablets of 10, 25, 50, 100, and 200 mg. Long-acting capsules of 30, 75, and 150 mg, suppositories of 25 and 100 mg, a syrup containing 10 mg per teaspoon, and an injectable with 25 mg per cc.

Controlling psychotic symptoms may require several hundred milligrams, but 25 every four hours helps nausea and vomiting.

Translating the label

Generic Thorazine is chlorpromazine. Dozens of related major tranquilizers exist. I list those useful for nausea and vomiting in the Compazine section (49.). The most popular antipsychotics are Mellaril (thioridazine), Prolixin (fluphenazine), Stelazine (trifluoperazine), Haldol (haloperidol), and Navane (thiothixene).

Side effects

A few doses for the stomach flu rarely causes problems, but long-term use is a different matter.

Standing in the supermarket checkout line, you may notice someone with a peculiar tic. Her tongue moves in and out, her lips purse, her cheeks puff, her jaws chew. You may believe she's just an eccentric who doesn't realize how bizarre she looks. The truth is she is either taking a major tranquilizer or has taken one in the past because she is suffering a side effect called tardive dyskinesia. Usually beginning after long treatment, it's more common in the elderly and in women. Most distressing, it may not disappear after stopping the drug, and there's no good treatment.

Thorazine and other major tranquilizers clearly affect the brain in ways we don't yet understand, because other "movement disorders" also occur after chronic therapy. One resembles Parkinsonism, a common neurological disorder that produces a tremor, rigidity, and a shuffling walk. Another is the alarming dystonia I described in the Compazine section. Finally, many patients become uncontrollably restless. They pace endlessly; when sitting or trying to sleep, they cannot keep their legs from shifting and moving. Luckily, these reactions respond to drugs or a change in medication.

On a more mundane level, Thorazine causes drowsiness, especially during the first weeks of therapy. If this is intolerable, the psychiatrist can substitute a less sedating drug such as Haldol or Stelazine. Thorazine also tends to cause dizziness, a dry mouth, and constipation; other antipsychotics may or may not do this less often. Women's breasts occasionally swell and produce milk, and their periods may stop, an effect of antipsychotics on the brain, not the ovaries.

This is only a partial list of side effects of these very important but dangerous drugs. They should be used when they'll help, but never without close medical supervision.

Interactions

Food. None.
Alcohol. Thorazine intensifies the effect of alcohol.
Drugs. Intensifies action of tranquilizers, anesthetics, and narcotics.

Pregnancy. No evidence that Thorazine causes birth defects, but newborns show neurological side effects when their mothers are taking antipsychotics. Sometimes that can't be avoided.

Nursing. Low doses are O.K., but women taking large amounts probably shouldn't nurse.

Sex. Tends to inhibit ejaculation without interfering with erection, although impotence rarely occurs.

Allergies

Itchy hives aren't rare, and all drugs in the Thorazine family produce photosensitivity, so patients should stay out of the sun.

Wholesale cost

Cosit is 3 cents for 25-mg tablet, 4 cents for 50 mg, 6 cents for 100 mg; 25 mg of injectable costs about 60 cents.

Antidepressants

51 Tofranil • 52 Prozac

Ten years after synthesis of Thorazine, researchers testing a related compound, imipramine (Tofranil), found it useless for relieving psychotic symptoms but unexpectedly good for depression. Since then a score of antidepressants have appeared, none superior to imipramine although many offer different or fewer side effects. Unlike the case with major tranquilizers, family doctors often prescribe antidepressants, but they should prescribe them more. A great deal of untreated and undertreated depression exists.

Tofranil and Prozac are good for:

1. *Depression.* Not all the grief, misery, and disappointments of life require medical treatment, and even severe depression usually goes away al-

though 15 percent of patients commit suicide before that happens. On the other hand it's not true (as I was taught in medical school) that drugs are only useful for the worst cases. As with any illness, if depression interferes with your normal life, it's worth a trip to the doctor.

2. *Bedwetting.* For children over six with a stubborn problem, they often help. In fact, imipramine is FDA-approved for this. Bedwetting in older children is not rare; I did it occasionally as late as age 12. My parents never made a fuss, although changing the sheets was my responsibility, and I eventually stopped. Drug treatment benefits parents more than the child; perhaps they should take the pills.

3. *Preventing migraine.* Every victim should have a trial.

4. *Chronic pain.* No one is certain why antidepressants can help persistent low back pain, tension headaches, neuralgias, irritable bowels, and other stubborn pain disorders. Their antidepressant effect is probably not the answer, because we use lower doses.

How they work

Although we don't know for sure, our leading theory is probably on the right track. To understand antidepressants you must first unlearn the popular description of the human brain: a huge switchboard or (lately) computer that works by electricity. Although it's true nerves transmit a signal from one end to the other by electric current, that's a boring explanation. A nerve either fires or it doesn't. Unlike man-made devices, the voltage or current never changes. All nerve impulses are the same.

Interesting things happen where one nerve meets another. In the brain one nerve may connect with 50 others, but unlike circuits in a "hard-wired" computer, living nerves don't touch. A gap called a synapse separates every nerve from its neighbor, and that's where the body exerts control and where drugs can interfere.

No electricity passes between nerves. When a signal reaches the end of one nerve, it generates a gush of a chemical "neurotransmitter" that floats across the gap and sticks to receptors on nearby nerves. Depending on the type and quantity, the neurotransmitter may (1) do nothing, (2) cause the next nerve to fire, (3) inhibit it (prevent it from firing for a while) or (4) make it more or less sensitive to future shots of neurotransmitter.

Different areas of the nervous system use different neurotransmitters. You may have heard of norepinephrine, serotonin, acetylcholine, and dopamine; we have known these for decades, but more turn up all the time. It's an area of intense research.

Cocaine and amphetamine ("speed," diet pills) force nerve endings to pour out their norepinephrine. That makes you feel wonderful—until the supply runs out. Then you feel terrible. Sigmund Freud performed the first antidepressant research before turning his interest to psychoanalysis. Freud believed that the newly isolated drug, cocaine, was a brilliant advance and prescribed it liberally to patients, friends, and himself. He later changed his mind.

Depressed people have low levels of norepinephrine and of another neurotransmitter, serotonin. Antidepressants increase that level, but not as violently as amphetamines and cocaine. In fact, antidepressants take weeks to work and don't produce the euphoria that makes cocaine so popular. No one takes antidepressants for fun.

How dispensed

Tofranil comes as 10-, 25-, and 50-mg tablets and long-acting capsules containing 75, 100, 125, and 150 mg plus an injectable containing 25 mg per 2 cc. Starting dose is 75 mg per day, but it usually takes 150 to treat depression. Chronic pain and bedwetting respond to 25 to 50 mg.

Prozac comes only as a 10 mg and 20 mg capsule/5 cc solution.

Translating the label

Tofranil and Janimine are the two brands of imipramine.

Prozac is the only brand of fluoxetine.

Plenty of rivals exist. Despite a great deal of hype, all relieve depression equally well. Newer ones offer fewer annoying side effects in exchange for a wildly high price.

Old:
- amitriptyline (Elavil, Endep)
- doxepin (Sinequan, Adapin)
- trimipramine (Surmontil)

· desipramine (Norpramin, Pertofrane)
· nortriptyline (Aventyl, Pamelor)
· protriptyline (Vivactil)
Newer:
· amoxapine (Asendin)
· maprotilene (Ludiomil)
· trazodone (Desyrel)
Newest:
· bupropion (Wellbutrin)
· paroxetine (Paxil)
· sertraline (Zoloft)

Side effects

Despite their similarity to major tranquilizers, these are more dangerous. Although it's difficult to kill yourself with Thorazine, antidepressants rank among the leaders in overdose deaths, although Prozac and others in the newest group seem to be exceptions. The safest treatment for severe depression, especially among the elderly, is electroshock, but that has such a terrible reputation in the popular imagination that it's hard to get.

In the past we scanned tables as complex as a Chinese restaurant menu trying to pick the antidepressant that wouldn't make the patient even more miserable. Was the patient depressed and tired? If so, we'd avoid Tofranil or Elavil that would make them more tired. Vivactil or Aventyl wouldn't. Was depression accompanied by insomnia and agitation? Then Tofranil or Elavil was just the ticket. Did the patient have heart disease? That was tricky because older antidepressants weakened the heart. Doxepin was the best choice although it made patients very sleepy. A choice for older patients was the trickiest of all because they are more sensitive to constipation, dizziness, dry mouth, and blurred vision produced by most of the drugs. Aventyl was probably the best but not by much.

Despite all these annoyances, the older drugs work as well as the newer ones, and most patients do fine. Tofranil is my choice for depression accompanied by restlessness. It makes most patients drowsy, but a dose before bedtime helps them sleep. I mention the other side effects (constipation and so on), but most patients don't find these too upsetting.

If patients are already fatigued, I suggest Prozac, but Aventyl or Vivactil are good alternatives and much cheaper. Prozac's spectacular media attention has probably faded by the time you read this, but that will be no great loss. Its major advantage is that most patients are not aware they're taking an antidepressant, which isn't the case with Tofranil. I suspect that Prozac has become so popular because people believe they're depressed at least part of the time (and I'm not sure they're wrong), and a harmless treatment seems wonderful. Many who wouldn't dream of seeing a psychiatrist are asking the family doctor for Prozac. But it is not entirely benign. Ten to 15 percent of patients become anxious and insomniac, about 10 percent feel queasy. Weight loss is fairly common. Other drugs in the "newest" class also have fewer side effects.

Interactions

Food. None.

Alcohol. Antidepressants increase its effect.

Drugs. Older antidepressants increase the effect of many hypertensive drugs, as well as major and minor tranquilizers. Prozac does this less often.

Pregnancy. After 30 years of use, no one is certain if Tofranil causes birth defects; no one knows what to make of the few reported cases. No defects are reported from Prozac, but it is too new to draw any conclusion.

Nursing. Probably excreted in the milk, so nursing is inadvisable.

Sex. Depressed people lose interest in sex, so antidepressants have a positive effect. But a few percent of both sexes notice breast swelling, and a few men become impotent. These occur less often with Prozac.

Allergies

Four percent of Prozac users develop an allergic rash, and there's no evidence other drugs do better. Photosensitive rashes are also not rare.

Wholesale cost

Tofranil: 1.4 cents for 10-mg tablet, 2 cents for 25 mg, 2.5 cents for 50 mg. Other old antidepressants cost about the same.

Prozac: $2.20 for single 20-mg tablet.

53
BuSpar

In their perpetual search for tranquility, humans have consumed drugs and alcohol for thousands of years. With the rise of chemistry in the nineteenth century, doctors discovered bromides and prescribed them until well past World War II. Cheap and toxic, bromides faded slowly with the arrival of phenobarbital after the turn of the century. As a student 25 years ago, I heard older doctors claim phenobarbital produced tranquility as well as that newfangled and expensive Valium. They were right. Phenobarbital's disadvantages are that large doses cause undignified behavior similar to drunkenness, very large doses are fatal, and withdrawal after long-term use is dangerous. Valium is safer, but not otherwise superior.

The modern age of psychopharmacology began in the 1950s with Miltown (meprobamate), which caused a media splash as intense as Prozac's today. Although still on the market, Miltown turns out to be no safer than phenobarbital, so there's no reason to use it.

A genuine advance occurred with the benzodiazepine family (Valium, Librium, Dalmane, Ativan, Xanax) in the early 1960s. These are genuinely safe; suicide with an overdose is almost impossible. With effort one can become addicted, and during the 1970s I chuckled over articles and TV news spots in which patients described how the family doctor forced Valium prescription after prescription into their hands until they became hopeless junkies. In fact, although doctors overprescribe tranquilizers, and patients often exert pressure to get them, addiction rarely occurs.

On the other hand, it's wrong to call these tranquilizers. They're also sedatives. The more you take, the sleepier you get. As I tell patients, "If you prefer being sleepy to being nervous, then you're tranquil." Thorazine is a genuine tranquilizer. Large doses control wild behavior better than small doses without producing much more sedation. Trying to quiet a hallucinating schizophrenic with Valium won't work no matter how drowsy he or she becomes.

In truth, benzodiazepines have some genuine calming properties and relieve short-term anxiety disorders. The problem is that patients enjoy the slight euphoria they produce as well as their sleep-inducing action. That sleep is not very refreshing, but unhappy people dread lying awake at night.

The mid-1980s saw the release of BuSpar (buspirone), the first pure tranquilizer. Unlike many useful new drugs, it hasn't become a best-seller, and patients don't ask for it. In fact, when I switch patients accustomed to Valium and so forth, they don't like it. "It isn't working," they complain. What they mean is that they miss the euphoria or sedation. The best candidate for BuSpar is someone who has never taken a tranquilizer, so a generation may have to pass before it's popular.

BuSpar is good for:

Anxiety: excessive and unrealistic worry. This is a tricky definition. My wife worries excessively about her artistic career, and she complains that I grumble unrealistically about problems with writing or medical practice. But neither of us takes tranquilizers. As with any disorder, if it becomes painful enough to interfere with daily living, you need professional help.

BuSpar and other tranquilizers are not good for:

Unhappiness. The saddest visit I make is to a hotel guest after a tragedy— often the death of a child or spouse. The guest is weeping, and relatives urge me to "give her something" or "put him out." Although I'm liberal with tranquilizers in these circumstances, they don't work. No drug safe enough to use outside an operating room will put anyone to sleep. No matter how much drowsiness a drug causes, it won't drive a terrible memory from your mind or blunt the misery of losing your job, a broken love affair, or the diagnosis of a serious disease. I try to provide a sympathetic ear—the best therapy for anyone going through a bad time.

How it works

So far no satisfying explanation exists. This is so for all the benzodiazepines from ancient Librium through the latest (new ones continue to pour onto the shelves). Benzodiazepines act on areas deep in the brain, affecting receptors for certain neurotransmitters; a calming action results. BuSpar doesn't act that way, although it may act on different receptors. Benzodiazepines also relax muscles and suppress seizures, but BuSpar doesn't. Clearly, there's much we don't know about how emotional stress affects the brain. Learning how BuSpar works will open many doors.

How dispensed

Five and 10-mg tablets.

Usual dose is 5 mg three times a day, and it's rarely necessary to give more than 10.

Translating the label

BuSpar is the brand name of buspirone. Sooner or later, competitors in the same class (azaspirones) will appear, but I doubt there will be many unless BuSpar catches on. Benzodiazepines continue to dominate the market. The most popular:
- Librium (chlordiazepoxide)
- Valium (diazepam)
- Ativan (lorazepam)
- Xanax (alprazolam)
- Tranxene (clorazepate)
- Dalmane (flurazepam)
- Serax (oxazepam)
- Centrax (prazepam)
- Doral (quazepam)
- ProSom (estazolam)
- Restoril (temazepam)
- Halcion (triazolam)

Side effects

Three percent of users stop the drug because of dizziness, nervousness, or insomnia. One percent have nausea.

BuSpar's advantage are the side effects it *doesn't* share with benzodi-azepines: sedation, confusion, and difficulty concentrating.

Interactions

Food. Probably none.

Alcohol. Unlike other sedatives, BuSpar doesn't seem to potentiate alco-hol's action.

Drugs. Few interactions have turned up, although it's a bad idea to com-bine BuSpar with a class of antidepressant known as MAO inhibitors, but family doctors rarely use them.

Pregnancy. No reported problems in animal studies but not recom-mended.

Nursing. No human studies, but it's excreted into rat milk.

Sex. Now and then someone reports increased or decreased sexual drive. Impotence is rare.

Allergies

One percent suffer itching or a rash.

Wholesale cost

Sixty cents for 5-mg tablet, $1 for 10 mg.

Generics of many benzodiazepines such as Valium are only a few cents a pill.

54
Lithium

Nineteenth-century doctors used lithium bromide as an anticonvulsant and sedative (see bromides in phenobarbital section 57.), and some of their patients probably suffered mania, but lithium fell out of fashion when safer drugs arrived.

During the late 1940s an Australian researcher, J. F. Cade, noticed lithium salts made his guinea pigs lethargic. Everyone who studied lithium knew that, but Cade made the sort of simple but brilliant observation that wins Nobel prizes. He not only tried it on agitated mental patients, but kept track of who benefitted. It turned out manic patients responded best. Within a few years others confirmed his findings (which doesn't always happen—be patient when anyone announces an amazing discovery). By the 1950s, lithium was accepted throughout most of the world.

But not in the U.S. During the 1940s, doctors tried lithium chloride as a salt substitute (lithium is closely related to sodium). This was disastrous because it's toxic, and some patients died. The experience prejudiced American doctors against lithium, keeping it off the market for 20 years. FDA approval didn't arrive until 1970.

Lithium is treatment of choice for:

1. *Manic-depressive disorders* (also known as bipolar disorders for obvious reasons). If anyone doubts that mental illness is a brain disease, bipolar disorders are convincing evidence. During the first phase the victim feels enormous self-confidence and energy. If he or she can function (hold a job, show good judgment) this is called hypomania, and everyone enjoys that feeling. In frank mania, a patient can go without sleep for days and either work without cease at a particular goal or become so restless work is impossible. Although amusing when they joke, boast, and chatter endlessly, these people are profoundly disabled. A manic victim can ruin his life by selling his property for a silly business venture, engaging in a massive buying spree, or (feeling threatened) become violent. A young manic male is the most dangerous mental patient.

   About 1 percent of the population suffers a bipolar disorder, so it's not rare. It also runs in families, affecting 20 percent of close relatives of a patient.

   No one sees a doctor for hypomania, and isolated mania is rare. Almost all patients have periods of profound depression, often more frequently than periods of mania. Although antidepressants relieve this depression, they are poor treatment because they increase manic episodes. Lithium is better.

2. *Depression*. Just as mania without depression occurs, the reverse is possible, so some depression may be manic-depression without mania. Lithium is a fairly effective antidepressant.
3. *Cluster headaches*. A type of migraine that mostly affects men. Not a primary treatment, it's worth a try when others fail.

How it works

Unlike all other psychiatric drugs, lithium has no effect on a normal person's mood, and (surprisingly since it's such a simple atom) no one knows how it works in mood disorders. Lithium probably inhibits release of norepinephrine and dopamine from nerve endings in the brain. Amphetamines and cocaine produce a gush of neurotransmitters, so the reverse action seems a reasonable explanation for controlling mania.

How dispensed

As lithium carbonate in capsules and tablets of 300 mg, a slow-release tablet of 300 mg, a slow-release capsule of 450 mg, and a lithium citrate syrup of 300 mg per teaspoon.

Healthy adults begin with 600 mg twice a day. The dose can be increased every week to over 2,000 mg if necessary, and the doctor must check blood levels during treatment. Mania usually fades within two weeks after which dose is reduced to maintenance level, usually between 900 and 1,200 mg per day. This is also the dose for cluster headache.

Translating the label

Brands are Eskalith, Lithane, and Lithobid. Cibalith-S is the syrup.

Side-effects

Nausea occurs at beginning of treatment but usually diminishes. Most common persistent effects include fine hand tremor, increasing urination, and mild thirst. Vomiting and diarrhea occur less often. In normal doses, lithium does not cause sedation, so drowsiness is a sign of toxicity.

Interactions

Food. Take after meals.

Alcohol. None reported but it's never a good idea to take more than one mood-altering drug.

Drugs. Lithium becomes more toxic when body's sodium level is low, so we advise patients not to restrict salt intake. Diuretics also lower sodium, so we don't prescribe them (treating high blood pressure and mania together is tricky). Aspirin and all NSAIDs (see Motrin, 62.) elevate a lithium level. Sodium bicarbonate and theophylline can lower it.

Pregnancy. Lithium probably causes birth defects, so the dilemma is similar to anticonvulsants.

Nursing. Excreted in milk and toxic to infants.

Sex. Impotence and premature ejaculation occur rarely.

Allergies

Pure allergies are rare; acne and generalized itching occur slightly more often.

Wholesale cost

Six cents for 300-mg capsule.

55
Clomipramine

In my profession, being called "obsessive" or "compulsive" does not offend. Getting through medical school is not easy without such qualities, and you probably want that sort of doctor—one who according to the definition thinks single-mindedly and works persistently in pursuit of a goal.

Although useful in problem solving, single-minded thoughts and persistent acts in pursuit of a meaningless goal make life miserable for 2 percent of Americans. Drugs can help.

Clomipramine is treatment of choice for:

1. *Obsessive-compulsive disorders.* For five years before and during medical school, I lived in a fifth floor walk-up on the Lower East Side of New York. Leaving the building, I sometimes wondered if I had locked the door. Unobsessive people would decide they had done so by habit and walk on. Others would rack their brains, trying to remember, but it's hard to remember habitual acts. If you were like me, you'd curse and retrace your steps. The door would be locked.

   Hurrying back to climb four flights became a persistent annoyance until I devised a solution. Instead of walking off each day, I locked the door deliberately while saying loudly to myself "I have locked the door!" Then, several blocks away, when I wondered about the door, a distinct memory of my thought reassured me.

   That illustrates a touch of obsessive-compulsive behavior (obsession is the thought; compulsion the action). Most of you can recall similar inconveniences. Like periods of depression or anger, these are evidence that no one is perfect. We don't call them sickness unless they make life difficult.

   A victim of OCD leads a miserable life. Obsessions about contamination or disaster are common, so washing and checking are the leading compulsions. Unable to avoid the thought that disease germs are everywhere, a man may wash his hands after every contact with a doorknob, handshake, and so forth. He may spend hours a day washing, arrive late for appointments, and be under a dermatologist's care for stubborn hand dermatitis. Another may be unable to sleep without getting up 50 times to make sure the oven is off.

   Friends aware of this problem do exactly the wrong thing. They reassure the patient ("So what if the oven is on; it'll raise the gas bill, but the house won't burn down") or use common sense ("I shake hands all the time, and I never get sick..."). Faced with any emotional illness, laymen and even doctors can't resist the urge (it verges on obsession) to point out defects in the patient's reasoning. The explainer is always correct, and it never helps.

   Before the late 1970s, we assumed this was a rare disorder, the result of suppressed childhood conflicts. Treatment was long-term psychoanalysis to bring these conflicts into the open. It didn't work.

Unlike patients with schizophrenia or severe depression, most victims of OCD are not obviously sick and have a realistic view of their problem. Well-adjusted in other areas, they are terribly upset at the single, crazy thought that forces them into a silly action again and again. Their behavior seems so irrational most are ashamed to see a doctor. This is too bad because we now know that OCD is a "real" disease—i.e., distinct abnormalities of the brain are present, and it's strongly hereditary. Even better, we have good treatment, so we don't have to rely on psychoanalysis (like prescriptions for rest, avoiding stress, and a nourishing diet, we often recommend psychoanalysis for incurable problems).

That doesn't mean psychiatric therapy isn't essential, but we now focus on the actual problem, not hidden conflicts. Therapists guide the patient through behavior exercises in which he confronts the unreasonable urge and practices not obeying it. But these obsessions are so strong behavior therapy alone is too stressful for most who try. Clomipramine suppresses intrusive thoughts so a patient can more easily deal with them.

2. *Trichotillomania.* Compulsive hair-pulling. Another disorder more common than we believed, it affects women almost entirely. Psychiatrists have begun to wonder if other compulsive behaviors such as nail-biting may respond as well.

Clomipramine is good for:

Depression. Chemically similar to Tofranil, it probably works as well, but there's no reason to go to the extra expense.

How it works

Like Tofranil and Prozac, clomipramine works on the brain, increasing neurotransmitters that pass between nerve endings. As you read in Tofranil, section 51., norepinephrine and serotonin are the transmitters. Clomipramine increases serotonin much more than norepinephrine, and that may explain why it relieves OCD, but the evidence is not overwhelming. Prozac also leans toward serotonin, but so do other antidepressants that don't work as well.

How dispensed

Capsules of 25, 50, and 75 mg. We begin with 25 mg per day and work up to 100 mg over the first two weeks then to a maximum of 200 to 250 over the next several weeks. As with other antidepressants, depression should lift within a month, but obsessive-compulsive symptoms take two or three times longer.

Translating the label

Clomipramine comes as Anafranil. The antidepressants Prozac and Zoloft are not quite as effective but have fewer side effects. Similar drugs are in the FDA pipeline. Long available in Europe (as was clomipramine for 20 years before approval here), they probably work.

Side effects

This is a difficult drug, probably slightly more unpleasant than the Tofranil family. Twenty-five percent of users complain of dry mouth. Fifteen percent have either drowsiness, dizziness, or tremor. Twelve percent suffer constipation, 10 percent nausea, and 5 percent abdominal pain. Ten percent sweat excessively. Five percent complain of increased appetite and weight gain, but this is probably more common. Women often switch to Prozac for this reason. Seizures occur in 1.5 percent of those treated for a year with at least 300 mg. Overall, about 20 percent of users stop treatment because of side effects.

Interactions

Food. Taking after meals may avoid digestive upsets.
Alcohol. Same as Tofranil.
Drugs. Same as Tofranil.
Pregnancy. No human birth defects reported, but we use it only if essential.
Nursing. No obvious problems, but we'd rather not use it.
Sex. Five to 10 percent of patients notice increased or decreased sexual

desire. About 30 percent of men have delayed ejaculation. Fifteen percent become impotent.

Allergies

Two percent suffer rash, itching, or hives.

Wholesale cost

Cost is 75 cents for 25 mg, $1 for 50 mg, $1.30 for 75 mg.

56
Antabuse

The chemical disulfiram was long used in rubber manufacture, and rubber workers quickly lost their taste for alcohol. No one thought much about that until the 1940s when a Danish drug company suspected disulfiram killed intestinal parasites and assigned two researchers to find out. It seemed to work on animals. Human testing came next, so researchers tried it on themselves. It seemed safe, but after several days each began to feel ill. Now and then they suffered a throbbing headache with nausea, dizziness, and flushing that passed in a few hours. At first they blamed the flu. Then they blamed spoiled food. Finally, they wondered about the drug. Weeks of trial and error passed before they realized drinking wine or beer while on disulfiram made them sick.

Naturally, everyone was disappointed. No matter how well the drug killed parasites, this side effect made it unmarketable. Alcoholism wasn't a big problem in Denmark, so the company didn't pursue that avenue. They dropped the project.

Medical science only learned about the study later when one researcher mentioned the curious experiment during a talk. A reporter was in the audience, and the newspaper article that followed created a surprising stir (alcoholism, needless to say, was a bigger problem in Denmark than anyone thought).

Disulfiram (Antabuse) is good for:

Making alcoholics sick. That sounds wonderful. Give Antabuse to Uncle Charlie, and after one lapse, he knows better than to touch the bottle. In the past doctors were fairly generous in urging patients to take it, and an occasional alcoholic asked for it. Some treatment programs still use it.

Antabuse works—that's why it's in this book. But by "works," I mean it performs as advertised: making anyone who drinks dreadfully ill. If you want to know how well it cures alcoholism here are the statistics: zero. No long-term study shows that Antabuse improves the outcome. It may be good for short-term use in a highly motivated alcoholic beginning a treatment program as a discouragement to momentary temptations. I refuse prescriptions to anyone not in a program and then only if the counselor agrees.

How it works

When you drink, your body breaks down alcohol to acetaldehyde, then to water and carbon dioxide in a few steps that you learned in high school chemistry. Antabuse blocks the step after acetaldehyde, a relative of formaldehyde, so it accumulates in the blood and makes you sick.

How dispensed

Tablets of 250 and 500 mg; 500 mg is maximum daily dose, although doctors sometimes reduce that after a few weeks.

Translating the label

Antabuse is the only brand of disulfiram.

Side effects

In the absence of alcohol, Antabuse is safe although a small number of patients complain about drowsiness, upset stomach, or metallic taste. The alcohol reaction is sufficiently dangerous that we don't like to prescribe it to anyone with a serious medical problem, especially liver disease, heart disease, or diabetes.

Interactions

Food. Avoid anything containing alcohol such as sauces, vinegars, and ciders.

Alcohol. Remember that aftershaves, massage lotions, and innumerable medications contain alcohol.

Drugs. Antabuse often greatly increases the blood level of Dilantin and isoniazid (a tuberculosis treatment). Taking Flagyl and Antabuse together can lead to a psychotic reaction.

Pregnancy. Alcohol definitely causes birth defects, but we're not certain about Antabuse.

Nursing. No one has studied the matter; probably not a good idea.

Sex. Impotence occurs, although alcoholics also do poorly in this area.

Allergies

Itchy and acnelike rashes are not rare although they usually disappear after a few weeks.

Wholesale cost

Seven cents for 250-mg tablet; 12 cents for 500 mg.

57
Phenobarbital

A venerable family, barbiturates date from the nineteenth century and served as a physician's leading tranquilizer, sleeping pill, and antiseizure medication as late as the first half of the twentieth. Treacherous as sleeping pills (overdoses kill, withdrawing from addiction is far more dangerous than from narcotics), they remain available, but I suspect addicts consume most of today's production. Only older doctors or the most stubborn aged insomniacs continue to rely on Seconal or Nembutal. Our grandparents took small doses of barbiturate as tranquilizers; phenobarbital dominated the market until the 1950s when Miltown took over, soon followed by Librium, Valium, and the like.

Aside from a role in general anesthesia, barbiturates have almost dropped out of medical practice with the exception of phenobarbital. Discovered early in the century, it quickly became the leading drug for epilepsy, a position it held for 50 years. It still works.

In case you're interested, phenobarbital supplanted the leading nineteenth-century epilepsy drug: bromides. Although toxic, bromides worked both for epilepsy and as tranquilizers. Like so many toxic drugs, they stayed around for too long, and I still remember radio jingles extolling Bromo-seltzer.

Phenobarbital is good for:

1. *Epilepsy.* A family of neurological disorders, all are characterized by sudden, short-lived abnormal electrical discharges in the brain. When the discharge spreads everywhere, the brain cannot function so the victim loses consciousness and falls down. But a discharge over part of the brain won't cause the popular image of a seizure, and in some forms of epilepsy it takes an acute observer to realize anything is wrong. Although they may begin after a brain injury or infection, most seizures are "idiopathic," meaning no one knows the origin.

During grand mal epilepsy, the victim loses consciousness, falls, and suffers vigorous muscle contraction and spasm for a short time. Grand mal is the most common form, and phenobarbital is a good treatment although no longer the choice. It's most often used in combination with Dilantin and Tegretol. Phenobarbital also helps simple partial seizures that affect part of the body or brain without loss of consciousness.

2. *Insomnia and anxiety.* Still FDA-approved, newer drugs work better.

How it works

Although all barbiturates suppress seizures, phenobarbital and a few obscure relatives work in doses that don't put patients to sleep. They suppress electrical conduction generally but more strongly at junctions between nerves by reducing the action of neurotransmitters. You can read more about nerve conduction in the Tofranil section (51.).

In the presence of enough phenobarbital, a wild electrical discharge dies out before spreading widely enough to produce a seizure.

In an unrelated action of phenobarbital, it stimulates important liver enzymes that break down drugs passing through, so doctors must keep an eye on the blood level of other medication. See below under drug interactions.

How dispensed

Tablets of 15, 30, 60, and 100 mg, an elixir of 20 mg per teaspoon, and an injectable. Sixty to 120 mg a day is the usual dose for seizures although a stubborn case may require as much as 200.

Translating the label

All phenobarbital is generic today.

Side effects

One in three patients complains of sleepiness although that often improves after a few weeks. Children occasionally become agitated. Excessive doses make patients appear drunk and unsteady, and that sometimes happens with normal doses.

Interactions

Food. None, but phenobarbital as well as Dilantin can interfere with absorption of calcium and action of the vitamin, folic acid. Rarely, that results in a form of the bone disease rickets (from low calcium), or anemia (from low folic acid).

Alcohol. Alcohol greatly increases the depressant action.

Drugs. A big problem with anticonvulsants. Phenobarbital decreases the effect of anticoagulants, cortisone, griseofulvin, quinidine, tetracyclines, estrogens, progesterone, and birth control pills. It may increase or decrease the level of Dilantin and a few other seizure drugs. Sedatives, tranquilizers, and some antihistamines make sleepiness worse.

Pregnancy. An even worse problem than drug interactions. A grand mal seizure can severely damage a fetus, so women can't stop treatment while pregnant. Furthermore, children of women with epilepsy have more birth defects even when no drugs are involved—but the risk is only 4 to 6 percent, so most babies are normal. Seizure drugs, unfortunately, also increase birth defects, and none is preferable.

Nursing. 100 mg per day causes sedation in a nursing infant; less may not.

Sex. No reported problems.

Allergies

A 1- to 2-percent risk but higher in those already suffering asthma, hay fever, hives, or other allergic conditions.

Wholesale cost

Old drugs are cheap. Phenobarbital costs 0.5 cents for a 15-mg tablet, 0.7 cents for 30 mg, and 0.9 cents for 60 mg.

58
Dilantin

Bromides and phenobarbital made patients drowsy, so everyone yearned for an anticonvulsant that wouldn't. During the 1930s researchers took up the search among relatives of phenobarbital, and the discovery of phenytoin (Dilantin) became one of the early triumphs of scientific pharmacology. Introduced in 1938, it became the best-selling seizure drug, a position it held until the 1980s when Tegretol (next section) took over.

Despite a distant chemical resemblance to barbiturates, Dilantin behaves differently. It suppresses seizures in a different manner and has its own collection of side effects which are, unfortunately, no less unpleasant. But Dilantin helps a wider variety of problems, probably because it suppresses abnormal nerve discharges so effectively.

Dilantin is good for:

1. *Epilepsy.* It's better than phenobarbital for grand mal and simple partial seizures, although we sometimes combine the two.

   Dilantin also suppresses another type known as complex partial seizures (formerly temporal lobe or psychomotor seizures). These are simple partial seizures in which the patient loses conscious contact with the environment. A simple partial seizure may include hallucinations or strong emotions such as fear or anger, but patients remain aware of what's happening. In complex partial seizures, patients stop what they are doing and engage in a new behavior. It may be as simple as standing quietly for a few minutes or walking aimlessly, but some victims perform activities that require great skill such as traveling a long distance.

2. *Trigeminal neuralgia* (tic douloureux) and other episodic pain attacks as well as some chronic pain disorders. Tegretol works better, and I discuss these in the next section.

3. *Abnormal cardiac rhythms.* The best treatment for abnormal rhythms caused by digitalis toxicity, it's not superior for long-term rhythm disorders and rarely used outside the hospital.

How it works

Doesn't affect neurotransmitters but acts on the cell itself, stabilizing the membrane (i.e., making it less sensitive). Experts compare Dilantin's action to a local anesthetic like Novocaine. This anesthetic action works on all cells, which explains its use for cardiac and other nerve disorders.

How dispensed

Tablets of 50 mg, long-acting capsules containing 30 and 100 mg, suspensions containing 125 and 30 mg per teaspoon, and an injectable with 50 mg per cc.

An average adult dose is 300 mg per day. A rule for seizure drugs is to increase the dose until either seizures disappear or side effects become unacceptable. Few Dilantin users tolerate more than 600 mg.

Translating the label

Surprisingly for a 50-year-old drug, only one brand of phenytoin exists along with the inevitable generics: Dilantin. A number of experts disapprove of generic Dilantin and Tegretol because FDA standards for approval accept blood levels that vary too much to make neurologists comfortable. Almost all advise patients to stick to Dilantin (or Tegretol) made by the same company to avoid sudden changes in blood level. Finding the same company is almost impossible when using a generic because pharmacists change their suppliers, and large HMOs switch regularly to whoever gives the lowest bid. Your doctor will have a strong opinion on the subject.

Side effects

Because they rarely feel drowsy, patients prefer Dilantin to phenobarbital at first. Whether they prefer it over the long haul depends on their tolerance of several side effects.

After a few months, 20 percent of patients notice swollen gums. Although vigorous brushing three times a day minimizes swelling, it's a tiresome annoyance especially in adolescents. Swelling of other connective tissue occasionally causes coarsening of facial features. Five percent of patients suffer acne or excessive hair growth, so women sometimes complain. These reactions knocked Dilantin out of first place among seizure drugs once experts decided Tegretol was not as dangerous as they thought (see the next section).

Unlike phenobarbital, high doses don't cause drowsiness, but may produce the same unsteadiness and slurred speech that resembles drunkenness. That rarely happens at the average dose.

Interactions

Food. Same problem with folic acid and calcium as phenobarbital.

Alcohol. Alcohol increases blood level of Dilantin, but long-term abuse (with liver damage) decreases the level.

Drugs. As many as other anticonvulsants. The following drugs may (or may) not increase blood level of Dilantin: blood thinners, Antabuse, Tagamet and other H2 blockers, many tranquilizers, Thorazine, Compazine, and other phenothiazines, estrogens, aspirin, and older antidiabetic pills.

The following may decrease blood level: Tegretol, sucralfate, and antacids.

Phenobarbital may either increase or decrease Dilantin's blood level.

Dilantin impairs action of the following drugs: blood thinners, digitalis, tetracyclines, estrogens, Lasix, oral contraceptives, quinidine, and theophylline.

Older antidepressants sometimes precipitate seizures in patients on Dilantin.

If that sounds hopeless, don't worry too much. Plenty of patients on other drugs get along fine with Dilantin.

Pregnancy. The same danger as with phenobarbital.

Nursing. Probably O.K.

Sex. No reported problems.

Allergies

Two to 5 percent of patients experience a spotty, measleslike rash within two weeks of starting treatment. It's mild and goes away in a few days without stopping the drug. A less common but more serious reaction consists of fever, puffiness around the lips and eyes, swollen lymph nodes, and a more intense itchy rash. That requires cortisone and no more Dilantin.

Wholesale cost

Four cents for a 100-mg capsule. Eighteen cents for brand name 100-mg Dilantin.

59
Tegretol

When you consider that anticonvulsants suppress brain function, it's amazing their side effects usually remain tolerable. Eventually we'll develop seizure drugs as benign as the new antihypertensives, but until then patients must settle for Tegretol.

Synthesized in 1953 by a drug company searching for a competitor to Thorazine, it didn't pan out, and its anticonvulsant action wasn't discovered until the 1960s. Europeans quickly adopted Tegretol as their drug of choice, but our FDA, as usual, worried more about safety than its overseas counterparts. During this period, a few reports surfaced of patients suffering bone marrow suppression leading to anemia, a low white count, and occasionally death. As a resident 20 years ago, I remember lectures extolling the superiority of Tegretol, but warning us to use it only when other drugs failed because of the small risk of deadly complications. In case we forgot, we could read a terrifying warning in the package insert and PDR.

By the 1980s neurologists had seen so little serious marrow suppression they began to doubt the original reports, and we now believe Tegretol is as safe as Dilantin or phenobarbital and less risky than drugs we prescribe routinely like penicillin. In 1988, FDA softened the warning in the PDR from terrifying to merely anxiety-provoking. By this time Tegretol had become America's best-selling anticonvulsant as well as the world's.

Tegretol is treatment of choice for:

Trigeminal neuralgia (tic douloureux). In this agonizing disorder, flashes of excruciating facial pain occur when victims move or touch their face—while eating, shaving, talking, or brushing their teeth.

A few percent of victims have multiple sclerosis or a brain tumor compressing the trigeminal nerve that supplies the face. In the past no one knew the usual cause, but today we're fairly sure a small artery in the brain has moved slightly, pressing on the nerve, making it hypersensitive. An operation can correct that, but it's major surgery, and patients prefer drugs if they work. If not, they yearn for surgery.

Because of tic douloureux's resemblance to a seizure disorder, doctors tried anticonvulsants and found they helped. Tegretol helps the most.

Tegretol is good for:

1. *Epilepsy.* It works as well as Dilantin for the same seizure types: grand mal, simple partial, and complex partial. Choosing between them doesn't depend on effectiveness or safety but cost, convenience, and side effects. Tegretol costs three to four times more and, unlike Dilantin, must be taken twice a day. Women and children prefer Tegretol, but there's no reason to switch if Dilantin is satisfactory.
2. *Other episodic pains beside trigeminal neuralgia as well as some chronic pain disorders.* Dilantin works for these, too, but Tegretol is usually better. Examples are glossopharyngeal neuralgia (like trigeminal neuralgia except that pain affects the throat), pain occurring after nerve injury, or "phantom limb" pain after amputation. It also helps postherpetic neuralgia, the nagging ache that occasionally remains after an attack of shingles (see Zovirax acyclovir, section 16., for discussion of shingles).
3. *Restless leg syndrome.* This mostly affects middle-aged women who feel an uncomfortable sensation in their legs, especially at night.
4. *Withdrawal from addictive substances.* Tegretol decreases withdrawal symptoms of benzodiazepine (Valium, Librium, Xanax) addicts. As good as other drugs for alcohol withdrawal and some studies show it reduces the craving for cocaine. Now and then patients ask for a prescription to "help" in withdrawing from their addiction at home. I always

refuse, and no sensible doctor agrees. Giving drugs to drug addicts to manage their addiction is ridiculous; if they were competent to handle drugs they wouldn't be addicts. When used, Tegretol must be part of a supervised treatment program.

5. *Psychiatric disorders.* Manic-depressives who don't respond to lithium should try Tegretol. Although not as effective as other antidepressants for pure depression, it works half the time. There are encouraging signs it helps patients with explosive personality disorders—those who suddenly become aggressive or launch into another unstoppable behavior.

How it works

For suppressing seizures, Tegretol's action is identical to Dilantin. That may explain its other uses, but no one is certain.

How dispensed

Tablets of 200 mg, chewable tablets of 100 mg, and a suspension of 100 mg per teaspoon.

Treatment begins with 200 mg twice a day, increasing by 200 mg per day every week until best response occurs or side effects become too great; 800 to 1200 per day usually works.

Translating the label

Tegretol is the brand name of carbamazepine.

Side effects

Most common is nausea, one reason the dose starts low and slowly increases. Dizziness, unsteadiness, and vomiting are less common and tend to diminish as therapy continues. Drowsiness occurs, but no more often than with Dilantin.

We still worry about bone marrow suppression, so the doctor will take a blood test every six months or yearly. This is no inconvenience because everyone on anticonvulsants should see a doctor regularly.

Interactions

Food. Take with meals to minimize digestive upsets.

Alcohol. No obvious interaction, but we don't like to give to anyone with liver disease, because liver damage is a rare reaction.

Drugs. As complex as other anticonvulsants. Drugs that increase Tegretol's blood level: H2 blockers, Danazol, calcium blockers, erythromycin, lithium, niacin, and Darvon. Tegretol reduces effect of following drugs: acetaminophen, tetracyclines, theophylline, blood thinners, and antidepressants. When other anticonvulsants are given with Tegretol the interaction is unpredictable.

Pregnancy. As risky as Dilantin and phenobarbital.

Nursing. Probably safe.

Sex. Rare report of impotence.

Allergies

Five percent of patients develop rash at beginning, but we continue treatment unless it's persistent or too unpleasant.

Wholesale cost

Sixteen cents for 200-mg tablet, double that for brand name Tegretol.

60
Caffeine

Physiology was the bane of my first year in medical school. Although I enjoyed the class, lectures took place after lunch, and soon after sitting down in the warm lecture hall I became drowsy. This was a serious problem because taking good notes is essential in medical school (medical books are enormous; you can't use them to study for exams). After a few sleepy weeks, I remembered someone had given me a present of a "Campus-Pak"—small samples of aftershave lotion, toothpaste, shampoo, and so on. Included was a packet of something called "No-Doz" that was supposed to restore alertness. I took two at the end of lunch and forgot about them.

Unlike most college students, we arrived early for lectures. Waiting for the professor, I normally socialized with friends, but this time I noticed something peculiar. I was not only talking with friends but with everyone. Too restless to sit, I paced the aisles, chattering and telling jokes. I felt wonderful. What was going on? . . . Then I remembered the No-Doz. Since I never drank coffee, I was probably hypersensitive to caffeine.

"This is terrific stuff," I thought and immediately bought several bottles. Sadly, the exhilaration faded as my body adjusted after a few weeks, but No-Doz continued to eliminate my drowsiness after lunch. I still don't drink coffee. Later, I discovered caffeine's limitations. It didn't work for serious drowsiness. After a sleepless night in the hospital during my residency, two No-Doz perked me up for about five minutes. Taking more produced no effect except queasiness. Other students took huge amounts before tests, but they were never the best students: They appeared jittery and desperate but not particularly awake.

Caffeine is good for:

1. *Relieving mild drowsiness.*
2. *Vascular headaches.* As I'll mention in the ergot chapter further on, the caffeine in many headache remedies helps because it constricts cerebral blood vessels.
3. *Pain except for vascular headaches.* Many pain remedies contain small amounts, but I doubt caffeine adds much to the other ingredients. I list some below.
4. *Asthma.* Strong coffee was the treatment of choice during the nineteenth century. We don't use it today because a close relative, theophylline, works better.

How it works

Caffeine probably stimulates norepinephrine release from nerve endings. If you recall in the Tofranil/Prozac section 51. and 52., that's how amphetamines and cocaine work. Although its action is much milder, caffeine influences the same chemical path but in complex ways researchers have yet to unravel.

How dispensed

As 100- and 200-mg tablets. A strong cup of coffee contains about 100 mg.

Translating the label

No-Doz and Vivarin are popular over-the-counter stimulants.

Cafergot and Wigraine are ergot-caffeine mixtures that help vascular headaches. Pain remedies that combine caffeine with aspirin, acetaminophen, or tranquilizers include Anacin, Fiorinal, Excedrin, Vanquish, Esgic, Norgesic, and Darvon Compound.

Side effects

Mostly what you'd expect of a stimulant: anxiety, nervousness, insomnia, palpitations. Less often it causes nausea and loss of appetite. Although abdominal pain is not a side effect, caffeine stimulates gastric acid secretion so don't take it if you have an ulcer. It's also a mild diuretic.

A few years ago, a debate raged on whether caffeine aggravated painful, fibrocystic breasts. The consensus today is it doesn't.

Interactions

Food. Avoid foods that contain caffeine: cola drinks and tea. Chocolate contains a similar ingredient, but it's rarely a problem.

Alcohol. No interaction. Despite the popular belief, caffeine doesn't reverse the depressant action of too much alcohol.

Drugs. Although no help with drunkenness, caffeine does antagonize both the depressant and painkilling action of narcotics. Don't combine caffeine with oral asthma drugs because both have similar actions.

Pregnancy. In 1980, the FDA issued a warning advising pregnant women to "limit their exposure." Experts today doubt that caffeine poses a threat.

Nursing. Probably O.K. in modest amounts.

Sex. No problems.

Allergies

Rare.

Wholesale Cost

Cost is $5.70 for 60 tablets of 100 mg.

PART V
Drugs for Pain

The nonsteroidal anti-inflammatories

Over the past 20 years, these drugs (called NSAIDs for short) have captured much of the painkilling business from codeine, aspirin, and acetaminophen (Tylenol, Datril, Panadol, Anacin-3). NSAIDs are superior in most ways and more dangerous in a few. That seems peculiar when you realize the FDA approved over-the-counter sale of the most popular NSAID, Motrin (ibuprofen) during the mid-1980s.

How they work

Easier if you understand the title of this section. Nonsteroidal means "not cortisone." Cortisone turns off inflammation like a switch, but you'll learn why it's no competition to NSAIDs in the discussion of drug 74. Anti-inflammatory means what it says, but you should know plenty of pain remedies are not anti-inflammatory: acetaminophen (remember the brand names from earlier—I won't mention them again) and narcotics like codeine, morphine, oxycodone, and propoxyphene (Darvon).

"Inflammation" is what happens when your body responds to an injury. Blood vessels dilate; more blood flows in, so the damaged area becomes red and warm. These vessels also become leaky; fluid, cells, and body chemicals pour into the area, so it swells. Swelling produces pain, but the cells and chemicals themselves cause pain as they deal with injured tissue. Inflammation is a tricky concept because many body chemicals (prostaglandins, bradykinin—you don't have to remember these) that cause inflammation participate in other painful conditions (headaches, menstrual cramps) that don't involve tissue injury. Anti-inflammatories help these, too.

The cardinal signs of inflammation, as medical students learn, are redness, warmth, swelling, and pain. Naturally, you'll only notice all four if inflammation is superficial, but NSAIDs help most deep pains, the major exception being those in the digestive tract.

"Redness, warmth, swelling, and pain" may remind you of something else: infection. That's an injury, too, and the body responds in the same way. Fortunately, NSAIDs don't suppress your ability to fight an infection. Cortisone is not so discriminating.

No drug company feels part of the big leagues until it develops its own NSAID. No doctor can remember them all, and only rheumatologists need to know the subtle differences among them. For your purposes and mine, you should remember two: one old, one new.

An Old NSAID

61
Indocin (indomethacin)

Appearing from the 1940s to the early 1960s, these were never best-sellers because they routinely caused unpleasant side effects and occasionally deadly ones. Many are off the market, and several remaining should probably go the same route.

Among the newest of the old, indomethacin appeared in 1963. Its side effects are no less unpleasant but rarely fatal, and it remains superior to newer drugs for several important indications.

Indocin is NSAID of choice for:

Gout. An ancient, common affliction in men (rare in women—only 5 percent of victims), gout is a form of arthritis, inflammation of a joint. Many men have high levels of uric acid in their blood, and occasionally, for unclear reasons, uric acid crystals suddenly appear in a joint, producing excruciating pain, redness, and swelling. Untreated, this lasts a few days to a few weeks, and 93 percent of those having a first attack will have more.

Most first attacks occur in the base of the big toe. Sooner or later, 90 percent of victims suffer there, so the diagnosis springs to mind quickly in a man with severe big toe pain (but chronic pain is probably arthritis or a bunion). Other gout sites are the instep, ankle, heel, knee, and wrist, but almost never the back or shoulder.

All NSAIDs help gout, but doctors have the most experience with Indocin, and it may work quickest. Relief usually begins in less than a day. After a few attacks, most victims yearn never to have another, and medical science can oblige. You can read about a drug that should prevent 100 percent of gouty attacks in the Zyloprim section 81.

Indocin is good for:

1. *Arthritis, bursitis, tendinitis, injuries, headaches.* No NSAID stands out for injuries or general aches and pains, so it's appropriate to begin with either of the two in this chapter, but others work as well.
2. *Fever.* Fever forms part of the inflammatory response, and all NSAIDs suppress it, but there's no reason to use them unless aspirin or acetaminophen don't work.

How dispensed

Capsules of 25 and 50 mg, a long-acting capsule containing 75 mg, a suspension containing 25 mg per teaspoon, and 50-mg suppository.

Doctors treat gouty attacks with large doses for a limited period. One course would be 50 mg three times a day for three days followed by 25 mg three times a day for four days.

For other conditions, 25 mg two or three times a day is a reasonable starting dose, although one can go as high as 50 mg three times a day.

Translating the label

Indocin is the only brand of indomethacin.

Side effects

Indocin gives nearly half its users a headache, an equal number queasiness and abdominal pain. Most patients persist despite these; only one in five discontinues the drug. NSAIDs not only irritate the stomach, they cause bleeding, although not as frequently as aspirin. Perhaps 3 percent of patients bleed, but the rate is probably higher in the elderly. Diarrhea and dizziness are not rare. Like aspirin, NSAIDs also decrease the blood's ability to clot, but the effect is not as severe or long-lasting.

Interactions

Food. Always take after eating.

Alcohol. None known.

Drugs. Lithium: increases lithium blood levels by 50 percent. Also increases blood level of methotrexate, an anticancer drug also occasionally used to treat rheumatoid arthritis and psoriasis. Diuretics: Sometimes reduces both diuretic and antihypertensive action.

Pregnancy. Forbidden. Causes fetal deaths in animals. Also speeds cardiac maturation late in pregnancy—a useful quality in premature infants with certain heart defects but not desirable in a healthy pregnancy.

Nursing. Not advisable.

Sex. None known.

Allergies

Pure allergies to Indocin are uncommon, but all NSAIDs distantly resemble aspirin, so those who suffer rashes, hives, or asthma after taking aspirin might do the same with Indocin. Then again, they might not.

Wholesale cost

Four cents for 25 mg, five cents for 50 mg, and one dollar for 75-mg extended release capsule.

A Newer NSAID

62
Motrin (also Advil, Nuprin, Medipren, Rufen—all ibuprofen)

The mid-1970s saw a pleasant advance with the appearance of ibuprofen followed by an avalanche of similar drugs (all, of course, long available in Europe). Although not superior to Indocin and its relatives, they are much easier to tolerate.

In 1984, the FDA approved ibuprofen for sale without a prescription. As soon as that happened, patients began to look disappointed when I recommended it. Didn't I have something stronger? I had to explain—as I have earlier in this book—that FDA uses safety, not strength, to determine eligibility for over-the-counter sale.

Ibuprofen's competitors are probably as safe, and many doctors routinely prescribe them, but ibuprofen should be your first choice. It may be the oldest in its category, but none of the newer is better.

Motrin is NSAID of choice for:

Menstrual cramps. Birth control pills were the mainstay of treatment for cramps until well into the 1980s. If they weren't acceptable, doctors recommended aspirin and rest—a much inferior remedy. Relieving menstrual cramps wasn't a high priority for the medical profession 20 years ago, so a decade passed before doctors realized how well NSAIDs worked. They're so effective that if they don't help, you should see a gynecologist to find out if another condition is responsible.

Motrin is good for:

1. *Arthritis, bursitis, tendinitis, injuries, headaches.*
2. *Fever.*

How dispensed

Tablets of 300, 400, 600, and 800 mg; over-the-counter ibuprofen comes in 200 mg. There is also a suspension containing 100 mg per teaspoon.

Taking 400 mg every four hours is a reasonable starting dose, but 600 may work slightly better. There's no benefit in going higher than 3,200 mg per day.

Translating the label

Prescription ibuprofen comes as Motrin, Rufen, and Ibu.

Over-the-counter ibuprofen includes Advil, Nuprin, Ibu-tab, Medipren, Pamprim-IB, Ibuprin, Haltran, Trendar, and Midol-200.

Related NSAIDs available by prescription:
- naproxyn (Naproxyn, Anaprox)
- fenoprofen (Nalfon)
- ketoprofen (Orudis)
- ribiprofen (Ansaid)
- diclofenac (Voltaren)
- piroxicam (Feldene)
- oxaprozin (Daypro)
- etodolac (Lodine)
- nabumetone (Relafen)
- meclofenamate (Meclomen)
- mefenamic acid (Pontsel)
- tolmetin (Tolectin)
- sulindac (Clinoril)—a relative of Indocin but properly a member of this group.

Side effects

Only 10 percent suffer digestive upsets, and headaches aren't significant. On the other hand, internal bleeding is no less common than with Indocin. Elderly seem more susceptible to bleeding, and doctors are growing reluctant to allow them to take NSAIDs for extended periods.

Interactions

Food. Take it with food.

Alcohol. None known.

Drugs. Same as with Indocin.

Pregnancy. Animal studies show no problems, but it may also speed up cardiac development late in pregnancy.

Nursing. Probably O.K.

Sex. No problems reported.

Allergies

Rashes and itching occur at least 3 percent of time. Again, some risk exists of cross-reaction with aspirin allergy.

Wholesale cost

Three cents for 200 and 400 mg. Four cents for 600 mg. Six cents for 800 mg.

63
Acetaminophen (Tylenol)

Tylenol is a public relations triumph—a brand name that has entered the common vocabulary. Just as your mother looked for Jello rather than "flavored gelatin dessert" at the market, you probably won't ask for acetaminophen when you have a headache. To the chagrin of other manufacturers, you're much less likely to request Panadol, Anacin-3, Datril, Tempra, or Liquiprim, either.

Although available without a prescription only since 1955, doctors knew about acetaminophen a hundred years ago. It didn't catch on because a similar pain remedy, phenacetin, was already popular—so popular that doctors suspected it was a mood stimulator. Europeans consumed huge quantities, but Americans also enjoyed it; the "APC" tablets handed out freely during my army service were aspirin-phenacetin-caffeine. After World War II, doctors began noticing a rare catastrophic kidney disease turning up more and more. Some concluded that it affected those taking large amounts of phenacetin and named it "analgesic-abuse nephropathy." Others doubted a drug used by so many for so long could be so poisonous. The debate continued for decades before medical opinion shifted firmly against phenacetin, and it's now off the market.

Acetaminophen is good for:

1. *Fever.* As effective as aspirin.
2. *Pain.* Equal to aspirin for headaches, muscle aches, and injuries but not for conditions in which inflammation plays a role: arthritis, bursitis, tendinitis. Inflammation also figures in menstrual cramps, so you should prefer Motrin, Advil, Nuprin, and so forth.

How it works

When the body breaks down phenacetin, one product is acetaminophen, which lacks the poisonous side effects of phenacetin but also provides no mood elevation. Unlike aspirin, acetaminophen has no effect on inflammation, so it's inferior for arthritis, tendinitis, bursitis, and menstrual cramps but it provides some pain relief. Although we're not certain, most likely acetaminophen works on the brain (where fever and pain are controlled) but has no effect on the "periphery" where inflammation takes place. Aspirin effects both brain and periphery.

How dispensed.

Many sizes and forms. An adult dose is two 325-mg tablets every four hours, but three may work a little better. "Extra strength" tablets are 500 mg, so the dose is two every four hours.

Translating the label

The popular acetaminophens are Tylenol, Panadol, Anacin-3, Datril, Tempra, and Liquiprim. Innumerable combinations exist, so read the fine print listing the ingredients. You should also be careful of the main label. Anacin is aspirin (plus caffeine), but Anacin-3 is acetaminophen. St. Joseph's Aspirin and St. Joseph's Aspirin-free are not the same.

Side effects

Almost no one complains. Huge doses cause liver damage that is often fatal, but this isn't a risk for the average user.

Interactions

Food. None.

Alcohol. No real interaction, but anyone with liver disease must avoid it—and that includes alcoholics still drinking.

Drugs. None significant.

Pregnancy. We recommend acetaminophen if a pregnant woman wants something for pain or fever.

Nursing. No problems.

Sex. None known.

Allergies

Very, very rare.

Cost

One cent for 325-mg tablet, 1.4 cents for 500 mg.

64
Aspirin

The bark of the willow served for centuries to treat "agues," fever. Noting the bitter taste, eighteenth-century doctors decided it contained quinine, another bitter drug that lowered fevers (see quinidine, section 25.). When nineteenth-century chemists began isolating active chemicals from the bark, they found salicylic acid, still used in wart and corn removers, but too toxic to take internally. The first safe drug, sodium salicylate, reached the market in 1875, and its success encouraged a chemist with the Bayer Company to develop acetylsalicylic acid: aspirin. Bayer began selling it in 1899 and still does, but plenty of other manufacturers have joined them. Americans consume about 25 billion tablets per year.

Aspirin is good for:

1. *Fever.* But not in children. Use acetaminophen. A rare but devastating liver inflammation called Reye's syndrome seems to strike a few children given aspirin during a viral infection.
2. *Arthritis, bursitis, tendinitis, injuries, headaches.*
3. *Preventing heart attack.* We've known since the 1970s that aspirin works for "secondary prevention." It lowers the chance of a second heart attack in patients who've had their first or who are otherwise at a high risk with severe angina, hardening of the arteries, or after bypass surgery.
   Whether healthy people benefit wasn't answered until 1987. Since 1983, 22,000 doctors including me have taken a pill a day containing either aspirin, vitamin A, or placebo to discover if (1) taking aspirin prevents heart attacks and (2) taking vitamin A prevents cancer. After four and a half years, those taking aspirin had half as many heart attacks as those on placebo, so researchers stopped that part of the study. The vitamin A–cancer part continues because no clear results have appeared.
   Aspirin probably helps men over 40 and women over 50 with any in-

creased risk: smoking, cholesterol above 220, diabetes, family history of a heart attack before age 50. It won't help as much as eliminating the first two risk factors, and anyone who can't tolerate aspirin shouldn't take it even though the dose is only one every other day.

4. *Preventing stroke.* Here studies show benefit only for those already at very high risk: people who have had small strokes, early strokes or "transient ischemic attacks," and those with narrowing of their cerebral arteries. Studies may never show that healthy people can prevent strokes with aspirin. Although clots in the brain cause most strokes (aspirin should, in theory, prevent these), a minority result from bleeding, and aspirin encourages bleeding. The doctors in my study who took aspirin suffered a slightly higher risk of hemorrhagic stroke.

How it works

Aspirin and other members of the "salicylate" group are nonsteroidal anti-inflammatory drugs (NSAIDs) like those in sections 60 and 61. Compared to those, aspirin—

1. Suppresses fever as well.
2. Treats arthritis as well and perhaps better, provided a patient can tolerate huge doses.
3. Isn't useful for gout.
4. Is inferior in relieving menstrual cramps.
5. Probably damages the stomach more strongly.
6. Thins the blood more and for a longer period—a risky side effect when treating pain but useful in other circumstances.

How dispensed

Too many sizes and forms to list. An adult dose for ordinary pain or fever is two 325-mg tablets every four hours. Many patients take only one and feel virtuous because they disapprove of taking drugs for minor ailments. While there's no harm in this, one aspirin may not work. "Extra-strength" preparations contain 500 mg. Taking three regular-strength gives the same effect.

Translating the label

Plain aspirin comes labeled as aspirin except in innumerable combinations where you must search the label.

Timed-release, buffered, or enteric-coated aspirin (Ecotrin, Easprin, Anacin-coated) are supposed to cause less stomach irritation. Despite their popularity, it's not certain that they do so, and they're much more expensive. Try them if plain aspirin upsets your stomach but not otherwise.

Other salicylates:

- Sodium salicylate—as irritating to the stomach but with less effect on blood clotting.
- Choline magnesium trisalicylate (Trilisate), magnesium salicylate (Masal), and Salsalate (Disalcid, Salflex, Mono-Gesic). Underused prescription salicylates, they produce no effect on clotting and less stomach damage than any other NSAID.

Side effects

If aspirin appeared today, the FDA would classify it as a prescription drug: too dangerous to sell over-the-counter. Despite this, doctors are only modestly concerned and patients show little fear of a drug that causes more unpleasant side effects, dangerous reactions, and poisoning deaths than any other. Europeans take it more seriously; they prefer acetaminophen and consume it with the same abandon we reserve for aspirin. As a result they see less aspirin hemorrhage and overdose (but far more acetaminophen liver and kidney failure; in large doses acetaminophen can be equally nasty).

Everyone taking aspirin suffers stomach irritation whether or not he or she notices. Perhaps 20 percent suffer so much pain or nausea they avoid aspirin. An equal number feel the benefit outweighs their discomfort. Everyone taking aspirin regularly has a small amount of bleeding and sooner or later a few percent bleed massively.

Aspirin interferes with blood clotting. You can demonstrate that by performing a bleeding time, a simple but inaccurate test that doctors rarely use. You perform a bleeding time by sticking your finger with a clean lancet then wiping away the blood until bleeding stops, perhaps after five minutes. Two ordinary aspirin doubles bleeding time for up to seven days—not a minor effect. Despite that, aspirin doesn't cause a bleeding tendency in healthy people, but you should stop taking it a week before any surgery, including dental surgery. No one with a bleeding problem or a medical condition that predisposes them to bleeding such as ulcers should take aspirin.

Black readers should recall my warning about glucose-6-phosphate dehydrogenase deficiency from the sulfa chapter. Aspirin sometimes provokes a reaction.

Large doses cause "salicylism:" ringing in the ears, dizziness, diminished hearing, headache, nausea. You may remember this combination because it's similar to "cinchonism" caused by quinine. Ringing in the ears signals you're taking too much aspirin unless you're on high doses to treat severe arthritis. Then it means that you're on the maximum therapeutic dose.

Interactions

Food. Always take aspirin with food in your stomach.

Alcohol. Combination increases stomach damage. Also taking aspirin with alcohol increases blood level of alcohol.

Drugs. Never use with a drug that interferes with clotting. Any doctor prescribing such a drug will warn you but you must learn to read labels and stay away from other drugs containing salicylates. Aspirin may interfere with the action of antidiabetic and blood pressure medication, but this is usually tolerable if the doctor remains alert.

Pregnancy. A study of 50,000 women failed to find a risk of birth defects in those taking aspirin during the first four months of pregnancy, but we still don't recommend it. Use acetaminophen if you must take something for pain or fever. Salicylates late in pregnancy are forbidden for same reasons as the NSAIDs in the previous section.

Nursing. O.K. when used occasionally.

Sex. No problems.

Allergies

These are not rare. Rashes occur, but the typical aspirin allergy resembles hay fever and asthma. Sensitive individuals develop itchy eyes, a stuffy, runny nose, and difficulty breathing after exposure to tiny amounts. In addition, aspirin provokes wheezing in 10 percent of adults with ordinary asthma. The "acetyl" portion of the acetylsalicylic acid molecule seems responsible because allergic patients can safely take other salicylates listed above.

Wholesale cost

Less than a penny for plain 325-mg aspirin. Enteric coating costs a dime.

---

65 Demerol • **66** Morphine

As mentioned in the Lomotil section (44.), humans have consumed opiates for thousands of years, mostly for their constipating action. Smoking and swallowing opium produced some pain relief, too, but that wasn't predictable or convenient until chemists isolated pure narcotics in the nineteenth century.

The first appeared in 1809, named after Morpheus, the Greek god of dreams. With the invention of the hypodermic needle soon after, doctors realized they had something that really worked. Drugs that worked were uncommon in the nineteenth century, a time when doctors enormously increased their knowledge of disease but made much less progress in treatment. As with all miracle drugs (and morphine is that) doctors vastly overprescribed it although, to be fair, buying and injecting yourself with morphine remained legal until the present century. Addiction may have been more common then than now.

Since then researchers have tried to improve on morphine by developing a narcotic with no addicting properties, fewer side effects, and longer action. Dozens of candidates have come forth; not one is superior.

Demerol appeared in 1939 with the usual enthusiastic predictions that turned out wrong. Ever since then Demerol has crushed a dozen competitors to far-outsell morphine for treating severe pain outside the hospital and to rival it for inpatients. No explanation except brilliant promotion by the Winthrop Company accounts for this success. Equal to morphine as a pain reliever provided the doctor gives an adequate dose (not always the case), Demerol's action doesn't last as long: two to three hours compared to four to five.

One reason for its popularity may be simply that it's called "Demerol" and not morphine, which has a disreputable association with addiction. When I want to help someone with severe pain from a kidney stone or fracture, I usually ask for morphine. Taking my request, the nurse often eyes me suspiciously, a reaction I never see when I ask for Demerol.

How they work

Narcotics bind to receptors in cells in areas of the brain that regulate pain perception (also, unfortunately, respiration and emotional behavior) as well as receptors in the digestive tract) inhibiting release of neurotransmitters. I explain neurotransmitters in the Tofranil-Prozac section (51. and 52.).

The medical term for narcotic action, *analgesia,* means relief of pain without loss of consciousness. Narcotics are not anesthetics; they won't put anyone to sleep except in near-fatal doses. They don't work as local anesthetics, either. If I tried to suture a laceration after giving morphine, the patient would complain bitterly. For the same reason, a surgeon couldn't give you a large narcotic injection, then take out your appendix painlessly.

Narcotics work best at relieving pain that's already present. Equally important, they also dull your emotional response to it. Most doctors don't realize that, but when I visit a hotel guest in extreme pain, I don't like to collect my money and leave until he or she feels better. So I wait. After about fifteen minutes I often hear the patient say, "the pain is still there . . . but it doesn't matter so much . . . ."

Morphine and Demerol are treatment of choice for:

1. *Severe acute pain.* Examples are postoperative pain, injuries, burns, kidney stones, and heart attacks. It's a bad idea to use narcotics for severe pain that keeps recurring such as migraines, backaches, and irritable bowels, but they work so well doctors are tempted.

2. *Severe chronic pain in someone who will die.* Traditionally that means someone with terminal cancer. Doctors have been criticized for skimping on pain relief for fear of turning dying patients into addicts. Experts agree that anyone with terminal cancer should receive enough narcotics to remain pain free—and so often the patient must never ask for relief. This is easily done, although it may require increasing doses.

Morphine and Demerol are good for:

1. *Pain of childbirth.* Keep an open mind if you've never experienced labor. Obstetricians prefer Demerol to morphine because it seems to depress the infant's respiration less.
2. *Severe heart failure.* When a patient is gasping for breath, a small amount of intravenous morphine often provides dramatic relief. No one is certain why; one theory explains that it relaxes blood vessels and thus reduces the heart's workload.

How dispensed

Injectable morphine comes in individual ampules containing from 5 to 15 mg as well as a vial containing 15 mg per cc. Fifteen mg is a reasonable adult dose. Taken orally, only a fraction is absorbed. Tablets, oral solutions, and suppositories exist, but doctors rarely use them outside of hospitals and hospices.

Injectable Demerol comes in individual ampules containing from 25 to 100 mg plus large vials of 50 or 100 mg per cc; 100 mg is equal to 10 mg of morphine. Unlike morphine, oral Demerol is fairly well absorbed and available as 50- and 100-mg tablets and a syrup containing 50 mg per cc.

Translating the label

After almost 200 years, most morphine is sold as morphine, but it's also called Roxanol, Duramorph, Astramorph, Oramorph, and MSIR.

Generic Demerol is meperidine in the U.S., but pethidine throughout most of the world.

Other powerful narcotics:

· Hydromorphone (Dilaudid)
· Oxymorphone (Numorphan)
· Levorphanol (Levo-Dromoran)
· Butorphanol (Stadol)
· Methadone (Dolophine)
· Pentazocine (Talwin)
· Nalbuphine (Nubain)

Heroin is illegal over most of the world. Similar to morphine, it offers no advantage.

Side effects

We worry most about respiratory depression, an action on the brain, not the lungs, so victims don't feel difficulty breathing. We breathe without thinking when the brain signals our lungs; narcotics weaken that autonomic signal. Rarely a problem when a patient is alert and healthy, this can be disastrous in someone very drowsy (after surgery or a head injury) or with severe lung disease (like emphysema or asthma) who requires more lung stimulation. Given a large dose of narcotics, these patients may quietly stop breathing.

More common side effects include dizziness, drowsiness, nausea, vomiting, and sweating. Strangely, these are not a big problem in patients with severe pain, becoming more common when patients are not so uncomfortable. Most healthy people without pain find an injection of morphine or Demerol an unpleasant experience.

Nausea is so common that most doctors mix a phenothiazine [see Thorazine (50.) and Compazine (49.)] in the same syringe and inject them together. That also increases the painkilling effect. The most popular are Phenergan and Vistaril.

Constipation occurs so regularly that some opiates are sold only to treat diarrhea [see Lomotil (44.)].

Interactions

Food. None.
Alcohol. Narcotics increase drowsiness and respiratory depression.

Drugs. All sedatives, sleeping pills, anesthetics, and other narcotics as well as most tranquilizers and antidepressants have the same action as alcohol.

Pregnancy. No known problems although they depress a newborn's respiration if given near childbirth. We are more generous in treating pregnant women for recurrent problems such as migraine because so many oral medications are riskier.

Nursing. Small amounts appear in milk, so one shouldn't nurse for a day after an injection.

Sex. Long-term use diminishes libido. Addicts have little interest in sex except as a source of income.

Allergies

Although rare, itching, flushing, hives, and other itchy rashes occur fairly often, possibly because narcotics release histamine (allergies do the same) and dilate blood vessels in the skin. Most of my patients who insist they're allergic to morphine or Demerol have had one of these nonallergic reactions.

Wholesale cost

One adult injection of Demerol or morphine costs about 75 cents.

67
Codeine

Almost identical to morphine (chemically it's methylmorphine), codeine possesses one tenth the strength. Ten times the dose would match morphine, but injectable codeine offers no benefits; I don't know anyone who uses it. Codeine's big advantage is good absorption when taken orally, so it's a common ingredient in prescription remedies for moderate-to-severe pain. Although less addictive than stronger narcotics, the FDA doesn't make this distinction, so a doctor who wants to prescribe plain codeine must write on a special "triplicate" prescription. Doctors must buy these special prescriptions and use them for strong narcotics, amphetamines, diet pills, and barbiturates; a copy goes to some government agency to monitor our prescribing habits. Dealing with triplicates is a bother, so we do it as little as possible. Fortunately, when combined with another drug, usually aspirin or acetaminophen, the FDA allows us an ordinary prescription, so that's how you'll get codeine.

Codeine is good for:

1. *Injuries, muscle aches, headaches.* Like acetaminophen, it's less effective than NSAIDs for arthritis, bursitis, tendinitis, and menstrual cramps.
2. *Cough.* Narcotics suppress coughing along with respiration, and codeine is the most popular ingredient in prescription cough remedies.
3. *Diarrhea.* Although almost never prescribed, it works as well as other narcotics, Lomotil included.

How it works

Same as morphine.

How dispensed

Tablets of 15, 30 and 60 mg and an injectable containing 30 and 60 mg per cc. 30 mg orally equals one or two aspirin or acetaminophen.

Translating the label

Codeine is so old, cheap, and tiresome to prescribe on a triplicate that drug companies have given up promoting it, so you'll only find it as a generic. Combinations are a different matter. Innumerable products exist containing codeine with aspirin (Empirin 2, 3, and 4), acetaminophen (Phenaphen and Tylenol 2, 3, and 4), barbiturates (Fiorinal), and muscle relaxants (Soma).

Side effects

Dizziness, drowsiness, nausea, and vomiting are so common that I rarely prescribe codeine unless a patient hasn't had a reaction in the past. For moderate pain, Motrin works as well. For a day or two of severe pain I give Percodan or Vicodin (next section). The only exceptions are patients with a stomach disorder who can't take aspirin or an NSAID. Although codeine upsets the stomach, it doesn't cause bleeding.

Interactions

Food. Take after a meal.

Alcohol. Codeine potentiates the sedative action of alcohol.

Drugs. Same as morphine.

Pregnancy. Codeine is an ancient drug with no birth defects reported and no problems in animal studies.

Nursing. Probably O.K.

Sex. It's possible long-term use causes the same diminished libido as strong narcotics, but that would be hard to achieve.

Allergies

As with stronger narcotics, itching and itchy rashes are common although rarely a genuine allergy.

Wholesale cost

About a nickel a pill. Strangely, combining codeine with aspirin or acetaminophen has little effect on the price.

68
Percodan

Seeing a hotel guest with a painful backache or sprained ankle, I give the usual advice and Motrin, but I often add a small box of four Percodan I carry in my bag. The first day of most ailments feels the worst, so this guarantees quicker relief. It also saves a few calls, because I tell guests to contact me if their discomfort persists, and the number I leave is my home phone.

Percodan is good for:

1. *Severe but short-lived pain.* Doctors undertreat this in healthy patients with codeine, a useful but overrated drug. In the dose most patients can tolerate, codeine is slightly stronger than aspirin.
2. *Pain in someone terminally ill.*

How it works

The same as other narcotics. Oxycodone, the major ingredient in Percodan, equals morphine's strength when given by injection. Given orally, it's half as strong.

How dispensed

As a tablet containing about 5 mg of oxycodone combined with 325 mg of aspirin. This is more reasonable than most drug combinations, but 325 mg is one adult aspirin, so you'll get a slightly better effect by taking another aspirin along with one Percodan. Every four to six hours is a reasonable interval.

Translating the label

A newer combination called Percodan-Demi contains half as much oxycodone with the same amount of aspirin.

Percodan is a brand, so a generic label gives only the ingredients, oxycodone and aspirin, although one generic has a name: Roxiprin. Plain oxycodone is available as Roxicodone.

Many companies sell oxycodone in which acetaminophen replaces aspirin: Percocet, Tylox, Roxicet.

All oxycodone combinations require a triplicate prescription. Hydrocodone resembles oxycodone with the enormous advantage that we can order it with an ordinary prescription. No logical reason exists for this. You'll find hydrocodone mixed with aspirin or acetaminophen in Vicodin, Zydone, Lortab, Lorcet, Anexsia, Hyco-Pap, Azdone, Co-Gesic, Damason-P, Duocet, and Hydrocet.

Side effects

Although there's no reason why Percodan should be easier on the stomach than codeine, I don't hear as many complaints. Other side effects resemble those of typical narcotics—plus, of course, aspirin.

Interactions

Similar to other narcotics plus aspirin.

Allergies

No different.

Wholesale cost

Twelve cents a tablet.

69
Xylocaine (lidocaine)

The first local anesthetic, cocaine, is still used by ear-nose-throat surgeons for minor procedures. Newer, less irritating anesthetics such as Xylocaine have superseded cocaine in other areas.

Although known in South America for centuries, it was only in 1884 that a scientist launched a thorough study of cocaine. You read about Sigmund Freud's conclusions in the Tofranil-Prozac section. Besides proclaiming cocaine a useful stimulant, he thought it cured morphine addiction, not a rare problem among colleagues. He turned out to be wrong on both counts, which did not help his career. At the same time, to Freud's chagrin, another Viennese researcher revealed cocaine's local anesthetic properties, and both the medical and dental profession quickly adopted it. If Freud had made that discovery, he might not have switched to another field.

Xylocaine is good for:

1. *Painful conditions on the skin and mucus membranes.* Xylocaine won't penetrate the dead layer of skin that protects your exterior unless it's damaged, but Xylocaine ointment helps superficial burns, abrasions, and insect bites. Applied to a mucus membrane, it relieves pain in a few minutes, so I prescribe it for severe sore throats and canker sores. Xylocaine gargle is superior to over-the-counter sore throat remedies, so ask for it if your doctor doesn't bring up the subject.
2. *Pain of childbirth, dental work, and minor surgery.* Injected beneath the skin, it numbs a small area. Injected near a large nerve by someone skilled in "regional" anesthesia, Xylocaine deadens that nerve and the large area it supplies.
3. *Pain of major surgery.* Injected into or around the spinal canal, it numbs the entire body below. "Spinal" anesthetic is safer than general anesthetic with fewer unpleasant after-effects. Get it if you can.
4. *Dangerous cardiac rhythms.* Local anesthesia numbs the heart, too, but

you won't encounter this use outside an intensive care unit. Doctors give it intravenously.

How it works

Xylocaine blocks the ability of nerve cell membranes to conduct an electric current. Many chemicals do the same—but only by damaging the nerve. Alcohol is an example. Local anesthetics do their work, then wear off, leaving the nerve as healthy as before.

How dispensed

You'll find it as a 5 percent ointment or a 2 percent solution for gargling. A 2.5 percent ointment is available without a prescription. Adults should use it as needed but never more than half the 5 percent tube or 150 cc of solution daily.

Translating the label

Xylocaine is the only brand of lidocaine you can buy. In case you're interested, the "Novocaine" used by dentists is a brand of procaine, a relative of lidocaine.

Side effects

Given intravenously, high doses cause nervousness and dizziness and even higher doses cause seizures, but these are unlikely when used topically. Numbness is the usual effect of Xylocaine in the mouth; unless you're careful you can chew your tongue or lip without realizing it. A numb throat makes swallowing dangerous, so don't eat during this time.

Interactions

Food. None, but don't eat within an hour after a gargle.
Alcohol. None, but don't drink within an hour of a gargle.
Drugs. Not a problem in topical use, but don't use another topical at the same time.
Pregnancy. No known human or animal problems.

Nursing. Probably none if used topically.
Sex. None reported.

Allergies

Rare with Xylocaine. Reactions occur more often with procaine (Novocaine), but those allergic to procaine aren't usually allergic to lidocaine. If your doctor doesn't realize that, tactfully suggest that he look it up.

Wholesale cost

Cost is $2 for 50 grams of 5-percent ointment; $3.20 for 100-ml bottle of lidocaine gargle.

70
Ergot (ergotamine)

Another natural drug, produced by a parasitic fungus that grows on rye. When the sacred books of the Parsees, written 2,500 years ago, denounced contaminated grain that made pregnant women "drop the womb and die in childbed," they meant ergots, still a good migraine treatment. The Greeks and Romans disliked rye so they didn't write about it, but it returned to the European diet in the middle ages and quickly produced frightening epidemics of St. Anthony's fire, a curse that produced intense burning of the hands and feet, sometimes ending in gangrene and loss of limbs. Abortions were another consequence, and medieval midwives made liberal use of ergot.

The medical profession didn't take it up until the nineteenth century (doctors didn't concern themselves with childbirth until the eighteenth century). Busy men, they administered ergot to speed up childbirth. It does this very well, even violently, and with a fair amount of injury to both mother and child. Nowadays we have safer drugs.

So far, migraine hasn't entered the picture, but no one dreamed of using this dangerous potion for a nonfatal condition until the twentieth century when researchers discovered the active ingredient, and doctors learned to prescribe it without risking life and limb. They isolated ergotamine, the first pure "ergot," in 1920.

Ergotamine is good for:

Vascular headaches. Migraine is an example; no one knows its cause. Drugs, irritating chemicals, allergies, and even stress produce other vascular headaches. Vascular means "pertaining to a blood vessel," and arteries are the source of pain, most often the temporal artery that flows vertically just in front of your ear. You can feel its pulse. With each heartbeat, the tender artery stretches, so a vascular headache pulsates and throbs. Remember that when I discuss how ergotamine works.

Migraine (from the Greek meaning, roughly, half-head) is a recurrent affliction attacking mostly women that begins in childhood or adolescence and usually fades in middle age. Commonly affecting half the head (as the name implies), it starts fairly slowly, rises to a crescendo of throbbing pain, often with vomiting and intolerance of light, and rarely lasts more than a day. You've probably heard of the flashing lights and other peculiar symptoms that precede a migraine, but only 20 percent of sufferers experience them. Most migraines are one-sided, but some aren't, and many one-sided headaches spread after a few hours.

Finally, you've certainly heard of muscle tension headaches, which are supposed to result from stress and produce a more generalized, dull ache that lasts hours to days. Many victims of tension headaches insist they have migraine because they feel any bad headache must be a migraine; a tension headache, they believe, is evidence of a neurosis but migraine is a real disease.

I once disapproved of mixing these two types, but lately I'm not sure it matters. Experts are coming to believe most headaches are a mixture of tension and migraine, especially after being present for a few hours. Some treatments (antidepressants, NSAIDs) help both. Ergotamine isn't supposed to help a tension headache, but it's worth a try.

How it works

Ergotamine vigorously contracts smooth muscle: the muscle that lines your blood vessels, internal organs, and digestive tract. If you recall, muscles you use to move around are called skeletal muscles. Ergotamine doesn't affect those.

It relieves throbbing headaches by constricting and stiffening arteries in the scalp. Muscle contraction also explains why ergots caused abortions and speedy childbirth as well as the side effects below.

How dispensed

1. *Sublingual tablets containing 2 mg.* I prefer this form because it works fast. Treatment should begin at the first sign of an attack with one tablet under the tongue. If necessary take another in a half hour and a third a half hour later, but no more than three a day or five a week.
2. *As an inhaler.* You squirt a puff into your mouth, breathe deeply, then hold your breath as long as possible. The dose is one puff every five minutes to a maximum of six and no more than 15 puffs per week.
3. *Tablets containing 1 mg.* All available pills add 100 mg of caffeine, also modestly effective for vascular headaches (which is what you experience a few hours after skipping your morning coffee; caffeine works wonders for that). Take two at the onset, then one every half hour until relief occurs, but no more than six. No one should take more than ten tablets per week.
4. *Rectal suppositories containing 2 mg plus caffeine and sometimes a tranquilizer.* You can take a second an hour after the first, but no more than five per week.
5. *Dihydroergotamine, a related ergot, is the injectable form.* Dose is 1 mg every hour to a maximum of 3 and no more than 6 mg per week. An injection seems to work better than other techniques for a full-blown attack.

Translating the label

Sublingual ergotamine may be called Ergostat and Ergomar.

The inhaler is Medihaler-Ergotamine.

Tablets are Cafergot and Wygraine. Another popular brand is Bellergal-S, a mixture of phenobarbital (an old tranquilizer) and 0.6 mg of ergotamine.

Although not useful for acute migraines, I prescribe it for garden-variety vascular headaches. The dose is one twice a day with no weekly limit.

The suppositories are also Cafergot and Wygraine.

Side effects

Obviously, St. Anthony's fire occurred when ergots constricted arteries enough to cut off the blood supply. We don't see this today, but numbness or tingling in the hands or feet is a sign you're sensitive to ergots. Ten percent of patients experience nausea and vomiting. Since this also accompanies migraine, it's difficult to blame the drug in every case, but plenty of my patients refuse to take ergotamine after a few experiences.

Ergots are addictive. Patients who ignore the limits on intake and treat themselves too often discover that stopping produces a flare in headaches.

Interactions

Food. None.

Alcohol. None, but alcohol relaxes arteries, so it provokes vascular headaches.

Drugs. An occasional interaction with other drugs that act on arteries, especially beta blockers, leading to too much constriction.

Pregnancy. Absolutely forbidden for obvious reasons.

Nursing. Unsafe.

Sex. Surprisingly, I haven't found any.

Allergies

Very rare. Itching and tingling are fairly common but that's the result of arterial constriction.

Wholesale cost

About 40 cents for an ergotamine-caffeine tablet, $2 for a suppository, 70 cents for a sublingual tablet. The inhaler is $30.

PART VI
Hormones and Drugs for Metabolic Disorders

71
Thyroid Hormone

The first hormone used in medicine (in 1891), thyroid remains a very satisfying drug because doctors enjoy curing disease, and curing thyroid deficiency is usually easy. Like most of the best drugs, doctors use thyroid hormone too often. If you're taking it the odds are better than 50/50 you don't need it. You'll read more about the overuse of thyroid later on.

Thyroid hormone is treatment of choice for:

1. *Thyroid hormone deficiency.* When thyroid hormone declines, most patients feel lethargic and have trouble concentrating, but they also become sick—meaning they lose their appetites. So, despite the popular belief, they don't gain much weight, although their skin appears puffy. Other common symptoms are heavy menstrual bleeding, constipation, dry skin and hair, and a cold feeling. Most adults notice a "goiter," an enlarged gland in the lower neck. If you suffer like this, have your thyroid tested. If the doctor tells you it's underactive and prescribes thyroid, you should feel much better in a few weeks.
2. *Goiter with normal thyroid function.* An inactive thyroid swells because the pituitary, the master gland at the base of the brain, pours out extra thyroid stimulating hormone (TSH) to force the gland to increase production.

Sometimes TSH fails, but when it succeeds in forcing adequate hormone production, you have a goiter without hypothyroidism. Some thyroids grow amazingly large, but even if they don't, doctors don't like to see a gland overstimulated for long periods. Some overstimulated glands eventually fail completely; others may turn malignant. Provided the goiter doesn't have an obvious cause (iodine deficiency is one, but very rare in the U.S.), giving thyroid inhibits pituitary secretion of TSH, so the gland shrinks.

How it works

Early in life thyroid hormone regulates growth and development. In its absence a tadpole won't turn into a frog, and a human grows up dwarfed, listless, and severely retarded (one in 6,000 newborns has a deficiency; hospitals should test for it routinely at birth). Once a human reaches adulthood, thyroid continues to regulate heat production, oxygen consumption, and the overall speed of bodily functions ("metabolism").

Two thyroid hormones exist, identical except for the number of iodine atoms. Thyroxine contains four (so we call it T4), and we consider it the most important. The gland also makes a small amount of triiodothyronine (T3), but to complicate matters the cells throughout your body produce a good deal more T3 as they break down thyroxine. T3 is actually four times stronger than T4 and works more quickly, but this is no advantage. T3 costs more, and using it as treatment makes blood thyroid tests difficult to interpret, so it's not popular.

How dispensed

Drug companies still buy cow, pig, and sheep thyroids from slaughterhouses, extract a powder with a high content of hormone, and convert this into pills called "thyroid." The exact amount varies from pill to pill but not by much when companies are careful. This was acceptable when synthetic hormone cost much more, but it's not today.

The best treatment is L-thyroxine in tablets of 25, 50, 75, 100, 112, 125, 150, 175, 200, and 300 micrograms, or µg (one-thousandth of a milligram), as well as an injectable containing 200 or 500 µg per 10 cc. 100 to 200 µg is the average daily adult dose.

Translating the label

Brands of L-thyroxine (also called levothyroxine) include Synthroid, Levothroid, and Levoxine.

No one gives a brand name to plain thyroid but the Armour meat company does a good business with its animal glands and would like you to ask for Armour thyroid. You can also buy an extract of pig thyroid called Proloid.

Side effects

None if used properly. Even used improperly it's safe *provided* you don't take more than your body needs. Your pituitary senses this extra hormone and releases less TSH, so your thyroid slows. If you take exactly as much as you need, your thyroid shuts down completely, and you survive on your pills. This works fine.

Too much causes side effects. One that seems positively desirable is weight loss, and people with too much thyroxine burn fat and get thinner. But victims of hyperthyroidism burn *everything*. They burn off muscle and get weak. They burn off bone and get osteoporosis. Their hearts beat too fast, their bowels move too much. They are sick.

Interactions

Food. Thyroxine is better absorbed on an empty stomach.

Alcohol. None known.

Drugs. Estrogens and oral contraceptives increase thyroxine requirements in someone with hypothyroidism. Cholestyramine (Questran) binds thyroid hormone in the digestive tract, so four hours should elapse between taking one and then the other.

Pregnancy. O.K.

Nursing. O.K.

Sex. If you're deficient, it will improve your sex life.

Allergies

None.

Wholesale cost

Cheap. About a penny for 100 µg, 1.4 cents for 200 µg. The equivalent of plain thyroid costs the same.

72
Insulin

Located behind your stomach, the pancreas mostly secretes digestive enzymes into the small intestine, but scattered throughout are clumps of cells that manufacture the hormone insulin, which diffuses directly into the blood. The action of insulin is discussed below. This section and the next summarize the two forms of diabetes, a disease of insulin deficiency. In the "adult" form, the pancreas still excretes some insulin, so the patient can lead a normal life on the proper diet and, if necessary, take drugs to stimulate the pancreas. You'll read about those drugs in the next section.

In the "juvenile" form (which sometimes affects adults) there is little or no insulin, and until well into the twentieth century victims died a slow, miserable death. In 1889, scientists showed that an animal without a pancreas developed diabetes, but over the next 30 years efforts to isolate the active agent failed. The obvious tactic—grinding up the pancreas and injecting extracts into diabetic animals—never worked.

After World War I, a Canadian researcher, F. G. Banting, considered the problem. Realizing the pancreas manufactures digestive juice, he suspected grinding it up released the juice, which then digested the antidiabetic hormone. Banting, assisted by a medical student, C. H. Best, devised a simple but Nobel-prize-winning method to avoid that difficulty: tying off the pancreatic ducts of a group of dogs and waiting a few months. Deprived of an exit for their juices, pancreatic cells died and withered away (insulin-producing cells don't require an exit; they secrete directly into the blood). The extract from these organs worked.

The first patient was 14-year-old Leonard Thompson. Despite an impossibly strict diet his blood sugar was astronomical, and he was drinking and urinating 3 to 5 quarts of liquid a day. Wasting away, he would have died in a few months. As soon as the injections began, his thirst and excessive urination stopped, he felt better, and he stopped losing weight. Along with Albert Alexander, who received the first penicillin, Thompson goes down in history, only with a better outcome. Fortunately, chemists quickly discovered ways to extract insulin from fresh organs, so slaughterhouses provided a cheap source.

Although Banting and Best were not well known, news of their discovery spread quickly around the world. You should doubt stories claiming that a humble scientist in Romania or Tijuana has developed a miracle cure for cancer or old age, but that everyone is ignoring it. The history of medical miracles is that they spread like wildfire—along with plenty of flops.

Insulin is treatment of choice for:

Insulin-dependent diabetes ("juvenile diabetes" is less accurate). No one really knows why diabetes develops, but the leading theory blames the immune system. Something, most likely a viral infection, triggers production of antibodies that destroy insulin-producing cells. Inheritance plays a role, but only to make a person susceptible. If one identical twin has juvenile diabetes, the risk of the other is only 50 percent, so there must be an "insult" that brings on diabetes. Giving immune suppressants has delayed onset in a few patients on the verge of diabetes, but these drugs are poisonous and experimental. The future will bring better preventatives, but for the moment insulin is the choice.

It's not the choice for most adult-onset diabetes because these people aren't deficient in insulin—often they have too much. See the next section.

How it works

Although insulin has many actions, an essential one enables cells to take in glucose (sugar) from the blood. Without glucose, cells have no energy source, and they starve. With no place to go, glucose piles up in the blood, then spills into the urine. The insulin-deficient body breaks down fat and muscle to produce other energy sources, so the patient loses weight. When insulin is very low and breakdown very high, the blood becomes more acid (a doctor can smell acetone on a diabetic's breath). When acid becomes dangerously high, patients go into "ketoacidosis" or diabetic coma.

Fortunately, brain cells don't require insulin to obtain nourishment; neither do your red blood cells, kidney, heart, or liver. All animals need insulin, and the closer an animal is related to us, the more its insulin resembles ours, but even fish insulin works in humans.

A regular insulin injection begins working in less than an hour, peaks at 4 to 6 hours, and fades out in half a day. Almost from the beginning, researchers began attaching proteins and metals to the insulin molecule to slow absorption. They developed an intermediate-acting version (called NPH or lente insulin) that works about half as fast, and long-acting (PZI or ultralente) that is a third as rapid.

How dispensed

Bottles usually containing 100 units per cc; 500 and 40 units per cc are also available. You don't need a prescription, but your doctor should tell you exactly what to buy.

Until well into the eighties, diabetics used a mixture of pig and cow insulin obtained from slaughterhouses. These worked fine despite the slight difference from human insulin. Occasionally a patient developed "resistance" to that insulin or suffered what seemed like an allergic reaction. If that happened, a doctor would try more expensive pure pork insulin.

By the mid-1980s genetic engineers succeeded in changing a common germ so it can't lead a normal germ's life but lives permanently in a large vat, manufacturing human insulin. Although not superior to earlier insulins, being identical to the natural hormone causes less resistance and fewer allergies. If someone is doing fine there's no reason to switch, but we usually start new diabetics on human insulin.

Twenty years ago, patients gave themselves a single injection before breakfast and were supposed to check their urine several times a day. "Spilling" a little sugar was considered wise because hypoglycemia was definitely dangerous, but we weren't as worried about an elevated sugar. Long-term diabetics have a much higher incidence of kidney failure, eye disease, and heart attacks than non diabetics, but no proof existed that strict control of blood sugar prevented these. Proof was hard to find because practically no one was strictly controlled. No technology existed to check blood sugar at home, so doctors didn't have a good reason to exhort patients to follow a rigid diet and inject themselves many times a day.

That has changed. Today, almost all doctors believe the disastrous complications of diabetes result from chronically high blood sugar. Good home glucose monitors are available. The standard therapy is two injections, before breakfast and dinner, with regular home blood-glucose monitoring. Urine tests are almost useless. I advise diabetics to consider a more rigorous program of three or four injections.

Translating the label

Some insulins are called Humulin, Novolin, Insulatard, Iletin, Mixtard, Velosulin, Lente, Semilente, Ultralente.

Side effects

None when insulin is secreted naturally into the bloodstream, which will be the case in the next century when we perfect today's crude implantable pumps. Today, even the purest human insulin can cause problems because it's injected where it doesn't belong—under your skin, saturating a small area of fat and connective tissue that isn't accustomed to it.

A common side effect is fat atrophy—a depression in the skin where the insulin has eliminated local fat. Occasionally, the opposite occurs—fat swells, forming a small, soft mass.

Hypoglycemia can occur for many reasons. Common ones include too much insulin, failure to eat enough, and unexpected exercise that decreases insulin requirements. Every diabetic should learn the symptoms and what to do. This is not a complete list, but headache, rapid heartbeat, hunger, sweating, trembling, and confusion are signs of low blood sugar.

Hyperglycemia occurs after too little insulin, too much eating, and from illness and emotional stress. Thirst and excessive urination usually appear first. Very high levels lead to nausea, vomiting, and abdominal pain followed by shock and coma.

Interactions

Food. No interactions, but a diabetic diet makes glucose control easier.

Alcohol. Alcohol tends to lower blood sugar in everyone, but it's all right in moderation.

Drugs. No real interaction, but beta blockers are risky because they may eliminate symptoms of hypoglycemia.

Pregnancy. A high blood sugar causes abnormally large babies and increased infant mortality and may cause birth defects. Any diabetic woman considering pregnancy should strictly control her glucose *before conceiving* by meticulous diet and multiple injections.

Nursing. O.K.

Sex. None, but diabetics frequently suffer impotence, and strict control may prevent it.

Allergies

Common, although the culprit is usually the chemicals attached to the insulin molecule or (less commonly these days) impurities. When itching, swelling, or redness occurs at the site of an injection, we call this a local allergy; patients should continue and expect the discomfort to diminish in a few weeks. Generalized reactions of hives, swelling, and shock were once rare; they are even rarer today with pure human insulin.

Wholesale cost

Cost is $15 for 10-cc bottle of 100 units per cc.

73
Micronase

Another accidental discovery, antidiabetic pills, saw the light in the forties when a French doctor noticed that several patients given sulfa for typhoid fever developed alarming low blood sugar. Other drugs occasionally do the same so this was not great news—until a French researcher made an important connection by feeding sulfa to diabetic animals lacking a pancreas and discovered it did not lower their sugar.

Soon after, the first oral antidiabetic (tolbutamide—Orinase) reached the market. Along with several relatives, it remains available and works fine, but a "second generation" appeared during the eighties, a modest but not dramatic improvement. Micronase is the most popular of the second generation. All antidiabetic drugs are distantly related to the sulfas (but current sulfas don't cause hypoglycemia).

Antidiabetic pills are good for :

Non-insulin-dependent diabetes. A different disorder from that in the last section, it's even more strongly hereditary. If your identical twin falls victim, your risk is 100 percent. Your chance is 30 percent if a parent or other sibling has it. Almost all non-insulin-dependent diabetics are adult, weigh too much, and secrete too much insulin. Despite the excess, they have less insulin than they need because their blood sugars remain elevated.

For reasons we don't understand, patients with non-insulin-dependent diabetes resist insulin. Their pancreases strain throughout adult life to maintain a normal blood sugar until advancing age and obesity produce so much resistance the organ can't keep up, and blood sugar begins to rise. Unlike juveniles who often reveal their diabetes suddenly with severe illness or coma, most adults learn the diagnosis after a routine blood test, but if they wait too long they'll get sick. Simply losing weight diminishes insulin resistance, often returning blood sugar to normal. Dieting, not an antidiabetic drug, is the treatment of choice.

How they work

They stimulate the pancreas to produce more insulin. Giving insulin is another way of getting more insulin. Pills offer no advantage except that patients prefer them to injections.

How dispensed

Glyburide comes as 1.25-, 2.5-, and 5-mg tablets, and the usual dose is 2.5 to 10 mg per day. A more finely ground version of glyburide (Glynase) sells as 1.5 and 3 mg tablets; 3 mg of micronized drug equals 5 mg of the regular form.

Another second generation antidiabetic, glipizide, comes as tablets of 5 and 10 mg. Most patients require 5 to 15 mg per day.

Translating the label

Micronase, Glynase, and DiaBeta are the brands of glyburide.
  Glucotrol is the brand name of glipizide.
  First-generation antidiabetics still popular:
  · Tolbutamide (Orinase)
  · Chlorpropamide (Diabinese)
  · Acetohexamide (Dymelor)
  · Tolazamide (Tolinase)

Side effects

As with insulin, taking too much leads to hypoglycemia. Otherwise, side effects tend to be less frequent than with the first generation, and this is their advantage. About 2 percent suffer some digestive upset: nausea, diarrhea, constipation, or bloating.

Interactions

Food. Taking on an empty stomach is not essential but makes for quicker absorption.
  Alcohol. As with insulin, antidiabetic drugs may increase alcohol's hypoglycemic action.
  Drugs. Although not forbidden, some drugs tend to augment hypoglycemic action, so doctors should be aware of them: aspirin and other NSAIDs, sulfas, and beta blockers.
  A larger number may do the opposite (or they may not): diuretics, cortisone, phenothiazines, thyroid, estrogens, birth control pills, and calcium blockers.
  Pregnancy. Although there is no evidence of birth defects, pregnant diabetics should go on insulin to control their sugar as strictly as possible.
  Nursing. Probably safe.

Allergies

Not terribly rare. Between 1 and 2 percent of patients suffer itching and hives. If not severe, we continue the medication, hoping it will go away. As with sulfas and another related family, thiazide diuretics, an occasional patient suffers sun sensitivity.

Wholesale cost

Glyburide: 30 cents for 2.5 mg, 45 cents for 5 mg.
Glipizide: 30 cents for 5 mg, 60 cents for 10 mg.

For long-term therapy these are not cheap (but you really should be dieting). The 1994 expiration of Micronase's patent means lower-price generics will be available by the time you read this. But if saving money is essential, a day's supply of first-generation Diabinese costs 2 cents.

74
RU486

Taken orally, RU486 causes an abortion. The only drug among my hundred not approved in the U.S., it's such a significant advance I must include it. The reasons for RU486's nonapproval have nothing to do with usefulness or safety.

It was another accidental discovery. In 1980, researchers at a French drug company, Roussel-Uclaf, were synthesizing drugs to block the action of cortisone. Routinely, they also tested each for its effect on other hormones. RU486 turned out to be a good cortisone antagonist but even better against progesterone, a hormone essential in early pregnancy.

News spread, and both the company and other scientists explored its use to interrupt pregnancies. It worked in animals, and in 1985, the first human tests succeeded—but only 80 percent of the time. Doctors suspected it succeeded the remaining 20 percent, but that the embryo and lining of the womb weren't expelled. This problem diminished when a Swedish researcher gave a prostaglandin (a natural substance that stimulates uterine contractions) a day or two after RU486. Now the success rate was 96 percent. Although not perfect, that's not bad for a new therapy.

In 1988 the French FDA approved its use in the first seven weeks of pregnancy, and several other countries followed. Roussel-Uclaf sells plenty of drugs in the U.S., and abortion opponents have made it clear they'll sponsor a boycott if it tries to obtain FDA approval for RU486. This had the desired effect, but equally effective was pressure on the FDA from the Reagan and Bush administrations. Under this pressure the FDA discouraged all research on RU486, including that unrelated to abortions. Remember that once the FDA approves a drug for one indication, a doctor can prescribe it for anything, so it would have been awkward if RU486 had turned out to be useful for, say, cancer treatment.

With the Democrats in office and pressure off the FDA, several RU486 studies are in the works, but years will probably pass before women have access to RU486 in the U.S. Abortion opponents must fight desperately against approval because once a woman can buy a pill and have an abortion their cause is lost.

Besides ending pregnancies, RU486 might be a good treatment for:

1. *Cancer.* Some breast cancers contain "estrogen receptors" on their cell surfaces. This means estrogens stimulate their growth, and drugs that antagonize estrogens do the opposite. Good antiestrogens exist, and doctors prescribe them to slow growth of breast cancers and to prevent recurrences after treatment.

   Breast (and a few other) cancers also contain progesterone receptors. So far we have no approved antiprogesterones. If research on RU486 pans out, this will be good news for cancer patients but, like antiestrogens, not a cure.

2. *Cortisone excess.* Several rare glandular diseases result in overproduction, so RU486 would help. But the body also produces extra cortisone in response to stress, and there are times when doctors want to counteract its action. As you'll learn in the prednisone section, cortisone slows

wound repair. Rubbing an anticortisone cream on a burn or other skin injury might speed healing.

How it works

Secreted by the ovary, especially after ovulation, progesterone increases the blood supply to the uterus and prepares the lining to accept a fertilized egg. If the egg isn't fertilized, progesterone secretion declines at the end of the month, the blood supply to the uterus drops, and its lining sheds, producing menstrual bleeding.

Soon after a fertilized egg implants in the uterus, it sends a chemical signal to the ovary to prevent this drop in progesterone, so secretion continues until the developing placenta takes over after two months. Blocking the action of progesterone makes it impossible for the uterine lining to nourish and support the pregnancy.

How dispensed

The dose is 600 mg in a single oral dose followed by a prostaglandin vaginal suppository or injection 36 to 48 hours later.

Translating the label

RU486 is also known as mifepristone. No brand name exists.

Side effects

Most women report some abdominal pain after receiving the prostaglandin. Eighty-six percent have their abortion within 24 hours of receiving prostaglandin, but persistent bleeding is common, lasting an average of nine days. Four percent require surgery to control bleeding or remove retained fragments.

Allergies

Allergies and interactions undoubtedly exist, but too few women have been tested in the English-speaking world to reveal them. This will change in a few years with the completion of studies in Great Britain.

Wholesale cost

Until FDA approval, any drug you receive as part of a legitimate clinical trial is free.

75
Prednisone

This is the most popular synthetic form of cortisone, a hormone produced by the adrenals, two small glands sitting on top of your kidneys. If you've heard of Adrenalin, that's a brand name of epinephrine, another adrenal hormone. You can live without epinephrine, but not without cortisone, hydrocortisone, and a few other "corticosteroids."

Insulin and thyroid deficiencies are common; not so with corticosteroid deficiencies. Most family doctors have never seen a case. Also unlike other hormones, huge doses of cortisone aren't poisonous (over the short term) and are spectacularly effective in relieving several medical problems including inflammation (which I discussed in the Motrin section).

Isolated and tried in the mid-forties, cortisone's actions seemed miraculous. Within days, inflamed, swollen arthritic joints became normal, and crippled victims found themselves without pain for the first time in years. Miserable psoriasis and eczema vanished. Asthmatics breathed easily. A cure for cancer could not have produced more excitement. The Nobel committee, which prefers to wait 10 or 20 years before honoring a discovery, rewarded cortisone on the spot. Even then the sad news was spreading that long-term cortisone was not a cure for arthritis, but positively dangerous. A short-term course also ends badly because joint pain flares worse than ever when the drug is stopped. The same flare usually occurs with asthma, psoriasis, and many other disorders.

But it's a near-miracle for some conditions. I use it most for poison ivy, and I suspect most family doctors do the same. A large dose for two weeks relieves the burning rash within a day, and by the end of the course the toxin has worn out.

You can take cortisone by mouth, but the natural hormone has an important role in salt retention, and large doses cause a great deal. Synthetic corticosteroids have eliminated that property.

Prednisone is good for:

1. *Inflammatory diseases.* Prednisone works better than aspirin or Motrin for run-of-the-mill arthritis, tendinitis, and bursitis, but we rarely use it for reasons mentioned above and elaborated on below. A corticosteroid injection into locally inflamed tissue is safe if not done too often.

   Prednisone works dramatically where inflammation is agonizing but short-lived. Poison ivy and other "contact" dermatitis rashes are a good example ("cortisone creams" work fine on small areas but aren't practical otherwise; they are discussed in a separate section). We use large doses to treat an exacerbation of severe asthma or ulcerative colitis, then hope to taper slowly to a small or zero maintenance dose without provoking a flare.

2. *Autoimmune diseases.* A family of diseases results when the body stupidly attacks its own tissues as if they were an intruders such as a germs. They have names like rheumatoid arthritis, lupus, polymyositis, pemphigus, arteritis, and autoimmune anemias and nephritis.

   As I wrote in the NSAID section, much overlap exists between inflammation and the immune response to a foreign invader. Unlike NSAIDs, prednisone suppresses both.

3. *Preventing organ transplant rejection.* Obviously the immune system doesn't welcome a large piece of foreign tissue.

4. *Allergies.* Like autoimmune disease, allergies are another instance of the body making an unnecessary fuss. We don't use prednisone for ordinary allergies, but if pollen is particularly heavy, a short course makes life tolerable for a hay fever victim if nothing else works. We don't like to prescribe it for other chronic allergic conditions such as asthma, eczema, and allergic conjunctivitis, but it's occasionally necessary. Corticosteroid inhalers have proven useful and safer in asthma and nasal allergies.

5. *Certain cancers.* Because they suppress and possibly destroy lympho-
cytes, corticosteroids form part of the chemotherapy of lymphocytic
leukemias and lymphomas.
6. *Adrenal insufficiency.* In this case doctors want the sodium-retaining
properties of the natural hormone, so prednisone and other synthetics
aren't the best choice. We prefer hydrocortisone.

How dispensed

Tablets of 1, 2.5, 5, 10, 20, and 50 mg and a liquid containing 5 mg per teaspoon. Adult adrenals produce the equivalent of 5 mg a day, but suppressing a violent inflammation requires from 50 to well over 100 mg. I use 60
mg a day for two weeks on poison ivy.

Translating the label

Deltasone, Prednicen-M, and Sterapred are brands of prednisone.
  Other common oral corticosteroids:
  · Hydrocortisone (Hydrocortone)
  · Prednisolone (Prelone, Pediapred)
  · Methylprednisolone (Medrol)
  · Triamcinolone (Aristocort, Kenalog)

How it works

Your natural corticosteroids are the preeminent hormones governing home-
ostasis: i.e., the ability of your body to function in response to a changing
environment. In their absence, you can stay alive only by eating every few
hours, consuming large amounts of salt, remaining in a constant warm temperature, and staying healthy.

  For example, corticosteroids permit your body to store glucose for future use and to manufacture it when needed. This is why blood sugar remains normal even if you stop eating for a few days. Without this action,
your blood sugar would plummet. Too much cortisone has the opposite action—your blood sugar would rise and you would get fat.

  Corticosteroids also regulate use of fats, proteins, salts, and blood elements in ways you don't have to know. In huge doses, prednisone suppresses protein synthesis and thus cell division in many tissues. This largely explains why it's useful; immunity, allergy, and inflammation all require quick action: rapid protein production and fast division of the immune cells. This also explains why it's dangerous.

Side effects

A week or two of high-dose prednisone is safe, but as more weeks pass we begin to worry. Genuine side effects (upset stomachs, rashes) are rare. The only exceptions are mood changes. Many patients on long-term, high doses become euphoric, a smaller number anxious and depressed and a few frankly psychotic. Other toxic reactions are a direct action of the drug.

1. Blood sugar rises, resulting in temporary or permanent diabetes (if permanent, patient was probably already at risk).
2. Increasing susceptibility to infections as well as masking one already present. High-dose corticosteroids can suppress the fever, pain, and general illness that accompany an infection.
3. Weakness because of muscle breakdown.
4. Osteoporosis and fractures because of increased bone breakdown (and decreased calcium absorption—another action of the drug).
5. Acne, easy bruising, and fragile skin.
6. Cataracts and glaucoma.
7. Salt retention, high blood pressure, and edema—but these are rare with prednisone and other synthetics.
8. Fat deposition, especially in the face and central body. After a few months most patients show a "moon face" and "buffalo hump" plus a fat central body with thin limbs.

This is not a complete list, but you're not likely to receive high-dose long-term prednisone unless you really need it.

Interactions

Food. None.
Alcohol. None.
Drugs. Since it increases blood sugar, prednisone worsens control of dia-

betes. Synthetic corticosteroids have a slight tendency to lower serum potassium, so a doctor should be cautious when combining them with a diuretic.

Pregnancy. Risky because large doses suppress developing adrenal, so the newborn may have a temporary deficiency. There's no strong evidence it causes birth defects.

Nursing. Probably safe.

Sex. No reported problems.

Allergies

Since it suppresses allergies, you'd expect these to be almost unknown.

Wholesale cost

About 1.5 cents for 5-mg tablet, 3.5 cents for 10-mg, 6 cents for 20-mg.

76
Estrogens

Only in 1900 did scientists prove that the ovary controls female sexual development. They removed both glands from animals, saw the sexual organs wither, then reversed these changes by putting the ovaries back. Another 25 years passed before anything useful came from this study because scientists couldn't isolate whatever it was the ovary produced. We call it estrogen.

Then they discovered a huge source in the urine of pregnant women. The first application was testing for pregnancy—a messy, expensive procedure that would horrify any woman today but was considered wonderfully high-tech at the time. A technician injected a woman's urine into a small animal, waited a few days, then killed it to examine the sexual organs.

Urine from a nonpregnant woman contains little estrogen, but a pregnant woman's urine made the animal's gonads enlarge.

Other early uses proved disastrous, especially giving estrogens to prevent miscarriages. At the time it seemed sensible: Since a normal pregnancy requires large amounts of estrogen, a failing pregnancy might require more. Common sense is a poor way to discover the truth, but doctors and patients find it comfortable, and 20 years passed before studies convinced most of us that estrogens didn't help, so we stopped using it. Later when a few children of these mothers turned up with genital abnormalities and vaginal cancer, we realized how much harm we had done.

Estrogens are treatment of choice for:

1. *Estrogen deficit.* You can say this about any hormone, so these are no exception. Congenital defects in estrogen production are rare; so is spontaneous "ovarian failure," but surgical removal of the ovaries is not so rare. Estrogens work perfectly for all. Many women believe a hysterectomy affects their hormone level, but it doesn't.

2. *Symptoms of menopause.* Mostly this means hot flashes that are not caused by lack of estrogen, but by a drop. Women born without estrogen never have hot flashes; when the level drops suddenly after surgical removal of the ovaries, symptoms are rapid and severe. Estrogen decline also shrinks the sexual organs, but this causes symptoms only when thinning of the vaginal wall makes it dry, fragile, and susceptible to minor infections.

   I doubt that a drop of estrogens causes fatigue, anxiety, depression, weakness, or general aches and pains, but I have no objection to a trial of therapy. When I see the patient a month or two later and ask "Did it work?" I occasionally receive an enthusiastic reply. More often I hear "I think so." That's a placebo response because estrogens work brilliantly against genuine menopausal symptoms.

3. *Preventing osteoporosis.* Both sexes suffer osteoporosis (thinning and weakening of bone) beginning about age 35. Women suffer more, partly because their bones are smaller to begin with and they exercise less than men, but mostly because the drop in estrogens around menopause causes an acceleration in bone loss. One in three women suffers a verte-

bral fracture after age 65 and one in three breaks a hip if she lives long enough. These are devastating injuries: one third are dead within a year of a hip fracture and many of the rest remain permanently disabled.

A popular belief exists that extra calcium slows this loss, but it doesn't. Only estrogen succeeds. Women on treatment suffer less than half as many fractures, and this protection remains as long as they continue. Once they stop, bone loss resumes.

Estrogens are good for:

1. *Preventing heart attacks.* Women on estrogens have less than half as many according to several large studies. Combined with their protection against osteoporosis, this swamps the risk of certain cancers and makes estrogens positively beneficial for almost every menopausal woman. That sounds too good to be true, so universal estrogen use after menopause is not generally accepted. But we're thinking about it.
2. *Acne; excessive hair.* Only a fair treatment, it takes a high dose and a long time to see a result, but it's worth a try.
3. *Temporary relief in advanced breast and prostate cancer.* High doses often shrink these malignancies; routinely prescribed for breast cancer, estrogen for prostate cancer has declined in recent years with the development of drugs causing fewer side effects.

Unreliable for birth control by themselves, estrogens are excellent combined with a progestin. Oral contraceptives are discussed later.

How it works

Although the ovary makes most estrogens (there are three), other tissues such as adrenal, liver, fat, and muscle also synthesize them by acting on male hormones that resemble female hormones chemically and are produced by both sexes. These other tissues make up the sources of estrogen in men and also in women after menopause—not an insignificant amount.

Estrogens are largely responsible for puberty in girls. They cause growth and development of the vagina, uterus, and breasts as well as reshaping of the skeleton and body fat to produce an adult woman. Pubic and armpit hair require male hormone, although only a small amount. Male hormone also stimulates development of the sebaceous glands of the face that leads to acne.

In almost all adult animals, a cyclic increase in estrogens produces periods of "estrus" in which the female is intensely interested in sex. It may occur monthly or only once every few years; at other times the female rejects any male advance. The human female's estrogen cycle doesn't seem to influence her sexual desire. Using the scientific term, she is always "receptive."

During the first half of the menstrual cycle estrogen thickens the lining of the uterus to prepare it to receive a fertilized egg. Estrogen declines during the last half of the cycle. The thickened uterine lining shrinks and sheds, producing bleeding provided the estrogen rises high enough and drops far enough.

Women have lower cholesterol than men until menopause when the difference diminishes. This is probably an action of estrogen and is responsible for her lower risk of heart disease.

How dispensed

Premarin, the most popular, comes as tablets of 0.3, 0.625, 0.9, 1.25, and 2.5 mg as well as a vaginal cream and injectable. A good starting dose for replacement therapy is .625 mg daily.

The cream relieves postmenopausal vaginal thinning, but pills do just as well. Some women receive a monthly estrogen injection. Although no advantage to the patient, the doctor benefits because he can charge for an injection. If he writes a prescription for tablets, the pharmacist gets your money.

Translating the label

Premarin is the only brand of "conjugated estrogens," which, boasts Wyeth-Ayerst, comes exclusively from natural sources (i.e., horse urine).

Other popular estrogens:
- Esterified estrogens (Estratab, Menrium), another natural estrogen
- Estrone (Ogen), also natural
- Ethinyl estradiol (Estinyl) a synthetic also used in birth control pills
- Quinestrol (Estrovis), a close relative of the above

- Estradiol (Estrace, Emcyt), another synthetic that also comes as a skin patch
- Chlorotrianisene (TACE), another synthetic.

Side effects

In "physiological" doses as replacement, side effects are the normal actions of an estrogen: breast swelling, mild water retention, occasional vaginal bleeding. High "pharmacological" doses produce the same side effects I discuss under birth control pills.

Some of the more alarming actions of birth control pills (blood clots, heart attacks, strokes) don't occur with replacement doses, but neither does the protection against ovarian and uterine cancer. In fact, women on estrogen replacement have a much higher incidence of uterine cancer. Although almost always curable, it's still not desirable, and most experts believe giving progesterone for a week at the end of each monthly cycle or even continually eliminates this risk. Women on estrogens also have double the risk of gallstones.

Interactions

Food. None.
Alcohol. None.
Drugs. None significant.
Pregnancy. Forbidden.
Nursing. Probably O.K. in replacement doses, larger doses are less safe.
Sex. Reports of both increasing and decreasing libido. Given to men, it eliminates the sex drive.

Allergies

Rare.

Wholesale Cost

Premarin (conjugated estrogens): 35 cents for .625 mg. Thirty dollars for vaginal cream. A twice-a-week estradiol skin patch costs about $2.

77
Progesterone

At the turn of the century, scientists not only discovered the ovary controls female development, they found pregnancy depended on a small area of the ovary called the corpus luteum. When the ovary ejects an egg halfway though the menstrual cycle, a patch of yellow tissue remains behind (corpus luteum means "yellow body"). When researchers destroyed the corpus luteum of a pregnant rabbit, it miscarried. During the late 1920s, other scientists prevented the miscarriage by injecting an extract from the corpus, so obviously a hormone was involved. This was progesterone.

It was tedious work to process corpus luteums of ovaries collected from slaughterhouses, so progesterone remained scarce and expensive until the 1950s when cheap synthetics appeared and launched the golden age of birth control. You'll read about The Pill itself in the next section.

Progesterone and its synthetic derivatives ("progestins") are good for:

1. *Endometriosis.* This is a common and undertreated condition in which the lining of the uterus seems to migrate to other parts of the body, usually nearby in the low abdomen. Just as the uterine lining grows, sheds, then grows again with each menstrual cycle, so do these stray implants. Since there's no place for the shed tissue to go, it may accumulate in a mass that a doctor can feel during an exam. Even worse, cyclic bleeding inside the pelvis is painful.

For reasons we don't understand, endometriosis is uncommon in women who have been pregnant and symptoms usually improve after pregnancy, but any woman who hasn't been pregnant and who suffers severe or worsening "menstrual cramps" and pain during sex should be evaluated. In severe cases, the gynecologist must surgically remove the implants, but suppressing the menstrual cycle relieves milder cases. Giving a large dose of progestin daily does this.

2. *Dysfunctional menstrual bleeding (DUB).* DUB is heavy bleeding *not*

caused by disease of the uterus such as cancer or fibroids. Mostly it results from a hormonal abnormality—either too much estrogen (so the uterine lining grows too thick and becomes fragile) or too little progesterone (remember that a drop at the end of the cycle makes the lining shed cleanly). DUB occurs most often in teenagers before their cycle becomes organized or around menopause when it nears the end. Giving a progestin for ten days near the end of each cycle creates a normal period a few days afterward.

3. *Avoiding unwanted pregnancy.* Several "mini-pills" contain progestin alone with no estrogen. Taken every day with no monthly interruption, they are a good contraceptive although slightly less good than combination pills—97 percent effective as opposed to almost 100 percent. Because daily progestin produces a fair amount of unpredictable spotting, they have never caught on.

An injection of long-acting progesterone (Depo-Provera) provides contraception for three months. Doctors in many European countries have used it since the 1970s with no serious problems, and some American doctors offered it during the early 1970s despite lack of FDA approval (remember—doctors can use an available drug in any way they think best). Then a few studies found tumors in beagles and the FDA issued a warning that doctors could not ignore. Almost all experts doubted that Depo-Provera caused cancer in humans, but in America's malpractice climate no doctor would dare use it in the face of that warning. After considering the matter for 20 years, the FDA changed its mind in 1992, so now doctors have resumed prescribing it.

In December 1990, the FDA approved an implant (Norplant) that releases progestins into the blood for five years. Inserted under the skin of the upper arm, it can be removed at any time. Norplant works as well as birth control pills (and better than the mini-pill), but causes more irregular bleeding—in about 15 percent of users.

Finally, one of the few IUDs still available in the U.S., the Progestasert, slowly releases progesterone while in place. This has a local action on the uterus; practically none reaches the bloodstream. It's much superior to the old coils and loops.

How it works

Just before ovulation, the corpus luteum surrounding one egg sharply increases progesterone production. This acts first to hold back maturation of other eggs (hundreds are waiting), then to stimulate small arteries and glands in the uterus to make the lining hospitable to a fertilized egg. Without fertilization, the corpus luteum withers after ten days, and progesterone production drops. This constricts the arteries supplying the uterine lining, cutting off the blood supply and causing it to slough.

A fertilized egg takes seven days to reach the uterus and settle in. Almost immediately it secretes another hormone, human chorionic gonadotrophin (HCG), which prevents the corpus luteum from withering. Sensitive pregnancy tests detect HCG almost as soon as it appears. Progesterone from the corpus luteum is essential for maintaining the pregnancy for two months until the developing placenta begins producing its own.

How dispensed

Medroxyprogesterone, the most popular oral progestin used for bleeding and other gynecological disorders, comes as 2.5-, 5-, and 10-mg tablets. Depo-Provera is a long-acting injectable form.

Five to 10 mg per day for the last part of the cycle is reasonable for DUB. Endometriosis requires 40 to 60 mg per day; some doctors give 150 mg of Depo-Provera every one to three months.

Translating the label

Medroxyprogesterone can be Provera, Amen, or Cycrin.
Other oral progestins:
- Norethindrone acetate (Norlutate, Aygestin)
- Norethindrome (Norlutin)
- Megestrol acetate (Megace)
- Progestin mini-pills contain either norethindrone (Micronor, Nor-Q.D.) or norgestrel (Ovrette)

Side effects

Low doses for contraception produce almost no side effects except intermittent bleeding that occurs fairly often. Larger amounts occasionally cause nausea, weight gain, edema, or depression.

Interactions

Food. None.
Alcohol. None.
Drugs. None significant.
Pregnancy. Forbidden. Some evidence exists that it causes birth defects.
Nursing. Probably O.K.
Sex. Estrogens affect the libido, but it's doubtful that progesterone does.

Allergies

Hives and other itchy rashes occur but rarely.

Wholesale cost

Eleven cents for 10 mg of medroxyprogesterone.
150 mg of Depo-Provera costs about $36.
One Norplant costs about $76.
One month of mini-pills costs about $22.

78
Birth Control Pills

As soon as sex hormones appeared, scientists knew they could suppress fertility. Estrogens and androgens do this in both sexes, but only after unpleasant and unsafe doses. The older progestins were not much better, but by the 1950s researchers had combined progestins and estrogens in huge doses that today's women would not tolerate and today's FDA would not approve, but which seemed like a scientific marvel at the time. The first "pill" was approved in 1960 and quickly swept the country.

As with most new drugs, side effects that slipped by after a few thousands treatments came to our attention when the number rose to several million. A major scandal broke around 1970 when studies confirmed that women on the pill suffered a higher incidence of blood clots in veins that sometimes led to clots in the lungs (pulmonary emboli) and brain (strokes) as well as a higher incidence of heart attacks. Congressional hearings denounced doctors for foisting a dangerous drug on the public. A torrent of lawsuits descended on pharmaceutical companies. Newscasts and magazine stories told of women dying in the prime of life. Sales dropped sharply.

As years passed, sales recovered and continue to rise. Although today's pills contain one quarter or less hormone than the original, they remain under a cloud. Polled, most women on the pill believe it's bad for their health and increases the risk of cancer. The truth may be the opposite.

Combination oral contraceptives are good for:

1. *Preventing pregnancy.*
2. *Suppressing mild endometriosis.*
3. *As a morning-after pill.* Taken within 48 hours of unprotected intercourse, a high-estrogen pill twice a day for three days usually keeps a fertilized egg from implanting, but there are no guarantees.

How they work

Since estrogens and progesterone prepare the lining of the uterus to accept a fertilized egg, too much might interfere. While that happens, the major action of combination pills is to suppress ovulation—the release of an egg from the ovary. The pituitary, not the ovary, governs ovulation, and a precise cycle of two pituitary hormones must occur to cause a dormant egg to mature, move to the surface, and leave the ovary. The smooth rise and fall of estrogen and progesterone feeds back on the pituitary to control its secretion; oral contraceptives scramble this rhythm.

How dispensed

The original Enovid of 1960 contained a whopping 150 mg of estrogen. By the mid 1960s this had dropped to 80 to 100 mg. Today's contain 20 to 50 mg; 35-mg brands are the most popular. Higher doses don't protect better; lower doses may protect less. During most of this time, women took the same pill daily for three weeks, none for a week, then resumed. If the packet contained a pill for the last week, it was either inert or included something harmless such as a vitamin or iron. The 1980s saw the introduction of pills in which estrogen remained constant throughout the cycle but progestin increased either once or twice. The pharmaceutical companies explained that this resembled more closely the natural hormone cycle. Like so much common sense, it seems reasonable at first but silly on further thought. Birth control pills are supposed to be unnatural. That's why they work. These newer pills are not superior, but they work fine.

Translating the label

Dozens of brands plus many generics exist.

Oral contraceptives are drugs, so a responsible user knows the name. As a hotel doctor, I'm regularly called by frantic women, usually on a honeymoon, who have lost their packet and explain: "They're pink . . . and come in a round box." Switching pills is probably all right but not the best course.

Side effects

Oral contraceptives contain more hormone than we prescribe after menopause so estrogen-associated side effects occur more often: breast discomfort, weight gain, nausea. We suspect the progestin causes two other common complaints, depression and fatigue. Doctors routinely tell women that minor symptoms diminish after a few months. If not we may switch brands because current pills contain several different estrogens and half a dozen progestins, so a new combination may be tolerable.

Spotting and irregular bleeding are not signs the pill isn't working, and changing to one with more estrogen eliminates them, but we don't like to do this unless that patient insists. Spotting also tends to diminish after a few months.

Older pills tended to raise blood pressure, blood sugar, and cholesterol, as well as increase the risk of gallstones. Today's low-dose combinations do that only slightly or not at all.

The massive studies that uncovered blood clots, strokes, and so forth, took place during the 1960s and 1970s when pills contained more estrogen. These risks probably remain, but they are concentrated in women over 35 who smoke. Risks are slight in others—so slight they may be more than canceled by the *good* side effects.

Oral contraceptives prevent ovarian and uterine cancer. Users have about 40 percent less ovarian cancer than nonusers and 50 percent less uterine cancer. Although hardly desirable, cancer of the uterus is almost always curable, so one can't argue that using the pill saves many lives. Ovarian cancer is a different matter. It's hard to diagnose and usually fatal—causing half of all deaths from gynecological cancer. Reducing your risk by 40 percent is not a trivial benefit.

Pill users also suffer fewer ectopic pregnancies, ovarian and breast cysts, tubal infections, toxic shock, menstrual bleeding, anemia, ulcers, and menstrual cramps. No one has weighed all the good and bad effects, but it's possible the average woman on birth control pills enjoys better health and a longer life.

Interactions

Food. None.

Alcohol. None.

Drugs. As mentioned in the antibiotic section, I keep reading warnings that antibiotics reduce the action of oral contraceptives and increase the risk of pregnancy. I read the same about drugs for epilepsy, tranquilizers, and NSAIDs (aspirin, Motrin, Advil, etc.). If that happens it must be rare, and I don't know of a doctor who warns women on the pill before prescribing these. The PDR gives its usual indecisive warnings. It's possible this is all nonsense, but no one knows for sure.

Pregnancy. Forbidden.

Nursing. Low-dose pills are probably O.K.

Sex. Unpredictable—they increase, decrease, or have no effect on libido.

Allergies

Rare. Not rare is a brownish rash over the cheeks and forehead. Called chloasma, it also occurs during pregnancy so estrogens provoke it, but sunlight is required. Although not an allergy, no one knows much about it.

Wholesale cost

Cost is $7.50 for a month's supply.

79
Testosterone

The dawn of endocrinology occurred before the dawn of history when primitive man observed that castration makes a eunuch. Formal research began in the nineteenth century and, as anyone could predict, scientists took up male hormones first. While male prejudice played a role, one can't ignore the universal belief that men grew old because their testicular function declined. Reputable nineteenth-century scientists gave themselves extracts of animal testicles and reported wonderfully increased vigor; these remained popular into the 1930s, and the belief hasn't entirely died out in many segments of the population and among a few doctors. In fact, testicular function decreases slightly after middle age but not very much. The brutal truth is that having lots of male hormone shortens life. Eunuchs and women live longer.

Early testicular extracts contained no useful hormone because the glands secrete only tiny amounts, and processing the testes destroyed even those. Only in the 1930s did scientists isolate the first male hormone—a barely visible pinch extracted by a heroic effort from 15,000 quarts of male urine. Soon after, we isolated testosterone, the principal human androgen, and chemists invented others that were effective orally. By that time, fortunately, the rage for taking male hormones had diminished. Although they have important uses, giving male hormones to males is more dangerous than giving female hormone to females.

Testosterone is treatment of choice for:

Testosterone deficiency. A few boys are born without the ability to make testosterone, and that doesn't become apparent until puberty. Parents of normal boys begin to worry when no signs of change appear by junior high. Family doctors feel the pressure, and it's hard to convince parents that a small minority of normal boys don't begin puberty until age 15 or later. I suspect that most testosterone given to teenagers treats the parents, not the patient. No boy should receive male hormones without a thorough endocrinological evaluation to make sure he doesn't have brain or pituitary disease—which probably causes more absent puberty than testicular failure.

Testosterone is good for:

1. *Impotence.* At medical school in the 1960s we learned that psychological stress caused 90 percent of impotence with medical problems making up the rest. Dutifully, we tested men for diabetes and a few neurological

diseases, and if nothing turned up, we offered reassurance and sent them off for psychotherapy that didn't work.

Research gradually turned up more medical causes of impotence, and by the 1990s experts considered stress responsible for well under half of cases. Nowadays an affected man deserves a thorough evaluation that includes studies of testicular and pituitary hormones.

2. *Building muscle.* The medical profession gave itself a black eye around 1980 when we noticed athletes taking extra male hormone to build muscle strength and bulk. Not only was that dangerous, experts proclaimed, *it didn't work.* Training produced the larger muscles, the weight gain was water retention, the increased strength placebo effect, they explained. I worked at a college student health service at the time and remember the skeptical expressions of the gigantic football players who came in a vain attempt to get the drugs legally and were forced to listen to my lecture.

   We were wrong. Huge doses of male hormone (the medical term is "anabolic steroid") plus training grow muscles better than training without hormones. Lied to about the good effects of steroids, athletes were skeptical of warnings about their dangers, but these are true. Anabolic steroids in the necessary amounts are far more dangerous than the earliest birth control pills. Users are guaranteed a shorter life.

   As for the morality of using drugs to enhance performance, that's cheating, and users deserve punishment, but we shouldn't moan too much about the decline in morality. Athletes have used performance-enhancing drugs for thousands of years; the only difference is that we have better ones today.

3. *Some advanced breast cancer.* High doses slow the growth.

4. *Endometriosis.* Progestins and birth control pills have fewer side effects, and other drugs are more effective.

5. *Some severe anemias.* High-dose androgens stimulate red blood cell production in patients with severe blood disease or kidney failure that suppress the bone marrow (the source of red cells). This treatment is fading fast now that genetic engineering is pouring out formerly very rare hormones that directly simulate red cell production.

How it works

Males have a high testosterone level at three stages in their lives. The first surge occurs when the developing embryo is about two months old, declining before birth. This stage converts the primitive "urogenital tract" into male genitals. The female embryo doesn't require extra estrogen to develop, so a male that fails to produce testosterone is born looking like a girl.

The second rise occurs after birth and drops again several months later. No one knows why, but the leading theory explains that it encourages the developing brain along male lines.

Finally, a permanent increase occurs at puberty to produce the changes you're familiar with. Besides maturing the genitals, this testosterone speeds bone growth and height, greatly increases muscle mass (especially around the shoulders), and eliminates the layer of fat under the skin, which is why male skin is rougher and shows prominent veins. Skin becomes thicker, hairier, and more oily, the larynx enlarges, and (if baldness runs in the family) hair begins to fall out. Despite the popular belief that it's a sign of aging, baldness is a sign of sexual maturity because it begins at the end of puberty.

As every athlete knows, male hormones are strongly anabolic—meaning they build up tissue. The opposite is catabolic. Cortisone is strongly catabolic because it breaks down tissue. Estrogens are somewhat anabolic but less so than androgens.

Don't assume anabolic means "good" and catabolic "bad." In a healthy adult both are in balance; when they aren't we call that "disease." Increasing muscle tissue is one anabolic action of testosterone, but it builds up other tissues that are less desirable, as you'll learn later.

How dispensed

Plain testosterone isn't well absorbed orally, but slightly modifying the molecule to methyltestosterone changes that. It comes in tablets of 10 and 25 mg as well as sublingual tablets of 10 mg.

The dose to bring on puberty or treat impotence is 10 to 40 mg per day of the tablet or half that amount of the sublingual. Breast cancer and anemia may require five times more.

A popular injectable form is testosterone in an oil base. The oil delays absorption, so a 100-mg injection every two weeks may work.

Translating the label

Methyltestosterone might be called Android, Metandren, Testred, and Virilon. Brands of testosterone in oil include Depo-testosterone and Virilon-IM.
Other oral androgens:
- Fluoxymesterone (Halotestin)
- Oxymetholone (Anadrol)

Side effects

Replacement doses are benign. Larger amounts produce effects males would expect such as more acne and faster hair loss, but a few surprises turn up. Excess male hormone is actually feminizing: testes shrink, sperm production drops, sometimes breasts enlarge. This occurs because the pituitary gland senses the presence of too much androgen, so it reduces secretion of its own sex hormones. Pituitary hormones (not testosterone) govern male fertility and testicle size. Most likely, breasts grow because the body normally converts some androgen into estrogen, so someone with too much male hormone also has too much estrogen.

The anabolic action encourages tissue activity that is definitely not desirable. Cholesterol production rises sharply, so premature hardening of the arteries, heart attacks, and strokes are not rare in young male anabolic steroid users. Every prostate swells as the years pass; extra male hormone speeds that up, and probably encourages prostate cancer as well as liver cancer. Other liver abnormalities and jaundice are fairly common side effects.

Interactions

Food. None.
Alcohol. None.
Drugs. Androgens increase insulin requirements. Like so many drugs, they may increase anticoagulant action (see Warfarin, 38.), but androgens are particularly risky.

Pregnancy. Forbidden. As you might expect, male hormones masculinize a female embryo.

Nursing. Probably not a good idea in large doses.

Sex. Male hormones increase sexual desire in women. It often does the same in men, but occasionally the opposite occurs. Androgens restore male potency if androgen deficit is the cause, but not otherwise.

Allergies

Very rare. Although common, acne is not an allergy.

Wholesale cost

Methyltestosterone: 5 cents for 10-mg tablet, 10 cents for 25-mg.
Testosterone in oil costs about $9 for 10-cc vial containing 100 mg per cc.

80
Proscar

Approved in 1992, finasteride (Proscar) is the newest drug in this book. Useful in itself, it's also a significant advance, the first drug to block action of a male hormone without miserable side effects. Besides its approved use, it offers the potential to relieve several tiresome disorders that affect women as well as men.

Proscar is treatment of choice for:

Prostatic hypertrophy. This is discussed in the section on antihypertensive Hytrin (36.). Because prostatic tissue contains alpha receptors, alpha blockers like Hytrin produce a modest shrinkage, but Proscar produces more.

Proscar is good for:

Nothing else at the moment, but too little time has passed for me to hear rumors of useful non-FDA-approved uses. Theoretically, blocking the action of male hormone should improve acne, male-pattern baldness, and excessive hairiness in women. Research will confirm or refute this, but well before studies appear doctors will prescribe it on their own, so the grapevine will generate hints. Scientists are also exploring Proscar's role in treating prostate cancer.

How it works

Finasteride blocks conversion of testosterone to dihydrotestosterone (DHT). Produced mostly in the testes, testosterone acts as the basic male hormone in humans, but once it reaches target tissues (genitals, prostate, skin), an enzyme converts it to DHT, a more powerful hormone that does most of the work.

Treatment with finasteride lowers tissue dihydrotestosterone levels by 85 percent. The prostate begins shrinking within a few weeks, reaching a maximum reduction of 28 percent after three months. Up to 90 percent of men urinate more easily provided they continue taking the drug. DHT levels return to normal two weeks after discontinuing.

How dispensed

A 5-mg tablet. Dose is 5 mg per day.

Translating the label

Proscar is the only form of finasteride.

Side effects

Surprisingly few. For decades doctors could shrink the prostate with estrogens or with drugs that suppressed the pituitary, the master gland at the base of the brain that secretes half a dozen important hormones. We could do this, but we tried not to. Used in men, estrogens eliminate sexual drive and increase the risk of heart attacks. Pituitary suppressors also suppress sexual function, and they're spectacularly expensive.

Interactions

Food. None.
Alcohol. None.
Drugs. Many studies show no important problems.
Pregnancy. Forbidden; boy fetuses need male hormone.
Nursing. No studies at this time.
Sex. Only an occasional report of diminished sexual drive, impotence, and lower ejaculate volume.

Allergies

So far nothing significant.

Wholesale cost

About $1.80 for 5-mg tablet.

81
Allopurinol (Zyloprim)

In the Indocin-Motrin section (61. and 62.) you learned that excruciating attacks of gout occur when uric acid crystals appear in joints. Although NSAIDs relieve attacks, anyone suffering several of them becomes anxious never to repeat the experience. Victims have an elevated blood uric acid; lowering it prevents attacks. Until the 1950s, doctors prescribed diets, forbidding alcohol and organ meats. This worked even less well than other dietary treatments because almost all uric acid is manufactured in the body, not consumed in food. During the 1950s, researchers developed two drugs that increase urinary excretion of uric acid: probenecid (Benemid) and sulfinpyrazone (Anturane). Still available, they work fine provided the patient has normal kidney function and no uric acid kidney stones that are not rare in gout.

Ten years later, allopurinol appeared and immediately become more popular, partly because it was newer and worked in a clever way, but also because it prevents gouty attacks as well as other complications of gout in the kidney and other organs.

Zyloprim is treatment of choice for:

Preventing hyperuricemia (high blood uric acid) from cancer treatment. As you'll learn below, uric acid is a normal product of tissue breakdown. When chemotherapy or radiotherapy kills cancer tissue, a torrent of uric acid pours into the blood. This can damage the kidneys, so doctors routinely give Zyloprim before beginning.

Zyloprim is good for:

Preventing gouty attacks. It's no good for treatment. In fact, it often provokes attacks during the first weeks of therapy. Then attacks should disappear forever as long as uric acid is kept low—which means treatment never stops.

Zyloprim is NOT appropriate for:

Hyperuricemia (high blood uric acid). While gout victims almost always have hyperuricemia, the reverse isn't true. Almost everyone with a high uric acid doesn't have gout and never will have it. Furthermore, a high level is common, especially in men of middle age or older where the incidence nears 10 percent. One percent or fewer of these men develop gout each year, and all authorities disapprove of giving allopurinol to prevent this. Yet, I constantly see patients on the drug because "my uric acid was high."

They are not taking it for their own benefit, but to treat the doctor. An abnormal lab test makes many doctors uneasy, and they feel an irresistible urge to do something about it. Zyloprim corrects an abnormal uric acid in a week or two. When that happens, the patient doesn't notice any change, but the doctor feels better.

How it works

Your body builds up and breaks down tissues constantly. Uric acid is one of many waste products. Although it normally passes out harmlessly in the urine, uric acid has a tiresome property: it doesn't dissolve well in body fluids. If the level rises modestly, the fluids can't hold it, so crystals settle out. In the joint, this is a painful gouty attack. In the kidney they cause stones, and in the worst cases (rare today because of allopurinol) they pile up as chalky deposits under the skin. Allopurinol solves this problem in an ingenious way that partly explains why we like it. As the body breaks down complex molecules, allopurinol simply blocks the last step that converts two substances called hypoxanthine and xanthine into uric acid. Unlike uric acid, those dissolve easily even at high concentrations.

How dispensed

Tablets of 100 and 300 mg; 300 mg is an average daily dose to prevent gout. Cancer therapy requires double or more.

Translating the label

Zyloprim is the only brand of allopurinol available.

Side effects

Some patients suffer more frequent gouty attacks during the first few months. Otherwise it is remarkably benign for a drug that blocks an important chemical reaction. Only rarely do patients complain of headaches or digestive upsets.

Interactions

Food. Take it with meals.

Alcohol. None reported.

Drugs. Amoxicillin and ampicillin probably increase the chance of a rash (see under *allergies*). Thiazide diuretics plus Zyloprim are a tricky combination, as discussed below.

Pregnancy. Causes birth defects in animals, so we discourage use.

Nursing. Excreted in milk, but no one knows what this means.

Sex. A rare report of impotence.

Allergies

Hypersensitivity reactions occur 1 percent of the time, but are sometimes nasty and may not occur until months have passed. Most commonly, patients suffer an intensely itchy rash that may form blisters and peel. Several studies report a rare severe reaction with fever, liver damage, and kidney failure. Most occurred in patients taking thiazide diuretics. Experts suspected that kidney disease was present before therapy began, so diuretics are probably safe with Zyloprim provided the doctor makes sure your kidney function is normal.

Wholesale cost

Three cents for 100-mg tablet, 8 cents for 300 mg.

PART VII
Drugs for Respiratory Conditions and Allergies

Antihistamines: Benadryl and Seldane

French researchers synthesized the first antihistamine during World War II, so it did not make a big splash. Soon after, Americans produced diphenhydramine (Benadryl), launching a gush of similar drugs that has not stopped and has even produced improvements over earlier ones. Like all useful and safe drugs, antihistamines are overused and used for the wrong conditions by both doctors and patients.

Benadryl remains the most popular of the old, Seldane the best of the new, but there really are no bad antihistamines.

Antihistamines are treatment of choice for:

Blocking the action of histamine on your skin and upper respiratory tract. Histamine needs blocking in:

–Allergic rhinitis ("hay fever")

–Allergic conjunctivitis (itchy, watery eyes that accompany hay fever but can occur alone in response to foods or something inhaled)

–Urticaria ("hives"—itchy, pink welts that wax and wane over large areas of the body)

–Allergies to food and drugs that cause other itchy rashes

Histamine is a chemical produced by your immune system in response to a harmful invader such as a virus or germ. It dilates blood vessels (so the affected area turns red) and makes vessels leaky so that plasma carrying defensive chemicals and cells pours into the area, making it swell, hurt, and itch. Essential in fighting infections, histamine becomes a nuisance in the face of a harmless intruder such as a pollen, food, or drug. Your immune system is no more perfect than the rest of your body and sometimes attacks by mistake.

ANTIHISTAMINES ARE GROSSLY MISUSED THROUGH IGNORANCE OF THREE USEFUL RULES.

A. *Allergies itch!* At least they do on the skin and in the upper respiratory tract. A stuffy, runny nose makes all laymen and many doctors think of allergy, but they are usually wrong unless itching is part of the picture. If the nose doesn't itch, I ask about itchy eyes or an itchy tickle over the roof of the mouth. If the answers are negative I assume I'm dealing with a cold or a hypersensitive nose ("vasomotor rhinitis") that runs or clogs in response to minor irritations. A substantial minority of patients who complain of an allergy really suffer from vasomotor rhinitis—a tiresome and underdiagnosed condition that antihistamines don't help.

B. *Histamine doesn't damage the skin.* The intense itch of poison ivy, eczema, chemical irritations, contact dermatitis, and sunburn arises from skin injury, not histamine, and antihistamines don't help much. Many doctors routinely prescribe them, but cold compresses and bland creams work better. For severe cases I give cortisone creams or pills.

C. *Histamine is not involved* in colds or other upper respiratory infections.

For less important uses, older and newer antihistamines differ, so I discuss them separately.

How they work

They block action of histamine on many tissues (but not all; see Tagamet, 39., for another class of antihistamine). Most important, they keep capillaries from dilating and leaking.

Blocking is not the same as *reversing*, so if you wait for a full-blown attack before taking a pill, you'll wait several more hours until the histamine already working wears off. For best results during an allergy episode, take an antihistamine around the clock.

Older antihistamines block part of the autonomic nervous system, depress some areas of the brain, and stimulate others, which produce annoying side effects but also mildly useful actions that sell a great deal of Benadryl.

82
Benadryl

Take Benadryl first for hay fever or an allergic rash.

If it doesn't help, make sure you have the right diagnosis before switching. If it works, but you can't stand the drowsiness, try chlorpheniramine (Chlor-Trimeton), another old antihistamine.

Besides blocking histamine—

Benadryl is good for:

1. *Motion sickness.* But scopolamine is better (see 48.).
2. *Insomnia.* The most popular ingredient in over-the-counter sleeping pills, it works if you're particularly sensitive.
3. *Anxiety.* As I explained in BuSpar (53.) section, most tranquilizers are sleeping pills in a lower dose. Doctors who object to prescription tranquilizers are often happy to recommend Benadryl. Tranquilizers work better.
4. *Parkinsonism.* A distressing neurological disease that mostly affects the elderly, producing slowing of movements as well as a tremor. When you see an older person with a hand tremor who walks with slow, shuffling steps think of parkinsonism. Several powerful drugs help; Benadryl is not among them, but it reduces tremor in mild cases.

How dispensed

Capsules of 25 and 50 mg and an injectable of 10 and 50 mg per milliliter. You can buy 25-mg capsules over-the-counter as well as an elixir containing 12.5 mg per teaspoon.

A reasonable dose is 25 to 50 mg every four hours.

Translating the label

For allergies and motion sickness, Benadryl is by far the most popular form of diphenhydramine, although plenty of generics exist.

As a tranquilizer or sleeping pill you'll find it as Sominex, Unisom Dual Relief, Nytol, Sleep-eze, and Miles Nervine.

Other popular antihistamines of the older generation:
- Chlorpheniramine (Chlor-Trimeton, Teldrin)
- Brompheniramine (Dimetane)
- Dimenhydrinate (Dramamine)
- Hydroxyzine (Atarax, Vistaril)
- Promethazine (Phenergan)
- Tripelennamine (PBZ)
- Cyproheptadine (Periactin)
- Meclizine (Antivert, Bonine)

Side effects

Half of everyone taking Benadryl feel drowsy, but half feel fine so don't assume either will happen to you. Some older antihistamines produce drowsiness less often, but it's always a risk. More rarely, especially in children, Benadryl causes jitteriness and insomnia. A few patients report fever, dry mouth, or upset stomach.

Interactions

Food. None.

Alcohol. Increases sedative action.

Drugs. Tranquilizers and sedatives also increase Benadryl's sedative action.

Pregnancy. No problems reported after almost 50 years of use, but no one knows for sure.

Nursing. Babies are very sensitive to antihistamines, so we discourage their use.

Sex. No problems.

Allergies

Surprisingly, oral antihistamines cause allergic rashes 1 to 2 percent of the time and sun sensitivity more rarely. This happens more often when applied as a cream—a useless use.

Wholesale cost

Cost is 1.5 cents for a 25-mg capsule; only slightly more for 50-mg; $1.50 for 4 ounces of elixir.

83
Seldane

Antihistamine drowsiness was so common and tiresome that companies introducing a new product into the overcrowded market knew their only hope was to convince us theirs wasn't so bad. Advertisements invariably boasted of this aspect and were always wrong, so doctors grew cynical. But researchers persisted, and in the mid-1980s the Merrell Dow Company hit the jackpot with Seldane. Studies showed that 8 percent of users complained of sleepiness—but so did 8 percent of those given placebo, so it's possible Seldane causes no drowsiness at all.

As an antihistamine, Seldane is a treatment of choice for allergies, but—

Seldane is good for:

Nothing else. So far there's no evidence that it helps the other complaints I list in the Benadryl section.

How dispensed

As 60-mg tablets, taken twice a day.

Translating the label

A gold mine, you won't find terfenadine under any name but Seldane.

Other companies are working frantically to come up with a rival; so far two have appeared:

Astemizole (Hismanal) and loratidine (Claritin). Advertisements boast that they stay in the blood so long that a once-a-day dose works fine. Unfortunately, they also take longer to build up in the blood and provide relief, so I don't recommend them except for long-term therapy.

Side effects

Because they don't penetrate into the brain or block the autonomic nervous system, newer antihistamines don't cause drowsiness, jitteriness, or dry mouth. The incidence of upset stomach is probably the same.

Interactions

Food. None.

Alcohol. None, but you should avoid the combination.

Drugs. Both erythromycin and ketoconazole (a relative of miconazole) slow the breakdown of Seldane; high blood levels of Seldane by-products occasionally produce dangerous cardiac rhythms.

Pregnancy. A new drug, so I don't advise it.

Nursing. Not recommended.

Sex. None known.

Allergies

Probably the same as Benadryl. Fewer are reported but that's because Seldane is so new.

Wholesale Cost

Cost is 90 cents a pill; you could buy 60 Benadryl for one Seldane.

84
Pseudoephedrine (Sudafed)

Like amphetamines and cocaine, Sudafed stimulates the sympathetic nervous system. Other drugs in this book (Catapres, Hytrin, Inderal) block parts of this system, so they lower blood pressure, and sometimes they slow the heart and make you sleepy. Stimulators do the opposite. Much weaker than amphetamines, you can buy Sudafed without a prescription, and I don't know anyone who takes it for pleasure.

Sudafed is good for:

Relieving stuffiness. Violently stimulating sympathetic nerves constricts arteries and makes blood pressure skyrocket. Gently stirring the nerves with Sudafed rarely does that, but it may constrict the dense clump of vessels in your nose enough to relieve a stuffy nose and congested sinuses.

The eustachian tubes connecting the middle ear to the outside world open into the back of the nose, so taking Sudafed before a plane flight may assure that air can get in and out of the middle ear as cabin pressure changes. However, everyone bothered by ear pain during a plane flight should keep a nasal spray (Afrin, Dristan, Neo-synephrine) handy and use it before takeoff and before descent.

Sudafed is not so good for:

Suppressing your appetite. Since amphetamines work, you might predict that weaker sympathetic stimulators do the same but more gently. Acting on this theory ten years ago, drug companies began promoting over-the-counter diet pills containing an almost identical decongestant, phenylpropanolamine. Although still available, they probably don't work except in people terribly sensitive to side effects.

The only difference between over-the-counter diet pills and ordinary decongestants is the packaging and hugely increased price. If you want to experiment, use ordinary cold medicines.

How it works

Drugs stimulate the sympathetic system by increasing the neurotransmitter, norepinephrine, that carries signals between nerves. How amphetamine does that is explained in the Tofranil (51.) section. Caffeine's action is distantly related; so is Sudafed's.

How dispensed

As 30-and 60-mg tablets, a long-acting capsule containing 120 mg and a syrup with 5 mg per teaspoon. Adults take 60 mg every four hours or a long-acting capsule every 12.

Translating the label

Sudafed is the most popular brand. Afrin tablets and many generic forms of pseudoephedrine exist.

Phenylephrine and phenylpropanolamine act similarly to pseudoephedrine, but they are almost impossible to find except as part of a combination cold remedy.

I couldn't possibly keep up with cold remedies that contain pseudoephedrine as one of a combination. All seem clever and logical (a drug for fever, a drug for cough, a drug for congestion), but they usually contain too little of one or another (drug companies are far more worried about side effects than curing you; no one sues a drug company if the drug doesn't work, but if there's a bad reaction . . .), so you're always better off buying individual drugs.

Decongestant-antihistamine combinations are the exception. Take Sudafed first if your nose is stuffed from a viral infection, take an antihistamine if it's an allergy. If you're not satisfied, try a combination. Some good antihistamine-pseudoephedrine mixtures:

- Actifed
- Drixoral
- Chlor-Trimeton Decongestant
- Sudafed Plus
- Benadryl Decongestant
- Pediacare-2

· Bromfed
· Dorcol

Side effects

The same as caffeine—nervousness, jitteriness, insomnia.

Interactions

Food. None.
Alcohol. None.
Drugs. You shouldn't take pseudoephedrine with an infrequently used class of antidepressant called MAO inhibitors. The label contains an ominous warning about taking Sudafed if you are on high blood pressure medication. It's appropriate to let your doctor know, but I don't know of anyone who has forbidden it.
Pregnancy. No known problems.
Nursing. Probably O.K.
Sex. None.

Allergies

Extremely rare. A closely related drug, adrenalin, treats allergies.

Wholesale cost

Cost is 1.2 cents for 30-mg tablet, 33 cents for long-acting capsule.

Decongestants like Sudafed work better for stuffiness and won't make you drowsy.

Antihistamines like Benadryl work better for a runny nose, but cause drowsiness (except for the newest which aren't sold over-the-counter.)

85
Dextromethorphan

Despite the unfamiliar name, you've taken dextromethorphan because it's the usual anticough ingredient in over-the-counter cold medicines.

Civilized countries throughout the world allow small amounts of codeine in nonprescription remedies. While you can't buy any form of codeine without a prescription in the U.S., this is no great loss because dextromethorphan works as well for coughs.

You should never see a doctor simply to get a cough medicine.

Dextromethorphan is good for:

Suppressing a cough. Treating cold symptoms does no harm although it doesn't speed recovery. It's all right to take a cough medicine for a few days.

Some health enthusiasts frown on treating symptoms. Fever, runny nose, and cough are signs the body is trying to eliminate the infection, they insist, so suppressing the symptoms is harmful. Although sensible, that implies the body is perfect, so whatever it does must be right. The truth is the human body is an ingenious organism that often goes haywire and behaves stupidly.

How it works

Although chemically similar to other narcotics, dextromethorphan lacks addicting or painkilling properties, but retains a narcotic's ability to suppress cough centers in the brain.

How dispensed

Mostly as an ingredient in innumerable over-the-counter liquids, tablets, and lozenges. If you look hard, you can find a product that contains nothing else.

A reasonable adult dose is 30 mg every six hours.

Translating the label

Here are remedies that contain only dextromethorphan:
- Benylin-DM syrup
- Delsym syrup
- Hold lozenges
- Sucrets cough control lozenges
- Robitussin cough calmers
- Vicks Formula 44 cough medicine

Side effects

Dextromethorphan doesn't share narcotic effects on the digestive system and brain although very high doses produce drowsiness.

Interactions

Food. None.

Alcohol. Theoretically, interactions resemble other narcotics, but I haven't noticed problems.

Drugs. None significant.

Pregnancy. No one knows.

Nursing. Probably O.K.

Sex. No known problems.

Allergies

Again, even less common than with other narcotics.

Wholesale cost

Cost is $4.25 for four ounces of Benylin-DM, $10 for 96 Robitussin cough calmers.

86
Adrenalin

If you recognize the name, Parke-Davis is pleased because it's their patented brand of epinephrine, one hormone produced by the adrenal gland (cortisone is another).

Stress provokes epinephrine release, so you experienced its action the last time a careless driver almost ran you down or your boss bawled you out. Your heart raced, your breathing rate increased, your skin turned pale (because blood concentrated in your muscles), and you felt tense and alert. If necessary, you could have run faster and farther or defended yourself more aggressively.

In psychological terms, Adrenalin produces the "fight or flight" reaction, but except for the occasional dishonest athlete who takes a similar drug before a meet, we consider these undesirable side effects. Taken one by one, however, some of Adrenalin's actions are lifesaving.

The original member of a family of drugs that can clear up a stuffy nose (see previous section), kill your appetite (amphetamines or diet pills) or stop premature labor (ritodrine—not part of my 100), Adrenalin remains the most useful.

Adrenalin is treatment of choice for:

Anaphylaxis. This is the immediate, catastrophic allergy that can kill. Occurring within minutes after exposure (mostly to insect venom, foods, and injected drugs), the most dangerous symptom is sudden difficulty breathing sometimes accompanied by a profound drop in blood pressure. Less ominous signs are florid, itchy hives, cramps, vomiting, and diarrhea. Every doctor who gives injections keeps a syringe of epinephrine on hand; so do patients with known sensitivity, especially to insect stings.

Adrenalin is good for:

1. *Asthma.* Adrenalin powerfully relaxes bronchial muscles whether they're

constricted by anaphylaxis, drug action, allergy, or asthma. For a patient sick enough to see me, I give an injection. Adrenalin works as well by inhalation through a nebulizer but the action is short, perhaps half an hour. Newer relatives that last four to six hours such as Alupent, Ventolin, and Proventil have replaced it. Doctors also give these in metered-dose inhalers for use at home during less severe attacks. You can buy an epinephrine inhaler without a prescription. It works fine, although newer drugs work better.

You can't take Adrenalin orally. Tablets of the newer drugs work fairly well but produce a good deal of tremor and jitteriness. Inhalers rarely do that, so doctors prefer them.

2. *Constricting blood vessels.* Although it relaxes bronchial tubes, epinephrine does the opposite for superficial blood vessels. Local anesthetics with epinephrine last longer because the constricted vessels don't carry away the anesthetic. In eye drops, epinephrine gives a pleasing cosmetic affect by eliminating redness, again by constricting blood vessels.

3. *Glaucoma.* In glaucoma, pressure in the eyeball fluid rises too high. Epinephrine eyedrops lower it.

4. *Stimulating the heart.* Normally, we don't like this action, but we make an exception if death is the alternative. You won't encounter this unless you have a cardiac arrest.

How it works

In the Catapres and Inderal sections (31. and 32.) I mentioned the sympathetic nervous system, its alpha and beta receptors, and drugs that lower pressure by blocking them. Epinephrine does the opposite, stimulating both alpha, beta one, and beta two. Stimulating B2 receptors relieves asthma. Stimulating B1 receptors makes the heart pound, not a symptom asthmatics appreciate.

Epinephrine doesn't penetrate the brain as well as the amphetamines. Sympathetic stimulation of the brain causes alertness and intense emotion (not always pleasant; some people feel unbearable anxiety) while suppressing appetite, nausea, and motion sickness. Amphetamine's actions wear off in a few weeks, but people who enjoy the feeling find it hard to stop.

Killing the appetite, even for a few weeks, seems a reasonable way to start a weight loss program, but it doesn't work. During the first weeks, everyone on diet pills loses 10 to 20 pounds—but I don't call this "dieting"; anyone can lose 10 to 20 pounds; a bad case of the flu will accomplish that. For taking off a significant amount of weight, diet pills fail 100 percent of the time.

B2 stimulation also relaxes the uterus. Epinephrine isn't selective enough, but the newer stimulators probably work despite lack of FDA approval. Ritrodine (Yutopar) might help asthma, but it's only approved for stopping premature labor.

How dispensed

Ampoules and vials containing 1 mg per milliliter (1:1,000); 0.3 to 0.5 mg is the usual adult dose for allergies or asthma. We use epinephrine ten times more dilute (1:10,000) for injection directly into the heart during cardiac arrest.

Drops contain 0.5 percent, 1 percent, and 2 percent.

Translating the label

Adrenalin and EpiPen are brands of epinephrine for injection.

Inhalers are Primatene Mist, Bronkaid, and AsthmaHaler. You can buy them over-the-counter.

Better inhalers include albuterol (Proventil, Ventolin), metaproterenol (Alupent, Metaprel), terbutaline (Brethaire), pirbuterol (Maxaire), and bitolterol (Tornalate). These require a prescription.

Epinephrine eyedrops are called Eppy-N.

Side effects

What you'd expect from sympathetic stimulation: pounding heart, jitteriness, anxiety, headaches. B2 stimulation causes a tremor—rare with Adrenalin but not so with oral sympathetic stimulators.

Adrenalin must never be injected near the fingers or toes where constricted vessels may cut off the blood supply entirely.

Interactions

Food. None.

Alcohol. None.

Drugs. Your doctor should know if you're taking another sympathetic stimulator such as Sudafed or a diet pill. There's also a risk in combining epinephrine with a sympathetic blocker such as the Inderal family and Catapres. Antidepressants and antihistamines may increase epinephrine's action.

Pregnancy. Large doses cause birth defects in rats; none has appeared in humans.

Nursing. Probably O.K.

Sex. No problems reported.

Allergies

No one should be allergic to epinephrine although sulfites in the solution might cause a reaction.

Wholesale cost

Cost is $9 for 30-cc vial; $1.40 per ampoule containing 1 cc.

87
Aerobid—Cortisone Inhaler

Asthma sufferers have twitchy, hyperreactive airways, so insults from nature (temperature changes), the atmosphere (pollen, dust), or infections (colds) trigger an excessive response. Almost any change in a narrow airway makes it narrower, so an asthmatic can lead a miserable life. Good drugs expand a tight airway (see Adrenalin section), but patients are better off if narrowing never occurs.

As you learned in the prednisone (75.) section, adrenal steroids shrink swollen, inflamed tissue, constrict blood vessels, suppress allergies, and inhibit the action of histamine and other "mediators" of immunity. All these actions work wonderfully to keep touchy airways open. Steroids are life-saving for the worst cases and the only means to make life bearable for moderate-to-severe asthma.

The prednisone section also points out the dangers of long-term use. Doctors agonize over beginning steroids, worrying that "weaning" the patient will be impossible, exchanging the miseries of the disease for the side effects of treatment.

Cortisone cream is safer than pills. "Why shouldn't that be true for inhaled cortisone?" doctors wondered 40 years ago when its miraculous properties and catastrophic side effects burst on the world. They tried it, and it didn't work. When you inhale a drug, more than 90 percent never reaches the lung, settling in your mouth and throat, so you swallow it (provided you use the best technique; if you inhale wrong, you swallow 100 percent). Asthmatics who inhaled early steroids got better, but suffered the same bad effects after chronic use. So researchers spent 20 years searching for an inhaled cortisone without "systemic" action, and they succeeded.

Aerobid is treatment of choice for:

Preventing asthma—not only in the worst cases but in all but the mildest. Although new inhaled steroids are safe, all take a few days to work, so they are useless in treating an attack. Like blood pressure medication or migraine prophylaxis, they only help when used regularly.

How it works

Swallowed steroids remain in the blood a long time, allowing them to work but also giving them the time to do bad things. A good inhaled steroid doesn't have to stay around. Ideally, the body should destroy it as soon as it enters the bloodstream, and this is what happens. Blood from your digestive tract passes through the liver, and almost no Aerobid that flows in appears at the other end. The fraction that settles on your bronchial tubes acts locally with only a tiny amount absorbed. Long use of these inhalers causes essentially no systemic side effects.

How dispensed

As an inhaler. Two puffs in the morning and two in the evening prevent most asthma attacks. An occasional patient requires twice that amount.

Translating the label

Aerobid is the brand name of flunisolide.

Other steroid inhalers work as well but require four treatments per day instead of two. You may think this is a trivial difference, but long and sad experience has taught me that patients who feel well are very bad about taking medicines—and that includes me. I have no trouble remembering morning and night doses but usually forget those in the middle of the day. An asthmatic who begins to wheeze after forgetting a few doses quickly resumes, but it's too late.

Other good corticosteroid inhalers:

· Beclomethasone (Vanceril, Beclovent)

· Trimacinolone (Azmacort)

· Dexamethasone (Decadron) is not in this class. It stays in the body and produces the same side effects as prednisone. Use it only if a specialist gives a good reason (perhaps all the others have failed).

Side effects

Inhaled corticosteroids occasionally suppress immunity where they settle in the mouth and throat, producing an overgrowth of candida, the common fungus that produces vaginal infections. This shows up as white patches that are most unpleasant to look at. Occasionally, patients notice hoarseness or throat irritation.

Interactions

Food. None.

Alcohol. None.

Drugs. None, but switching a patient from oral steroids to inhalers is a tricky business requiring close attention and frequent visits.

Pregnancy. Since little is absorbed it should be safe, but steroids are very bad for a developing fetus, so we try not to use them.

Nursing. Probably safe.

Allergies

A theoretical possibility to the solution carrying the steroid. Rare.

Wholesale cost

Cost is $44 for inhaler containing 100 puffs.

88
Beconase (or Vancenase)— Cortisone Nasal Sprays

A major advance in allergy therapy occurred around 1980 with the appearance of locally acting cortisone sprays, but family doctors don't use them enough, partly from reluctance to give cortisone for a minor ailment and partly because patients don't complain enough. If your nose makes you miserable for more than a few weeks of the year, you should know about them.

Beconase spray is treatment of choice for:

1. *Nasal allergy (allergic rhinitis).* If your nose itches and runs for more than a few days, and you feel fine, think of allergy (colds make you ill). If this becomes a chronic problem, it's almost certainly an allergy. If your doctor agrees, the first step is to find the cause and get rid of it. Medical science can't overcome an obvious source such as a cat or wool rug.

If you don't know the source, resist the urge to ask for skin tests and "shots." Like oral steroids for asthma, allergy hyposensitization is a last resort when life is miserable despite the best therapy. A solid minority of victims achieve comfort with antihistamines, and a majority notice improvement. Nevertheless, doctors stick with antihistamines too long. Speak up if you'd like to feel better or don't like antihistamine side effects. Cortisone nasal sprays are safe; they bring relief more quickly than allergy shots, and almost everyone benefits.

2. *Vasomotor rhinitis.* If your nose is persistently stuffy and runny without itching, this is the likely cause. Although more common than allergic rhinitis (many people have hypersensitive noses), doctors tend to misdiagnose it. Since it's not an allergy, antihistamines don't work well.

How it works

Identical to the locally acting asthma corticosteroids in the previous section. In fact, Beconase and its relatives are the same drugs. As soon as doctors realized how well they shrunk inflamed bronchial tubes, they suspected they would do the same for similar tissue higher in the respiratory tract, and they were right.

How dispensed

In both plastic or glass bottles containing 25 cc of liquid together with an atomizer and nasal adapter. Both are also available as inhalers.

Dose is one or two sniffs in each nostril twice a day. Don't expect immediate relief, but you should feel better in a few days. Give up after three weeks if there's no improvement.

Translating the label

Beconase and Vancenase are brands of beclomethasone. Both come as cans of aerosol as well as spray.

Nasalide is the brand of flunisolide nasal spray.

Nasacort is a triamcinolone spray.

Side effects

One fourth of patients suffer nasal irritation, and 4 percent have sneezing attacks—a reaction to the vehicle, not the beclomethasone because subjects using a spray minus the steroid have the same complaints.

Interactions

Food. None.

Alcohol. None

Drugs. Stay away from other nasal sprays, but if you're completely plugged, use a decongestant spray first to allow the steroid to enter.

Pregnancy. Same warnings as for asthma inhalers.

Nursing. Probably O.K.

Allergies

Wheezing, hives, and allergic rashes occur, but they are rare and usually from the vehicle.

Wholesale cost

Cost is $30 for spray, $28 for inhaler.

PART VIII
Drugs for the Skin

89
Cortisone Creams

The smelly era of dermatology disappeared during the 1950s. Previously, a patient with a serious skin disorder wielded tubs of tar and jars of sulfur, painting his or her body with colorful, odoriferous goos. Today, a white cream from a tube serves the same purpose although not always more effectively. Tar and other old remedies are messy but helpful, and they are underused. Cortisone creams are vastly overused, but when they work, they work.

Cortisone cream is good for:

Itchy, inflammatory rashes, including poison ivy and other chemical irritations, eczema, hand dermatitis, seborrhea (pink, flaky skin—including dandruff), insect bites, and dry skin. Be careful here. If a fungal or bacterial infection causes itching, cortisone relieves it (cortisone is wonderful for itching), but the infection will spread faster because even topical steroids suppress immunity.

They work for some nonitchy eruptions such as psoriasis, but not as dramatically. Treatment requires stronger concentrations and perhaps occlusion (covering the skin with a plastic wrap overnight). Don't use cortisone on a nonitchy rash without a doctor's advice.

How it works

Like oral corticosteroids, cream suppresses inflammation. It constricts superficial blood vessels, so fluid and blood cells pass through without leaking out. When skin vessels constrict, redness disappears; more important, lack of this "inflammatory exudate" eliminates the swelling and itching that accompanies it.

As noted in the prednisone section (75.), corticosteroids suppress protein synthesis and cell division. Rubbed on the skin they do the same, so they help disorders in which cells multiply too fast (psoriasis, seborrhea) but delay healing and weaken normal skin.

How dispensed

Tubes, bottles, and jars containing ointments, creams, lotions, and gels in many concentrations. A thin coating twice a day works fine.

Creams are most popular because they rub on easily and disappear, but they are not the choice for all conditions. Ointments (greasy like Vaseline) work best, and they are also the most moisturizing, so you should prefer them for a rash on a dry area. Lotions and gels are drying, so they work best on wet, oozing skin. Use a lotion in hairy areas. Creams are a compromise between ointments and lotions, but they usually work fine.

Translating the label

Perhaps 50 brands of dozens of synthetic and natural corticosteroids exist. Experts classify all into seven categories from weakest to strongest, but no doctor can keep track of them. I use three of the most popular, and you'll do well to remember them.

1. Weak: 1 percent hydrocortisone (Hytone, Carmol, Synacort, Nutracort, Eldecort, Caldecort)
2. Medium: triamcinolone cream (Kenalog, Aristocort)
3. Strong: fluocinonide (Lidex, Fluonex)

You can buy 1 percent hydrocortisone cream without a prescription. It's too weak to do much harm unless your self-diagnosis is wrong.

Side effects

Now and then I see a sad case, usually a young woman, who has been applying cream to her face. Pleased at the quick improvement, she continues to use it. Her skin looks fine for a few months, then pimples and a few pink blotches appear on her cheeks. Perhaps she's developing resistance, she thinks. She needs something stronger. Her doctor obliges, and the rash vanishes only to reappear in a few weeks, so she appeals to the doctor again. Caught in a vicious cycle, the patient applies more and stronger cortisone until someone, usually a dermatologist, realizes that her skin is badly damaged—not from an obscure disease but from the treatment.

Cortisone is deceptive because it works so well: It makes every rash feel better, and it may make it look better, but it doesn't cure anything, and long-term use of medium and strong steroids guarantees trouble.

A week or two does no harm on a susceptible rash. As more weeks pass, cortisone's ability to suppress immunity, protein synthesis, and cell reproduction begin to show. Skin grows thin and fragile. Small blood vessels become visible. Bruises emerge for no apparent reason. Redness, itching, pimples, eczema, oozing, and flaking appear. Rashes caused and cured by cortisone look the same, so all bets are off if one appears during treatment.

Never use anything but weak creams on your face, armpit, and genitals. Skin is thin there, so cortisone penetrates well with a small risk of skin damage. Medium and strong creams are positively dangerous in these areas. Never use a strong cream on any part of the body without regular visits to the doctor.

Interactions

Food. None.

Alcohol. None.

Drugs. No oral drugs interfere.

Pregnancy. O.K. in small amounts, but not when extensive treatment is required. A tiny amount penetrates into the blood.

Nursing. O.K.

Allergies

You can't be allergic to cortisone because it suppresses allergies, but it's not rare for the other ingredients ("vehicle") in the cream to provoke itching, burning, or a rash. Changing preparations can help and should be discussed with your doctor.

Wholesale cost

· 1-ounce tube of 1 percent hydrocortisone: $1.30.
· 15-gram tube of 0.1 percent triamcinolone: $1.35.
· 15-gram tube of fluocinonide: $6.40.

90
Retin-A

This is tretinoin, a form of retinoic acid related to vitamin A. Although vitamins are supposed to be safe and natural, this is definitely not so with retinoic acid. Even rubbed on the skin, it's potent and unpleasant but excellent for several common problems.

Retin-A is treatment of choice for:

1. *Acne.* But only acne dominated by blackheads and whiteheads. Antibiotics, benzoyl peroxide, and Accutane work better for pimples.
2. *Wrinkles.* Despite my skepticism when the announcements appeared during the late 1980s, Retin-A does eliminate fine wrinkles that are usually the result of sun damage. Don't confuse these with the large wrinkles of aging that don't originate in skin but in deep connective tissue where no cream can penetrate.
3. *Preventing skin cancer and precancerous conditions.* Although not universally accepted, a growing number of dermatologists believe that it works through the same mechanism (see below) that relieves acne and sun damage.

How it works

By increasing the speed of skin cells' multiplying and shedding. Skin originates in a "basal layer" a fraction of an inch below the surface. Cells in that layer multiply, then move upward and die, forming a protective layer that sloughs continually to be replaced by other dead cells moving up.

Under the influence of Retin-A, cells shed more rapidly, so they are less likely to plug pores (leading to comedones: whiteheads and blackheads). Solar radiation thickens and wrinkles the surface, but Retin-A-treated skin is thinner because of increased cell turnover, so areas of sun damage are shed before that happens.

How dispensed

As 20- and 45-gram tubes of cream in three concentrations: .025 percent, .05 percent, and .10 percent. As 15- and 45-gram tube of gel in two concentrations: .01 percent and .025 percent. As 28-cc bottle of .05 percent liquid.

Apply every other day for several treatments to make sure you're not too sensitive, then increase to daily. Improvement in acne and wrinkles may take a month or two.

Translating the label

Retin-A is the only brand of tretinoin, and it's sold by prescription. Watch out for vivid magazine ads extolling wrinkle creams with similar names. They contain zero tretinoin.

Side effects

Retin-A irritates, so skin may burn after application. Some patients can't tolerate this, but irritation isn't necessarily a good sign, so it's all right to try to prevent it. Patients assume they must wash their face before applying, but that makes skin more sensitive. Try applying Retin-A to unwashed skin before deciding you can't stand it. Also, creams and low concentrations are gentler than liquids, gels, and higher concentrations.

After a few weeks of Retin-A, expect your face to look worse as comedones and precancerous skin becomes inflamed and red. This should disappear in a few more weeks.

Interactions

Food. None.

Alcohol. None when taken internally.

Drugs. Don't combine Retin-A with other drying or abrasive topicals such as strong soaps or cleansers or anything containing alcohol, salicylic acid, resorcinol, or sulfur.

Pregnancy. Applied to the skin, retinoic acid is probably harmless (but see Accutane, section 92.).

Nursing. Probably O.K.

Allergies

Skin reactions are almost always from its irritating properties. Genuine allergies are rare, although Retin-A makes skin more sensitive to sunburn, so patients should apply a sunscreen and avoid sun exposure. But everyone should avoid sun exposure. It isn't required for your health and causes premature skin aging, wrinkles, and cancer.

Wholesale cost

About $45 for 45-gram tube, $38 for bottle of liquid.

91
Benzoyl Peroxide

Although I write prescriptions for benzoyl peroxide, it's also sold over-the-counter so I spend a good deal of time persuading patients it works. You can buy plenty of useless acne soaps, scrubs, astringents, and lotions over the counter, but if you buy benzoyl peroxide you're getting something good.

Benzoyl peroxide is good for:

Acne. It's my treatment of choice for mild and even near-moderate acne.

How it works

You'll find a discussion of acne in the Accutane section. Peroxides like benzoyl peroxide kill germs by a powerful oxidizing action. Destroying germs in your follicles is probably its major action although it also seems to reduce sebum production and cause peeling of the skin surface.

How dispensed

As creams, gels, lotions, washes, and bars with concentrations of 2.5, 5, and 10 percent. Begin with 5; there's no evidence 10 percent works better. Try a gel first. If it's too drying, use a cream.

Rub over the entire face (not just the pimples) daily for a week, then increase to twice a day.

Translating the label

Brands include Benzac, PanOxyl, Desquam-X and -E, Persa-Gel, Benzagel, Clearasil, Clear by Design, Oxy-5 and 10, Vanoxide, Xerac, and Theroxide. Ignore other ingredients such as alcohol, sulfur, resorcinol, zinc sulfate, or salicylic acid.

Side effects

Expect some drying and irritation. Ten percent of patients find that too unpleasant.

Interactions

Food. None.
Alcohol. None.
Drugs. Applied with an antibiotic cream (also an acne treatment), ben-

zoyl peroxide neutralizes the antibiotic, but it's all right to use one in the morning, the other at night.

Pregnancy. No data on either animals or humans.

Nursing. No one knows if it's excreted into milk so the PDR, always helpful, advises us to "exercise caution."

Allergies

Rare. Direct damage, not allergy, causes most skin irritation.

Wholesale cost

Cost is $2.50 for 1.5 ounces.

92
Accutane

Related to Retin-A (tretinoin), Accutane (isotretinoin) isn't effective on the skin, but is a major advance in acne treatment when taken orally. It's also the most unpleasant drug we use for a nonfatal condition, but those who need it are usually miserable enough to bear with the side effects.

Accutane is treatment of choice for:

Cystic acne. This is the worst, most disfiguring form; large pimples and boils cover the face. Not terribly rare, it was once treated with large doses of antibiotics or oral cortisone with fair to poor results. Accutane cures almost everyone.

Accutane is good for:

Moderate acne. Some doctors use lower doses to treat extensive pimples that aren't responding to antibiotics and creams. When my patients' pimples don't respond, it's usually because they're bored taking pills and applying creams several times a day. With persistence, most acne improves.

How it works

Suppresses sebum production. The "pores" in your face are openings through which sebaceous glands just underneath secrete an oily substance—sebum. Under the influence of male hormones at puberty, the glands become more active. Too often they become overactive, pouring out sebum and other material that obstruct the opening, producing a comedone (whitehead or blackhead). Material accumulates. Bacteria in the pore feed on the sebum, producing irritating substances. If the gland ruptures into the tissue beneath the plug, a pimple appears. A more extensive ruptures produces a large cyst.

Under the influence of Accutane, sebum production may drop to 10 percent of normal, and cysts melt away. After treatment, the glands return to normal, but cysts usually stay away, so a permanent change occurs that we don't yet understand.

How dispensed

Capsules of 10, 20, and 40 mg.

Fifty to 100 mg per day is average adult dose and four months the usual treatment period. Most patients remain free of cysts, but 30 percent require a second course.

Translating the label

Accutane is the only brand of isotretinoin.

Side effects

Accutane is poison—and its toxicity resembles a massive vitamin A overdose. We occasionally see this in vitamin enthusiasts, but it was more common in Arctic explorers who ate polar bear liver, a tremendous source of vitamin A.

Accutane not only dries up sebaceous glands (present over much of your body), it dries everything. Ninety percent of patients have painful, cracked lips. Eighty percent suffer dry skin with itching, peeling, and cracking or a dry, bleeding nose. Forty percent have dry eyes with persistent tearing. Sixteen percent have muscle and joint pains.

Other reactions are headaches, hair loss, nausea, and vomiting. Diminished night vision is common. Also common are liver damage and elevated cholesterol and triglycerides. Almost all side effects disappear after treatment, but everyone on Accutane must have regular blood tests.

Interactions

Food. None.

Alcohol. Modest drinking is allowed but no one with liver damage should receive Accutane.

Drugs. Most acne is best treated by a combination of drugs, but you must use Accutane alone. Users must religiously avoid vitamin A pills or any supplement containing the vitamin.

Pregnancy. Accutane almost guarantees birth defects. Despite extensive warnings from doctors and a frightening package insert, women still take the drug, get pregnant, fail to return to the doctor, and give birth to a deformed child. This happens so often some experts advise taking it off the market for everyone.

Nursing. Forbidden.

Sex. Surprisingly, none reported.

Allergies

Although rashes are common, most are from dry skin, not allergy. Sun sensitivity occurs as often as with Retin-A, so every patient should use a sunscreen.

Wholesale cost

Very high: $3, $3.50, and $4 for the 10-, 20-, and 40-mg capsule. Count on spending over $1,000 for a four-month course.

93
Minoxidil

The strongest antihypertensive in this book, minoxidil is so powerful I never use it. I can control blood pressure with less unpleasant drugs.

One side effect makes it particularly offensive to women. On the other hand, men have known and secretly taken advantage of this side effect since its discovery in the 1960s.

Minoxidil is good for:

1. *Severe high blood pressure.* But not for routine or even fairly bad hypertension because the drug is too strong to use alone. Minoxidil reduces pressure in the kidneys so much those organs assume that something is dreadfully wrong. As I mentioned in the diuretic section, the kidneys regulate blood volume, so they retain salt and water when volume is low. Although a lifesaver when you're bleeding heavily or dehydrated, fluid retention defeats our efforts when we're treating high blood pressure because it brings pressure back up. To prevent this, we give minoxidil with a diuretic.

   If that isn't enough, the heart reacts to the lower pressure as if there weren't enough blood; it beats faster. Since patients with hypertension often have heart disease, making the heart work harder is not a good idea, so we also give a beta blocker when we prescribe minoxidil.

2. *Growing hair.* We knew minoxidil grew hair from the beginning. That's why we rarely prescribed it for high blood pressure. By the 1970s we noticed that a few of our balding colleagues weren't so bald. Knowing these men were not suffering high blood pressure, we made sly jokes about their drug habits, but they seemed pleased enough to continue. By 1980, the Upjohn Company knew of this underground use of its product. Researchers knew the FDA was unlikely to approve such a powerful drug as treatment for baldness, but they wondered if rubbing it into the scalp had commercial possibilities. Studies showed a modest effect, and the FDA gave its nod a few years later.

How it works

Minoxidil lowers blood pressure by directly relaxing arteries. Although that increases blood flow to the skin, it's probably not responsible for hair growth because plenty of other drugs have the same action. No one knows why minoxidil grows hair.

Men don't grow bald because hair "falls out" permanently. Every human hair lives for two to three years, then drops off to be replaced by another growing up from the same follicle. Only the skin on the top of a man's head behaves differently. If he is destined to become bald, those follicles slowly shrink. Each new replacement hair is smaller than the one before, but even scalp as naked as a billiard ball grows a thin fuzz. Minoxidil definitely slows follicle shrinkage but reverses it only a slight amount. You should use the lotion at the first sign of thinning hair and never stop. Follicle shrinkage quickly resumes once you do. Minoxidil doesn't work as well once scalp is obviously bare.

I think a 2 percent solution is too weak. In the old underground days, pharmacists earned extra income grinding up pills and making their own solution. Five percent was common, and I obtained some myself. It may have worked, but I grew bored after six months and stopped. I was surprised when the company pushed for a 2 percent solution, but it was probably anxious to avoid side effects.

How dispensed

Tablets of 2.5 and 10 mg. We begin with 5 mg per day and gradually increase. Most blood pressure responds to less than 40 mg.

The solution comes in 60-ml bottles. Patients rub it into the scalp twice a day.

Translating the label

Minoxidil has never been popular so no rivals have appeared. Loniten is the only tablet. The solution is Rogaine.

Side effects

Except for unwanted hair, minoxidil has surprisingly few side effects for such a powerful drug (diuretics and beta blockers should prevent fluid retention and rapid heartbeat). Three percent of patients accumulate fluid around the heart ("pericardial effusion"), which may cause no symptoms or some shortness of breath. If mild, it may respond to increasing the diuretic.

Rubbed into the scalp, minoxidil rarely causes problems.

Interactions

Food. None.

Alcohol. Alcohol also relaxes blood vessels, so it may drop blood pressure temporarily.

Drugs. Except for diuretics and beta blockers, it's unwise to take other blood pressure medications at the same time.

Pregnancy. No reported problems in humans, but we use it only if there's no alternative.

Nursing. Only if treatment is essential.

Sex. No problems noted, but the patient will be taking a beta blocker, too.

Allergies

Fewer than 1 percent experience rash severe enough to require discontinuance.

Wholesale cost

Twenty cents for 2.5 mg; 35 cents for 10 mg.
Rogaine costs $57 a bottle—only a few months' supply.

94
Tar

The same material that covers city streets, tar is the black residue that remains after heating wood or coal at a high temperature. In medicine, coal tar remains an excellent but underused drug for several skin disorders that also respond to cortisone. Cortisone creams are more fragrant, convenient, and easier to apply but also more dangerous and sometimes less effective. Patients prefer cortisone. Many family doctors never use tar, but dermatologists know its value.

Tar is good for:

1. *Scalp seborrhea.* This means dandruff, although other conditions like psoriasis (see below) also produce flaking and itching. Tar treats them all. I tell patients to begin with widely advertised nontar shampoos such as Head and Shoulders, Zincon, Purpose, or Selsun Blue. Only mildly effective, they are also much cheaper. If they fail I prescribe tar shampoos. Easy to find, they are black, thick, and smelly, although today's products are not unpleasant.
2. *Chronic itchy skin disorders.* These include common eczema and dry skin that affects large areas of the body as well as localized contact dermatitis and hand eczema. Family doctors universally prescribe cortisone creams, and so do I, but I never forget that cortisone only relieves itching. It doesn't cure anything, and applying all but the weakest concentration daily for more than a few weeks is a bad idea. If you have a long-standing itch problem, learn to use tar. Tar baths are soothing. Tar ointments and pastes relieve itching without cortisone's side effects.
3. *Psoriasis.* I explained how skin grows in the Retin-A section. A cell normally takes four weeks from birth in the basal layer before its dead shell drops off (your skin surface sheds constantly but you don't notice). Psoriasis is a disorder of intense overactivity. Skin cells in psoriasis take

only *four days* to turn over. Overactivity makes skin bright pink, and the intense shedding means psoriatic skin is covered with white scales and flakes.

Until 40 years ago sufferers spent a great deal of time in tar: not only bath water containing tar but the pure goo. They plastered it over their bodies and left it there. When the eruption seemed out of control, they entered the hospital to be tarred from head to foot. After a day, attendants removed it—a tedious job requiring scrubbing with mineral or vegetable oil—and the patient lay under an ultraviolet light. Then tar was reapplied and the process repeated. After a few weeks, the worst eruptions melted away and often stayed away for a year.

Patients never liked this, so they happily accepted newer creams and procedures that are more convenient and almost as good. Tar treatments are still available in less expensive psoriasis "day-care centers," and you should ask about one if you're not satisfied with your condition. You should also consider tar as a supplement to cortisone creams, but it takes an enthusiastic doctor to persuade a patient to tolerate the mess and smell.

How it works

No one knows. Coal tar is a complex mixture of chemicals with antiseptic, irritant, anti-itching, skin softening, and cell toxic properties. It's also photosensitizing. Cells exposed to tar are hypersensitive to ultraviolet light which damages and probably kills them. That's how tar-light treatment counteracts the overactive cell division in psoriasis.

How dispensed

As shampoos, gels, creams, pastes, and bath oils. Many dermatologists and a rare family doctor have personal favorites and ask pharmacists to prepare a special mixture from crude coal tar.

Translating the label

Tar shampoos include Sebutone, Pentrax, Zetar, Polytar, Tegrin, X-Seb T, and Denorex Extra Strength.

Tars for direct skin application or bathing include P&S Plus, Balnetar, Pragmatar, Zetar, Fototar, Tegrin, and Estar.

Side effects

Shampoos are benign. Applied directly to the skin, tar can be irritating.

Interactions

Food. None.

Alcohol. None.

Drugs. Don't use other drugs that cause photosensitivity such as Retin-A, tetracyclines, or griseofulvin.

Pregnancy. Coal tar is full of chemicals that cause birth defects, but it's probably safe applied to the skin in modest amounts.

Nursing. Probably O.K. in small amounts.

Allergies

Rashes, burning, and pimples are not rare, but these are mostly from direct damage rather than an allergy.

Wholesale cost

Cost is $2.50 for 4 ounces of generic tar shampoo. Generic shampoos are not easy to find, but it pays to look because brands cost three times more. Twelve ounces of tar bath oil cost $15.

PART IX
Nutrients

95
Potassium

A close relative of sodium, potassium in the body occurs mostly inside your cells. Sodium is mostly outside in blood and tissue fluid. Their exchange across your cell membranes controls nerve excitability and muscle contraction. During the firing of a nerve, for example, a burst of potassium exits the cell and sodium enters. Afterward, the nerve must expel the excess sodium before it can fire again. Sodium and potassium are also essential for your body's fluid and acid balance. Fortunately, they are so abundant in the diet that no healthy person should worry about consuming too little.

Too much is a different matter. Too much of either is poison, but the margin for error is much smaller for potassium. Blood is mostly salt water (sodium chloride) with very little potassium. Normal blood sodium is 140 mM (millimoles) per liter. Normal potassium is 4.0. Taking in enough sodium to raise your level from 4 mM to 144 is harmless; raising your potassium from 4 mM to 8 will kill you. A blood potassium of 2 mM would probably do the same, so doctors spend a fair amount of time thinking about potassium.

Potassium is treatment of choice for:

Potassium deficit. Short of starvation, dietary deficiency doesn't cause this, but it does occur from:

A. *Excess excretion through the kidneys.* Diuretics are the leading cause. The remainder include rare kidney and hormone disorders as well as the action of some drugs not included here (although large doses of intravenous penicillin lower potassium). Licorice contains a substance that causes potassium loss, so people who consume huge amounts get into trouble. We learned that in medical school; it's one of those strange facts no one forgets, but no one has ever seen a case either.

B. Excess excretion through the digestive tract. This means through vomiting, diarrhea, surgical drainage, and uncommon intestinal disorders that interfere with absorption.

C. Excess excretion in the sweat. But this requires days of hard work in a hot climate. Never take potassium supplements to prevent this.

Potassium is good for:

Preventing potassium deficit. In the past we treated high blood pressure with a diuretic plus potassium chloride. Potassium chloride liquid is cheap and sickening; tablets are palatable but more expensive, and an adequate dose requires a large number, so doctors prescribed too little, and patients took even less. Even with a proper dose, potassium levels had the frustrating habit of drifting downward. When that happened, increasing potassium didn't seem to work. The level stayed borderline or even slightly low. It made doctors nervous, although patients didn't mind.

Did it matter? Probably not if the patient was in good health and following a low-salt diet (sodium and potassium complement each other; the more sodium you eat, the more potassium you lose; the less sodium you eat. the less potassium you lose). Today, when we treat high blood pressure with lower doses of diuretics, potassium loss is even less important, and I don't prescribe potassium for most patients. Exceptions are those with heart disease (low potassium makes muscles more irritable), those on high doses of diuretics—usually for heart failure—and everyone on digitalis (see explanation in digoxin section, 24.). Even here I prefer Dyazide.

Patients often ask if they should eat foods rich in potassium—mostly bananas and other fruits. I always encourage them because everyone should eat more fruit, but a diet to overcome a deficit or counteract a diuretic would soon become as disgusting as liquid potassium. I love bananas, but ten a day would strain my affection.

How it works

See introduction.

How dispensed

In liquids, powders, effervescent granules, tablets that do and don't dissolve in water, capsules, and extended-release capsules and tablets. Many liquids and dissolving forms are flavored, but always taste before you buy. If it tastes fine *make sure it's potassium chloride!* Potassium citrate, bicarbonate, and gluconate are sold for the same conditions, but they don't work as well, and few doctors prescribe them.

A reasonable daily dose to prevent potassium loss is 20 to 40 mEq (that's milliequivalent if you remember high school chemistry; if you don't, it's not important). We give 40 to 100 when trying to increase a low potassium. If you're taking less or hate the taste, discuss it with the doctor. He might substitute a potassium-sparing diuretic or decide you can do without it. Don't make this decision on your own.

Translating the label

Someone in every pharmaceutical company earns a salary thinking up brand names, a job that apparently demands little creativity because the chemical symbol for potassium ("K") satisfies their employer's requirements. Potassium chloride comes as Kato, Kaon, K-Dur, K-Lor, K-lease, K-Lyte, K-Norm, K-Tab, Kay Ciel, Klor-Con, Klorvess, Klotrix, Kolyum, Micro-K, Rum-K, Slow-K, and Ten-K.

Side effects

Aside from the foul taste, potassium chloride is positively corrosive to the digestive tract, so you must take liquids and powders with large amounts of water and after meals. In the past companies tried to avoid this with slow-release capsules that occasionally settled into one spot, released their potassium, and burned a hole. This is rare with newer products, but a minority of patients still complain of nausea, abdominal pain, or diarrhea.

Interactions

Food. Take after meals.

Alcohol. None reported.

Drugs. Never take with drugs that prevent potassium loss such as Dyazide or with angiotensin-converting-enzyme inhibitors.

Pregnancy. Probably safe as long as it doesn't produce a higher than normal blood level.

Nursing. Normal milk is rich in potassium, so there should be no problems.

Allergies

I don't think you can be allergic to potassium.

Wholesale cost

For 20 mEq of powder: 13 cents. For 10-mEq extended-release tablet: 7 cents. For 16 ounces of 10 percent liquid: $2. One tablespoon, half an ounce, contains 20 mEq.

96
Iron

When massive doses of niacin lower cholesterol, it's not acting as a nutrient but a drug. I include only a few nutrients as nutrients because deficiencies aren't important in the U.S., so most vitamins and minerals aren't useful enough to number among my hundred. Iron is one exception.

In past centuries doctors knew that driving a dozen nails into an apple, then eating it several days later relieved chlorosis or "green sickness," a common ailment of young women that made them pale, weak, and slightly green. Mild jaundice probably caused the color (nowadays jaundice turns you yellow, but perceptions change).

Iron is treatment of choice for:

1. *Iron-deficiency anemia.* Despite the universal belief, the average American diet contains all the essential nutrients. In fact, it contains far more than you need of good things (vitamins, minerals) as well as those you could do with less of (fat, cholesterol, salt, sugar, protein). Iron is an exception. The typical diet contains enough iron—but not a great excess. Fortunately, the body is fiercely efficient in conserving it. Once inside the body, 90 percent is recycled and only 10 percent lost, mostly through shedding of surface cells plus a little in bile that escapes in the feces. If we eliminate pregnant women and nursing infants, almost all iron deficiency is the result of bleeding. By far the most common and benign iron deficiency occurs in premenopausal women. Blood is full of iron, so the average menstruating woman needs twice as much as a man. Ten percent of women bleed heavily enough to require three or four times as much iron. Except for the heaviest bleeders, women can take in enough by diet if they make an effort, but young women tend to avoid foods richest in iron: meat, eggs, nuts, and beans. The end result is that 30 to 40 percent are deficient and half of these are deficient enough to become anemic. We usually learn of this anemia by a blood count, not because a patient complains. Most iron-deficiency anemia is mild, and mild anemia doesn't cause symptoms.

   Iron deficiency in men and in women no longer menstruating is almost always a sign of bleeding from some organ that shouldn't bleed, so a doctor must always find the source.

2. *Preventing iron-deficiency anemia.* A pregnant woman on the best diet loses iron stores during the last half of pregnancy, although she might not become anemic. It's good practice to give iron supplements during pregnancy. Deficiency isn't dangerous to the fetus, which extracts the iron it needs even if the mother has too little, so babies are rarely born anemic. Newborns should receive iron supplements after three months of age if breastfed or fed unfortified formula until the time they begin solid food. It's also a good idea for women with heavy periods to take iron (iron—not vitamins with iron).

How it works

Although iron takes part in many body functions, over 80 percent serves to make red cells in the bone marrow with the excess stored in the liver and spleen. Iron forms an essential part of the huge molecule, hemoglobin, which transports oxygen from lungs to tissues and carbon dioxide in the reverse direction. When intake is low, the body uses iron stored in the liver and marrow as long as it lasts (biopsies show absent iron even before anemia appears). Then the iron level in the blood drops. Anemia develops when too little iron is present to make the normal number of cells, but before this happens red cells begin to shrink. As anemia progresses, a doctor examining a blood smear will see red cells grow smaller, thinner, and become misshapen. Pieces and fragments of cells also appear. To make matters worse, the red cells don't live as long; normal life is four months.

When iron is replaced, the marrow can increase red cell production to five times its normal rate, so iron therapy corrects mild anemia in a few weeks, severe anemia within two months.

How dispensed

As ferrous sulfate (the cheapest) in 325-mg tablets, 200- and 250-mg sustained-release capsules, 160 and 525 mg of sustained-release tablets, and a liquid containing 220 mg per teaspoon.

As ferrous gluconate in 300- and 320-mg tablets and 435-mg capsules as well as a suspension of 300-mg per teaspoon.

As ferrous fumarate in 100-, 200-, and 325-mg tablets, a suspension containing 100 mg per teaspoon, and drops of 75 mg per ml.

Taking 325 mg of ferrous sulfate three times a day is the usual dose to treat iron deficiency. Ferrous gluconate contains half as much iron, so the dose must double. Ferrous fumarate contains 50 percent more iron than sulfate.

Translating the label

Ferrous sulfate: Feosol, Ferrocon, and Slo-Fe. Ferrous gluconate: Fergon and Ferralet. Ferrous fumarate: Ircon, Feostat, Hemocyte, Ferro-Sequels.

Ignore innumerable combinations of iron with vitamins and other minerals. They offer no advantage in treating or preventing iron deficiency, but are popular with those who take supplements as a general health measure. Patients who have experienced pure iron often prefer mixtures because side effects are much less. Combinations reduce side effects by containing less iron, so they are the treatment of choice for those who don't need treatment.

Side effects

Ferrous sulfate is hard on the stomach; 25 percent of patients suffer cramps, constipation, diarrhea, or nausea, and 10 percent have severe symptoms. When that happens we try the gluconate or fumarate or perhaps the sustained-released forms, but they are often no improvement.

Iron turns the stool black and may give you a black tongue.

Interactions

Food. Iron is absorbed best on an empty stomach. Taking it with food diminishes the side effects at the expense of less absorption, but there's often no choice.

Alcohol. No obvious interactions.

Drugs. Adding vitamin C to an iron pill increases the amount absorbed but also the side effects; I don't recommend it. Antacids greatly reduce iron absorption, and iron prevents tetracycline absorption.

Pregnancy. Necessary.

Nursing. Also useful.

Sex. No problems.

Allergies

Very rare.

Wholesale cost

One penny for 325-mg ferrous sulfate tablet. Five cents for 200-mg timed-release capsule.

Twelve cents for 320 mg of ferrous gluconate (equivalent to half the dose of ferrous sulfate).

Eleven cents for 325 mg of ferrous fumarate.

97
Calcium

Although essential for nerve and muscle function (see the calcium blocker section 34.), bones contain over 90 percent of body calcium and are the site of the only calcium disorder most of you will encounter.

Calcium is treatment of choice for:

Calcium deficiency. Rare. Congenital deficiencies are so uncommon most doctors have never seen one. Another cause, now fairly rare, is surgical removal of the thyroid. The thyroid has nothing to do with calcium, but tucked behind it are four tiny (and unrelated) parathyroid glands that secrete parathyroid hormone essential for calcium metabolism. You can get along without a thyroid, but life is difficult without parathyroids, and surgeons occasionally took them out along with the thyroid. Today they are more careful.

Calcium is good for:

1. *Preventing osteoporosis.* Be careful here. Osteoporosis is inevitable as you age, so the most you can do is prevent it from proceeding faster than necessary. Women should make an effort because calcium disappears from their bones far too rapidly after menopause. As you read earlier, estrogens are the treatment of choice. It's all right to take calcium, too, but good studies prove calcium alone after menopause doesn't slow bone loss.

   The time to pay attention is *before* bone loss begins. Although you can't pack more into your bones than they normally take, you can end up with less by consuming too little. Once calcium loss begins, it's best to start out with as much as possible. Diet can provide the minimum 1,200 mg per day provided it contains plenty of dairy products, the leading source. Women who don't drink a quart of milk a day should take supplements.

2. *Neutralizing acid.* Some antacids (Tums, Titralac) contain calcium carbonate, but we prefer products with aluminum or magnesium because calcium also stimulates stomach acid flow.

How it works

Provided you have adequate amounts of vitamin D and parathyroid hormone, calcium is easily absorbed through the small intestine. It's carried in the blood to the skeleton where special cells add calcium to bone—and other special cells extract it and carry it away. Bone is never stable—calcium is always going in and coming out. Bone buildup predominates from birth until growth stops. After age 35, breakdown occurs slightly faster than buildup.

How dispensed

Mostly as calcium carbonate in tablets containing 250 to 600 mg and as a powder dissolved in water. Chalk is calcium carbonate, so the taste is not attractive. The current RDA is 1,200 mg. Calcium gluconate and calcium lactate taste better but each tablet contains much less calcium so you must consume three to four times more.

Translating the label

Brands include Os-Cal, Cal-Lactate, Calciday, Calcet, Caltrate, Cal Plus, and Calci-Chew. Antacids like Tums, Rolaids, Alka-Mints, and Titralac also work fine as supplements. I recommend a large bottle of generic calcium carbonate.

Side effects

Few except an occasional upset stomach. Although calcium stimulates gastric acid secretion, this doesn't seem to cause problems.

Interactions

Food. None.

Alcohol. Alcohol lowers intestinal calcium absorption.

Drugs. Calcium interferes with absorption of tetracycline.

Pregnancy. Requirements increase by 50 percent, but supplements aren't necessary on a good diet. Enormous doses of calcium cause birth defects, so don't get carried away.

Nursing. Requirements also increase by 50 percent during nursing, but the same advice applies.

Allergies

Almost unheard of.

Wholesale cost

Less than one penny for 600-mg tablet of calcium carbonate. Slightly more than a penny for calcium gluconate or lactate.

98
Fluoride

Ten percent of America's water is naturally fluoridated, but no one paid attention until someone noticed a massive increase in tooth decay among children in Bauxite, Arkansas. Searching for a cause, researchers discovered the city had changed to a new water system a decade before. The only difference in the new supply was lack of fluoride.

A quick look around the country revealed tooth decay was less common where water contained fluoride, so public health workers drew the obvious conclusion, and communities began adding fluoride to their water.

Almost immediately (in the 1940s) a movement sprang up to insist that fluoride was a dreadful poison. As aggressive as today's animal rights or antiabortion fighters, they stalled fluoridation for several decades. I remember vicious election campaigns featuring more fervent debate than the presidential race—and fluoridation always lost. In the 20 years since the antifluoridation movement's decline, fluoridation has spread to about half the water supply although dietary supplements and topical applications have exposed more of the population.

Cancer and brain damage predicted by the movement haven't come to pass, but fluoridation has harmed one segment of the population: dentists. A grave shortage existed during the 1960s, and the American Dental Association urged students to enter the profession. You won't hear that campaign today. The decline in tooth decay has been an economic disaster. No one worries about a shortage of dentists today, and many dental schools have shut their doors.

Fluoride is treatment of choice for:

Preventing tooth decay. I still remember a statistic from high school science in the 1950s: Five percent of the population reached adulthood with no cavities. That number had stood for a century, but today it's over 50 percent and declining. Although epidemic over most of the world, tooth decay is declining in the U.S. Fluoridation is the great unsung public health triumph of our time.

How it works

Fluoride is incorporated into the crystals of enamel, the hard outer layer of the tooth, making it even harder.

How dispensed

Tablets of 0.25, 0.50, 1, and 2 mg and drops containing 0.125 and 0.25 mg per drop.

Your water supply should contain one part per million. The local water board will know. If it contains less than 0.3 parts per million, an infant should receive 0.25 mg until the age of two years, 0.50 mg until age three, then 1 mg until age 15. There's no evidence fluoride helps after permanent teeth are completely formed. Believe it or not, evidence is conflicting that brushing with fluoride toothpaste helps, but most experts believe it does.

Translating the label

Some brands are Pediaflor, Fluoritab, and Luride.

Side effects

About 10 percent of those taking normal amounts of fluoride continuously show slight pale mottling of the teeth. This is of no consequence but your dentist should know about it. Higher doses produce more intense mottling.

Fluoride is poisonous in high doses, but all current bottles contain 120 mg or less, which is not dangerous.

Interactions

Food. None.
Alcohol. None.
Drugs. None.
Pregnancy. None, and some experts believe that taking fluoride during pregnancy strengthens the baby's developing teeth.
Nursing. No problems.

Allergies

Rare.

Wholesale cost

Cost is 0.6 cents for 1-mg tablet.

99
Folic Acid

A useful vitamin, folic acid is one of the few in which supplements are important in otherwise healthy adults. There are also hints that it helps women with an abnormal pap smear.

Folic acid is treatment of choice for:

1. *Folic acid deficiency.* This causes anemia, but it's rare in America because folic acid occurs widely in green leafy vegetables, grains, beans, nuts, and liver. We occasionally see deficiency in malnourished alcoholics, drug addicts, and the poor elderly as well as victims of diseases that interfere with intestinal absorption.

   A few months after entering practice, I saw a young woman who had felt increasingly tired for months. A blood count showed severe anemia, but I couldn't find a reason (almost always bleeding, if you remember the iron section). It occurred to me she was taking oral contraceptives, and a quick look in a medical text reminded me the pill can interfere with folic acid absorption. A few weeks of supplements cured her, and we both felt very pleased. Although I haven't seen a case since, I keep it in mind.

2. *Preventing certain birth defects.* Within the past few years evidence has become overwhelming that women who take folic acid supplements early in pregnancy have a much lower risk of delivering a child with a neural tube defect—a devastating defect that can result in either a stillbirth or permanent paralysis. The critical period occurs during the first few weeks, so a woman planning a pregnancy must begin supplements before impregnation.

Folic acid is good for:

1. *Preventing folic acid deficiency.* We routinely supplement patients with digestive diseases that cause "malabsorption" and occasionally do so for

healthy people on drugs that interfere with folic acid—most often birth control pills and anticonvulsants.

2. *Correcting a mildly abnormal pap smear (maybe)*. When my wife's pap turned up slightly abnormal, her gynecologist told her to take folic acid, and several months later a repeat pap was normal. This proves nothing; my patients' repeat paps are also usually normal, and I don't give folic acid, but some gynecologists do. I researched the subject and discovered that several studies over the past 20 years have found that women with abnormal but not cancerous cells on pap smears improved on folic acid. Most were taking birth control pills. Experts consider these findings "interesting," but no one has drawn firm conclusions although I'm leaning to the opinion that women on the pill should take folic acid

How it works

Folic acid participates in the complex process of synthesizing DNA, the material that makes up your chromosomes. Mostly, a cell synthesizes DNA when it divides because it must duplicate its chromosomes before that can happen. All cells need folic acid, but those that divide rapidly need more. Since the bone marrow giving rise to blood cells is the fastest dividing tissue of the body, anemia marks the first sign of deficiency.

How dispensed

Tablets of 0.1, 0.4, 0.8, and 1.0 mg. The normal dose is 1.0 mg per day; treating an abnormal pap smear requires 10 mg.

Translating the label

Folvite is one brand, but generics are common.

Side effects

None reported for oral folic acid.

Interactions

Food. None.

Alcohol. None.

Drugs. High doses may weaken action of anticonvulsants.

Pregnancy. None in normal doses.

Nursing. None.

Allergies

Not reported.

Wholesale cost

Cost is $7.50 for a thousand 1-mg tablets.

100
Vitamin B₁₂

A famous rock singer wants a B_{12} shot before every performance, and when he stays in my Los Angeles hotels, I give the injection. It is a formal ceremony. I walk through the large anteroom of the suite, past managers and hangers-on to an inner room where I assemble my syringe. Then an attendant conducts me to the bedroom where the singer waits. He drops his jeans and I inject. Then I retrace my steps, collecting my money from the manager. I love it. Patients often ask for B_{12}, and I have no objection to giving it provided they have no medical problem requiring treatment. In 20 years of practice, I remember only a few occasions when I gave B_{12} to someone who needed it.

A little history reveals why laymen and some doctors look on vitamin B_{12} as a great energizer. As recently as the 1920s, family doctors like me cured practically no one. Surgeons in the 1920s cured patients routinely by repairing defects and chopping out diseased tissue, but what could a medical doctor do? We knew how to prevent a few infections by immunization, relieve pain and diarrhea with narcotics, suppress seizures with phenobarbital, and fever with aspirin. Dramatic cures were rare, and doctors enjoyed them as much as patients.

Then two Harvard physicians discovered a cure for pernicious anemia: liver—in large amounts; liver is a rich source of B_{12} although that discovery occurred later.

A nasty disease and not rare, pernicious anemia results from vitamin B_{12} deficiency despite a normal diet. For unknown reasons, victims lose the ability to produce stomach acid. Without acid, the stomach can't produce a substance known as intrinsic factor. Without intrinsic factor, your intestine loses almost all ability to absorb vitamin B_{12} (known as extrinsic factor before it was named).

The liver stores huge amounts of B_{12}, so years pass before a patient runs out. Progressive weakness brought the majority to the doctor, but the body adapts amazingly well to anemia that develops slowly, so these patients lived on with frighteningly few red blood cells, perhaps 10 percent of normal, before they finally died. Pernicious anemia also damages nerves, so patients suffered numbness of the arms and legs and difficulty walking. They were often bedridden for years.

Within days of beginning liver therapy, red cell production increased, and within weeks weakness disappeared. It was a miracle. Only when antibiotics appeared ten years later did a similar miracle enter the popular imagination.

Just as everyone knows antibiotics cure "infections," they assume B_{12} restores energy. That's why patients often suggest they need these—and why doctors happily prescribe them for ailments they don't help (but which nothing else helps either).

Vitamin B$_{12}$ is treatment of choice for:

Vitamin B$_{12}$ deficiency. Besides pernicious anemia, deficiency occurs if a surgeon removes your stomach (the source of intrinsic factor) or the far end of your small intestine (where B$_{12}$ is absorbed). Less often it occurs following removal of smaller parts of the stomach or intestine, probably because that allows bacteria to grow in the small intestine, and they consume the B$_{12}$ passing through.

It's almost impossible to become deficient by diet alone because B$_{12}$ is universally present in animal and dairy products. This means vegetarians who don't eat dairy products are at risk, but even this is rare because legumes (peas, beans, nuts) are often contaminated with germs containing vitamins. However, we advise vegetarians to take B$_{12}$ unless they drink milk.

How it works

Like folic acid, B$_{12}$ is essential for the synthesis of DNA. All growing cells require it, and blood cells require a great deal.

How dispensed

As an injectable containing 30, 100, and 1,000 micrograms, or µg (one thousandth of a milligram—a tiny amount), per milliliter. The maintenance dose is 100 to 1,000 µg per month, which is far larger than the normal requirements of 1 µg per day.

Most drugs are colorless, but not vitamin B$_{12}$, and seeing a vivid red liquid injected into your body certainly adds to B$_{12}$'s magical qualities.

Tablets of 25, 50, 100, 250, 500, and 1,000 µg. Many medical books insist injections are the only reliable treatment for pernicious anemia and similar disorders, warning that oral B$_{12}$ is positively dangerous because it's so poorly absorbed.

Some doctors disagree. Without intrinsic factor, the intestine absorbs less than 1 percent of swallowed B$_{12}$, but B$_{12}$ is cheap. If you swallow enough, enough will get through. A thousand times your daily requirement of 1 µg often works; less is dangerous. Many physicians are coming around, but you may have to bring up the subject.

Translating the label

The injectable is known as cyanocobalamin. All popular oral preparations are multivitamins, so you'll have to look hard to find B_{12} alone. If you need B_{12}, your doctor will guide you.

Side effects

Not a problem.

Interactions

None.

Allergies

Only a rare reaction to the vehicle in the injection.

Wholesale cost

Cost is $3.50 for a hundred 1,000-µg tablets, $1.50 for vial containing ten injectable doses of 1,000 µg.

PART X
Drugs You Should Know More About

Ten Underused Drugs

1. Sucralfate

Unlike their use of H2 blockers, doctors don't prescribe sucralfate for vague digestive complaints. Yet it's a better placebo because it isn't absorbed, so side effects are minimal.

Sucralfate is also a fine but neglected ulcer treatment, so mention it if you have an ulcer.

2. Amantadine

Doctors are so accustomed to prescribing an antibiotic for viral infections they forget another drug that actually works. Review the amantadine section (17.), and be prepared to bring up the subject if you think you have the flu.

3. BuSpar

Despite the popular impression, most doctors dislike prescribing tranquilizers. One good reason is that they are inappropriate for most emotional problems. Another reason, this one fair to poor, is that tranquilizers are supposed to make you feel good. Although we take pleasure from making sick patients feel normal, we frown on making them much happier than normal or euphoric. This is also why doctors are stingy with powerful pain drugs even in dying patients.

From bromides to phenobarbital, Valium, and Xanax, tranquilizers provided pleasure along with tranquility, so they acquired a bad reputation. The BuSpar (53.) family doesn't have this action, and I expect doctors to become more generous once the news spreads.

4. Salsalate and other nonacetylated salicylates

Related to aspirin, it's less powerful, but we compensate by a higher dose (1,500 mg twice a day).

Reports of massive GI bleeding from NSAIDs are making us more and more uncomfortable. No one takes them for a fatal disorder, so even a rare disaster is unacceptable—and these aren't rare.

Many doctors don't realize that Salsalate and other "nonacetylated salicylates" mentioned in the aspirin section (64.) are easier on the stomach than all popular anti-inflammatories including Motrin, Indocin, and aspirin, but this ignorance won't last as pressure mounts against NSAIDs. Salsalate is already my anti-inflammatory of choice for patients over 65 who are at highest risk of bleeding, but I'm leaning toward it for everyone.

5. Calcium

The epidemic of osteoporotic fractures deserves action as vigorous as the anticholesterol campaign that began pouring out of magazines and the media in the late 1980s. Wheels are slowly creaking in this direction as doctors lose their inhibition toward giving estrogens after menopause, but I would like to see more emphasis on calcium. Only a minority would benefit, but it's not a small minority; every woman should take a gram of calcium carbonate a day from high school on.

6. Nasal spray

Travelers suffering ear pain after a plane trip are the bread and butter of a hotel doctor, but I'm surprised at how many flight attendants and pilots call for the same problem. You'd think they know what to do.

They assure me that they've chewed gum, swallowed decongestants, and (I wince) pinched their nose and blown to "clear" their ears. *Don't* do that. The other methods are feebly effective. A nasal spray

(Neo-synephrine, Dristan, 4-Way, Afrin, Otrivin) works better.

The eustachian tube, the only connection between your middle ear and the outside world, exits deep in your nose. Swelling from a cold or allergy seals this opening, trapping air in the ear. Changes in pressure while flying or even driving over a mountain force this air to expand and contract, stretching the eardrum painfully.

The best preventative is to spray your nose before the plane takes off, wait five minutes, then spray again. This carries the spray deep inside where it can reach the eustachian tube outlet. If your ears hurt while flying, spray again. Spray before the plane begins its descent an hour before landing. All travelers should carry a spray; don't expect the plane's first aid kit to stock one.

7. Griseofulvin

Patients complain quickly when their fingernails turn yellow, but they seem less concerned about toenails. Many assume that thick, crumbly toenails are another sign of age, but nails can't age because they're already dead. Only disease makes them ugly, and nail funguses are as common as athlete's foot. Griseofulvin usually cures them provided you take it long enough.

Doctors don't like extended drug treatment for a cosmetic problem, so they rationalize by claiming it doesn't work well. I've read estimates that only 20 percent of toenail treatments succeed. My experience is better; over half of my patients are cured—at least initially.

I may be prejudiced because I treated my own toenails successfully—on the third attempt. During the first two, I took griseofulvin for eight and twelve months, and the infection returned within a year. Fifteen months in 1983 did the trick, and my nails have looked fine since. Don't try this unless you're prepared for a long haul.

8. Antidepressants

Undertreating depression once verged on a scandal, but family doctors take it more seriously now. They are more likely to neglect antidepressants for common pain disorders. If beta and calcium blockers don't reduce the frequency of migraines to a tolerable level, we should add an antidepressant, first alone, then in combination with one of the blockers.

An antidepressant at bedtime is worth trying in most chronic pain disorders such as tension headaches, low back pain, or irritable bowels. It often diminishes attacks; try one for several months.

9. Beconase or Vancenase

Although cortisone inhalers for asthma caught on quickly, family doctors have been slow to prescribe them for nasal disorders. Allergists know their value. They are probably the treatment of choice for any but the mildest hay fever and the only remedy for a hypersensitive nose (vasomotor rhinitis).

10. Placebo

Sold in bottles of 100 colorful capsules, they are grossly underused. Unfortunately, using them may involve telling a lie, which doctors hate. If a doctor says truthfully, "Take this and you'll feel better in a few days," as he hands a placebo to someone with "bronchitis," there's a chance the patient will ask:

"Is this an antibiotic?"

Lying is out of the question, and evasions like "It's as good as an antibiotic for bronchitis" sound suspicious, so doctors avoid placebos in favor of drugs with genuine value (but not for the disorder for which they're given).

While our reluctance to pretend a fake pill is real may be admirable, why don't doctors feel bad when they give a real drug as a placebo? The truth is they do suffer a twinge of guilt, but it's easy to suppress because most doctors do the same, and patients are grateful.

Ten Overused Drugs

If, after listening to a description of your illness, the doctor announced that a spirit from the local mall had taken up residence in your liver you would not feel reassured. If he asked you to lie on the floor while he sang hymns pleading with God to cast it out, your confidence in his ability would drop still lower. Yet patients from many cultures consider this normal medical practice.

Closer to home, if your doctor's prescription produced a day of cramps and diarrhea, you would certainly complain. But until late in the last century, everyone looked on a good "purge" as appropriate treatment. A physician took pride in his cathartics, and when patients discussed a doctor's reputation, they gave high marks for the violence of his purges.

This illustrates an ancient truth. A sick person who visits a doctor expects certain behavior. Although modern Western patients don't expect dances, songs, bleeding, or potions that make them miserable, this is not a mark of superiority because modern patients expect a drug. It must be one only a doctor can prescribe; over-the-counter drugs don't count. Pills are acceptable, but a shot acts faster. Of course, modern drugs really work, but this is a minor element besides the deep human desire that a doctor "do something."

Many readers would deny coming to a doctor for a drug; they just want to feel better, they would insist. If nothing will help, they won't be upset. Such patients exist, but they are a minority. I am slower than most doctors to pull out my prescription pad, so I endure more pain than most. I see the disappointment in my patients' eyes when they learn than I can't "give them something." Doctors genuinely want to help you, and we feel bad if we can't. We also feel bad if we've done our best and the patient doesn't feel "helped." So we sometimes add a prescription. Doctors also prescribe unnecessarily when they're fairly certain no treatment is required but feel uneasy doing nothing. They're really treating themselves.

My candidates for the ten most overused drugs:

1. Erythromycin

Several times a week, a hotel guest phones to assure me he doesn't require a housecall. Could I do him a favor and phone an antibiotic into a pharmacy to nip his bronchitis before it ruins his trip?

These are stressful calls. The guest is never happy to hear my discussion of aspirin, fluids, cough medicine, and the incurability of viral infections. Sometimes I hear a hint that I'm holding back in order to make a visit and collect a fee. In fact, I don't look forward to seeing these people. Office patients rarely make a scene when I explain they don't need an antibiotic, but hotel guests show less restraint. At the conclusion of my visit, the guest—often a busy businessman—must reach into his wallet and pull out a good deal of cash. If he feels he's not getting his money's worth, the visit ends on a very unpleasant note.

2. Tetracycline

Tetracycline comes as a two-color capsule. Erythromycin is usually a red tablet, so choosing which placebo may be a matter of the doctor's color preference that day. Tetracycline upsets the stomach less, but it's easy to avoid erythromycin upsets by giving too little. Taking 250 mg three times a day of either is always inadequate for an adult and four times a day is marginal except for small people. A five-day course is also worthless. Remember that strep throat requires ten days (and that you shouldn't get tetracycline for strep) and pneumonia or serious chronic bronchitis requires at least ten days of 500 mg four times a day.

3. Amoxicillin

Doctors hardly ever misuse plain penicillin because of its reputation as the original miracle antibiotic. Instead, they give amoxicillin. Although useful for ear and bladder infections, patients mostly receive amoxicillin as a placebo for viral coughs, sore throats, and sinus congestion.

To repeat my warning from the amoxicillin chapter: if you need penicillin (to treat strep, for example) you should never receive amoxicillin. It works no better, costs much more, and doesn't avoid penicillin reactions.

4. Ceclor

A public relations triumph but also a good drug, Ceclor differs from the above drugs in two important ways:

A. It's spectacularly expensive and—

B. You'll often get Ceclor for an infection it cures (although cheaper antibiotics are the choice).

Just as you don't want a placebo, you don't want Ceclor when an antibiotic at a tenth of the price works as well. Study the appropriate chapters before seeing the doctor and decide if you want to suggest an alternative. Remember that your doctor may not realize how expensive it is.

5. Cipro

Ciprofloxin has three qualities doctors love. It's new. Even better, it's the first member of an important new class of antibiotic called fluoro-quinolones. Finally, it kills a broad spectrum of bacteria; few oral antibiotics kill more. Miles Pharmaceuticals has spent a fortune in free samples and glossy journal advertisements, but it has paid off in an avalanche of unnecessary prescriptions.

Despite being the fourth most-prescribed antibiotic in the U.S. (after amoxicillin, Ceclor, and Augmentin), Cipro is not a treatment of choice for common infections. Now and then I use it as an alternative for prostatitis, gonorrhea, or traveler's diarrhea, but for respiratory, skin, and bladder infections, half a dozen older antibiotics work as well or better at a tenth of the cost (Cipro rivals Ceclor in the price department). I hardly ever see disorders for which Cipro is a real advance: severe intestinal infections (such as typhoid or shigellosis) as well as bone and urinary tract infections by unusual bacteria.

Don't make the mistake of believing that Cipro's very broad spectrum is a sign of superiority. If you recall my discussion of broad versus narrow spectrum in the Ceclor section (7.), narrow is better. In many ways, "broad spectrum" is a weasel word (like "exceptional child" or "senior citizen"). It sounds good but isn't.

6. Thyroid

Nowadays that means pure hormone, L-thyroxine (Synthroid, Levoxine). If you're taking plain "thyroid" it's even more likely you don't need it.

Some experts estimate that one in 50 to 100 adults suffers an underactive gland, and this is true if you count everyone taking thyroid. However, one doctor studied 1,500 patients during a routine exam and found six (one in 250). Another took patients off their thyroid to see how many didn't need it. Sixty percent didn't.

Most worthless thyroid goes to women complaining of chronic fatigue or difficulty losing weight. Although these are frustrating problems, conscientious doctors have a modest success rate. However, a quick exam, a few sympathetic words about a "slow metabolism," and a thyroid prescription save the doctor a good deal of time (at least on the first visit), and patients never complain. Many are convinced they feel better within a few days although thyroxine takes two weeks to work.

It's cheap, small doses are harmless, and many patients look uncomfortable when I suggest stopping for a month to check their natural hormone level (testing for thyroxine while taking thyroxine won't help). So I don't insist, but everyone on thyroid should review the thyroid hormone section (71.) and give the matter thought. You might be healthier than you think.

7. Zantac

The H2 blockers broke all speed records in leaping from approved drug to folk remedy. Within a few years, Americans discarded their baking soda, Alka-Seltzer, Pepto-Bismol, and antacids, relying on a Tagamet for every bloat, cramp, and belch.

Although less common than garden-variety dyspepsia, gas, and irritable bowels, ulcers and reflux are much easier to treat, so doctors passed out Tagamet, Zantac, Axid, or Pepcid for every gastrointestinal problem hoping for equally satisfying results. Doctors did this not only because they were lazy (treating irritable bowels and nonulcer dyspepsia takes time—see my book *The Complete Book of Better Digestion*) and ignorant (they didn't know how) but also because patients were genuinely pleased. Just as laypeople know that antibiotics cure "infections," they know that Zantac cures ulcers. If it relieves one bellyache, why not another?

Common digestive disorders come and go unpredictably, so it's easy to give Zantac credit. If life remains tolerable there's no rush to make a change. If not, let the doctor know. You don't need a gastroenterologist for most digestive disorders, but if your doctor doesn't want to spend time talking about diet and lifestyle changes and is tired of telling disappointed patients that some over-the-counter medications really work, that's who you'll see.

8. Darvon

Along with lesser known Dolene, this is propoxyphene, a mild pain reliever. As easy on the stomach as acetaminophen and lacking aspirin's anti-inflammatory action, it's equally effective at three times the cost. I rarely prescribe it unless patients ask, but they ask fairly often. I suspect it provides a slight buzz, but perhaps being a prescription drug gives Darvon a charisma that aspirin or Tylenol lacks. In the past, doctors worried about codeine addiction; we considered Darvon less risky. But it turns out that both have the same tiny abuse potential.

Once available as 32-mg capsules that worked as well as placebo, 65 mg is the smallest dose sold today. It equals one aspirin or Tylenol. Nowadays almost all Darvon is combined with aspirin (Darvon Compound) or acetaminophen (Darvocet), a reasonable mixture.

9. Zovirax tablets

Don't confuse this with the ointment discussed under "drugs that don't work." Although the tablets work, most genital herpes victims don't need them. Zovirax helps when sores are painful or extensive. Taken within two days of onset, it gives quick relief.

Almost every case I see consists of a few sores that may or may not itch, and I explain these will disappear within a week without treatment. Patients worry about recurrences, but Zovirax won't prevent them.

A few patients are pleased a drug isn't necessary; most aren't. Seeing their unease, I quickly add that I'll prescribe something, and I give an inexpensive antibiotic ointment as a placebo. This satisfies those who haven't heard of Zovirax. For those who have, I explain that the ointment doesn't work and that pills speed healing if taken early but have no affect after two days. I can't remember a patient who refused treatment after listening to me. The yearning for "something" is too intense. Doctors know this, so most give Zovirax without my explanation.

10. Micronase

As you read in its section, Micronase (73.) and other oral hypoglycemics treat non-insulin-dependent (adult-onset) diabetes. They are fine for thin patients, not for the overweight majority. If you're overweight and taking a pill for your diabetes, this may be unnecessary or positively harmful. If blood sugar remains elevated, the correct treatment is insulin or less food. If your sugar is normal while taking Micronase, it would be normal without pills if you ate less—a much healthier course.

The cells of an adult diabetic resist insulin action, so the pancreas work overtime. Oral hypoglycemics force the pancreas to work even harder. More than any tissue, fat encourages insulin resistance. The less fat, the less resistance. As weight drops so does blood sugar. If the patient loses enough, sugar may return to normal, so the pancreas stops straining. You should appreciate this because eventually an overworked pancreas exhausts itself and stops producing, making insulin essential.

Ten Drugs That Don't Work

The FDA has been reviewing over-the-counter drugs for 20 years, eliminating those that don't work, but they're not through and tend to pass over questionable drugs that do no harm.

The mere fact that a drug is sold only by prescription does not guarantee quality. Many turn out to be surprisingly feeble, but until they stop making money or reveal dangerous side effects, they remain on the market.

This list is far from complete.

1. Simethicone

A gas remedy. Used by veterinarians for a bloating disease in cattle, it's present in many antacids, digestive remedies (Flatulex, Digestrol), and in pure form as Mylicon-80. Purported to work by breaking up gas bubbles and dispersing foam, this wouldn't eliminate gas even if it were true. Simethicone is harmless, but you're better off with activated charcoal. For more advice on gas, read the chapter in my *Complete Book of Better Digestion*.

2. Kaolin and 3. Pectin

Treatment for diarrhea, you'll find them in Kaopectate, Donnagel, and Parapectolin.

If you like natural remedies, these qualify. Kaolin is powdered clay, pectin a gluelike carbohydrate extracted from citrus peels or apples. They are supposed to thicken watery bowel contents, but there's no evidence they do.

4. Guaifenesin (glyceryl guaiacolate)

An expectorant—something to force the respiratory tract to produce more mucus. You'll find it in innumerable cough remedies (Robitussin, Entex, Hycotuss, Naldecon, Novahistine, Quibron, Triaminic).

A dry cough is terribly unsatisfying. "I can't get anything out," patients complain. "If I could just cough it up . . . " I explain that this is how one feels when a virus irritates the bronchial tubes. *Nothing is stuck down there!* Nothing needs loosening. Cough remedies (codeine, dextromethorphan) and cough drops help modestly.

This is one of many truths that few patients believe, and I have no objection to guaifenesin, a safe drug. I don't prescribe good expectorants for minor infections because they're too toxic. The last time you threw up, you may have noticed mucus filling your throat as the moment approached; good expectorants cause nausea. Syrup of ipecac works fine; so do potassium iodide and ammonium chloride.

Researching this section, I was impressed with the number of experts who informed me the best expectorant is several glasses of water. "Drink lots of water," I hear my colleagues advising. "It will loosen your mucus."

Like so much traditional advice, it's wrong. Mucus is a thick chemical produced by special cells lining your respiratory tract. Swallowing extra water won't change its chemistry. You're better off dripping water on the mucus after it's secreted into your bronchial tubes. Try breathing steam from a vaporizer or hot shower. But remember—there's probably no excess mucus down there.

5. Zovirax ointment

Now history, the genital herpes panic of the early 1980s produced as much distress as AIDS today along with the usual worthless cures. Respectable researchers found that ether, dimethyl sulfoxide, and several live viral vaccines healed herpes nicely; nutritionists prescribed the amino acid, lysine, as well as various combinations of vitamins with superb results, and doctors used common sense in prescribing idoxuridine or vidarabine, drugs useful for herpes eye or brain infections. Everyone now agrees these were useless, but you would have heard plenty of arguments at the time.

Zovirax (acyclovir) produced spectacular media attention as well as scientific excitement not only because it worked but because it was a major advance—the first nonpoisonous antiviral drug. Because of this furor no layperson and many doctors didn't realize the ointment doesn't work. This was no secret. The manufacturer announced it publicly, and every journal article pointed it out. Although Zovirax tablets work nicely, the ointment has *no* affect on a recurrence. Used for first attacks (which are much less common) it shortens the course by a day or two.

Unfortunately, ointment was all we had for a year until the pills appeared. Patients with sores on their genitals begged for treatment, and doctors yearn to help patients even if nothing helps, so Zovirax ointment became a smash hit. Even today doctors prescribe it for a host of skin conditions including fever blisters for which it is also useless.

6. Antispasmodics

A huge class of remedies, they are supposed to relax the digestive tract, relieving the pain of an irritable colon, dyspepsia, bowel cramps, and gas bloating. Examples are Donnatol, Librax, Bentyl, Robinul, Darbid, Kinesed, Belladenal, Pathilon, and Pro-banthine. An ancient equivalent, tincture of belladonna, is still available.

Some antispasmodics include a tranquilizer (usually phenobarbital, the cheapest; Librax has Librium), but all contain an "anticholinergic" for the spasm. Cholinergic nerves belong to the parasympathetic nervous system (see scopolamine, 48.), the counterpart of the sympathetic system discussed in the Clonidine section (31.). As you'd expect, cholinergic nerves stimulate the digestive tract. Blocking this action is easy; belladonna, atropine, and scopolamine have worked for centuries.

Although an adequate dose puts your bowels to sleep, one experience with complete cholinergic blockade will persuade you a spastic colon isn't so bad. Besides the GI tract, cholinergic nerves supply other organs including the bladder, salivary glands, sweat glands, and eye muscles. If you can't remember all these, a large dose of anticholinergic will remind you because you'll suffer from difficulty urinating, a dry mouth, dry skin, dizziness, and blurry vision.

Manufacturers solved this problem neatly by reducing the dose until most patients don't notice side effects. This is also too low to work.

7. Muscle relaxants

Victims of back and neck pain wonder if something to "relax the muscles" would help, and doctors oblige with carisoprodol (Soma), metaxalone (Skelaxin), cyclobenzaprine (Flexeril), and methocarbamol (Robaxin). I don't prescribe them unless a patient asks.

Useful drugs exist for spasticity as the result of disease (strokes, multiple sclerosis), but they are fairly toxic. Experts are skeptical that a safe drug can relax normal muscles without relaxing the rest of you. Valium works fine. Twenty years ago it was the leading muscle relaxant, but its role as a tranquilizer tainted it slightly, so everyone was happy when newer drugs took over. They are not superior.

None of these relaxes muscles directly. All slow nerve transmission in the brain or spinal cord; if they worked mostly on nerves supplying skeletal muscles, they would do what advertisements claim, but they seem to affect all nerves equally. If you want to relax, take a tranquilizer.

For muscle injury, try heat, massage, and an NSAID—but remember that minor injuries heal without treatment.

8. Antiseptics

These include alcohol, Mercurochrome, merthiolate, tincture of iodine, hydrogen peroxide, betadine, and other brightly colored or smelly chemicals. Used more vigorously than most people can tolerate, some disinfect intact skin, so they're useful before surgery, but don't put antiseptics on abrasions, cuts, or other injuries. They do more harm than good.

9. Antibiotic creams

Neosporin, Bacitracin, Polysporin, Mycitracin.

A good rule on skin injuries is: don't try to kill germs. Germs are tough. They live in the same world as you and I, exposed to pollution, heat and cold, bad food, and dangerous neighbors. Germs are accustomed to living around irritating chemicals, so it takes powerful poisons to discourage them. Compare this to living skin cells that spend their lives bathed in soothing tissue fluid whose temperature and salt concentration hardly change. Plain tap water kills them. Applied to injured skin, antibiotic creams are occasionally irritating. Antiseptics kill your cells more efficiently than the average germ. Don't use them. Wash off dirt under a tap and clean the area around (but not in) the wound with soap and water. Your body is accustomed to dealing with germs, but it can't handle dirt. See a doctor if you can't get dirt out of a wound. Otherwise, leave it alone. A dry, nonstick dressing will protect against accidental bumps; that's all it accomplishes.

This advice is impossible to follow because humans have an uncontrollable desire to put something on damaged skin. Patients always rush to the medicine cabinet after an accident. Family doctors routinely give in to the urge (but not plastic surgeons who are careful to minimize skin damage). When I work in emergency rooms, nurses look deeply uncomfortable when I ask them not to dunk every laceration or abrasion in a bowl of antiseptic.

Follow my instructions for getting rid of dirt. Then if you can't resist the urge to apply something, use —

Mercurochrome. Although a weak antiseptic, it stains skin a brilliant red. The sight convinces most patients that something important has happened. If you prefer more action try —

Hydrogen peroxide, an unstable compound that foams on contact with the skin. This is harmless but gives a vivid impression of blowing germs to smithereens.

10. Drugs to revive the brain

Senility in someone you love may be more tragic than a visible disease because it destroys what we love most: an individual's personality. Clearly something terrible is happening in the brain.

Laymen have always believed that senility results from a declining oxygen supply, either generally or through "strokes." This seems reasonable, so doctors took it seriously, and they still do. Reasonable medical theories have amazing staying power despite lack of evidence. Somewhere in the U.S. as you read this, a researcher with an oxygen chamber has recruited the local nursing home for a course of treatment. Eventually a journal article will appear giving results of before-and-after mental testing, and scores will be higher after oxygen. Medical journals have published such studies for 50 years, yet no expert advises giving oxygen to your elderly relatives. It's impractical, expensive, and works feebly if at all.

Similarly, a host of drugs are supposed to increase blood flow to the brain. Among them are papaverine (Papavid), niacin, isoxsuprine, nylidrin (Ardilin), and ergoloid mesylates (Hydergine). Enthusiasts point to studies showing good results with their favorite, but taken together the evidence is flimsy, and most neurologists are not impressed. Alzheimer's, the leading cause of senility, is almost certainly a disease of nerves, not of diminished blood supply. As of 1993, Tacrine is the only drug proven to improve the senility of Alzheimer's disease, and it works by affecting neurotransmitters and nerve transmission in complex ways. Although the improvement is only mild, Tacrine may herald a more effective class of drugs; if so I'll include one in the next edition of this book.

Index

The United States and Latin American Wars

1932-1942

The United States
and Latin American Wars
1932-1942

BRYCE WOOD

Columbia University Press

NEW YORK AND LONDON 1966

Bryce Wood is an Executive Associate of the
Social Science Research Council.

327.7308

W 85 w

56259

Nov, 1966

Preface

THIS BOOK grew out of an interest in the experience of American countries in trying to prevent and limit the three international conflicts that broke out in South America in the decade beginning in 1932: the Chaco War between Bolivia and Paraguay; the Leticia dispute between Colombia and Peru; and the Marañón question between Ecuador and Peru.

These struggles compromised the belief that America differed from Europe in being a continent of peace; the Latin American states were weak, but they proved capable of ferocious fighting at their levels of firepower. The conflicts also broke a custom, for there had been no serious outbreak of interstate violence in South America since the War of the Pacific, a full half-century earlier. Further, these wars, declared or undeclared, brought into question the very existence of what had come to be called the "inter-American system."

The obligations and procedures of the system were refined and improved at the six major conferences of American states held from 1933 to 1942. It was, however, in these same years that three wars broke out and were fought to finishes that the inter-American system affected only in slight degree. It was in this era, also, that the Good Neighbor policy was developed by the United States.

If attention is given only to the ultimately peaceful settlements of these conflicts and to the documents produced by the conferences, it is possible to regard the system as an effective one. If, on the other hand, attention is given to the course of the conflicts and the negotiations accompanying them, the system appears as inadequate and as requiring radical transformation if future wars were to be prevented.

It is the discrepancy between the ideal and the real—between peace in aim and war in fact—that this study tries to explore. Why were clear obligations not respected? Why was "America" helpless when American states fought each other? If the United States had responsibilities as the single great power in the system, why were they not carried out? How far did the United States go in making influential its concern for peace?

In dealing with these questions, this book follows the intergovernmental negotiations, for they have not previously been set forth on the basis of comprehensive access to official documentation of the United States. In addition, an attempt is made to relate the roles played by governments to the scenario as written at inter-American conferences, and as influenced by impulses, ideas and aspirations of statesmen of American countries.

The unhappy experience of the American states in this period may have induced them to accept the obligations of peaceful settlement of disputes in the treaties of 1947 and 1948 that established the Organization of American States. The full story of these disputes cannot be told until the records of the contestants themselves become available, and there remain many unanswered questions. In what will probably be a long "meanwhile," so far as the Latin American countries are concerned, the view from Washington may be of interest to men who are puzzle-solving or community-building animals, or both.

Acknowledgments

TO Grayson Kirk of Columbia University I should like to express appreciation for encouragement at the outset of this study.

My thanks go to the Rockefeller Foundation and the American Philosophical Society for financial assistance and to the Social Science Research Council for a grant of time; and to Joseph H. Willits, formerly of the Foundation and Pendleton Herring of the Council for their personal interest in my research.

Access to the documents of the Department of State was greatly aided by John C. Dreier and Edward A. Jamison, and by G. Bernard Noble, former Director of the Historical Office, and E. Taylor Parks, Chief, Research Guidance and Review Division of that Office, whose own scholarly concerns place other scholars in their debt, because of their appreciation of the aims of research no less than of the Department's need to protect the frankness of despatches and memoranda.

My visit to Asunción in 1962 was made pleasant and memorable by the hospitality of James S. Cunningham of the United States Embassy, who showed me some of the Chaco's avifauna and terrain.

In Latin America, interviews were of great value in refining interpretations, and in learning of the availability of documents and maps. I wish to record my profound thanks for their courtesy in receiving me to Mauricio Nabuco, former Brazilian Ambassador to the United States and Secretary-General of the Brazilian Foreign Office in 1942; and to Julio Tobar Donoso, Foreign Minister, 1938--

1942, and at present a member of the Supreme Court of Ecuador. I am also deeply indebted to a number of other officials and private citizens in Latin America who in manifold ways aided an itinerant scholar but to whom personal thanks would be inappropriate in this place.

To the members of the staff of the Historical Office and of the Records Service Center of the Department of State I am grateful for their sustained concern in making pleasant a search for records that occasionally outran the scope of indices; Doris E. Austin, Margaret G. Martin, Marion Terrell, Dorothy A. Cross, Anna Vukovich; and Mary Ellen Milar and Clarence E. Holmes.

Herman Kahn and his colleagues of the Franklin D. Roosevelt Library aided materially in finding letters and other personal documents that added color to the official record.

To immediate and affiliated associates of Columbia University Press I wish to proffer thanks: Kathryn W. Sewny, for editorial advice; Vaughn Gray, for transforming my rough sketches into orderly maps; and Edwin N. Iino, for the index.

Virginia Staman Wood, substantive collaborator and procedural associate, has been, happily, largely responsible for keeping this volume from being longer and appearing later.

Contents

The United States and Latin American Wars

1932-1942

Introduction

ONE OF THE OLDEST, most cherished, and most consistently sought objectives of United States policy toward the countries of Latin America is the maintenance of peace among them. In every Latin American war during the past hundred years the United States has attempted to bring about peace. In all the cases during this period when border incidents led to sustained fighting, as in the Leticia affair in 1932 or the Marañón conflict in 1941, the United States took a leading part in finding paths to peaceful settlement. In the many lesser disputes the Department of State has aided in the restoration of amicable relations, often by participating in intricate negotiations for periods of several years. The creation and propagation of treaties of arbitration and conciliation have been the concern of successive administrations since the inception of the modern Pan American movement.

The lively interest of the United States in Latin American disputes has arisen from various sources, some of them more important than others at different periods. From the early days of the republic there has existed a feeling that the Americas should be, as distinct from Europe, a continent of peace; this feeling has, of course, been shared in Latin America. A sense of responsibility for guiding the Latin American states toward peaceful modes of international relationships has been manifested by the United States, particularly since 1900. Following its rejection of membership in the League of Nations, this sense of responsibility seemed to deepen, and the years from 1920 to 1942 mark the period of greatest peace-keeping activity by the United States. The peace movement in the United States numbered among its public adherents many men of affairs who, particularly after World War I, were moved by humanitarian motives and were willing to go to great pains to avert conflict between states in the Americas.

At the same time some of these men of affairs were ordering or supporting the use of force by the United States to overturn or to maintain governments in countries of Central America and the Caribbean. In Washington, however, approval of the use of force by the United States was not seen as inconsistent with condemnation of the use of force by Latin American countries. These two lines of conduct were really part of a single system of thought. The Marines were regarded as being an arm of the law—international law, in this case, as interpreted and upheld by the United States. In this view, certain standards of order and respect for property had to be observed by all governments as members of a civilized community, and the United States represented civilization north of the Panama Canal. Equally characteristic of a civilized community was the maintenance of peace among its members. The United States rarely undertook to enforce peace between states in the Americas, but it did feel a deep responsibility to assist morally, ceremonially, and institutionally in the maintenance of peace.

The compatibility of these two policies within the legal concept of a civilized community adequately accounts for their contemporaneous association. They later came to be looked upon as incompatible when the United States was persuaded that its unilateral enforcement of disputed legal standards of behavior was politically embarrassing, morally indefensible, and economically unrewarding. A new theory was then developed that united the traditional concern for peace among the Latin American countries with a renunciation of the use of force on the part of the United States itself. After 1931 fewer and fewer official references were made to the concept of a civilized community. The new concept was that of a good neighborhood, and, instead of law and force, the new methods found for settling disputes between the United

States and Latin American countries were the manifold ways of political compromise.[1]

Armed conflicts between countries in Latin America have not been of frequent occurrence. Since the War of the Pacific in the early 1880s, war has been declared only by Paraguay against Bolivia in 1933. On only two other occasions—in the Leticia affair between Colombia and Peru and in the Ecuador-Peru conflict, which will here be called the Marañón dispute—has organized fighting by national armies proceeded significantly beyond the stage of border affrays. The armies of Latin America have been engaged more often in civil wars than in wars between countries.

If the Latin American countries have only rarely been belligerent in the past hundred years, it cannot be denied that they have been disputatious. Of the approximately thirty boundaries demarcating the Latin American states, disputes over about twenty of them survived into the twentieth century. By 1942, however, nearly all controversies had been terminated in the sense that most of the boundaries had been formally established. The areas that remained undefined lay between the Dominican Republic and Haiti, between Honduras and Nicaragua, between Argentina and Chile in the Beagle Channel, and between Ecuador and Peru.

That these boundary disputes should have lasted so long is less remarkable than that they should have given rise to so few serious outbreaks of fighting. It should not be forgotten that only in 1955 was a boundary dispute between the states of Arizona and California finally settled nor that the United States and Mexico reached an agreement only in 1963 about the sovereignty over the Chamizal tract on the Rio Grande. The extended duration of boundary disputes in Central and South America was due in part to the vagueness of eighteenth and early nineteenth century legal documents on which claims were based and in part to the fact that many boundary areas were sparsely populated. In the Chaco, for example, as late as 1933, there were few if any Bolivian settlements other than military posts east of Villa Montes, and one of the most westerly Paraguayan villages was the Mennonite Colony, about seventy-five miles from the Paraguay River. Where the land was forbidding and contacts were few, boundary disputes for many years were little more than debates among lawyers. In the absence of a judge or of practical men who were more interested in drawing a frontier so they would know where they stood than in arguing the meaning of ancient manuscripts, the lawyers maintained their arguments, so notoriously indeed that they came to be called "doctors of boundaries." With the growth of population and improvements in overland transportation, governments finally found it necessary to know the exact limits of their dominions, as did Panama and the United States in defining a part of the boundary of the Canal Zone by starting from "a tack in a stake."

Although most of the disputes arose over fairly small areas where the general course of a frontier was mutually accepted, the Bolivia-Paraguay (Chaco) and Ecuador-Peru (Marañón) conflicts each involved an area of more than fifty thousand square miles. The dimensions of the prizes in these cases combined with other causes to make it impossible to find peaceful solutions without an intervening trial by battle.

Many Latin American boundary disputes were solved simply by negotiations between two countries. Brazil's statesman, Baron do Rio Branco, established an outstanding reputation as a diplomat by peacefully completing a series of boundary treaties with Brazil's neighbors. Other disputes were settled by arbitration. During the nineteenth century it was customary for Latin American states to name a European government or monarch as arbitrator; the king of Spain was chosen on several occasions, and the kings of Great Britain, Italy, the president of France, the government of Switzerland, and the Pope also served as arbitrators. In only one dispute, that between Bolivia and Peru in 1902, was a Latin American arbitrator, the president of Argentina, selected by the disputants. The Latin American states called infrequently on the United States in the nineteenth century for aid in the settlement of disputes by means of arbitration, but during the first four decades of the twentieth century the United States was formally asked for this type of assistance on four occasions.

Between 1914 and 1942 simple bilateral boundary agreements and arbitral awards were no longer being made in the Americas. They were largely, although not entirely, replaced by compromise settlements attained with the aid of mediators, either before or after a resort to armed force. It is significant that, on the one hand, in the seven years from 1902 to 1909 no less than five boundary disputes were settled by arbitration and six by bilateral negotiations; and that, on the other hand, between 1911 and 1942, of six boundary disputes terminated, only one, that between Guatemala and Honduras, was arbitrated. The plebiscite determined upon by the Coolidge arbitration in the Tacna-Arica case was never held, and the arbitration that followed the Chaco War was a mere formality, since it provided only a contrived judicial sanction for a diplomatically determined boundary. In the Guatemala-Honduras case, the arbitration by Chief Justice Charles Evans Hughes was preceded by intermittent mediatory efforts by the United States from 1917 to 1931. As to the other five settlements, mediation by the United States alone resulted in the settlement of three; in the remaining two, the conflicts over the Chaco and the Marañón, the United States played a leading role in mediatory groups which developed political formulas that made possible a return to peaceful relationships.

These figures should be interpreted with caution. Arbitration is a procedure commonly used when the difference is a minor one or, less commonly, when the two disputants are nearly equally confident of a favorable award. The very fact that certain boundary controversies were the last to be settled suggests that they may have been the most resistant to arbitral techniques. The Chaco and Marañón conflicts involved large territories, and treaties of settlement were not ratified until 1938 and 1942. However, the Bolivia-Peru frontier dispute also comprised an extensive region, and arbitration brought it to an end in 1909. The question remains whether, if the populations of the countries in the first two disputes had been in closer contact before 1910, arbitral settlements might not have been consummated. In this connection, it is of importance to note that, in the Ecuador-Peru controversy, the inhabited boundary zone between the Andes and the Pacific was fairly well recognized on both sides and was little changed in 1942; it was over the nearly empty spaces east of the Andes that the dispute endured.

It is at least arguable that the decline in numbers of arbitrations after 1914 was due in part to a new-found preference for political, as distinct from juridical, ways of drawing boundary lines. This contention—for it is no more than that—may be strengthened when it is recalled that the reduced use of arbitration for boundary disputes accompanied the gradual weakening of the idea that there was an international standard of justice that strong states were entitled to uphold against weak states, sometimes by the use of force.

The reasons for this phenomenon are not entirely clear, but contributory factors may be worth speculation. The institution of arbitration, which depends absolutely on the faithful fulfillment by governments of their previous commitments to accept the award—a rule as fundamental as the more general principle of international law that treaties shall be respected—suffered three damaging assaults in America during the years 1910–14. In 1910 Ecuador refused to continue with the nearly completed arbitration by the King of Spain in its dispute with Peru, as the result of the premature disclosure of a probable decision that was regarded as unacceptable in Ecuador. A further blow to arbitration was struck by the United States when it rejected the decision of the arbitral tribunal in the Chamizal dispute with Mexico in 1911. Three years later Panama declined to recognize the decision of Edward D. White, Chief Justice of the United States, in its boundary difference with Costa Rica. It may have been this experience that Ambassador Francisco Castillo Nájera of Mexico had in mind in 1938 when he told Sumner Welles in reference to Mexico's oil expropriations that Mexico had no great faith in arbitration.

In addition, strong as is the tradition of arbitration in the history of international relations in the Americas, it is notable that arbitration in the nineteenth century amounted principally to an appeal to European, that is, extra-American, judgment. After 1914 many factors combined to turn the American states away from Europe and toward the United States when disputes arose. The prestige of European states declined as a consequence of World War I, along with that of their rulers as individuals. This was an important consideration in Latin America, where it was realistically recognized that the acceptance of an arbitral award depended not only on the justice of the decision but also on personal respect for the arbiter. It was probably for this reason that heads of states, and not panels of jurists, were so frequently selected as arbiters by the Latin American governments, even though it was recognized that the substance of an award would probably be determined in fact by anonymous legal experts.

After 1910 no Latin American boundary controversy was settled by a European arbitrator, and it was no accident that in the only such dispute terminated by arbitration after 1910 the arbitrator was the Chief Justice of the United States. When Panama rejected Chief Justice White's award, as mentioned above, Secretary of State William J. Bryan wrote:

The United States could not, of course, be a party to anything which would cast discredit upon the Arbitrator, who is the presiding officer of the highest court in our land. Neither could we view with indifference the baneful influence which a rejection of its award by either party would have upon arbitration as a means of adjusting disputes between nations.[2]

Panama continued to reject the award until 1921, when Secretary Hughes, in the quaintly formal language of the day, informed the Panamanian government that, unless it transferred the disputed territory to Costa Rica, "the Government of the United States will find itself compelled to proceed in the manner which may be requisite in order that it may assure itself that the exercise of jurisdiction is appropriately transferred," and the boundary determined in accord with the "award of the Chief Justice of the United States," and, in another sector, with the award of former President Loubet of France.[3]

Secretary Hughes's earlier service on the United States Supreme Court may have added a bit of stiffness to this communication, which was nothing less than a threat to employ force if Panama did not comply within a "reasonable time." After agonized protests and the sending of a special mission to several countries in South America in a fruitless attempt to secure aid against Hughes's threat, Panama gave in. Therefore, in 1931, when Guatemala and Honduras chose Hughes, then Chief Justice, as arbitrator, each had the best of reasons to believe that the other would accept the award, and in the outcome that belief was fully justified. It was apparent that the

office of Chief Justice of the United States had acquired a respect
not exceeded by any other arbiter of the age. This is believed to be
the only instance in which the United States employed a threat of
force in the Americas to obtain acceptance of a previous arbitral
decision, and the only occasion after 1903 when the United States
interfered in like manner in any American international controversy.

The prestige of the United States as a center of power and therefore as a source of respected judgment in controversies among
Latin American states was greatly enhanced by the initiative taken
by the Department of State in expressing its concern that peace be
maintained; by the assurance felt by Latin American governments
that the Department would give serious and detailed consideration
to each case; and by the reputation for impartiality that it was
gradually conceded the Department deserved. This reputation was
among the Department's most zealously guarded and carefully culti-
vated possessions. It is remarkable that even in the 1920s, when
Washington was most severely criticized for its intervention in
Latin America, states of both South and Central America did not
hesitate to appeal to Washington as an impartial participant in the
settlement of international disputes. In the Tacna-Arica controversy, for example, President Calvin Coolidge was named as arbitrator to decide whether a plebiscite should be held, and President
Herbert Hoover was largely responsible for the ultimately successful compromise. One of the more convincing evidences of the
Department's objectivity was that its gloomy expectation that it
would become the butt of criticism from both sides in a dispute was
regularly fulfilled.

In addition, the rejection by the United States of the Covenant of
the League of Nations and its isolationist policies in the 1920s combined with the growth of closer inter-American relationships in the
slow rhythm of Pan American conferences to stimulate the seeking
of American solutions to American disputes. The League of Nations
formally interposed in both the Chaco and Leticia disputes, but it
did so in each case only after the American states, including the
United States, had made protracted, vain efforts to avert armed
struggles. In the Chaco dispute the League was even less successful
than the American states. In the Leticia affair the League's action

consisted of the appointment of a commission to direct what amounted to a reoccupation of Leticia by Colombian troops; this was an operation for which the American states were then organizationally unprepared and which neither Brazil nor the United States cared to undertake. The League served the dual function of barely saving face for the government of Peru and of freeing Brazil and the United States from responsibility for an action that would assuredly have been an historic and never-forgotten source of Peruvian resentment. This was certainly a useful function, but it was not one that Colombia and Peru were willing to recognize formally; in the protocol of May 24, 1934, terminating the dispute, no reference whatever was made to the League of Nations or its commission. The protocol asserts in its preamble that "the proscription of war" is a fundamental duty of states, and that "this duty is the more agreeable for the States which compose the American community, among which exist historical, social and sentimental ties which cannot be weakened by divergencies or events which must always be considered in a spirit of reciprocal understanding and good will." [4] It was the expression of pride in the achievements of the "American community" rather than gratitude toward or dependence on the League of Nations that was at that moment most characteristic of the frame of mind of Latin American diplomats.

In the course of inter-American relations since 1823, the use of the term "American community" in 1934 takes on considerable significance. There were alternatives to this expression, notably "Latin American community" and "world community." Whether or not the principal negotiators of the Leticia protocol, Roberto Urdaneta Arbeláez for Colombia and Victor M. Maúrtua for Peru, who were ably assisted by Afranio de Mello Franco for Brazil, gave anxious consideration to this choice of words, their reference to the "American community" is an important fact from the point of view of the United States. After the several failures of the Latin American states in the first half of the nineteenth century to form an international organization among themselves, the Pan American relationship became a reality, however tenuous, after 1889. That relationship was less important in 1934 for its positive achievements in international cooperation than in assuring the presence of the

United States as part of the American community in the minds of the statesmen of Latin America. The presence of United States delegates at official Pan American gatherings in the previous forty-five years had given the United States a secure place in the concept of an American community, whatever may be said of the accomplishments of the Pan American conferences in that period. So secure was that place that it was not destroyed, although it was shaken, by the United States interventions in the Caribbean states between 1900 and 1927.

The presence of the United States unquestionably was a deterrent to the fulfillment of desires for the formation of a Latin American community, although it would be difficult to demonstrate that the Department of State's policy was principally or even significantly motivated by this aim in the years before 1929. On the contrary, the United States government in the 1920s gave to the Latin American countries an excellent opportunity to forsake the American community either for a regional association of their own or for the League of Nations. Between 1920 and 1933, and particularly after the Havana Conference of 1928, the Pan American relationship was nearer to destruction than at any time after 1889. If the South American states had been given leadership by a combination of governments, including Argentina and Chile, and perhaps Brazil, a Latin American community might have been formed in the second half of the decade of the 1920s. Or, alternatively, if Brazil had not been given cause to withdraw from the League of Nations in 1926, it is possible that the South American states might have become sufficiently accustomed to working together at Geneva as to have formed their own community when the League of Nations began to dissolve following the Italo-Ethiopian conflict.[5]

However, Latin American leadership did not emerge, and Brazil resumed its traditionally close and friendly relationship with the United States. During this period of estrangement within the American community, the presence of the United States was most significantly manifested by its unremitting efforts to aid the Latin American states to live together in peace. Despite its own departures from what might be called the community spirit in imposing temporary armed interventions in Honduras and Nicaragua, the United

States continued to associate itself actively with the worthy cause of inter-American peace. Although the presence of the United States in the Americas after 1900 was always felt through its military and economic strength, neither military nor economic power alone could have held the Latin American states in the Pan American system nor prevented them from forming one of their own. The principal positive force exerted by Washington that tended, whether consciously or not, to keep alive the spirit of an American community during this period of strain was the leadership by the United States in attempts to maintain peace. If military interventions by the United States had been accompanied by indifference in Washington to disputes in the Americas, the impulse toward inter-American cooperation might well have become dormant, if not lifeless.

Through its sponsorship of the Central American treaties of 1923, through its support of the Gondra treaties, through its initiative in the Washington arbitration conference of 1928, the United States sustained the momentum of the Pan American ideal of association for peace. The custom of common striving, the reiterated adherence to common principles even in the face of admitted failures to realize them—these continued to be realities of the multilateral diplomacy of the American states that were not wholly without influence on the men who experienced them. The unceasing symbolic attachment of the United States to that ideal formed the stuff of the American community during the first half of the period between the two world wars. These achievements may appear insubstantial, but, like a bridge of gossamer, they spanned the time in the 1920s when interventions by the United States threatened to break the community asunder and when it was not inconceivable that the Latin American states might otherwise have formed an organization of their own. This bridge was not a chain; it could not hold the American community together. However, so long as it was kept open by the United States, it could sustain the faith of some Latin Americans and North Americans that the resuscitation of the American community might be achieved.

Although Secretaries of State Hughes, Kellogg, and Stimson defended their employment of coercion in Latin America, their attachment to the cause of peace in general was demonstrated by

their support of the movements toward disarmament and by the
Kellogg-Briand Pact. Such evidence of pacific intent in relations
among the great powers supplied ground for hope in the Americas
that the United States might ultimately renounce force as an instrument of national policy toward the small and weak nations of the
Caribbean area. This hope began to be realized as early as 1931 when
Stimson became disillusioned with intervention in Nicaragua and
embarrassed by his position there when he sought to curb the Japanese intervention in Manchuria.

The bridge of collaboration for peace was also a reminder of the
principal collective and honorable endeavor to which all the American states were still committed. More importantly, it kept alive a
feeling of responsibility and of concern about the American community on the part of an unbroken succession of Secretaries of State. It
was the tie that made inter-American affairs uniquely different from
the contacts of the United States with any other part of the globe.
Otherwise, relations with the Latin American states would have
degenerated to the level of completely bilateral military and economic interests, quite devoid of any conception of common purpose. Such a development would have meant the end of the
movement then known as Pan Americanism; a new association
might subsequently have been formed, but it would have been
different, and it would have had to cope with the disappointment
and suspicion created by the break with an aspirant past.

On the assumptions, therefore, that the preservation of the idea of
inter-American unity was desirable and that a continuity of active
collaboration in some form was necessary to such preservation, the
United States government's concern for peace played an important
and even a vital role in the survival of the series of inter-American
conferences. When Cordell Hull became Secretary of State, he
found that the seventh conference, scheduled for Montevideo in
1932, had been postponed by his predecessor for a year, "so poor was
the prospect of effective cooperation in the Western Hemisphere."
He records that he had decided long before he took office that "one
of our principles in dealing with Latin America would be religious
adherence to the principle of nonintervention." [6] Although he
added: "Actually, our task was to create a whole new spirit," this

statement was an exaggeration since the old spirit was not quite dead. A commission of five American states had for several years been struggling with the problem of peace in the Chaco, and Secretary Stimson had consulted with his colleagues in certain other American states to try to avert war between Colombia and Peru over Leticia. Hull's first action with respect to Latin America, he notes, was to continue the pacific moves begun by Stimson in the Leticia conflict.

Between 1910 and 1942 there was no sharp break in the policy followed by the United States government in exerting a pacifying influence on Latin American international conflicts. Beginning about 1932, however, that policy played a different role in the story of the development of inter-American institutions. Before 1932, as suggested above, the policy served to shield the flickering flame of the hopes engendered by Simón Bolívar and fanned by James G. Blaine. After 1932 the policy no longer stood alone as an element of inter-American unity, but it became one part of the broader policy of the good neighbor. Its importance diminished as the policies of nonintervention and of reciprocal trade agreements became major springs of inter-American collaboration and as the need for measures of hemispheric defense became imperative. In addition, the situation in which the policy of pacification had operated underwent a great change in 1932 when serious fighting broke out in the Chaco, and Peruvian irregulars took possession of Leticia. Violence on this scale among Latin American states had not occurred for decades. Secretary of State Henry L. Stimson, who had just a year previously proclaimed that military protection would not be afforded to United States citizens in the interior of Nicaragua, was in no mood to send Marines into the interior of South America to enforce armistices, and, in the depth of the economic depression, such crusading activity would certainly have come under severe criticism from the United States Congress.

Stimson vainly appealed to the combatants to cease fighting, and through mediation and conciliation he attempted, vainly, to bring about peace. Stimson's methods were followed by those of Hull, who, with equal unsuccess, exerted even less pressure on the contending states than did Stimson. When faith in the principles of the

Kellogg-Briand Pact was naively strong, Stimson spoke harshly and publicly to the Peruvians. In the long course of the Chaco War, the policy of the United States was less concerned with stopping the fighting than with the avoidance of charges that Washington was exerting pressure on either belligerent, and in the Marañón conflict in 1941–42 the United States did not lift its voice in public to condemn the Peruvian invasion of Ecuador beyond stating that the Peruvians were fishing in troubled waters.

In no comparable period in the century following 1830 were there so many conflicts between states in the Americas as in the fourteen years between 1928 and 1942. Confronted by a welter of unused and unusable treaties and a confused effort to apply principles of free enterprise in the settlement of disputes, the government of the United States did not find it possible to take the lead in the adoption of measures firm enough to prevent warfare in South America. The burdens that would have been shouldered had the United States undertaken to prevent fighting by the use of force or other effective means might have been onerous indeed. In addition, the initiation of such action by the United States would not have been in keeping with the noninterventionist principles that the United States government strove mightily to keep inviolate in other aspects of the good neighbor policy. Restrained by its tradition as well as by its new concept of policy toward Latin America and baffled by the absence of accepted procedures for the maintenance of inter-American peace, the United States in this period found itself limited to the expression of a maximum of good will amid a minimum of common effort—a policy that may be described as one of solicitude in anarchy.

All the American states, in this pre-institutional period of their society, shared the experience of failing to maintain peace. For some of them, this meant being invaded; for others, including the United States, it meant the long frustration of earnest and persistent negotiations.

In this sense, the following accounts of the Chaco, Leticia, and Marañón conflicts may be regarded as an educational process undergone by the American states. This, of course, is an interpretation after the fact and should not be taken as implying that the policy of the government of the United States had a pedagogical tinge.[7] It acted, as will be seen, primarily from other motives, but one long-range effect of its refusal to take forceful measures in these conflicts was to engender a keen appreciation in Latin America of the desirability of the organization of power in the interests of peace within the continent. Thus, the failures of the American states in the 1930s may have marked the start of a new political experiment in cooperative interstate relationships in the form of the Organization of American States.

However, between the conception and the development of American methods of cooperation for the prevention of war there was interposed an arduous and, in many ways, unhappy experience of trying to prevent, to stop, and then to settle several South American conflicts. It is this experience and the part played in it by the United States government that are the main themes of the following pages. A constant question facing Washington was a variant on the classic: "Am I my brother's keeper?" To what extent did a great power, associated with a group of weaker states, have a responsibility, either to avert the suffering attendant upon their wars or to impose settlements at the end of wars that judiciously compounded fairness and political realities? How broad were the duties that power bestowed? On the whole, the United States took a narrow view of the range of its obligations. Had it not done so, the Organization of American States might have taken quite a different form.

PART ONE

The Chaco War, 1928-1938

CHAPTER I

The Failure to Prevent War

THE CHACO WAR between Bolivia and Paraguay was the first serious conflict between states in Latin America in the twentieth century. Bolivia had lost its Pacific coastal province of Antofagasta to Chilean troops in 1879 and had given up its claim to the province in 1904. In 1929 Bolivia's hopes of getting a port on the Pacific were dashed when Peru and Chile divided the provinces of Tacna and Arica. Although Bolivian exports and imports could pass freely through the Chilean port of Arica, Bolivian political leaders considered themselves shut in without full control of a route to and a port on the ocean. Frustrated in the west, they looked from their high plateaus eastward, over the nearly uninhabited plain called the Chaco, to the Paraguay River. There, across the river from the Paraguayan capital of Asunción, some 800 miles above Buenos Aires, they fixed their extreme claims in a long territorial dispute.

In the first three decades of the twentieth century, the Bolivians moved southeastward along the Pilcomayo River and across the plain of the Chaco, building roads and a series of small forts. The advance was slowed in the rainy season when much of the land was drowned, and it was hampered in the dry season because of an almost total absence of water. In the north there was not much fighting because the terrain was a swamp the year round.[1] However, by 1928, Bolivian troops occupied outposts on a rough north-south line from about 120 miles west of Asunción on the Pilcomayo River northward for about 300 miles to a point not far northwest of Bahía

Negra, the head of barge navigation on the Paraguay River. The Paraguayan leaders, who regarded the Bolivian advances as a threat to the very existence of their country, gradually reacted by building a line of forts of their own. Regular armed forces then faced each other in more than fifty posts in territory where no boundary line had been agreed upon, which each country claimed as its own, and where the maximum east-west distance between the claims of the two countries was over 400 miles.[2] A group of Mennonites from Canada, seeking peace and isolation, had settled in the eastern Chaco in 1924; there were scattered ranches, a few bands of Indians, and some lumber camps, but the fighting took place in an area nearly uninhabited by civilians.[3]

The conflict was important not only because of its scale and duration but also because of the possibility that it might involve Argentina and Brazil. These countries bordered on Bolivia and Paraguay, as well as the Chaco, and had both economic and strategic interests to protect. Chile's concern was only slightly less great. The Chaco itself was not known to possess important mineral resources, but oil fields had been found in Bolivia close to the western Chaco, where wells of the Standard Oil Company of New Jersey had been producing small amounts of oil near Villa Montes since the early 1920s.[4]

To the government of the United States, participation in efforts to keep peace in the Chaco, as in other parts of the Americas, was no new responsibility. As far back as 1878, President Rutherford B. Hayes had made an arbitral award in a dispute between Paraguay and Argentina over a part of the southeastern Chaco. In 1928 Washington was engaged in helping Latin American states come to peaceful agreements in at least four other boundary disputes. In American conferences the United States had taken a leading part in creating an ideal of inter-American peace by exhortations, resolutions, and treaties. Since the United States was not a member of the League of Nations, the officials of the Department of State felt a special responsibility for helping in every noncoercive way to find pacific means for settling controversies among the Latin American countries. This attitude was in part attributable to the Department's view that the "fundamental concept" of the Monroe Doctrine was "the peace and safety of the Western Hemisphere through the absolute political separation of Europe from the countries of this Western World." [5]

In the early years of the Chaco dispute, the United States government resisted efforts by the League of Nations to bring about a peaceful settlement, and in this attitude the United States was supported by a number of Latin American countries that persisted in the desire to find an "American solution" to their family quarrels. Finally, the controversy was regarded in Washington as a challenge to North American leadership in the peace movement associated with the Kellogg-Briand Pact. That the Department of State took a serious interest in the dispute is demonstrated by its doggedly persistent efforts, in cooperation with other American governments, to prevent war (1928–32), to bring the fighting to an end (1932–35), and to secure a treaty of peace (1935–38). The Department's files contain over 6,500 separately numbered documents relating to the Chaco during this period, and the total number of documents may comprise an additional thousand.

The critical development of the struggle in the Chaco began with a frontier incident on December 5, 1928, when Paraguayan troops attacked and destroyed the Bolivian Fort Vanguardia [6] at the northern end of the lines of outposts. Bolivia replied by mobilizing its army and by taking Fort Boquerón near the southern end of the line. Bolivian planes dropped bombs on Bahía Negra in the first foreign aerial attack experienced by a South American town. None of the bombs exploded.[7] Paraguay immediately appealed to the Permanent Commission established in Montevideo in accordance with the Gondra Treaty of 1923. Paraguay had apparently planned to create the incident in the hope of drawing attention to the situation and bringing about diplomatic action by other countries; [8] the attack was timed to occur just before the meeting of the International Conference of American States on Conciliation and Arbitration, which opened in Washington on December 10. At the Conference, arrangements were made on January 3, 1929, for the suspension of hostilities and the appointment of a five-nation Commission of Inquiry and Conciliation. The members of the Commission were representatives of Colombia, Cuba, Mexico, Uruguay, and the United States.

The Commission arranged a settlement of the incident through a return of the two forts, but its efforts to solve the dispute as a whole by proposing arbitration met with no success. The Chairman of the Commission, General Frank R. McCoy, was reported to have maintained an attitude of impartiality "despite constant temptation to depart from it." "It was apparent throughout the negotiations that the United States was looked upon by the representatives of the Latin American countries who participated in the work of the Commission as a predominant influence even in the more remote region of South America directly affected." However, "the United States refrained from any attempt at domination or unwelcome control in a matter affecting the interests of Latin American Governments at least equally with those of the United States." [9]

McCoy himself reported that the neutral commissioners had told him that "the influence of the United States was the essential, and perhaps the only, means of settling the dispute; and, at the same time, the intimation was made that the Government of the United States should exert pressure to enforce its influence." However, he did not act on these suggestions and said that "any gesture which might imply the pre-eminence or dominance of the United States would be inconsistent and inappropriate." [10]

McCoy's position was not made easy by Bolivian requests that the Commission should force Paraguay to yield on certain points. "The refusal of the neutral Commissioners to comply even gave rise to the feeling on the part of the disappointed Delegation that the neutral Commissioners had adverse prejudice." [11]

General McCoy's impartiality set the standard for all future action of the United States in the controversy.

Aided by the Government of Uruguay, the two countries on July 24, 1930, restored the frontier situation as it was before December 5, 1928, with the return of Forts Boquerón and Vanguardia. However, attempts to reach a settlement of the dispute through direct negotiation as well as arbitration failed, and arms were purchased abroad by both disputants [12] in expectation of what began to appear as an inevitable conflict. General McCoy had earlier reported that the neutral commissioners regarded the Vanguardia and Boquerón incidents as "extremely grave symptoms and as sharp warnings that hostilities on a larger scale, and eventually war, would be the certain results, if the two countries were permitted to continue in the acute situation which had developed by the middle of December, 1928." [13]

Although Secretary of State Stimson had told the Bolivian Minister that he "had very much on his mind and heart" the situation concerning the Chaco,[14] he did not see his way clear during the following two and a half years to accept such advice as that given by President Augusto B. Leguía of Peru that "the United States should take matters in hand and address the Governments of Bolivia and Paraguay very firmly to the effect that this situation must cease and that the questions involved should be settled by arbitration with plenary powers to determine all matters in dispute once and for all." [15] Further, it does not appear that, at any time before the war began, Stimson contemplated action more forceful than cooperative participation with other American governments in friendly mediation. Feeling that the situation was "fraught with very grave danger," Stimson repeated again and again his desire to "have in being immediately some machinery which, through the exercise of friendly neutral good offices, can prevent outbreaks." Asserting that "the essential thing is the establishment of the machinery of conciliation," [16] he urged first the other neutral states, and then Bolivia and Paraguay, to get it in running order, but it was not until November 11, 1931, that representatives of Bolivia and Paraguay met in Washington with representatives of the neutral states. The purpose of the meeting was to discuss a pact of nonaggression, and it was arranged only after steady and patient efforts by the neutrals, moved by the cautious but persistent encouragement of Stimson and Francis White, Assistant Secretary of State for Latin American Affairs.

During the period of a year and a half the negotiations passed through many phases, of which only a few will be mentioned here. Throughout, the government of Paraguay made plain its desire to renew negotiations with the assistance of the neutrals.[17] The attitude of Bolivia was less clear, partly because three different governments held office in La Paz during this time. The position of the two countries differed in two important ways. First, the Bolivians had a definite goal for their troops, the west bank of the Paraguay River from Asunción north to Bahía Negra. Acquisition of the latter port at least was expected, particularly since it had been allotted to Bolivia by three negotiated but unratified treaties made by the two countries in the second half of the nineteenth century.[18] Paraguay's claim at this time to the whole of the Chaco involved a considerable land area, but no comparable essential goal at its extreme western border. Because the Paraguayans had long been in possession of the places most desired by the Bolivians, military action may have seemed necessary to Bolivians to assure getting them, since arbitration was a chancy procedure. Paraguay, while claiming all the Chaco, could readily afford to negotiate on the basis of a line somewhere in the largely uninhabited western Chaco beyond her river towns, including Bahía Negra, and west of the settled agricultural areas, particularly the Mennonite colony, which was connected by a ninety-mile railroad to Puerto Casado on the Paraguay River.[19]

In the second place, Bolivia's principal cities were either in the foothills or on the high Andean plateau. The heart of the country was a mountain fortress Paraguay could not hope to storm, while Asunción, on the plain, had no natural defenses other than the Paraguay River. A lost war could not vitally injure Bolivia, but it could end Paraguay's existence as an independent state. "To the Paraguayan citizen the war was a question of national existence; for the Bolivian it was a distant affair." [20]

These differences are reflected in the reports of the American ministers in Asunción and La Paz. The former wrote of the "anxiety" in Paraguay over the situation and stated that Paraguay was distrustful of Bolivia as a result of the "pressure of Bolivian troops upon areas which Paraguay has so long considered her own beyond question or argument." He added however: "There can be no doubt of the sincerity of the Government in its desire to maintain peace, and of the dread of the people of a war. . . . Her hope is that the efforts of the Neutrals . . . and the pressure of public opinion may make Bolivia sincerely desirous of an arbitration of the boundary." One of the Minister's diplomatic colleagues from a South American country said that he considered that "Bolivia's policy of continuous penetration and postponement of arbitration is a settled one." [21]

The atmosphere in La Paz was markedly different. Ambassador Edwin V. Morgan in Brazil reported the Brazilian Minister in Bolivia as saying that the Bolivian Chief of Staff had told him that the Bolivian army proposed "aggressive action against Paraguay, occupation of Chaco forts on Paraguayan frontier, and bombardment by airplanes of Asunción." [22] Ambassador William S. Culbertson reported that the Chilean Minister for Foreign Affairs received confirmation of the intention of the Bolivian Chief of Staff "to make war on Paraguay, latter's argument being that is cheaper than the armed peace." [23] Direct from La Paz, the Department had reports from Chargé Edward G. Trueblood that "there is a distinct cleavage in high Government circles, one group being aggressive and the other conciliatory" but that the newspaper *La Razón*, "regarded as the administration mouthpiece," had stated "that Bolivia's patience is exhausted, its optimism gone, and that 'we know that there is only one method, which sooner or later must decide.' " [24]

In Washington there was growing realization of the possibility of war, and the Department of State continued unremittingly its impartial efforts to find a way to peaceful settlement by collaborating with the informal group of neutrals composing the Commission. At this time, however, and later, the United States refused to be drawn away from an existing conciliation effort into acting alone or with other states. A Brazilian suggestion that the United States could bring about peace "more expeditiously alone" was not accepted.[25]

The attitude of the Bolivian government and of its minister in Washington appeared to be in accord with a general policy of postponing action or discussion about the basic question of sovereignty over the Chaco. This attitude apparently rested on the expectation that the United States would be the dominating influence in any decision made by the neutral Commission. The Bolivians, whose claims were based mainly on juridical interpretations of colonial documents, felt that "undue weight would be given to possession, occupation and colonization of territory rather than to legal titles," if the United States participated in the settlement. This prejudice apparently dated from the Hayes award in 1878.[26] It was also based upon Bolivian interpretations of the position of the Department of State in the then unsettled Guatemala-Honduras boundary dispute, and of the action of General McCoy as chairman of the Commission of Neutrals created in 1929.[27]

There also appeared to exist an impression on the part of some influential Bolivians that the United States had exerted pressure on both Chile and Peru, but particularly on the latter country, in order to bring about a settlement of the Tacna-Arica dispute. On this point, however, Dr. Alberto Salomón, former Foreign Minister of Peru, had assured Bolivian officials that the United States had not brought pressure on Peru but had employed its good offices in an impartial manner.[28]

The persistent labors of the Neutrals reached one of many climaxes on October 19, 1931, when a joint telegram, signed by all the other nineteen American countries, was sent to Bolivia and Paraguay, urging them to sign a nonaggression pact and to reach a final solution of their controversy.[29]

The conference to study a nonaggression pact held its first session on November 11, 1931, and its last in July, 1932. Despite Bolivian efforts to keep the five neutral representatives in the position of simple observers, they succeeded in playing the role of mediators and were able to produce a draft pact drawn up by the two delegations on May 6, 1932. The actual draft was prepared by Francis White at the request of the parties and was written after two weeks of almost daily informal meetings between White and the Bolivian and Paraguayan representatives. It represented the utmost amount of agreement then attainable.[30] Paraguay rejected the draft pact on the ground that "Paraguay requires that the pact of non-aggression be backed by a sufficient and effective international guarantee. The word or signature of Bolivia alone does not merit our confidence because we have the unhappy experience that for her pacts are 'Chiffons de papier.'" [31]

While the Paraguayan government did not specify the nature of a satisfactory guarantee, it appeared that there were two plans under consideration in Asunción. One, supported by certain civilians, including President-Elect Eusebio Ayala, favored a proposal by the Neutrals for substantial reductions in the armed forces of both countries.[32] The other, which shortly became firm Paraguayan policy, required the withdrawal of all Bolivian troops to a line in the

western Chaco at about the 62d parallel of longitude, the withdrawal of Paraguayan troops to the Paraguay River, and the subsequent arbitration of the dispute.

The Bolivian government gave informal approval to the draft
nonaggression pact, with minor modifications, on June 3. The Department of State repeatedly urged the Paraguayan government not
to make its rejection of the pact a final one, but the pact was forever lost to view in new clouds of war.

On June 15, 1932, there occurred in the Chaco a new incident at
Fortín Carlos Antonio López near Laguna Pitiantuta on the north-
central front.[33] This incident marked the beginning of heavy fighting during the summer of 1932 and may be considered as the starting point of the Chaco War. A Bolivian offensive in August
captured several Paraguayan forts on the central front; a Paraguayan counterattack, however, not only recaptured these but
pushed the Bolivian army back several miles from the advanced
positions they had held on June 1. During this period appeals from
the Department of State and the Neutrals that the fighting be
stopped were acknowledged but disregarded by both sides.

The negotiations during the summer of 1932 and the following
winter are instructive, but they cannot be followed here in detail.
From the point of view of the development of the policy of the
United States, however, there are a number of features of interest.

The concern of the United States government, as stated on more
than one occasion, was summed up by White: "The only interest of
the United States in the matter is to have this question settled and
have fighting and bloodshed cease. We are not looking for credit for
ourselves—we have settled enough matters to have plenty of credit
to our balance—and we are not looking for any glory in this
matter." [34] Washington's interest was not casual; it was intense, and
it does not appear that it was complicated by either strategic or economic considerations. The Standard Oil Company of New Jersey
held a producing concession from the Bolivian government in an
area close to the uttermost boundary of the Chaco as defined by
Paraguay, but there is no evidence that the Department of State
considered this fact as in any way affecting the position it adopted
toward the Chaco conflict.

That the United States was willing that others enshroud themselves in any glory arising out of peace efforts was clearly shown in
connection with the supreme effort for peace made in this early
stage of the struggle. This was the application of the so-called
Stimson doctrine of nonrecognition, first used against Japan in Manchuria and based on the Kellogg-Briand Pact. All the American
states except the combatants signed a joint declaration on August 3,
1932, declaring that "they will not recognize any territorial arrangement of this controversy which has not been obtained by peaceful
means nor the validity of territorial acquisitions which may be obtained through occupation or conquest by force of arms." [35] This
declaration was verbally approved by both Bolivia and Paraguay,
but no noticeable changes in policy resulted, nor any cessation of
hostilities. Not until after the rainy season, which began early in
November, was fighting gradually broken off; it was started again in
May, 1933, when the rains ended, and the central Chaco dried out.
The application of the Stimson doctrine as a way to peace appears
to have originated with Francis White, who began work on a draft
declaration on July 7, when he learned that Paraguay had decided to
withdraw its delegate, Juan José Soler, from the negotiations.[36]

Soler actually left Washington for New York about July 20,
apparently intending to sail for Asunción, but he returned on July
23. On the following day Bolivia informed the neutrals that its delegates could not continue to negotiate "in view of the repeated acts
of violence of Paraguay . . . without diminishing the dignity of
our country." [37]

Eduardo Diez de Medina and Enrique Finot at this point seemingly failed to act with their accustomed diplomatic finesse; if their
announcement had preceded Soler's return to Washington, they
might have forced the neutrals to center their attention on what
they could then have made to appear as Paraguayan intransigence.
Such a maneuver was all the more important since they presumably
knew even better than White that, as the latter wrote: "All reports
showed that Bolivia was preparing to make an attack by force in the
Chaco and to temporize with the Neutrals." [38]

Stimson agreed to the proposed declaration but preferred that the
initiative come from a Latin American country. White suggested to

the Argentine Ambassador, Felipe A. Espil, that Argentina might make the proposal. Espil thought this was possible but preferred that White should make the suggestion directly to Carlos Saavedra Lamas, Argentine Minister for Foreign Affairs. White did so, through Robert Woods Bliss, the American Ambassador in Buenos Aires, who discovered that Saavedra Lamas did not wish to take the initiative because a refusal to cooperate on the part of Brazil, Chile, or Peru, " 'would place Argentina in a very invidious position vis-à-vis Bolivia.' " [39]

Saavedra Lamas had proposed an appeal to Bolivia and Paraguay to be made by Argentina, Brazil, Chile, and Peru, a group which later worked together at certain times and became known as "the neighboring countries." Brazil, however, on July 30, objected to the plan on the ground that it would take negotiations out of the hands of the Neutrals, and it was consequently dropped. The Neutrals approved the declaration drafted by White, and it was sent to the American states by the Commission of Neutrals, after acceptance by the neighboring countries.[40]

On August 5, Bliss reported from Buenos Aires that the news of the declaration "was hailed here as a triumph of Argentine diplomacy, the credit being given to . . . Dr. Carlos Saavedra Lamas, for the formula 'No recognition of territory acquired by force.' " [41] Saavedra Lamas accepted without protest the acclaim given him in Argentina.[42] However, he was subjected to a vigorous attack by a prominent opposition senator, Lisandro de la Torre, of Sante Fe, not only for having taken credit for an action that originated in fact in Washington but also for having approved a declaration that expressed the same " 'peremptory tone' " as that used by Stimson to Japan with regard to Manchuria. Dr. de la Torre had obtained copies of telegrams exchanged between Buenos Aires and Washington, but, despite his documentation and the gravity of his charges, Saavedra Lamas successfully defended himself in terms of " 'generous collaboration' " with the other American states that were trying to bring peace in the Chaco.[43] Francis White added a conclusive comment on the subject on August 18:

Mr. Espil then said that he had been asked by Mr. Saavedra Lamas to inquire why the words "de este controversia" had been put in the joint telegram on August 3 and how they were to be interpreted. (This should definitely dispose of any claim on the part of Saavedra Lamas to having been the author of the declaration of August 3.) [44]

Concerning the authorship of the August 3 declaration, White soon found himself in an odd position. Having been principally responsible for its formulation and having failed to obtain Saavedra Lamas's consent to act as its official sponsor, White had remained silent when Saavedra Lamas accepted credit for it. On August 22, in a conversation with Diez de Medina and Finot, the Bolivian delegates to the moribund nonaggression conference, White was then faced with the statement that

one reason for public opinion in Bolivia being opposed to the August 3 declaration is that the Minister of Foreign Affairs of Argentina had claimed authorship of it and, as Argentina has been known always to be very friendly to Paraguay, it was felt that this was an Argentine suggestion directed against Bolivia and that Argentina had gotten the Neutral Commission to adopt a pro-Paraguayan and anti-Bolivian attitude. [White said he] could assure them most categorically that this suggestion did not come from Argentina. They said that they understood this; that they had received information which they thought was trustworthy which had showed that it did not come from there. I told them that I could assure them most unreservedly that such was the case. [45]

The spirit of the Department of State in participating in the efforts to keep the peace is illustrated by White's report of his conversation with the two Bolivian delegates. He noted that the Neutrals "had made suggestions to try to bring the Bolivian point of view into accord with the August 3 doctrine, but that we had had no help from Bolivia." He hoped Bolivia would now make some suggestion so the Neutrals "could try to be helpful." [46]

Although this solemn invocation of the principle of nonrecognition of territory obtained through occupation or conquest was ineffectual in stopping the conflict, it was taken seriously by the Department of State. There is little evidence, however, that the other American governments placed great confidence in the efficacy of the declaration or that they continued to impress its significance on the disputants. [47]

The view within the Department in November, 1932, was stated by Acting Secretary Wilbur J. Carr, who warned Paraguayans not to forget the declaration of August 3. He erroneously predicted: "The only way Paraguay can get title in the Chaco which will be recognized by the other American nations is through a peaceful settlement. The way to a peaceful settlement is now in Paraguay's grasp if she will be moderate and cooperate with the Neutral Commission." [48]

This affair was only the second of a long series of encounters between the Department of State and Saavedra Lamas, who remained in office until February, 1938.[49] The Argentine Minister for Foreign Affairs was a lawyer of considerable ability, a man of extraordinary personal vanity, and a devious and audacious diplomat, who managed to combine a capacity for antagonizing and enraging foreign diplomats with the compilation of a record of personal achievements unrivaled among American statesmen of his time. In the five years from 1932 to 1936 he became known as the author of an antiwar treaty, ratified by the United States and many other countries; he was awarded the Nobel Peace Prize in 1936 and was elected president of the Assembly of the League of Nations in the same year, three years after arranging for the return of his country to membership in the League. He was both hated and feared by many statesmen in America, and it is highly probable that but for his maneuverings the Chaco conflict would have been shorter and less costly in life and other resources. At the same time he was signally honored by the United States and by other countries in the Americas and in Europe. His influence on international political developments in the Americas during his term of office was greater than that of any other Latin American statesman, and on several important occasions he succeeded in obstructing policies espoused by the United States. The Department of State made every effort to gain Saavedra Lamas's good will with remarkable sincerity and persistence, but the results were less than meager.[50]

In a conference with Francis White, the Paraguayan delegate, Soler, reported that Argentina had suggested in Asunción that

the Neutrals wished to withdraw from the negotiations and leave the whole Chaco matter in the hands of Argentina. . . . He attributed Argentina's action to the vanity of Saavedra Lamas and his desire for publicity. Mr. Soler said that he knows Saavedra Lamas well and that he is a most vain man. He was afraid Saavedra Lamas would do considerable damage and thought it might be helpful if he could be flattered in some way to keep him from completely upsetting things.[51]

Whether or not White and Stimson were influenced by this talk, they later dealt with Saavedra Lamas as though they agreed with Soler's recommendation, and Cordell Hull followed suit.

If the United States was not seeking glory from the Chaco negotiations, it certainly did not obtain any. Bolivia and Paraguay each accused the United States of partiality toward the other.[52] The position of the United States was an exposed one in several ways. White, as Assistant Secretary of State and Chairman of the Commission of Neutrals, was both formally prominent and actually influential in the activities of the Commission. The United States could not claim, as it did in connection with the Commission headed by General McCoy in 1929–30, that its representative was not instructed by the Department of State. The other states members of the Commission were frequently represented by chargés d'affaires, who often did not attend the meetings, and White was the single permanent representative, familiar with the entire course of the negotiations in Washington. As chairman, White frequently carried on informal negotiations with the delegates of Bolivia and Paraguay alone or together, and as Assistant Secretary of State his sources of information about the activities of the neighboring countries were far more extensive than those of his colleagues. In addition, the Department of State repeatedly asked its ministers in Asunción and La Paz to appeal to the two governments to accept suggestions from the Neutrals or to withdraw from an intransigent position. These appeals were often made without simultaneous support from other American governments, except, of course, in the case of joint declarations such as that of August 3, 1932.

None of the Neutrals had a common border with Paraguay, and only one of them, Uruguay, was situated near the scene of the conflict. There existed, therefore, a tendency in several of the neighboring countries, especially Argentina, to consider that, since their interests were most directly affected, they, rather than the United States, should take the leadership in efforts to prevent war. This feeling had several effects, one of which was to give rise to attacks against the Commission of Neutrals and, therefore, indirectly against the United States as its leading spirit.

The United States was also attacked on other grounds. With funds obtained through a loan by American bankers in 1927, Bolivia had purchased arms and military equipment in the United States and elsewhere. In July, 1932, when the Paraguayan troops recaptured Fortín Carlos Antonio López, they found "a blouse apparently made in the United States for military purposes." [53] Paraguay later complained of shipments of war materials by private companies in the United States to Bolivia until, for other reasons, the United States declared an embargo on the shipment of such materials to either belligerent.

An additional handicap to the United States as a peacemaker was the inclination on the part of some South American countries, particularly Argentina and Peru, to oppose giving an important role in the settlement of South American controversies to the United States. This attitude was not often expressed openly by South American diplomats but was none the less apparent. In a report from Lima, the comment was made that the Peruvian government had apparently desired that the neighboring countries should take the Chaco dispute into their own hands "and walk away with it from the Commission of Neutrals, making it a purely South American matter. Here again peeps out the fundamental distrust of us in this part of the world and the irresistible impulse to handle South American questions without any participation from the United States." [54]

This distrust, which was to diminish in the later 1930s, was by no means universal in South America. Paraguayan statesmen, on more than one occasion, indicated that they had more confidence in the impartiality and good faith of the government of the United States than in that of other American governments.

This same note was heard in the request of the Bolivian Foreign Minister to Minister Edward Francis Feely that the latter use his influence "to prevent what he termed the 'intervention' of the four neighboring countries in the present negotiations," since the Bolivian government "feared that their participation in the negotiations could only redound to the prejudice of Bolivia's interests. He explained further that Bolivia had no confidence in the sincerity of intentions of either Argentina or Chile." [55]

It is also significant that, in spite of the existence of an underlying distrust or dislike, it was far more common for Latin American countries to turn to the United States for assistance in settling their boundary controversies than to other Latin American governments, although the latter recourse was by no means unknown. One of the features of this situation was that, in general, Latin American countries were not as willing as the United States to take the role of mediator, unless they were certain that they would be successful. They did not, as among equals, wish to give offense to a near neighbor; they felt they had a smaller margin of prestige to risk, and for some, the expenses of engaging in a mediation might represent a substantial part of restricted budgets for diplomatic activity.[56]

It is hard to find any kind of moral suasion or pacific diplomatic technique that Stimson and White failed to use in their sincere attempts to avert war, and there is no evidence that the Department of State seriously contemplated the adoption of coercive measures against either or both of the disputants. Minister Feely in La Paz reported on October 10, that there was "a grave fear amongst Bolivian bankers that as a last resort, the Neutral Commission may consider the attachment of the Central Bank's reserves held in New York, as a means of forcing Bolivia to accept an armistice," [57] but such action does not appear even to have been contemplated in Washington.

In a significant conversation with the Bolivian Minister, Luis O. Abelli, White noted that Abelli had tried to get him to say

that the United States would not intervene at all in case of war. I told him I would make no such statement whatsoever; that of course we had no intention of intervening by force in the Chaco matter but that our moral support would certainly be against a resort to arms and would be used against any country so resorting.[58]

In contrast to the Bolivians, who were anxious that the United States should not intervene by force of arms, the Paraguayans were hoping that the United States might, with other American states, consider sending troops to the Chaco as a guarantee against a Bolivian attack.[59]

To a Paraguayan inquiry about whether the Neutrals would provide "an effective guarantee" that the nonaggression pact would be carried out, White replied that "if they contemplated a guarantee that would be enforced by arms they certainly were wide of the mark because this Government certainly would not give any such guarantee and I felt confident that the other Neutrals would not do so either." [60] On June 3, White told Soler that "obviously we would not send any troops to the Chaco to enforce a pact." This did not mean, however, that Washington was averse to the use of force or other sanctions by other American states. White suggested that the neighboring countries might be willing to agree to stop any military supplies from reaching the belligerents and that Argentina and Brazil patrol and police the Ballivián-Vitriones line. This idea met with an interested response from Espil, but not from the two governments concerned.[61]

Another attempt to get action by the neighboring countries in the form of policing or sanctions was made in talks initiated by Secretary Cordell Hull during the Montevideo Conference in December. Mateo Marques Castro, of Uruguay, demurred, citing the difficulty of identifying the aggressor because minor incidents in the Chaco were "so difficult of examination." Brazilian Foreign Minister Mello Franco told Hull that he "was opposed to the application of sanctions—if such action should involve the participation or acquiescence of Brazil therein." In these discussions Hull made it clear that it would not be possible for the United States to participate in any sanctions for the purpose of bringing an end to the Chaco War.[62]

Although the United States restricted its influence to what White called moral support, it did not succeed in avoiding charges of what Latin American countries referred to less loftily as "pressure." As Bolivia and Paraguay took turns at being intransigent toward proposals by the Neutrals, the United States, acting directly and apart from the Neutrals through its diplomatic representatives in La Paz and Asunción, said various things to each government that were of varying degrees of pleasantness. In August, White told Minister Post Wheeler in Asunción:

It was Paraguay's failure to work through the Commission early in July that greatly aggravated the situation. It is hoped that you can persuade the Paraguayan Government that now is the time to exercise patience and calm, attempt to quiet and not to inflame the war spirit, and to cooperate with the Neutrals and through them with all the other nations of America.[63]

In response to a telegram from the Bolivian government asserting that it could not admit "foreign pressure" to the detriment of its rights, by the Neutrals or others, White said that "we have never brought any pressure to bear." Minister Luis O. Abelli replied that "the McCoy Commission had presented a pact of arbitration," to which White replied that, while that was true, "there had been no pressure brought to bear and it had not been accepted. Furthermore, we did not intend to bring any pressure to bear." White added that

in talking to the Bolivians there might be times when they might well think I was pro-Paraguayan, and in talking to the Paraguayans, they might think I was pro-Bolivian. It would be necessary for me to undergo this risk in exploring every possibility of a settlement. . . . I would naturally not make any proposal that I thought would be inimical to the interest of either party . . . every possibility must be explored and no avenue left closed to a possible settlement—but that certainly did not mean that we were doing anything which was considered hostile to the interests of either country.[64]

White was acting here in a dual role. As chairman of the Commission he could urge his colleagues to approve notes to the combatants. As Assistant Secretary of State he could communicate to both governments directly and use the prestige of his office and his government. Although willing to make use of both his positions, he was restrained in the first by the cooperating states and in the second by his unwillingness to appear so insistent as to be open to the charge of using "pressure." Writing to Wheeler in the hope of speeding action on negotiations for withdrawal of forces in the Chaco, he suggested that the Minister discuss the matter "discreetly" with the Paraguayan government "without giving the impression that this Government is pressing Paraguay too hard and hence cause resentment." [65]

By the end of 1932 Stimson was discouraged. The peace "machinery" he had succeeded in keeping in working order with the continuation of the Commission of Neutrals had not prevented fighting in the Chaco. He had little hope for the effect of the moral influence to which White referred, and he did not think sanctions could be useful. In a talk with the Minister of the Irish Free State, Michael MacWhite, who had come to see him on behalf of Eamon De Valera, President of the Council of the League of Nations, about possible action by the League on the Chaco, Stimson said that the Chaco had "given him very great concern." He added that "both Bolivia and Paraguay apparently care nothing for what others may say and that there is really no hold on them as they have no sea coast. It is very hard to exert any sanctions or pressure any more than one could do against two tribes fighting in the interior of Africa." Predicting accurately, he said he thought that "if the nineteen American countries had not succeeded in making the countries stop hostilities he did not think that all the League of Nations could do it either." [66]

In dealing with the Chaco, Stimson and White confronted some issues, occasionally encountered with non-American countries, that gained special forms and flavors on the American continent. One of these problems arose when the United States urged a course of action upon another government and was told that such action could not be taken for reasons of internal politics. Frequently it was said that the government would fall, either because of a popular revolution or because of a seizure of power by the army. When the Paraguayan delegates were withdrawn from the nonaggression conference, Ayala said "no other action was possible in the temper of the people." [67] In December Ayala told Wheeler that acceptance of a line of evacuation proposed by the Neutrals would mean " 'that I would not be able to remain in the Palace 24 hours.' " [68]

The problem created by imminent independent action by army leaders was recognized by Secretary Stimson in an instruction to United States representatives in the neighboring countries, when it became clear that the declaration of August 3, 1932, had not succeeded in bringing about agreement in the Chaco. Stimson wrote:

Argentina has supported this Bolivian thesis [that existing troop dispositions be maintained in the Chaco] on the ground that unless something of this sort is done there will be a revolution in Bolivia, [President Daniel] Salamanca will be overthrown and a military Government come in which will be much worse than the present one. On the other hand, information received from Asunción indicates that unless Bolivia gives back the four Paraguayan forts last taken by her the military there will get out of control.[69]

In addition to the army, the political opposition to the government in power was ready to seize opportunities to gain partisan advantage. When Eusebio Ayala, a Liberal, was elected President of Paraguay, Wheeler reported that bitter opposition could be expected from the Conservative party. While he considered that Ayala was one of the few "broad-minded, learned, traveled and experienced men this country possesses," he regretted that there was in Paraguay little evidence "of the spirit which puts national affairs above personal politics and is able to lay aside petty differences in face of crisis. . . . The signs indicate that popular feeling will continue to be played upon with a view to creating a revolutionary spirit which may later be utilized." [70] As will later appear, this was unfortunately one of the most accurate forecasts made during the conflict.

There is no question that the statement that revolution might be imminent was often simply a description of the actual political situation. In some cases, however, it appeared that this line of argument used by diplomats and home officials was no more than an excuse for not following policies recommended by the United States. The Bolivian delegate to the Commission said

that the real trouble is that the military has been in control in Bolivia all along and it was the military who had caused the rejection of the Neutral proposal of August 2 that both sides go back to the military positions of June 1. He said that the military had insisted upon undertaking the military operations in the Chaco and that when recently the military had threatened a *coup d'état* in La Paz the Government had simply transmitted to the General Staff the Neutral proposal of October 12 and had told the General Staff that the responsibility for the decision as to its acceptance was on it.[71]

Shortly afterward, however, Minister Feely reported from La Paz that "a most reliable source" had informed him that President Salamanca had ordered the Bolivian advance in July, 1932, which had captured three forts, including Fort Boquerón,

and thus precipitated open hostilities. At that time, the Chief of the General Staff, General Filiberto Osorio Téllez, protested against a Bolivian advance on the ground that the positions could not be held even if they were taken, because the army was not prepared . . . and further that transportation facilities were entirely inadequate.

General Osorio resigned, but his resignation was not accepted, and he was relieved of his position after the Paraguayans recaptured Fort Boquerón. Feely attributed the Bolivian failure to agree to peaceful settlement to the confidence of Salamanca that Bolivia could easily defeat Paraguay [72] and, later, "because of his fear that the acceptance by Bolivia of a suspension of hostilities would lead to the overthrow of his Government." [73]

Although the possible fall of a government was usually put forward with the expectation that it would be accepted as an "absolute" reason for avoiding a given policy, such great weight was not always given to it by the Department of State. When the Argentine Ambassador, Espil, told White he thought the Bolivian government would fall if the Neutrals insisted that the two governments withdraw their troops to the lines of June 1, 1932, White "inquired which was the most essential for the good of this continent—to maintain the doctrine enunciated on August 3—or to maintain the present individuals composing the Government in Bolivia?" [74]

This conversation could, of course, much more easily occur between two diplomats if they were talking about a third country than if one of them represented the government whose fall was here regarded with principled calm.

A second kind of problem met by the United States may be exemplified by several incidents involving relationships with members of the diplomatic corps of Bolivia and Paraguay and with other Latin American diplomats. In the discussion between White and Soler about the authorship of the draft nonaggression pact, it was clear that Soler was endeavoring to avoid any responsibility for its terms, since he had subsequently discovered that it had been badly received in Asunción. Both the Bolivian and Paraguayan delegations were composed of men with political pasts who hoped for political futures at home. They were terrified of being held responsible for failure and avid for credit for success. Soler and César Vasconcellos had been sent to the conference without instructions, perhaps because their government had not wished to assume responsibility for policies that might give the opposition a target.

When the Paraguayan delegates called on White in July to inform him that they would have to withdraw from the conference, White told Soler that he thought this action "extremely foolish" and asked him not to present the note. Soler said that his instructions were categoric, and White told him "that the value of a diplomatic representative is in telling his Government when he thinks they are doing something foolish in order to keep them from doing so." Soler replied that "the problem of getting the Paraguayan Government to change its position" was White's and not his own. White disagreed and said that all he was called on to do was to inform the Neutrals about the withdrawal, adding:

The Chaco is a matter of complete indifference to this Government and none of its interests suffer in any way whatsoever whether the conference stops or goes on. At very considerable inconvenience and trouble to ourselves we are trying to help two friendly nations to compose their difficulties and it is certainly not our job to straighten out rows between the delegates and their Government or between themselves, or to keep one Government from doing an act which is against its own best interests. I told him I thought this was a task that belonged to him and Señor Vasconcellos.

Soler said that there had been charges in Asunción that the delegation was trying to prolong the conference "and he wanted to keep well out of any definite action which would look as though he were reluctant to have the conference terminated." [75]

The experience of the United States government in this and many other cases showed that the quality of diplomatic reporting could be expected to be poor when career politicians served as negotiators for Latin American countries.

The fact that the power and influence of the United States were greater than those of any of the other American states created unique problems for Washington. The Latin American governments were quick to protest about intervention or pressure by the United States when they did not like a move by the Department of State. On the other hand, they were also quick to try to get the United States to exert pressure on other Latin American states. The Bolivian Minister, Luis O. Abelli, provided an unusually naive example of this practice in the spring of 1932, when some of the neighboring countries were trying to avert war. Abelli said to White that La Paz had informed Argentina, Brazil, Chile, and Peru that

any action on their part would be looked upon as contrary to the dignity and sovereignty of Bolivia. . . . He said he wanted to tell his Government that I was calling off the four countries named—he thought it would help the situation and make his Government more friendly toward the Department. I told the Minister that I appreciated his motive and that, while I of course would welcome greater confidence on the part of his Government in the impartiality of this Government I did not want to achieve that end by a statement which was not wholly accurate.[76]

CHAPTER II

The Search for Peace

THROUGHOUT THE AUTUMN OF 1932, the Commission of Neutrals, and particularly Francis White, its Chairman, was engaging in four distinct sets of negotiations. First, there were those with the neighboring powers, who at various times made suggestions for bringing peace to the Chaco. Second, there were negotiations directly with Bolivia and Paraguay. Third, there were those with the Council of the League of Nations, which felt impelled to assert its interest in the dispute. Fourth, there were those with Ambassador Espil and Foreign Minister Saavedra Lamas of Argentina, concerning the latter's individual proposals for settlement of the conflict. Some of the groups with which White dealt were more tractable than others from the point of view of the Neutrals, but it is not clear that Bolivia and Paraguay were the most intransigent of the entities involved.

The Neighboring Powers

The neighboring powers, also known as the ABCP group, were probably the easiest for the Neutrals to deal with. The neighbors did not have a meeting place, a staff, a history of cooperation, or, perhaps most important, a recognized chairman. However, their eagerness to propose plans and initiate negotiations for peace in the Chaco in competition or in cooperation with the efforts made by the Neutrals was a concern of the Department of State as early as the spring of 1932.

White told Espil that he did not feel that the forthcoming Conference of American States at Montevideo could effectively deal with the Chaco but that he thought "the most practical results would come from an agreement among the four states bordering on Bolivia and Paraguay, namely Argentina, Brazil, Chile and Peru, as to definite action." [1] The Neutrals were desirous of cooperating with the neighboring powers and asked their Washington ambassadors not to become members of the Commission but to associate themselves with a declaration of the Neutrals that viewed with concern the military preparations in Bolivia and Paraguay. Argentina, through Espil, indicated to White that it did not think it "convenient" that the neutral Commission should be enlarged, but Argentina would be glad to cooperate with it.[2]

With this action there commenced a long and chaotic period of joint, parallel, and individual negotiations, involving the Commission and the neighboring powers, as well as foreign ministers playing lone hands. All were futile in preventing war, and the number of choices available gave Bolivia and Paraguay opportunities of polite declination of any one by indicating that they were interested in a method or solution offered by someone else. These opportunities were taken by one or the other state as its momentary interest indicated; if its fighting chances were bright, it chose the least promising of peace overtures.

The confusing picture of intrigue was made vivid by word reaching the Department of State "that Argentina stated in Asunción that the Neutrals wished to withdraw from the negotiations and that these should be placed in the hands of Argentina." [3] This evidence of an attempt at deception by Saavedra Lamas was presumably only one influence affecting White's opinion that Saavedra Lamas was "a most vain man and a publicity seeker. Every diplomatic officer in Buenos Aires has complained that he has double-crossed him, misled him, and even directly lied to him." [4]

Secretary Stimson said, after these developments were known, that "the only way for the negotiations to succeed is to have them centered in one place only and if suggestions would be sent to the Neutrals before being discussed with Bolivia and Paraguay it would greatly help the task of the Neutrals and prevent any crossing of wires." [5]

A new effort at collaboration was made on August 25 by the Chilean Minister for Foreign Affairs, Miguel Cruchaga Tocornal, who proposed through Ambassador William S. Culbertson the calling of a conference to which would be invited representatives of Bolivia and Paraguay and of each of the four neighboring powers and one representative of the Commission of Neutrals, presumably the United States.[6] White told Espil that the Neutrals welcomed the cooperation of the ABCP group, but they did not favor this proposal, since it would exclude some of the Neutrals, and they wished to keep the Commission intact.[7]

This significant failure to bring the Neutrals and neighbors together demonstrated the very real difficulties of cooperation. There was a lack of communication of plans and intentions, partly because of time and distance, partly because of a desire on the part of statesmen to operate secretly so that, if their proposals were rejected, their prestige loss would be minimized, and, if their proposals were accepted, they could secure sole credit for a peaceful settlement. The neighbors were not united; Brazil preferred to work closely with the Neutrals, especially with the United States, and the others favored a South American way of settlement. On the other hand, the Neutrals showed that they were unwilling to abdicate their position. They formed the only recognized formal link between Bolivia and Paraguay, and, as Castle informed Culbertson, "The Neutral Commission is a unit and has been acting as a unit for four years and it desires to continue to do so." [8]

It is useless to speculate on what might have happened, but it seems clear that this moment was the most favorable opportunity ever offered the Neutrals to invite the neighbors to become members of the Commission or to throw their full weight behind a new organization, including the neighbors, and so to unify strong continental pressure against Bolivia and Paraguay. Through disunity on the part of the neighbors and through the adoption of an inflexible position by the United States and the other Neutrals, the opportunity, if it was there, was missed.

Negotiations with Bolivia and Paraguay

Finding that the declaration of August 3, 1932, had no immediate effect on preparations for war, the Neutrals tried to prove that they were not intransigent on insisting that troops be withdrawn to the June 1 line, by inquiring of Bolivia on August 17 what concrete proposal Bolivia might make which would lead to an agreement in the Chaco. Foreign Minister Julio A. Gutiérrez replied that Bolivia would agree to "a suspension of hostilities on the basis of the present position in the Chaco" and to a settlement of the dispute by arbitration or other amicable means.[9] This note included a strongly worded attack upon the Neutral Commission and on the Declaration of August 3. Charging that "the extremist attitude of the neutrals is what has brought us to this difficult point," Guitérrez claimed the declaration was retroactive in effect and applied "solely to the case of the Chaco, ignoring all past acts of violence and making allowance for all future injustices outside that territory." He blamed Paraguay for initiating attacks on forts on "Bolivian territory" and said in words probably intended to sting Washington: "It was then that 19 American nations appeared on the scene to proclaim the principle that might does not create right, a principle which all of them had forgotten in times which were unfortunate for many American nations which were the victims of force."

The response of the Neutrals was to call on both countries to agree to a truce for sixty days beginning on September 1. The truce proposal was rejected by Paraguay on August 29 and accepted for thirty days by Bolivia on August 30. The Paraguayan counteroffensive began in early September and met with rapid success.

The Paraguayan position was explicitly stated on September 26 by the Minister of Foreign Relations, Justo Pastor Benítez, in a note to the Neutrals. Paraguay would accept a truce if (1) both armies carried out an immediate and simultaneous withdrawal until the Chaco was "entirely demilitarized" under supervision by the Neutrals; (2) there was a reduction of "the military effectives" of each country to the minimum required for internal security, "to be

determined and supervised by the Commission of Neutrals";
(3) there was a "submission of the controversy to international
justice." [10]

Paraguay's military successes, and Bolivia's sudden wooing of the
Neutrals, caused the onus for hampering peace negotiations to be
shifted to Paraguay. White told Soler that his country's refusal to
accept an armistice made White unable "to escape the conviction
that . . . Paraguay would have to be considered the aggressor in
view of her refusal to accept." White told Soler he thought Paraguay was playing "a very dangerous game," since "the fortune of
arms may well turn against her," and "Paraguay will thus have lost
its opportunity and will have to take the consequences." [11] These
words had no visible effect in Asunción.

Finally, giving up hope of stopping fighting before the rainy season brought an enforced armistice, the Neutrals sharpened their
pencils for a long winter's exchange of notes. They first made a proposal to send representatives into the Chaco "to see that the agreement, if one is arrived at to stop hostilities, is respected." The
proposal was conditionally accepted, but the representatives never
took off for the Chaco. Noting that each of the countries demanded
guarantees that the other would not improve its military position,
White told the American press: "Obviously no guarantees can be
given to them except those of a moral sort." [12]

White's cable to Asunción that "the Mission of neutrals now
accepted by both parties is ready to start for the Chaco, with the
certainty that it can insure the reconciliation of the combatants"
was answered by Pastor Benítez's insistence on the prior establishment of "a régime of reciprocal security, consisting in the total
demilitarization of the Chaco and the reduction of the armies. Once
an agreement has been reached on these points the creation of a commission of neutral military men will be contemplated." [13]

The Neutrals on September 30 asked both countries to provide
definitions of the Chaco. The Paraguayans defined the Chaco as the
territory bounded by the Paraguay, Pilcomayo, Xauru (Jauru), and
Parapití rivers. The Bolivians defined the Chaco as "the area of the
Chaco which is subject to dispute or controversy," since the term
was inexact and "may embrace regions belonging to the unques-

tioned sovereignty of Bolivia." The Chaco, to Bolivia, was an area bounded on the north by lat. 22° S., on the west by long. 59° 50′ W., on the south by the Pilcomayo River, and on the east by the Paraguay River. Thus, to the Paraguayans the Chaco included somewhat more than 150,000 square miles; to the Bolivians, the "disputable Chaco" contained only some 20,000 square miles in the area immediately north and west of Asunción.[14] The western line of the Chaco, according to the Bolivians, was almost exactly the line of deepest penetration of Bolivian troops in the summer of 1932; its eastern border was the Paraguay River south to Asunción.

The Paraguayan delegation clarified its stand by saying that it was prepared "to submit to arbitration without reservations" the question of boundaries between the two countries, "as Paraguay does not admit any territorial dispute nor any question of recovery over the Chaco."[15] Minister Wheeler reported from Asunción that "Bolivia's reservation from the field of arbitration of the entire Chaco except the small portion covered by the Hayes Award has confirmed this Government in its conviction that no peaceful agreement can be arrived at with her and that Paraguay has no choice but to continue fighting till she [Bolivia] is in another mind."[16]

Baffled in this direction by the enormous disparity in the claims of the two countries, and in what they would agree to submit to arbitration, the United States government turned its attention to an attempt to arrange a withdrawal of troops by each side so that hostilities could not be precipitated by incidents between patrols. After ascertaining what he thought to be the views of both governments, Stimson, on December 2, 1932, informally proposed the withdrawal of Paraguayan troops to the Paraguay River, the withdrawal of Bolivian troops to a line west of long. 62° 30′ W. and north of lat. 22° S.—the so-called Ballivián-Vitriones line. The proposal included a plan for the definition of the Chaco by three geographers chosen by geographical societies in Great Britain, Spain, and the United States and for arbitration of the territorial limits of Bolivia and Paraguay within the Chaco as so defined.[17]

Secretary Stimson thought that this appeared to be "eminently fair" and that it had the advantage, from Paraguay's point of view, of bringing about "virtual demilitarization of the Chaco," while the advantage to Bolivia would be that hostilities would be stopped and demobilization could be achieved, with resultant economy.[18]

The Department of State was surprised when President Ayala flatly refused to accept the Ballivián-Vitriones line as a sufficiently distant withdrawal for Bolivian troops. Paraguay insisted that the Bolivians withdraw entirely west of long. 62° 30' W. throughout the length of that meridian in the Chaco. In a general review of the situation, vigorously upholding his proposal, Stimson urged Wheeler in Asunción to press Ayala for acceptance, noting that "Soler has led Neutrals to believe that a retirement to parallel 62° 30' would be acceptable." [19]

The Paraguayan government remained immovable, despite repeated efforts by Stimson and White, who pointed out that the withdrawal of Bolivian troops was to positions which at some points were farther west than the Pinilla-Soler line of 1907, which had prescribed positions beyond which the two countries agreed not to advance troops but which since had been disregarded. Noting that "Bolivia committed a costly error in not accepting the Neutral proposal last August to go back to the line of June 1," Stimson stated that the new plan "will put an end to the war," and that "Paraguay should learn from this lesson that when she can get her objectives by peaceful means it is much more to her advantage to do so than to trust to the uncertain hazards of war." [20]

Despite the near certainty of Paraguayan rejection of this proposal, the Neutral Commission formally presented it to Bolivia and Paraguay, with minor changes, on December 15, 1932. The Council of the League of Nations and all the other American states gave their support to the plan as drafted by the Neutrals. Paraguay promptly replied, stating that the plan left the Bolivian army in the center of the Chaco, while requiring the Paraguayan army "to abandon the Chaco entirely," and that the Paraguayan government, "while not questioning the intentions of the Commission, cannot consider the bases proposed as satisfactory or just." [21] The Bolivian reply of December 19 stated that Bolivia had "accepted in principle the main points of the proposal" but noted that the "absolute rejection by Paraguay" made it unprofitable to discuss any observations about the plan.[22] While the Bolivian government was thus able to appear to be willing to accept the proposal, it is by no means clear that it would have done so if the Paraguayan reply had been one that encouraged exploratory negotiations by the Neutrals.[23]

Behind the Paraguayan refusal there were several factors. One was the confidence of the army that it could ultimately defeat the Bolivian army. A second was that the loss of life in the 1932 campaign was regarded as heavy,[24] and this had heightened the intensity of the popular demand that guarantees must be absolutely reliable. Third, the line proposed by the Neutrals would still leave Bolivian occupation of a considerable area in the Chaco plain where concentrations of supplies and troops could be built up for a possible campaign beginning in May or June. This was an important consideration because, after the Bolivian defeat in 1932, with the loss of about thirteen Bolivian forts, the Salamanca government had engaged the services of General Hans Kundt, a German officer who had previously been an instructor in the Bolivian army and had served as chief of staff.[25] In the fourth place, the Paraguayan government did not place much faith in the Neutral Commission, either to understand Paraguay's position or to guarantee, by policing or other means, that Paraguay would be as secure as if there were a withdrawal of all Bolivian forces entirely behind long. 62° 30′ W.[26]

Following the Paraguayan rejection of the Neutrals' proposal, Soler was instructed on December 18 to return to Asunción, breaking off discussions with the Commission of Neutrals. He left Washington for New York but did not take the first boat south. It was announced in Asunción that he did so by his own choice and that he no longer represented the Paraguayan government. The Neutrals, however, chose to regard his withdrawal from negotiations as temporary, and his government's reply as less than an absolute rejection. The Neutrals described their plan as "just," "honorable," and as offering a "dignified" solution for both parties, and, in a note to both disputants on the last day of the year, they again made an appeal for peace, emphasizing that the approval of the proposal by the other American states and by the Council of the League of Nations "constituted a historic expression of the universal conscience and a most unusual verdict of civilized humanity on the Chaco question which the parties cannot ignore." [27] Ignore it, however, they did, and both sides prepared for new battles when the mud dried.

Soler's recall was greeted with approval by the entire press in Asunción.[28] President Ayala had to intervene to prevent a demonstration being organized "against the United States." [29]

It is doubtful that an armistice could have been arranged at this time in any case, but the Commission of Neutrals might have avoided antagonizing the Paraguayans had it not been led by Soler to believe that the proposal of December 15 was a fair one and therefore might be accepted in Asunción. Wheeler commented that Soler's view "seems to show an extraordinary ignorance of this Government's attitude and mind" and that Ayala had shown "recent distrust of his representations. . . . [Paraguay] has taken the defiant stand that she may lose the entire Chaco as a result of war but she will not lose it at the hands of the Neutrals and with her own consent." [30]

The governmental exchanges were enlivened in late December by the interposition of members of the "Committee of Americans resident in Paraguay," who sent a telegram to President Hoover protesting against " 'the manifestly pro-Bolivian proposals presented by the Neutrals and against the sale of arms to Paraguay.' " The telegram was published in the Asunción press, and the Paraguayan Minister of Justice, Worship and Public Instruction thanked the Committee for the telegram and said that Paraguayans would never forget the action.[31] Secretary Stimson instructed Wheeler to caution the signer of the telegram and other United States citizens involved "to refrain from any actions which might be considered as taking sides or a breach of the strict neutrality which they should maintain." [32]

The Paraguayan press went so far at this time as to make attacks on Francis White personally. *El Liberal*, the paper of the party of President Ayala, noted the above telegram to President Hoover from the American colony in Asunción and said:

"It is these noble citizens of the United States, set apart in this individual expression of theirs, and not Mr. White in his official character, who represent to us, in this crisis, the ideal procedure of their country, and the aspirations of the exalted North American democracy.[33]

The Neutrals and the League of Nations

The Council of the League of Nations, which had taken an interest in the Chaco dispute in 1928 during the Fort Vanguardia incident, was informed by the Bolivian government on July 21, 1932, of acts of alleged aggression by Paraguay in the Chaco. Throughout the rest of the conflict, the Council was concerned with the dispute and was active in various ways, notably in 1933 when it sent a commission of investigation to the Chaco. The story of the actions of the organs of the League has been told elsewhere.[34] From the point of view of the policy of the government of the United States, every effort was made to settle the dispute by cooperation among the American states, although these efforts proved unavailing.

In December, 1932, the Neutrals had suffered a fatal blow in their efforts to find an "American solution" for the Chaco dispute. They then turned southward, toward other American states, rather than eastward to the League of Nations, after tacitly admitting the failure of their four-year quest. The strength of the desire to obtain a continental settlement in the Chaco is underlined by the difficulties and embarrassments already experienced in trying to cooperate with the neighboring countries.

White, writing to Hugh Wilson in Switzerland, commented on rumors that Saavedra Lamas intended, when Argentina had rejoined the League of Nations, to present the Chaco dispute to the League, and stated that, in addition to Argentine and Chilean intrigues,

I do not think that Drummond or any of the European members of the League can possibly understand the political situations that exist in Bolivia and Paraguay and in the neighboring countries, the alignment of some of the neighboring countries with one or the other of the contending countries, and the jealousy between these neighboring countries, each one trying to spike the suggestions of the other and get support for its own. We have even had the anomaly of Argentina asking the Neutrals to exert influence on Brazil to have Brazil accept an Argentine proposal, and a similar request from Chile to exert our influence with both Argentina and Brazel to have them accept a Chilean proposal.

He added that independent suggestions from the neighboring countries "have made our task most difficult and have probably resulted in the rejection of at least one or two of our proposals. Brazil is the only country which has not done so." [35]

One attempt by the Council of the League to assert itself in the Americas was made after the Neutrals' proposal of December 15, 1932, had been rejected. Noting that fighting had again become intense in the Chaco and feeling that "in order to carry out action on the Manchurian affair, they must show continued interest and efforts towards a peaceful solution of this dispute." [36] the Council proposed in January, 1933, to send a small committee to attempt a solution. Stimson, however, stated that he was hopeful of results from a new move by the neighboring powers and that the Council should delay action for the time being. Significantly, he added: "It is the Department's view, on the basis of past experience, that the best chance of obtaining a settlement is through the cooperation of the neighboring powers and the Neutral Commission is doing everything possible at the present time to bring about such cooperation." [37]

In view of this suggestion, and of the expressed desires of Bolivia and Paraguay for delay, the Council decided to take no action for the time being.

Saavedra Lamas and the Neutrals

Shortly after the declaration of August 3, 1932, the Argentine government, on its own responsibility, proposed to Bolivia and Paraguay that they agree to a truce of one month, with each side to maintain its troops in the positions they then occupied. This proposal was inconsistent with the position of the Neutrals that Argentina was formally supporting, since the Neutrals considered that only a withdrawal to the positions occupied on June 1 would be in accordance with the principle of nonrecognition of territorial conquests. Furthermore, it gave Argentina's support to the position of Bolivia, which had not accepted the Neutrals' proposal for a withdrawal to the June 1 line, although such agreement had been obtained from Paraguay.

White felt that the reason for Saavedra Lamas's move was his desire

to try to show something which he had accomplished—he didn't much care how. He thought, as his Ambassador here said, that whatever Bolivia accepted and was supported in by the Neutrals and the neighboring countries, Paraguay would have to agree to. The Neutrals refused to agree to this and so did Paraguay.[38]

Bliss reported that Saavedra Lamas had instructed his ambassador in Asunción to tell the Paraguayan government that "Argentina was cooperating with [the] Neutral Commission; that [the] attempt to play [the] group of neighboring countries against [the] Neutral Commission was dangerous and futile and that Paraguay should treat loyally with [the] commission." [39]

This attempt of Saavedra Lamas to play a lone hand in the negotiations was a failure. White told Ambassador Bliss in Buenos Aires that, as a result of the incident,

there is a very strong feeling on the part of my Neutral colleagues against Argentina. I felt that the Neutrals and the neighboring countries should cooperate very closely and I regretted to see this bitter feeling develop—that I was doing what I could to keep the feeling as friendly as possible.

He said: "The Neutrals asked me to cable Mr. Bliss and ask him to go over Saavedra Lamas' head to President [Agustín] Justo and, while such a cable had been drafted, it had not been sent and I was not sending it." White felt that such a cable might embarrass both Bliss and the Argentine President "and would get us the ill will of Saavedra Lamas. Mr. Bliss said that was quite right and he was glad I had not sent the cable." [40]

Looking back, it may well be wondered whether White might not have felt later that the appeal to President Justo should have been made, in view of the subsequent efforts of Saavedra Lamas to settle the Chaco dispute in ways which would make him appear as principal peacemaker. It may be wondered whether the issue of the "ill will" of Saavedra Lamas was a real one, since it is at least open to question whether his motivations were based on good will or ill will, rather than on calculations of personal prestige and public credit for diplomatic victories. It may also be wondered whether the idea of gaining the good will or ill will of the Argentine government was, during this time, a valid one. There existed a rivalry between Argentina and the United States for leadership of the American states that went beyond personal characteristics peculiar to Saavedra Lamas and was evident in the policies of his successors in office. While this rivalry was not tinged with threats, nor were forcible measures even remotely in the background, during the 1930s the relationship between the two countries was such that attempts to promote good will as a means of enhancing collaboration were of extremely doubtful value.

Saavedra Lamas, of course, attempted to take advantage of the failure of the Neutrals to terminate hostilities, but he was unsuccessful. White learned from Espil that "there is a grave disagreement between Saavedra Lamas and Cruchaga. Each one is trying to bring about a settlement and get credit for it and is resentful of what the other is doing." [41] The Chilean Chargé told Francis White that "Saavedra Lamas would not support any proposal that was not his own." [42] White replied that it would be desirable to "wait and see what he is going to propose and perhaps humor and flatter his vanity a bit to see if we can not find some workable basis therein." [43] Then, and later, cajolery of Saavedra Lamas proved to be an utterly ineffectual technique of the foreign policy of the United States.

The Failure of the Neighbors' Efforts

A serious and concerted effort at bringing about peace was undertaken by Argentina and Chile, when the foreign ministers of these countries, Saavedra Lamas and Cruchaga Tocornal, on the invitation of the latter, met at Mendoza, Argentina, on February 1 and 2, 1933. A formula for the solution of the Chaco conflict was agreed upon at Mendoza, approved subsequently by Brazil and Peru, and foi mally presented in the name of the four countries to Bolivia and Paraguay, on February 25. The Mendoza formula provided for cessation of hostilities, withdrawal of troops by Bolivia to Forts Ballivián and Roboré and by Paraguay to the Paraguay River, reduction of armies to peacetime strength, and arbitration of the basic question.[44]

The outstanding feature of the Mendoza plan was that it was, at the outset, a strictly South American effort to obtain peace. The Act of Mendoza referred to "continental solidarity" and to the problems posed by the Chaco conflict to other countries, "especially the countries which are limitrophe neighbors." It made mention of "the lessons which flow from the continuous efforts previously made, with the most laudable purpose, by the Commission of Neutrals" and based the new proposal upon "the exploration carried out" by the Argentine government and the formula previously suggested by the government of Chile. If the plan were accepted by Bolivia and Paraguay, the four limitrophe states would then present the plan to the Commission of Neutrals, and the nine countries then would formally present the plan to Bolivia and Paraguay and ask the other American states to "second them in such action."

Noting that the Act of Mendoza appeared to have been written by Saavedra Lamas, Ambassador Bliss commented that the Argentine Foreign Minister cherished

the hope of giving greater, not to say predominating, influence to Argentina in the political development of the Latin American Republics.

This policy, or aspiration, is one which has imbued various Argentine statesmen in the past. It is a natural yearning of a proud, young and ambitious nation. In pursuing this policy, Dr. Saavedra Lamas assumes, as have his precursors, that the United States is the principal obstacle in his path and while I do not think he is, *per se*, anti-American in sentiment, he follows the line of others in endeavoring to counteract what he considers the preponderant influence of the United States throughout America and to prevent the United States from consummating its pan-American projects—such as the Neutral Commission in Washington—as the most effective way of guiding Argentina to the fore.[45]

Since the plan of the neutral Commission had failed of acceptance in December, an attempt on the part of the neighboring countries was not unjustified and was not opposed by the Neutrals. Hopes of success may have been encouraged also by the fact that Argentine influence in Paraguay was considerable and that it had been Paraguay which had rejected the Neutrals' proposal. However, the Argentine Foreign Minister revealed a lack of confidence in the Mendoza plan when, only three days after its submission to Bolivia and Paraguay, he requested the support of the United States to try "to force an armistice on Bolivia and Paraguay." Saavedra Lamas suggested that the United States "invoke the Kellogg Pact on Bolivia and also point out to Bolivia the 'incontestable value' of the aid which American bankers might lend to Bolivia." In reply, White said that the United States would wish to act only in conjunction with other members of the Neutral Commission and pointed out that Bolivia was not a party to the Kellogg-Briand Pact. Finally, in a significant statement, illustrative of his attitude on a general question of policy, White said that "despite charges to the contrary, this Government does not practice economic imperialism such as is envisaged by the mention of aid from American bankers." [46] White added that this proposal was "outside" the Mendoza formula now under consideration by the contending governments and that the neighboring countries "had best concentrate along that line."

This idea was brought up again by Saavedra Lamas in August. He said that

the best hope which he could see for a settlement was for the United States Government to bring financial pressure to bear on Bolivia . . . he thought that there were certain channels through which American money reached the Bolivians and which the discreet intervention of the United States Government might close. If Bolivia could no longer finance the war material he thought that the war would soon terminate.

In response to the report of this conversation, the Department instructed Ambassador Alexander W. Weddell that he "might appropriately take exception to any unsupported insinuation" by Saavedra Lamas "that the Bolivian Government is being assisted financially by Americans in carrying on its hostilities in the Chaco." The instruction stated that "as far as the Department is aware the Bolivian expenses of the Chaco conflict are being financed principally by heavy levies upon the Banco Central de Bolivia and by taxation." [47]

Again on March 7, Saavedra Lamas in a talk with Ambassador Bliss "stressed his desire that the United States Government should bring pressure to bear on the Bolivian Government to accept the formula. . . . Argentina could take care of Paraguay, on which Government it could bring pressure to bear." [48] In view of Paraguay's acceptance of the Mendoza plan, this pressure must have been considerable, since it was reported that President Ayala,

in spite of his bitterness since the Neutral proposal of December 15, has retained a strong desire that the United States figure in any agreement that may finally be arrived at. This from a distrust of individual jealousies among the Neighbor Powers and a dislike of any interference on American soil of the League of Nations.[49]

The neighboring countries optimistically but inaccurately informed the Neutral Commission that Bolivia and Paraguay had accepted in principle the Mendoza formula and suggested that the moment had come for the Commision and the four neighbors to undertake immediate negotiations for the cessation of hostilities for a period of sixty days.[50]

The Commission replied that it supported "cordially and decidedly" the formula and that the neighboring governments could so tell Bolivia and Paraguay, "in arranging the agreement of absolute cessation of hostilities." [51] In so doing, the Commission, in effect, rejected the proposal for joint negotiations made by the neighbors. The reason for this rejection was that it had information through the Department of State that Bolivia would accept an armistice only on the basis of the existing fighting lines and Paraguay would do so only if Bolivian troops were withdrawn to a Villa Montes–Roboré line,[52] and it did not wish in this unpromising situation to "make direct representations to the two countries."

In this connection, the Bolivian Minister in Washington, Finot, cabled La Paz that the Commission was not supporting the neighboring countries "with interest or enthusiasm and that the Commission would not be displeased if the present negotiations failed." [53] The Secretary of State immediately replied that there "was no justification for Finot's statement. The Commission supported fully the suggestions of the neighboring countries for an armistice" and would be glad to see their efforts succeed.[54] The United States ministers in Bolivia and Paraguay were instructed to join with their Argentine and Chilean colleagues in urging Bolivia and Paraguay to withdraw their reservations to the Mendoza formula on the points mentioned above.[55]

The result of this effort was that Paraguay withdrew its reservations to the Mendoza formula, but Bolivia refused to do so. An attempt then was made to bring renewed pressure on Bolivia, but it failed. As White described it: "Brazil apparently acted on its own a week or more before Argentina and Chile acted; then those Governments had acted, and Peru has taken no action whatsoever." Washington had received notification on April 19 of the terms of a strong Chilean communication to Bolivia, but White was ill, and no action was taken by the Department of State. White told Espil that he thought "there was no possibility of finding a solution as long as negotiations were carried on in the slipshod manner in which they have been carried on." [56]

The Chilean note stated that it was "now time to remind Bolivia of the responsibility she would assume for the eventual failure" of the Mendoza formula.[57] The Argentine note was in milder terms. The Peruvian inaction was consistent with its previous position that any armistice should be on the basis of existing troops' positions. The Bolivian government considered that this Chilean note was not compatible with the function of mediation engaged in by the neighboring countries, and its refusal to withdraw its reservations was not shaken by the note. In response to a formal memorandum from the Chilean Foreign Office, on April 27, that the United States associate itself with Argentina, Brazil, and Chile in bringing pressure to bear on Bolivia, White informed the Chilean Chargé that the United States would not wish to act independently of the Neutrals.[58]

The response of the Bolivian government to the strong representations made by Argentina and Chile was a circular telegram of May 5 to its diplomatic officers in the nine neighboring and Neutral Commission countries, suggesting that Bolivia was willing to hear any joint suggestions from these countries about the definition of an arbitrable zone.[59] The tone of this note was unconciliatory and was apparently regarded as "a slap in the face for Chile." [60]

The failure of the Mendoza plan left America incapable of concerted action, as is indicated by the following sequence of events. On May 9 the Commission of Neutrals suggested to the neighbors "an exchange of ideas" to determine what would be "useful and favorable to the interests of peace on the continent." [61] The next day

Paraguay declared that a state of war existed with Bolivia. On May 11 Bolivia informed the Council of the League of Nations that it considered Paraguay had, by declaring war, incurred sanctions under Article 16 of the Covenant. On May 20 the Council adopted a plan calling for the appointment of a commission to go to the Chaco. On the same day White suggested to Espil that the nine countries comprising the Commission of Neutrals and the neighbors should "agree to support the League's proposal." On May 23, White learned that Argentina would not accept the invitation to exchange ideas with the Commission, since the matter was in the hands of the League of Nations. On May 23 the Bolivian government urged on the neighboring countries that they join with the Neutrals in negotiations with Bolivia and Paraguay, and on the same day the British and French ministers in La Paz received instructions to urge Bolivia to accept the League of Nations plan. On May 25 the Chilean government informed White it did not propose to take any action in the Chaco, meaning that it would not exchange ideas with the Neutrals. On May 31 the Brazilian Foreign Minister stated that he did not approve of White's suggestion that the League plan be supported by the neighbors and Neutrals. He said that "Brazil feels that for reasons of continental policy and tradition the problem should, if possible, be settled by American means, but if these means fail then the American peace agencies should relinquish the task for the League to take on if it so wishes." [62]

The final peace effort in 1933 was made in mid-October. As a result of talks between Saavedra Lamas and Mello Franco, the presidents of Argentina and Brazil addressed telegrams to Bolivia and Paraguay on October 11, urging them to submit the dispute to arbitration. The flames of hope lit by this presidentially sponsored initiative were extinguished in two weeks by a Paraguayan rejection of the proposal.[63] This action by Saavedra Lamas was regarded by the Chilean Foreign Minister as a breach of the Act of Mendoza, in which the two countries had pledged common action in the Chaco. Cruchaga Tocornal was so embarrassed that he even presented his resignation to President Arturo Alessandri, who declined it.[64] This blow to the Act of Mendoza, which Saavedra Lamas himself had called "a new organ of pacification," was followed by a second, this time fatal. In July, 1934, Saavedra Lamas proposed a new formula for Chaco peace and asked Brazil and the United States, but not Chile, to give it their support in La Paz and Asunción. The political adviser of the Chilean foreign office said that "Chile was deeply offended that Saavedra Lamas had not consulted Chile in regard to this plan," since the Argentine government was not living up to the Pact of Mendoza.[65] Nothing more was heard about the Mendoza agreement; Saavedra Lamas's boasts about the "international personality" of South America were empty, at least with regard to its capacity to bring war to an end in the Chaco.

At the seventh Conference of American states in Montevideo, the United States participated in another peace effort. Although a short armistice was arranged from December 19, 1933, to January 6, 1934, no progress was made on the basic question, and hostilities were resumed. In the second week of December the Paraguayans had won the decisive victory at Fort Arce that marked the beginning of the long Bolivian retreat to the western Chaco.

The Failure of the Neutrals' Efforts

In view of the frustration of peace activities by the countries of America, the League's plan to send a commission to the Chaco appeared to be the one possible hopeful procedure that had been agreed upon by some responsible agency. Ambassador Bliss reported from Buenos Aires that Saavedra Lamas was "quite definitely committed to the attitude of not soiling his fingers further with the Chaco business."[66] The neighbors were chagrined, annoyed, and withdrawn. The Commission of Neutrals had no improvement on the December 15 plan to offer. Without Brazilian agreement, the Neutrals and neighbors together could not give official support to the League plan.

Accepting this situation, the United States obtained the cessation of the "four and a half years of patient endeavors" by the Commission of Neutrals, on June 27. The explanation of this step is given in a memorandum to President Roosevelt from Acting Secretary of State William Phillips, on the recommendation of Francis White.[67] In order "not to cross wires" with the League, Phillips suggested in a tone of satisfaction that the United States could "get out of the matter gracefully and leave it to the League and South Americans," who might form the entire membership of the League commission. The United States should not be a member of the commission because, if so,

we will surely run into conflict with Argentina, which is not a neutral and has openly supported Paraguay. It seems evident that Argentina will not work for the success of the League commission and failure, therefore, of such efforts is almost assured. We do not want to get into trouble with Argentina on account of American interests in that country. We have no interest in the Chaco.

The President apparently approved the action, the Commission of Neutrals ceased to exist, and Francis White resigned as Assistant Secretary of State on July 2, 1933. An additional reason for the adoption of this position by the United States, not explicitly referred to in this memorandum, was given by Francis White at the last meeting of the Commission, in saying that the Commission "had tried to get the neighboring countries to cooperate with us and they had refused to do so." [68]

The dissolution of the Commission of Neutrals caused disappointment in Brazil, which had withdrawn from the League of Nations. Foreign Minister Afranio de Mello Franco said that "he could not yet understand the action of Washington in abandoning the problem to the League, and he characterized that action as a blow to the Monroe Doctrine." He added that, if the League should attempt to apply sanctions, "he could not believe that the United States would view with equanimity such action by the League of Nations with respect to an American State." [69]

The Bolivian Minister, Enrique Finot, once more exploring ways of avoiding action by the League of Nations, asked if Assistant Secretary Jefferson Caffery "did not consider the present activities of the League in the Chaco matter to be somewhat in opposition to the Monroe Doctrine." Caffery replied in the negative.[70]

The United States was able to "get out of the matter" for exactly three months. As Ayala later remarked to Minister Meredith Nicholson, "the United States must be a party to any arbitration of the Chaco controversy because, in spite of what may be said in Latin

America, it is recognized that the United States is the only important world power in the western hemisphere." [71] In addition, as Joseph Avenol had remarked, "the jealousy felt for any Latin American state which played a leading role militated against successful common efforts within the Latin American sphere." [72]

The field was then open for the League of Nations Commission of Inquiry, which presented on February 22, 1934, a plan for arbitration of the dispute. The Council of the League requested support for this proposal from the American states, but the response was no more than lukewarm. Paraguay rejected the Commission's plan, and the Bolivian answer, while more responsive, was not a clear acceptance.[73] The Council of the League of Nations took no effective action on the report of its Commission in the spring of 1934, and the dispute was referred to the Assembly, at Bolivia's request, when it met in September.

Problems for United States Policy

The well-publicized failure to secure peace at the Montevideo Conference was followed by the failure of nearly forty other distinct attempts at peacemaking by individual statesmen and by formal and informal groupings of states. Finally, when the Paraguayan army could advance no more, nor the Bolivian army counterattack, the two governments accepted an armistice proposed by five American states in June, 1935. The intervening negotiations need not be described in detail, or even enumerated, but it may not be unrewarding to recount certain instructive episodes and to distinguish some outstanding features of the participation of the United States in this notable diplomatic struggle.

Efforts to stop the fighting continued in 1934 to occupy the attention both of the League of Nations and the major American states. The United States tried in vain to induce Argentina "through friendly counsel with the Government of Paraguay" to obtain a continuation of the truce arranged at the Montevideo Conference.[74] It was the view of Secretary Hull that the Argentine government could end the war by insisting on an immediate armistice and arbitration; he felt that the key to the situation was in the hands of President Agustín Justo and Saavedra Lamas.[75]

AN ARMS EMBARGO

Perhaps because of sensitivity to charges in Geneva and at home that the United States had obstructed the League of Nations in dealing with Chaco, and also out of a desire to take some constructive step after years of fruitless palaver, it was decided in Washington to prevent either belligerent from securing arms in the United States. As a preliminary move, inquiries were made of the neighboring powers whether they contemplated any action toward peace. In the telegrams of inquiry, the Department noted that

the attention of the entire world has recently been drawn very sharply to the continuation of war between Paraguay and Bolivia and to the moral responsibility of the neighboring countries and of the other powers of the American continent, in acquiescing in such prolongation without taking every possible effective and practical means of fostering pacific solution of the dispute.[76]

Replies were not received from all the states concerned, but, on May 18, a proposal for the prohibition of the sale of arms and munitions to Bolivia and Paraguay from the United States was introduced into the Senate on behalf of the administration.

Assistant Secretary of State Sumner Welles, in a press conference, said that, in view of uncertainty about the action of other American states, it appeared that the time had come for the United States to take action alone, although it preferred to work with

the other American states, particularly the neighboring republics, and with other nations of the world . . . we feel that we have done everything possible during these past few months to further the cause of peace between these two countries, and we also feel that the time has now come for us to take this action.[77]

The resolution authorizing the President to prohibit the sale of arms to Bolivia and Paraguay was unanimously passed by both Houses of Congress and signed by President Roosevelt on May 28, 1934, and a proclamation to this effect was issued on the same day.

This contribution to peace was protested by Bolivia as a violation of its commercial treaty of 1858 with the United States and also as favoring Paraguay which could import arms directly via the Paraguay River.[78] The Department of State countered with the interpretation that the treaty referred only to prohibitions of importation and exportation but not to the prohibition of the sale of articles in the United States. The resolution was regarded as fair to both parties since it applied equally to both so far as the United States was concerned. Finally, Secretary Hull brought the resolution into harmony with the good neighbor policy:

The Government of the United States, as you are well aware, has dedicated itself to the policy of the good neighbor. It would be in the highest degree inconsistent with that policy that arms and munitions of war manufactured in the United States should continue to be sold for the purpose of assisting in the destruction of the lives of the citizens of our two sister republics of Bolivia and Paraguay and in prolonging the warfare in the Chaco which has already resulted in such grave prejudice to the well-being and prosperity of those two republics.[79]

The Paraguayan government did not protest the embargo, probably because it had on order no munitions produced in the United States. The Foreign Minister did, however, issue a statement that the decision of the United States to make some exceptions to the embargo in the case of arms and munitions on which Bolivia had made payments prior to the proclamation had caused "painful surprise in Paraguay" and that such action "appears destined to stimulate a continuation of the war and to favor one of the belligerents." [80] The exceptions, for sales consummated before the proclamation, amounted to shipments valued at $615,071.38, although shipments arranged under contracts having a value of $2,065,421.79 were prohibited.[81]

It does not appear that the action of the United States had an important effect upon the course of the war.[82] Paraguay obtained its armaments mainly from Argentina and Europe. Bolivia was able to buy equipment in Europe throughout the conflict, except when, from November 1934 to February 1935, the League arms embargo applied to both belligerents. The action did, however, give the United States a special position among American states and relieved it of charges that its policy was contributing to the prolongation of the war by permitting the belligerents to purchase arms in its territory.

THE STANDARD OIL COMPANY

The Paraguayan press at various times during the war charged that the Standard Oil Company of New Jersey was aiding the Bolivian war effort. Paraguayans did not always distinguish between the Standard Oil Company and the Government of the United States in making these charges; as a result, as reported by Nicholson in Asunción, "the belief is deeply rooted and widely spread in this country, even among responsible and intelligent men, that the United States has aided Bolivia financially to carry on the War." [83]

An example of this attitude is found in an editorial in *La Tribuna* (Asunción) on February 15, 1934: "Bolivia is one of the countries of America which has been absorbed by the petroleum octopus and whose wealth has fallen into the hands of the Standard Oil Company, or, what is the same thing, of the United States of America."

Paraguayan prejudices were given new substance by speeches made by Senator Huey Long on May 30, June 7, and June 8, 1934, in the United States Senate, in which he charged that the Standard Oil Company was traditionally a promoter of wars and civil strife in Latin America and was aiding Bolivia in the Chaco war in order to obtain a port for the exportation of petroleum. President Ayala appeared to be influenced by these speeches to give more serious consideration than previously to the possibility that Standard Oil was aiding Bolivia financially.[84] The Standard Oil Company publicly and categorically denied that it was giving any aid to the Bolivian government or that it had in any way encouraged the Bolivian government to go to war to obtain a port or for any other reason.

However, in Paraguay, Nicholson reported:

There has . . . been such a campaign conducted by the press to attempt to prove that the Standard Oil is an ally of Bolivia and an enemy of Paraguay that even the most intelligent persons either are convinced of the truth of the sensational charges made or fear to express an opinion [opposed] to popular prejudice.[85]

A semi-official recognition of Senator Long's services to Paraguay was given, if not by the government, at least by the Commander-in-Chief of the Paraguayan field armies. *El Orden* (Asunción) of August 21, 1934, printed a large picture of Senator Long, with an announcement that, at the spontaneous and unanimous request of the soldiers, "the Bolivian Fort Loma Vistosa captured on August 16, has been renamed Senador Long" and that the name had been confirmed by the Commander-in-Chief. The paper added:

The Paraguayan Army in this fashion offers a merited homage to the defender of our cause, who, in an hour of moral disaster for the Continent, raised his voice in the dignified chamber of the Senate of his country, in protest against a criminal. The name of the great crusader for justice and right is heard today in the midst of the Chaco as a warning to usurpers and a challenge to Carthaginian gold.[86]

An opportunity to make a retort courteous was given to the Bolivian press six months later when Senators Marvel M. Logan of Kentucky and Joseph T. Robinson of Arkansas replied to Senator Long, with some kind words for Bolivia. *Tribuna* (La Paz), March 18, 1935, referred to these speeches and stated:

Today, the school teachers throughout Bolivia, during the hour for the study of geography, should gather their children around the map of North America and show them two states of the greatest republic of the north: Kentucky and Arkansas . . . which . . . ought to be known, in all their geographic and spiritual characteristics, to the children of Bolivia.

It was with little effect that Secretary Hull sent to Nicholson the statements of the Standard Oil Company declaring that none of the Company's oil properties lay within the Chaco as defined by Paraguay and that the Company's oil production was very small and "was sold locally in Bolivia." [87] The Department of State did not comment on the Company's statements except to say that it would be helpful if these and other facts "were made available to public opinion in Paraguay so that there may be no room for doubt as to the friendly and consistently impartial attitude of this Government as between the two belligerents." In reply, Nicholson reported:

The Paraguayan press has been assiduous in fostering the belief, now almost a national conviction, that the Standard Oil Company is sponsoring Bolivia in the Chaco war. The presumably spontaneous activities of the press in this respect have been supported by the utterances of foreign promoters of anti-American sentiment, and no incident is too trivial or irrelevant to serve as the basis for a renewal attack upon the Company.[88]

In these circumstances, the kind of evidence that might have had an effect on Paraguayan opinion was not forthcoming until 1937 when the Bolivian government confiscated the properties of the Standard Oil company.[89]

Saavedra Lamas and the League of Nations

In the summer of 1934, while the League of Nations was inactive, a new mediatory effort was started by Dr. Saavedra Lamas. Ambassador Weddell said that Saavedra Lamas considered "the Chaco conflict as being almost ripe for settlement, using the simile of a tree on which the fruit was mellowing, merely needing a delicate hand to shake the boughs." [90]

The first movement of Saavedra Lamas's delicate hand became apparent on July 14, when he submitted to the governments of Brazil and the United States a plan known as the Argentine Conciliation Formula. He told the two governments that the acceptance of the Formula by Paraguay was assured and asked their assistance in exerting "every possible influence" on the President of Bolivia to gain the latter's approval. The Formula provided for a conference in Buenos Aires for the conciliation of the belligerents, and for agreement for arbitration by the Permanent Court of International Justice if conciliation proved ineffective.

Secretary Hull stated his belief that "the question of promoting peace on the continent is one of continental responsibility" and expressed the hope that the government of Brazil would join in urging Bolivia to accept the Formula.[91] On receiving Brazil's expression of agreement, Minister Fay Allen Des Portes in La Paz was instructed to tell the Bolivian government that the United States government had been informed of the Argentine Formula "and believes it to be a method for arriving at a fair and equitable solution of this long standing controversy through direct conciliation." Secretary Hull expressed his government's "most earnest and sincere hope that the

Government of Bolivia will find it feasible to accept the invitation" to accept the Argentine Formula.[92]

There ensued a series of complicated negotiations, at the end of which the Bolivian government accepted the Formula with certain reservations. The Paraguayan government accepted the Formula without reservation but on September 13 desired to reconsider its acceptance on learning the Bolivian stand. There were several aspects of these negotiations that were of interest. One was the ability of Saavedra Lamas once more to guarantee Paraguayan acceptance of the Formula, a fact that indicated the extent of Argentine influence in Asunción.

A second feature was the concern of the United States with broadening the American base of the mediation effort. In correspondence with La Paz, Washington made it clear that the mediation was not "to be left to the 'sole auspices of Argentina' " merely because the initiative was that of Saavedra Lamas or because the proposed conference would be held in Buenos Aires.[93] The "eventual cooperation by the other republics of this continent" was suggested to the Argentine foreign minister on July 17. The first reaction of Saavedra Lamas was to say that "he was entirely willing that in the final solution all American Republics should be represented but that Argentina, Brazil and the United States must be careful to guard their dignity as first class powers in all negotiations." [94] The most specific implication of this remark was that Chile was not a first class power, in the opinion of Saavedra Lamas, and the exclusion of Chile from association in this peace initiative was one of its most notable features. The significance of this feature had been clear at an early date, as Secretary Hull noted on July 20 that "the Department has been confidentially informed by the Chilean Government that it is under the impression that it has been rigorously excluded from these peace negotiations and it has intimated that if this policy is persisted in the negotiations will necessarily prove unsuccessful." [95] It is not improbable that the Chilean government exerted influence on the government of Bolivia to reject the Argentine Formula. In any case, the Bolivian reservations succeeded in preventing the Formula from being accepted, and Chile was not brought into the mediating group of Argentina, Brazil, and the United States.[96]

The United States stand in this démarche is of some importance. Secretary Hull said:

This Government is decidedly of the opinion and has frequently so stated, that the furtherance of peace on the American Continent should be a matter of joint moral responsibility for all of the American Republics and does not believe that efforts in behalf of peace should be limited to any bloc or clique of American Republics. The latter procedure would be more likely to promote ill feeling than to further peace, particularly under present conditions. The precedent involved in this instance is one which this Government attributes the highest importance [*sic*].[97]

As a result of this strong stand, Saavedra Lamas finally accepted the view that other states would be invited when the belligerents' acceptance in principle had been obtained.

Such acceptance in principle was announced to the Department of State by Saavedra Lamas on August 11. However, no invitation was sent to other powers because it appeared that the announcement by Saavedra Lamas was premature. He was negotiating with the belligerents and with Brazil and the United States, and it appeared that he was saying different things to each of the representatives of the states involved. The Bolivian Foreign Minister was reported to be annoyed at "contradictory statements" he was receiving about bases for conciliation under discussion in Buenos Aires, and Brazilian Foreign Minister José Carlos de Macedo Soares also expressed "annoyance at the apparent discrepancy between statements made by Saavedra Lamas to the mediating countries on the one hand and the contending countries on the other hand, a course which may lead to serious complications." [98] However, on September 7 a response was given by La Paz, which was in the view of Saavedra Lamas " 'conciliable' " and in the view of Washington was "reasonable" although in need of some modification.

At this apparently auspicious moment for an American settlement in the Chaco, Saavedra Lamas made one of the most remarkable diplomatic moves of his career. His representative at Geneva, José María Cantilo, made a speech on September 12 to the League Assembly proposing that the Assembly attempt to solve the Chaco dispute. Cantilo gave the impression that he was speaking for Brazil and the United States as well as Argentina.[99]

This speech, however, was made entirely without consultation on the part of Argentina with Brazil and the United States, except that Saavedra Lamas had indicated that he had planned to send to the League "a bald statement of fact in order to guard his impartial position between the two belligerents." [100]

There was "distinct irritation tinged with discouragement" in Rio de Janeiro, not only at Saavedra Lamas's presuming to speak for his unconsulted colleagues but also at his abandonment of the joint mediation effort.[101] From Washington, Saavedra Lamas was told that the position of the United States could not be determined in Buenos Aires: "The position of Argentina with regard to the League is completely distinct from that of the United States and this Government reserves complete liberty of action with regard to what its policy may be in connection with the continuation of the present peace negotiations." [102] Nothing more; Saavedra Lamas's delicate hand received no more than a slap on the wrist for dexterously, and without warning, tossing the Chaco problem across the Atlantic.

The motivation of Saavedra Lamas in transferring the Chaco question to the League cannot be known with certainty, but it is possible to make some guesses about it that accord with available information. Cantilo told Ambassador Hugh Gibson and Wilson that Saavedra Lamas

felt that he had gone as far as he could in the Buenos Aires negotiations respecting the Chaco, that he does not wish to be left with the problem if the League will assume it, and that should the League adopt the Buenos Aires proposals as a basis for its efforts he would gain sufficient credit should the League succeed but that failure would be borne by Geneva. In a conversation with Avenol shortly thereafter he told me that he had just had a talk with Cantilo and related his impressions which were almost precisely what I have described above. Avenol added that this apparently fully accounted for Argentina's recent policy in Geneva.[103]

This suggests that Saavedra Lamas did not think that he could obtain Bolivian agreement to an armistice on his terms, but there were several other considerations that may have influenced him. One of these was his own prestige, which he defended and advanced with all ingenious resourcefulness. If he really despaired of his mediation at this time, the session of the League Assembly offered a graceful escape from a dilemma. Even if he believed the Bolivian position to be, as he had said, "conciliable," the Assembly offered another kind of opportunity; by placing the dispute in its hands he could show by a dramatic gesture that he could not be criticized, as Francis White and Hull had been, for refusing to allow the League a free hand in the Chaco. Further, this gesture could be interpreted as showing independence of the United States and as a praiseworthy attempt to strengthen the position of the League of Nations as having primary responsibility for keeping the peace throughout the world.

There is an additional possibility that might be regarded as unworthy of mention, except that the diplomatic record of Saavedra Lamas demonstrated a matchless capacity for successful personal intrigue. The suspicion is hard to down that Saavedra Lamas may have intended from the beginning that the League would not succeed in bringing peace to the Chaco. Ten days after Cantilo's speech at the Assembly, Consul Prentiss Gilbert reported from Geneva:

The League leaders in turning to Latin American representatives here for guidance or to solicit their consent to serve on a committee encounter diversity of opinion but discover little vital interest. Almost all are without instructions from their Governments. The situation is thus confused and the development of a definite plan is exceedingly difficult. From reasonably reliable sources I learn: Argentina is endeavoring to have the handling of the question left to Buenos Aires.[104]

Argentina's position, as stated privately by Saavedra Lamas, was "one of passive observance keeping in mind, however, the loyalty owed to the League." He added, prophetically, that he was "convinced that this [League's] Commission's efforts would fail." [105] In Chile, Argentina's position was differently viewed. Foreign Minister Cruchaga Tocornal "evinced considerable fear that Saavedra Lamas, through pique or personal ambition, may attempt in one form or another to impede the labors of the commission" planned by the League.[106]

Late in October it was stated that "Saavedra Lamas suggested to the Department that any further conciliatory action be postponed until the League had 'spent itself.' " [107] A rumor that Saavedra

Lamas had approached the governments of France, Great Britain, and Italy to try to obtain their collaboration with Argentina in the Chaco dispute was reported in November.[108] This rumor was not confirmed, and an official Argentine denial was not in itself convincing.

The League's effort at conciliation failed when Paraguay rejected its plan. On two previous occasions, in 1933 and in 1934, when a Saavedra Lamas plan was proposed, the Argentine foreign minister was able to guarantee in advance that Paraguay would accept the proposals and in each case his guarantee was fulfilled. It cannot, of course, be said that he could have obtained acceptance by Paraguay of the League report if he had tried to do so, but it is striking to note the contrast between his capabilities with respect to Paraguayan policy when a peace plan originated with him and when it originated elsewhere.

These considerations suggest that Saavedra Lamas's action at this time might be described as calling in the Old World to redress the balance of the New, and then going George Canning one better by proving the Old World incapable. He could in this way appear to be "the Great Peacemaker" (Spruille Braden's phrase) by neglecting no opportunity to restore peace to the Chaco. At the same time, however, he may have seen that he would be able, incognito because he could secretly arrange for Paraguay's rejection of any League plan, to give crashing emphasis to the necessity of an American solution to the Chaco War and, in particular, to the necessity for a solution that would give due recognition to the primacy of the role of Argentina, and of Carlos Saavedra Lamas. This is only speculation, and it cannot be documented, but it fits the known facts and is in harmony with characterizations of Saavedra Lamas's policy and personality as made by diplomatic observers at the time. If, as had been said, Saavedra Lamas would block any solution in the Chaco that was not his own, it was unlikely that he would voluntarily transfer the dispute to the League without the expectation that he would before long be able not only to block the League but also to play a major personal role in the settlement of the conflict. In this connection, it may be recalled that a Brazilian diplomat, commenting on the reasons why Foreign Minister Mello Franco of Brazil had succeeded in bringing about a peaceful solution of the Leticia dispute although none had been found in the Chaco, observed that Mello Franco "enjoyed the complete confidence of both parties to the controversy, and . . . there was no Saavedra Lamas in the case." [109]

The United States and the League of Nations

Although the field was now open for the League of Nations to try again to end this durable conflict, the League had to work without the active cooperation of the United States and Brazil. Washington informed League officials that it was "unable" to accept membership on any League Commission dealing with the Chaco.[110] Hull stated publicly that

this government's policy, as evidenced at Montevideo when the Commission of the League was considering the Chaco problem, was to act on it own individual judgment, and to furnish any and all cooperation to any peace agency which may be functioning or which is contemplating action designed to effect a peaceful settlement of the Chaco hostilities.[111]

As for Brazil, Foreign Minister Macedo Soares told Ambassador Gibson:

Comparing past League efforts with purely American efforts . . . experience has shown that we understand our own problems better than they are understood at Geneva and that we can settle American conflicts better and more expeditiously among ourselves than can be hoped for if duplicate negotiations afford the parties an opportunity to alternate between the two and thus complicate and prolong the discussion, as is being done at the present time.

Macedo Soares suggested that Hull make a declaration "stressing the importance we attach to settling American problems in America," and he added:

From the Brazilian-American point of view . . . "so long as Brazil and the United States are not members of the League of Nations we should not permit any intervention of non-American states in the handling of purely American problems." . . . The present problem is more fundamental than any question of procedure in handling the Chaco problem and [he] raised the question as to whether the Monroe Doctrine is to develop into an all American principle or whether we are going to allow it to be undermined by non-American handling of American affairs.[112]

In response, Hull said sympathetically that, while "it is the belief of the United States as it is of Brazil that American problems can be most advantageously solved through some form of cooperation between the American states themselves and not through the utilization of non-American agencies," the making of a declaration

would inevitably be construed as an attack upon the League of Nations or as a deliberate reflection upon its general utility. For that reason this Government believes it desirable to take no action now but will however undertake full and detailed consideration of the far-reaching policy suggested by the Brazilian Minister for Foreign Affairs.[113]

Such consideration does not appear to have been entered upon.

The League for its part began conciliation efforts in Geneva that by the end of October were admitted to be a "failure" by Avenol, largely because of "the absence of a Paraguayan representative." [114]

The "failure" of the League was authoritatively attributed to Argentina. The Argentine government, however, accepted membership on a new Advisory Committee appointed on November 24 by the extraordinary Assembly of the League, along with twenty-two other members. The United States declined to participate in the work of this Committee, although Gilbert was authorized "to maintain informal contact with the members of the Advisory Committee for purposes of information."

This decision differed markedly from the previous aloofness of the United States toward activities of the League and it was taken after careful consideration in the Department of State and after approval by President Roosevelt. On November 28 Secretary Hull had written to the President setting forth an account of the government's relation to the Chaco dispute. The Secretary noted that

the finding of a peaceful settlement has repeatedly been hampered by disagreement between the American mediating nations. The present report of the League provides the first occasion upon which all of the American republics (other than Brazil and the United States) have officially agreed upon a formal recommendation for the settlement of the dispute. There has likewise, as you know, existed on the part of certain of the American republics the suspicion that the United States might attempt through its major influence to dictate to the exclusion of other American nations the settlement of the controversy. Because of the special circumstances existing, I fear that were the United States to appear to adopt an attitude of passive opposition and refuse to cooperate, so far as it is able to do so, with the other American republics in this peace effort which has met with their official approval, the blame for the possible failure of the League efforts, or for the refusal of Bolivia or Paraguay to agree to the terms of the report, would be placed definitely upon the United States and that as a result thereof a very considerable amount of resentment might be created against this Government.

It was clear that the United States should not "take part in any committee" which would sit in Geneva, but Hull believed "that the wisest course for this Government to follow would be to . . . indicate its willingness to take part in the conference to be called by the President of Argentina, and in the work of the Neutral Supervisory Commission." [115] President Roosevelt replied: "I entirely approve the course outlined" in the above letter.[116]

Before sending its reply to the League's invitation, the Department of State consulted with the Brazilian government, and the two governments replied in similar terms to Geneva.[117]

American willingness to collaborate with the League of Nations was regarded in Washington as "necessarily contingent upon the acceptance by the two belligerents of the League Report." [118] Consul Gilbert did not, therefore, attend meetings of the Advisory Committee, although it was apparently contemplated that he should do so if the Report were accepted. The issue did not arise, however, because the Paraguayan reply of December 18 was regarded in Geneva as a rejection, although "the Latin Americans led by Argentina took the position that Paraguay's response was an 'interim reply' and left the door open for further consideration." [119]

A second rejection by Paraguay of the League plan resulted in the unanimous adoption, on January 16, 1935, by the Advisory Committee of a recommendation to League members that they lift the arms embargo on Bolivia, which had unconditionally accepted the Report of December 10, 1934, but maintain it against Paraguay. Anticipating this action, the Department of State had decided that it would not make any change in its policy of preventing the sale of arms in the United States to both belligerents. It was Mr. Welles's view that the effect of removal of the embargo on Bolivian purchases would in effect amount to a prolongation of the war. In addition, he stated that

we had no part in the formulation of the League recommendations and there is no reason why we should take punitive action against Paraguay, discriminating against her in favor of Bolivia, merely because Paraguay has refused to abide by the recommendations made by the League. If we took such action, we would incur the lasting enmity of Paraguay and obtain no advantage of any kind or description.[120]

Formally, the position of the United States government, approved by President Roosevelt, was that the Joint Resolution of Congress provided for the prohibition of the sale of munitions to both belligerents and that no change was contemplated in that policy which "will not, it is believed, interfere in any way with efforts which other governments may make toward restoring peace in the Chaco." [121] Although this formal position was readied in advance, it was not published, since no request for a statement of the attitude of the United States was made when the League action was communicated officially to Washington.[122]

In an attempt at the last minute to avert the imposition of the arms embargo against Paraguay, Argentina and Chile joined to try to bring Bolivia and Paraguay together in a new conciliation procedure. The attempt failed. Paraguay announced its intention to withdraw from the League on February 23, and the next day the Assembly's recommendation to members that they maintain the arms embargo against Paraguay alone went into effect; action by member states, however, remained to be taken by their governments. An American state was thus pilloried in world public opinion, to use a phrase of Saavedra Lamas's, by being the first country ever to be subjected to sanctions by the League of Nations for having violated the Covenant.[123]

An American Armistice

The application of the arms embargo by League members to Paraguay alone did not affect the course of the war, and it marked the last effort by the League to bring about peace in the Chaco. It remained for the American states to establish an agency that Bolivia and Paraguay could turn to when they felt further fighting was useless.

The record of the American states in the Chaco dispute had indeed been a dismal one, and it was made even sorrier by a thinly veiled attack on Saavedra Lamas by President Alessandri of Chile in the spring of 1935. Alessandri asserted publicly that the Chaco war was "unworthy of America" and that a peaceful solution was within the power of the foreign offices of Argentina and Chile, by which he presumably meant that Argentina's policy had been one of obstruction.[124] Probably by prearrangement, this declaration was followed by an interview given by Agustín Edwards, owner of *El Mercurio* of Santiago, on March 4. *El Mercurio*, the most influential paper in Chile and close to the foreign ministry, was usually most circumspect in its editorial comments on the policies of other countries. In this case, however, Edwards, formerly Chilean Ambassador in London, not only criticized the foreign policy of Argentina but attacked Saavedra Lamas by name, an extraordinary action for the proprietor of one of the most responsible of Latin American newspapers.

After charging Saavedra Lamas with Machiavellianism, and being animated with "a spirit of American discord," which was "anti-Argentine," the editorial asked: "What confidence . . . can Chileans have in the promises of Sr. Saavedra Lamas?"

On the previous day *El Mercurio* had stated editorially that the fighting in the Chaco was still going on

because the Chancellor of Argentina had not acted with the energy expected of him in the mission of peace, which is the first of the obligations that weigh upon the diplomacy of any country . . . there has not been in Buenos Aires the same resolute will that has existed in Santiago to call the belligerents to sanity with all the severity that their madness merits.

The incident passed off without a flare-up in Argentina. Saavedra Lamas made a general reply that was not contentious, and the Argentine press reacted calmly. The Brazilian Ambassador in Washington thought this might be "a good lesson to both sides. . . . It would teach Saavedra Lamas that he could not play fast and loose in inter-American politics and . . . it would be a warning to Alessandri to be more judicious as head of a large Republic." [125]

Later, Spruille Braden reported that he had heard various versions of the reasons for Alessandri's statement. One, from a Chilean diplomat, was that, when some progress had been made by Ambassador Felix Nieto del Río in his negotiations in La Paz in February, 1935,

Saavedra Lamas decided that a much more spectacular settlement of the Chaco War could be made if, on the occasion of President Vargas' visit to Buenos Aires, the Argentine and Brazil appeared together as the two leading mediators and the signing of the Peace Protocol be made a part of the program during Vargas' sojourn in Buenos Aires. Saavedra Lamas accordingly instructed his Ambassador Carlos Quintana to present a note to the Chilean Foreign Office stating that Nieto's negotiations in Bolivia were unsuccessful and had best be terminated. Alessandri, realizing that Saavedra Lamas' real objection was to push Chile to one side and substitute Brazil in the negotiations, was so enraged that he gave the famous interview.[126]

With regard to action by the League of Nations, the Uruguayan Minister in Washington said that, in his opinion, various European countries "were endeavoring to obtain League action applying sanctions in the Chaco matter in order to create a precedent which might be of value to them later in questions in which they were directly concerned." He thought Uruguay "could not agree that the League, which had been unwilling or unable to impose sanctions against powerful countries, e.g. Japan, should seek to impose them in the case of a conflict involving two small countries of Latin America." [127]

The situation at this time seemed no more propitious than in September, when Ambassador Hugh Gibson deplored the negotiatory procedures, saying that:

As matters now stand, there are American, Argentine, Brazilian, Bolivian and Paraguayan representatives negotiating in five different capitals. The two contending parties never want a solution at the same time or on the same terms. One or both of them are always afraid of a solution for fear of its effect upon their political fortunes and wherever they have seen danger of a settlement they have found in the negotiations carried on through numerous agents a maximum opportunity to create difficulties and diversions.

Gibson suggested agreement by the mediators on a formula, appointment by the mediators of one person in La Paz and one person in Asunción to obtain acceptance of the formula "in order to eliminate the necessity for endless checking and verification," and, if one party refused to accept the formula, the mediators should make it clear that it "would forfeit the sympathy of the other American countries who, as a last resort, might feel obliged to favor the country which accepted the formula." [128]

This suggestion was greeted sympathetically in Washington, but it was pointed out that

as a practical matter, because of the special relationship between Argentina and Paraguay, the elimination of Argentina from the mediation proceedings would in all probability jeopardize materially their successful outcome and so long as Argentina continues as one of the mediating powers the information received by this Government, as well as by the Government of Brazil, from its representatives in the capitals of the belligerent powers is invaluable as a means of confirming information emanating from Buenos Aires.[129]

This amounted to a delicately firm manner of expressing the distrust in Washington of the diplomatic activities of Saavedra Lamas, and this distrust may have influenced the Department of State in gradually reaching the view expressed about two weeks later: "This Government, in fact, believes that one of the fundamental needs of the American continent is the creation of a practical and effective American mechanism to be constantly available when disputes are threatened or break out between members of the American community of nations." [130] (The use of the word mechanism recalls Secretary Stimson's reference to the need for "machinery" some five years earlier.) It is probable that this conclusion was a powerful factor behind the proposal by President Roosevelt for the holding of the Buenos Aires Conference in 1936.[131]

In their desire to avoid the application of sanctions to Paraguay, Argentina and Chile continued their joint conciliation despite the Alessandri incident. However, they were obliged at the end of March to admit they could accomplish nothing in the Chaco, although they had managed in Geneva to arrange the deferment until May of further action by the League. This had been achieved by a joint statement to the Advisory Committee that they had reason to believe that their plan would be successful; that Brazil and Peru had been aware of the plan and that negotiations would be undertaken by the four nations concerned.[132] The Brazilian government, fearing that this statement might give the impression that it had not been cooperating closely with the United States, which it had in fact been doing, informed the League that it had not expressed any opinion about the Argentine-Chilean plan and that it would not engage in negotiations in any case without the participation of the United States. It was the view of the Foreign Minister, as expressed to Chargé Gordon, that "in order to avoid being called upon to participate in sanctions Argentina and Chile sought to ward off League action by making it appear that they had achieved much more success than was actually the case and he characterized their action as 'pure bluff.' "[133]

However, the bluff worked. The League deferred action on the Chaco, apparently because of the pressure of events in Europe, and a bit of international log rolling occurred. Gilbert reported that, at the time of the discussion of a resolution regarding German rearmament,

Simon, Laval and Aloisi most earnestly pressed the representatives of Argentina, Chile and Mexico to vote in its favor. . . . The whole atmosphere of the conversations which occurred at that time between the European and the Latin American Council powers was a partially expressed partially tacit understanding that in return for their support in the matter of the German question, Great Britain, France and Italy would accord Argentina and Chile a free hand in the League's disposition of the Chaco matter.[134]

The final phase of the negotiations for an armistice in the Chaco began early in April, 1935, with an invitation from Argentina and Chile to Brazil, Peru, and the United States to join in an attempt to end the war. Honors for the initiation of this culminative move may be shared by the League of Nations, the Department of State, and Argentina and Chile. The leading individual role, however, seems to have been played by Sumner Welles, who had initiated talks about a conference with the ambassadors of the neighboring powers in

December, 1934. Although Welles had then vainly hoped that a conference of these states might succeed in avoiding the imposition of sanctions by the League of Nations, the idea of such a conference was taken up later either by Cruchaga or Saavedra Lamas. Under the circumstances it was unavoidable that the conference be held in Buenos Aires, and this meant that the chairmanship of this, and the subsequent Chaco Peace Conference, would go to Saavedra Lamas. The enormity of the disadvantages of that decision was fully appreciated only in the course of the subsequent three years.[135]

Meetings of representatives of the five states began in May, after a month's delay caused by Brazilian irritation at having been left off a list of participants in a proposed economic conference between Bolivia and Paraguay that had been a part of the previous Argentine-Chilean peace suggestions. Saavedra Lamas said that Brazil's omission was the result of a typographical error, but the same mistake had, strangely enough, been made in Santiago as well as in Buenos Aires. The *Correio da Manha* (Rio de Janeiro) of April 12, 1935, said that international relations on such an important matter did not leave room for typographical errors, particularly when aggravated by "simultaneity."

With the mollification of this justifiable Brazilian annoyance, the five states, joined shortly by Uruguay, were represented at meetings in Buenos Aires during the month of May. The foreign ministers of Bolivia and Paraguay accepted invitations to meet, separately, with the mediatory group, which found both belligerents willing to be assisted in bringing the fighting to an end. A protocol was finally signed on June 12, 1935, providing for a cessation of hostilities, the holding of a peace conference to aid in mediation, and, if necessary, to arrange for arbitration of the fundamental question of the dispute. In this way fighting was ended after a war which had cost the lives of about 60,000 Bolivians and 40,000 Paraguayans. Over three years were to pass, however, before a peace treaty was ratified.[136]

Described in these general terms, the protocol seems to be such a reasonable document that the question might arise as to the reason for the great sacrifices made by each belligerent. However, the specific terms of the protocol registered the loss of the Chaco war by Bolivia. The Paraguayan army was in possession of the Chaco; what, then, was to be subject to arbitration? In article I(3) of the protocol it was stated that, in case no definitive settlement was reached by direct negotiation, "the parties shall proceed to draw up the arbitral *compromis;* the Peace Conference cannot relinquish its functions as long as the arbitral *compromis* is not definitively agreed upon." This left Paraguay capable of preventing any arbitration that would risk any of its territorial holdings and made it necessary for Bolivia to commence hostilities again if it hoped to secure any portion of the Chaco, even including those parts that its army had occupied in 1932. This meant that arbitration, which might have favored Bolivian claims, was in fact impossible, and a political solution, which could not ignore the military situation, was imperative.[137]

The situation was later explicitly recognized by Braden:

> The essential fact is that, since no agreement on the arbitral *compromis* was feasible, the peace treaty perforce had to be reached through direct agreement; the only alternative being another war. The inclusion of arbitration in an agreement once again had failed because loose ends flapped in a breeze of controversy; there was no time limit set for the drafting of the *compromis* and no obligation placed on the parties to accept an arbitration, the terms of which they each had not previously restricted entirely to their own liking.

Braden noted that the June 12, 1935, protocol contemplated the procedure of an "arbitration in law" but that the final arrangement was one of equity. The role played by arbitration in the Chaco dispute "was not merely—as might be supposed—that thereby the definitive boundary might be drawn within two limited zones. It is rather that arbitration supplied the procedure which enabled the mediators to obtain the agreement by both parties." Rarely in international disputes has arbitration been so flexibly interpreted.[138]

It is noteworthy that the technique utilized in this final peace effort was that of a meeting in one city of representatives of the neighboring powers, plus the United States. This action was a recognition of the mistakes of all past attempts at negotiations, except the feeble efforts in Washington in 1933 to bring the Neutrals and ABCP states together. However, more important was the fact that the capacity of Paraguay to win victories in the field had come to an end and that Bolivia saw no way to regain its former territorial position in the Chaco except through a military effort that its people were unwilling to undertake.

CHAPTER III

The Nature of the Conflict

SINCE, IN 1932, Bolivia was confident, and Paraguay was fearful, that the armed forces of no American state would repel aggression or provide a guarantee against fighting, both states felt that, if the dispute came to war, they would be left alone to fight it out. The government of Salamanca in La Paz confidently confronted war as the means of securing a deep-water port on the Paraguay River. The government of Ayala in Asunción dreaded a war but was resolved to fight, since the achievement of Bolivian ambitions, whether through war or arbitration on their terms, might well mean the end of Paraguay as an independent state.[1]

Throughout the four years before the war began in the summer of 1932, Bolivia behaved in a way similar to that of other states confident of winning an imminent armed struggle. Like Japan in Manchuria and like Italy in Ethiopia, Bolivia desired to be left alone by other states who made appeals for peace. Paraguay, on the other hand, like China and Ethiopia, tried repeatedly to secure the aid of other states in bringing about arbitration and in providing guarantees against fighting.[2]

In Bolivia there was little disposition to accept a solution by arbitration. The reaction in La Paz to a despatch from Washington in February, 1932, that the Bolivian minister, Luis O. Abelli, had favored arbitration by the United States aroused antagonistic comment in the press.[3]

In 1932 the Bolivian government refused to accept arbitration as a solution of the dispute, unless its scope were limited to that eastern part of the Chaco which was not occupied by its troops, which Bolivia referred to as the "disputable Chaco." Furthermore, Bolivia also refused to consider suggestions that recourse be had to the so-called "double arbitration" in which arbitral methods would be used to determine the questions to be put to an arbitral tribunal that would then determine the boundary line.[4]

A clear instance of this difference in attitude is shown by the responses of the two countries to the appeal of the Neutrals that, consistent with the declaration of August 3, 1932, concerning the nonrecognition of conquests, troops should be withdrawn to the positions they occupied on June 1, 1932, before the subsequent incidents in the Chaco. Paraguay accepted this proposal, and Bolivia, which had taken four Paraguayan forts in June and July, refused the suggestion and insisted that any cessation of hostilities should be on the basis of possessions as of the beginning of August. Although the Bolivian position was supported by the Argentine government, the United States took the view that acceptance of the Bolivian position would "definitely scrap" the declaration of August 3, since it would appear to confirm the Neutrals' acceptance of Bolivian conquests during the previous two months.[5]

The implication that may be drawn from these considerations that Bolivia was primarily responsible for the outbreak of the Chaco war is strengthened by a remarkably frank statement by Foreign Minister Julio A. Gutiérrez, in his reply of August 5, to the declaration of August 3:

Today she [Bolivia] is pursuing in the Chaco the recovery of what historically and juridically belongs to her. We are asked for peaceful settlement. We have proposed them several times in formal treaties which have not been ratified by Paraguay. We wish to terminate the Chaco question, the country being resolved to make even bloody sacrifices in defense of its territory. The nation needs to break the barrier which prevents access to its bank on the Paraguay River in order to have communication with the world. This is one of the bases for a solution which must be required for Paraguay to insure the peace of America.[6]

The fact that Paraguay was later declared by the League of Nations to be the aggressor does not affect Bolivia's primary responsibility. Paraguay had by then made gains in a war that it could reasonably regard as an invasion and was determined to drive Bolivian troops as far as possible from the Paraguay River. It is immaterial, in this view, whether the incident of June 15, 1932, at Fortín Carlos Antonio López was of Bolivian or Paraguayan origin. It is also immaterial that both countries might on more than one occasion be justifiably blamed for the continuation of the conflict. At the outset it was Bolivia that overconfidently offered battle, and Paraguay that desperately accepted the challenge. Such sympathy as existed abroad for either combatant was largely for Paraguay, at least among disinterested bystanders.

The causes of the war, as distinct from the responsibility for its onset, cannot here be examined fully, although two comments about them may be mentioned. Ambassador Alexander W. Weddell reported that General A. B. Robertson, the British member of the Chaco Commission of the League of Nations, told him that he thought

the fundamental issue in the Chaco has in the course of time become more psychologic than economic . . . the conflict which has been going on intermittently for more than fifty years has evolved into an issue where national pride is so much at stake that the original bone of contention—supposedly the Chaco—has really become secondary. The chief aim of both sides is to leave the field with their reputations enhanced and their colors flying.[7]

President Ayala, in a public address, viewed the war as neither a boundary question nor one of Bolivia's "need" to obtain an outlet to the sea.

At bottom, to Bolivia, the Chaco War is a matter of conquest. Bolivian statesmen have for some time called for the use of force against Paraguay, not in order to solve the boundary question, which never was insoluble, nor to satisfy necessities which they know to be nonexistent, but to find a remedy for serious weaknesses of internal morale.[8]

Fighting in the Chaco came to a standstill in November, 1932, after the rainy season began, with the Paraguayans temporarily victorious. They had driven the enemy out of the forts he had taken in June and July and had pushed him back in some places beyond the line of June 1, 1932. The Bolivians could barely maintain their

troops in forward positions, partly because of the marshiness of the
terrain in November and partly because the Bolivian supply line was
both long and weak. Fort Boquerón on the central front was only
about 120 miles from Puerto San Carlos on the Paraguay River,
which could be readily reached by ammunition scows from
Asunción, only 75 miles to the south. It was, however, almost 250
miles from Villa Montes, the principal Bolivian base at the eastern
foot of the Andes, which was itself about 500 miles from La Paz, the
capital, on the Andean plateau. The roads on both sides of Villa
Montes were bad and could only be used in certain seasons, and
there was a severe shortage of trucks. This factor of supply, apparently underestimated by the Bolivian government in 1932, was of
vital significance throughout the war, and it became one of the chief
limiting factors to the Paraguayan advance in 1935, which reached
at one point a distance of more than 150 miles northwest of Fort
Boquerón.

At the beginning of 1933, the Bolivian armed forces had been defeated and even humiliated; their own general had been dismissed;
General Kundt had been employed for 600,000 gold marks to return
to Bolivia, and it was obvious that a Bolivian offensive was planned
for April or May when the Chaco would be drying out. From Paraguay came news that General Kundt had "selected" about 120
"German officers" from other South American countries to go to
Bolivia.[9]

This decision to continue the struggle was not made in La Paz
without serious political complications. Minister Feely reported on
November 9 that, throughout the period of negotiations for a nonaggression pact, "all of the Ministers of Foreign Affairs have been
inclined toward a peaceful settlement, but the President [Daniel
Salamanca] has shown a mistrust of the Neutral Commission and a
stubbornness of attitude that has defeated all efforts to come to an
agreement." Salamanca was sure that Bolivia could win out in the
end, and he feared a revolution if he accepted a cease-fire agreement
after serious reverses in the field.[10]

Again, on December 6, Feely warned that the arrival in Bolivia of
General Kundt, new outlays abroad for munitions and the capture
by Bolivian forces of a few small Paraguayan forts were "clear indi-

cations that this Government intends to prosecute the war to the bitter end and I fear that the negotiations in Washington will be used only to delay a settlement and to gain time." [11]

From the point of view, therefore, of Bolivia's internal situation and its own resources, Feely saw no possibility other than a resumption of hostilities. However, he made one suggestion that seems to have received no attention in Washington, but that may have offered the only way to stop fighting in the last months of 1932. Noting that criticism of the government by Ismael Montes, a former President of Bolivia, had given momentary leadership to a "large sector of Bolivian opinion" critical of the government, he said:

Under the circumstances and because of the critical internal situation I am of the opinion that the Government would seize upon any pretext to extricate itself from the dilemma and that forcible measures by the neutrals would be welcomed as offering such a pretext although there would be a storm of protest.[12]

White had already told the Bolivian and Paraguayan representatives in Washington that coercive measures by the United States or the Neutrals were out of the question either as sanctions or as guarantees, and on October 18 Saavedra Lamas had expressed Argentina's opposition to anything beyond the moral influence of good offices. This opposition may be attributed to fear on his part that the actual sending of a commission to the Chaco would have meant that the Neutrals would be successful in solving the dispute, rather than to an attachment on his part to legal principles. Argentine disapproval of the action would have been enough to prevent it, however, even had the Neutrals been more strongly inclined to press the point than they showed themselves to be.

Feely's judgment suggests that, whatever Salamanca's intentions may have been, conquest of the Chaco was not a policy supported by all Bolivian political groups, particularly since Salamanca refused to accept the formation of a national cabinet. Feely implied that "forcible measures" by the Neutrals would be in the nature of a rescue mission, extricating Bolivia from a situation deplored by a substantial body of its influential citizens and saving it from a national disaster into which its willful president was driving it.

Feely's view was not dissimilar from that expressed earlier by Ayala, then President-Elect of Paraguay, that he thought "the only possibility of solving the boundary controversy between his country and Bolivia would be by strong pressure brought to bear on both governments to submit the matter to arbitration." Short of such action by the United States, Argentina, Brazil, and perhaps Uruguay, "he felt war was the only recourse left." [13]

If there were divisions in Bolivian opinion in the autumn of 1932, they disappeared by the spring of 1933. The government, expecting great things from General Kundt and having received assurances that Chile would not prevent the passage of arms and munitions through the port of Arica, was reported to be "determined to risk a military decision, or at least to inflict such a defeat upon Paraguay as will enable her to dictate terms of settlement." [14]

Arms shipments for Bolivia had been held up by the Chilean authorities at Arica early in February, perhaps as a means of bringing pressure on Bolivia to accept the Mendoza formula. On February 13 Finot had asked whether the United States would not do something toward getting the shipments released and was told that no action would be taken.[15]

A few days later, however, Chile permitted the shipments to go forward, and the Department of State was informed that this policy change had been attributed by the Paraguayan minister in Santiago, J. Isidro Ramírez, to pressure from the United States.[16] President Ayala of Paraguay had refused to credit this report. The Department of State declared it to be without foundation and stated that it probably referred to representations from the British Ambassador, who had requested entry to Bolivia for munitions of British origin that had been detained at Arica.[17]

The confidence on both sides in victory was the dominant element throughout the year 1933 in both the military and the diplomatic campaigns. This was the case despite the opinion expressed by President Ayala that "the present time is most propitious for a settlement as both peoples at heart desire peace; both are facing bankruptcy and smarting from losses and neither has won a sweeping victory." [18]

The Paraguayans had successfully thrown back the first Bolivian attacks and felt they had the enemy's measure; the Bolivians had recognized their weaknesses in communications but were sure that with more troops, bigger howitzers, better roads and more trucks, and newly imported leadership, it would not be long before they would break the Paraguayan defense line in the south near Nanawa and reach the Paraguay River near Concepción.[19]

Throughout the year both sides were able to import arms, ammunition, and other supplies. In January, 1933, however, Argentina stopped food exports to Bolivia. Paraguay's declaration of war on May 10 did not change the status of Arica as a free port for Bolivian imports of munitions from arms manufacturers in Europe and the United States. Paraguay also obtained some arms from these private sources, but it appears that the Argentine government itself was an important source of Paraguayan munitions. Francis White stated:

We have it from our Military Attaché in Buenos Aires that considerable quantities of munitions have been sent from the Argentine arsenals to Paraguay. There was an Argentine Military Mission in Paraguay which Argentina ostentatiously withdrew as a sign of its neutrality. The chief of this Mission was shortly afterwards appointed Military Attaché to Paraguay and is really the head adviser of the Paraguayan General Staff, making frequent trips to the front. Other members of the Mission drifted back secretly and are active in helping the Paraguayan army.[20]

More specific information was provided by Minister Wheeler in Asunción, who had received word from a source he regarded as worthy of attention, that "there arrived here five days ago two million rounds of machine gun and rifle ammunition with several thousand blankets and other accoutrements from Argentine arsenals, that more is to arrive this week and that the War Department here has assurance that it will be supplied to any extent necessary." [21] In another letter to Wilson, White said that the Bolivian delegate had told the Commission of Neutrals "that cartridges found on Paraguayan soldiers indicate that the cartridges belong to the Argentine army. He said this shows that Argentina is not neutral as it claims but is supplying war material to Paraguay. This conforms with information which we have had in the past from Buenos Aires." [22]

Less precise, although no less persuasive, evidence that the Argentine government had given material assistance to Paraguay was provided during the final negotiations for the peace treaty in 1938. Argentine Foreign Minister José Maria Cantilo assured Spruille Braden that he would warn Paraguay that it "must expect totally different attitude from Argentina than in the last war if another conflict occurs." [23] Later, Braden reported that President Roberto Ortiz, Cantilo, and the Argentine Chief of Staff had told the Paraguayan delegates that in the event of another conflict they must count on no help from Argentina.[24]

Uruguay provided a passive kind of assistance to Paraguay by facilitating the transshipment of munitions originating elsewhere, and Chile gave like aid to Bolivia. Neither of these countries, however, appears to have been an armament supplier, although the Paraguayans charged that Chile had helped the Bolivians. Wheeler referred to

antagonism which prevails in Paraguay toward Chile based principally upon the belief that Chile is in general favorably inclined toward Bolivia and that it facilitates the introduction of war material into that country and is even furnishing such supplies itself. This antagonism has been increased by the failure of the Paraguayan army to capture Villa Montes, the successful defense of which is locally attributed to the informed military counsel of Chilean military officers said to be serving in the Bolivian army and to the effective use of Chilean artillery manned by Chilean gun crews.[25]

Charges against Chile appeared in the Paraguayan press, and they were denied by the Chilean Minister in Asunción. At the very end of the war, Wheeler reported that the Paraguayans had gained a victory at Ingavi on June 8: "Among the 1200 prisoners captured by the Paraguayans was the Bolivian commanding officer . . . two Majors (one of whom, to the great satisfaction of Paraguay, is a Chilean) and twenty other officers." [26] The few Chileans who fought with the Bolivians seem to have been retired officers, whose participation was not authorized by the Chilean government.

During the summer of 1933 the Bolivians attacked with an army of about 60,000 men, of whom about 12,000 were in the supply services, without gaining a break-through. Then the Paraguayans counterattacked; catching their foe when his long communications system had broken down and his troops had insufficient ammunition, a major blow was struck at Fort Arce on September 15. A decisive victory was gained at Fort Gondra on December 11, when the Bolivian Fourth and Ninth Divisions were surrounded, and several thousand front-line troops were captured, with all their equipment.[27]

The Bolivians had made their supreme effort for victory with an offensive in early September, and Feely reported on September 5 that "the Bolivian Command has failed in its purposes."[28] In December the Bolivian army began a retreat westward across the Chaco, pursued by the Paraguayan army until toward the end of 1934. Then the Bolivians, aided by shorter communications and taking advantage of defensive positions in hilly terrain, were able to bring the Paraguayan advance to a halt. The Bolivians were not capable, however, of launching a new offensive, and the fighting lines were stabilized along a front approximately 200 miles west and north of the line on which the conflict had raged for the first year and a half of the war. It was on this line that the troops faced each other when hostilities ceased on June 14, 1935. It was not far from this line that the final boundary was laid down.[29]

For a full year, until his dismissal in December, 1933, General Kundt exercised a dominating political as well as military influence in Bolivia. Feely wrote to Francis White that "it is growing more apparent every day that General Kundt is handling the entire situation with an iron hand, and dictating policies to the government both political and military. . . . I feel that his influence will be opposed to a peaceful settlement at this time."[30]

In January, 1933, occurred the second instance of the aerial bombardment of a settlement by a Latin American air force. The Bolivians attacked with bombs and machine guns the Paraguayan town of Concepción, about 100 miles north of Asunción on the Paraguay River. This and later attacks on towns were justified by the Bolivian government on the ground that the towns "were Paraguayan military bases, and points of concentration of troops and military supplies."[31] The armies also employed such modern equipment as tanks and flame-throwers.[32] The Paraguayan army also had an air force, which was used to strike at Bolivian air fields and other military targets.

Feely reported that observers from the front, some of whom were Bolivian army officers, considered that in July the fighting had reached a stalemate, and added:

While the Bolivian Government no doubt realizes the futility of prosecuting the war under these circumstances, the sacrifices that have been made are so great, and the internal political situation so directly affected by the outcome of the war, that the government feels it has no alternative, if it is to remain in power.[33]

The stalemate continued until the Paraguayan victory at Fort Arce in September, 1933. Until this time Bolivian hopes seemed to remain fairly high, although they apparently turned from expectation of a military decision in the field to one of a Paraguayan collapse from internal economic and political difficulties. From September to the beginning of the retreat in December the Bolivian attitude was reported to be one of "strengthening . . . determination to continue at any cost the defense of her patrimony." [34]

The dismissal of General Kundt in December, 1933, returned power to another man whose reputation depended on a military victory, namely, President Daniel Salamanca. Before his election, Salamanca had publicly proclaimed on several occasions "the policy of force as the only means of settling the dispute." [35] Early in 1933 he had been criticized by ex-President Bautista Saavedra and by Dr. Luis O. Abelli, the former Minister of Bolivia in the United States. Dr. Saavedra charged that Salamanca, "to alleviate internal political complications," had brought the country into war for which it was not prepared "either diplomatically, economically, financially or in a military way." [36] Dr. Abelli criticized the government for having recourse to force in the Chaco and for "insisting on the prior delimitation of the arbitral zone." [37]

Having become involved in the war, however, Salamanca apparently saw no way of ending it except by victory or defeat. It is hard to interpret otherwise his failure to accept the advice of General Kundt given as early as July, 1933, "that if an honorable peace can be made, it would be advisable for Bolivia to accept it." [38] Even after the Paraguayan victory at Fort Arce, which was the prelude to disaster, the Bolivian government rejected the Brazilian-led neighboring countries in their proposals made under the auspices of the

League of Nations. The personal involvement of President Salamanca was enhanced by the fact that he had lost one son in the war in 1933, and another son was in the Chaco at the end of the year.[39]

In Paraguay, whose population of about one million was slightly less than a third that of Bolivia, the war effort was intense on the part of the people as a whole.[40]

After the Paraguayan victories late in 1933, it appeared that the power of the Paraguayan generals in determining national policy about the course of the war increased markedly and that of President Ayala and other civilians declined.[41]

The Bolivian army retreated about 130 miles between December 11, 1933, and February 20, 1934, when the main forces were reported to be at Forts Ballivián and Guachalla on the Pilcomayo River.[42] There was a serious shortage of officers in the Bolivian army after the disaster at Fort Gondra, and efforts at recruitment of officers were made in foreign countries. Minister Des Portes reported that in May "over 20 retired Chilean officers have come to La Paz to enlist in the Bolivian army" and that a group of Czech army officers arrived in June. The latter "in a moment of exuberance . . . did a large amount of damage to furniture of the Hotel Paris." [43] In addition to General Kundt and some German officers, there was also one Australian officer with the Bolivian army.[44]

The Paraguayan army also had the assistance of foreign military men, in addition to the advice of Argentine officers already mentioned. The Paraguayan minister in Washington admitted that "a few 'White' Russians were fighting as volunteers in the Paraguayan army." [45]

In pursuing the Bolivians, the Paraguayan army ran into difficulties of supply and communications similar to those that had hampered their enemy in the first year and a half of the war. As early as September, 1934, Minister Meredith Nicholson in Asunción reported that "high Paraguayan officials do not hope for a decisive victory in the field." [46]

While earlier reports of Paraguayan economic difficulties had given encouragement to La Paz, they had been proven to be unfounded. Early in 1935, however, Nicholson reported that "it is evident that Paraguay's situation is economically close to the desperation point." [47] Nevertheless, the Paraguayan army had by then driven the Bolivians back so far, that success gave rise to ambitions for the acquisition of territory even beyond the claims to the Chaco territory that had been previously officially announced. It was hoped, according to rumors, that the oil-bearing lands around Tarija might be added to the Chaco. Further, there was talk of uniting parts of the Bolivian departments of Chuquisaca and Tarija with the department of Santa Cruz de la Sierra in which there was alleged to be "separatist sentiment" to form "an independent republic—a sort of Manchoukuo—to serve as a buffer between Paraguay and Bolivia." [48] Early in March the Paraguayan army crossed the Parapetí River. Chargé Walter Thurston in Asunción stated that these actions "constitute actual invasion of Bolivia, inasmuch as the most extensive claims advanced by Paraguay bound the Chaco by the Parapetí River." [49]

The Paraguayan advance west of the river continued until April, when the oil town of Charagua was taken. The Bolivians then counterattacked, retook Charagua, and drove the Paraguayans southeastward across the Parapetí and back into the Chaco. [50] The Bolivian reaction was contained by the Paraguayans at Fort Ingavi in a battle on June 8, which was a serious defeat for the Bolivians involving the taking of 1,200 prisoners by Paraguayan forces. [51]

In the meantime, new mediatory efforts had been underway by a group of American states that succeeded in bringing about, on June 12, 1935, an agreement for the cessation of hostilities and the calling of a peace conference. Fighting ceased on June 14 and was not resumed.

The end of the fighting was greeted with relief and satisfaction in both Bolivia and Paraguay, although the mood in Bolivia was one of resignation and that in Paraguay was one of jubilation.

The three-year war ending a dispute over a century old had caused the deaths of about 60,000 Bolivian and 40,000 Paraguayan soldiers. The Bolivian army, which had been within 150 miles of Asunción, had been driven back about 200 miles westward, to the very edge of the territory included within the extreme limits of Paraguayan definitions of the Chaco. The Bolivians had lost 17,000 men as prisoners; the Paraguayans 2,500.

While the official position taken by other American nations was that there was no victor in the war and while this position was given some color by the fact that Bolivia had not sued for peace, it was evident to all that Bolivian aims had been frustrated and that Paraguay, in June, 1935, had won control of nearly the whole of the Chaco. The Paraguayans had achieved a great military victory, regardless of the question of the value of the territory involved. They had saved their country from a defeat that might well have resulted in the disappearance of Paraguay as an independent nation, and their troops stood on a line enclosing territory that approximately doubled the area previously regarded as unquestionably Paraguayan and that at some points was 100 miles beyond the lines of unratified treaties previously negotiated by the two countries for the division of the Chaco.

Dr. Luis A. Riart, the Paraguayan Foreign Minister, told Chargé Thurston that, by March, 1935, the war had entered a new phase:

The Chaco . . . belongs to Paraguay. Paraguay, however, was in the past willing to relinquish its title to a portion of that region as the price of peace. But since all its efforts to avert war, even at the expense of its territory, had failed there no longer could be any question of a partitioning of the Chaco. An effort had been made by Bolivia to take the Chaco by force, Paraguay had repelled the invasion and is in possession of the Chaco. The peace negotiations must take that fact into account and concern themselves with the question of peace, not territory. [52]

Bolivia, having given up the use of force to reach the Paraguay River, hoped through its own diplomacy and the efforts of mediating states, to win its original objective or some part of it. The mediating states, however, found themselves unable to overcome Paraguayan insistence on keeping nearly all of the land their troops had won, and they finally brought about a settlement that amounted to a ratification of Paraguay's military victory, since it completely excluded Bolivia from the Paraguay River, except in that small area bordering the extreme northeast corner of the Chaco, where Brazil, in the Treaty of Petropolis of 1903, had given Bolivia some 25 miles of river bank in a region where the river was useless for navigation.[53]

Compared to other wars, the Chaco conflict seems to have acquired a peculiarly low reputation. The Brazilian foreign office has referred to " 'the inglorious Chaco War.' " [54] A historian of the League of Nations has written that "the Chaco war may be regarded as the triumph of nationalist unreason over every sentiment of morality and common sense." [55] Historians in the United States join the refrain, and perhaps repeat each other, by calling the Chaco war "senseless." [56]

These are judgments made by nonparticipants—people who did not share the keenness of Salamanca's desire for an outlet to the sea or the sharpness of the fear of Ayala that a Bolivian presence on the Paraguay River might mean the loss of Paraguay's existence as a place where Paraguayans might make independent decisions about their fate. However, to Bolivians and Paraguayans in the 1930s this war meant life and death as individuals and as members of families, and honor and dishonor as men and women and as citizens of self-conscious societies. In comparable terms, it is as least arguable whether the World War of 1914–18 or the Spanish-American War would rate as less "senseless." Paraguayan and Bolivian criticisms of those wars have received less attention than foreigners' detractions of their own, but it does not follow that those wars were less senseless than that of the Chaco; it may merely indicate that possible peacemakers were less frustrated and less vocal, because less presumptuous. The Chaco war was a serious struggle between communities with lethal intent; it is a frivolous misjudgment to regard it as unreasonable, especially on the part of historians from countries whose martial record may be equally vulnerable.

CHAPTER IV

The Chaco Peace Conference—Frustration

The protocol of June 12, 1935, was drafted under urgent pressure and, unfortunately, contained many ambiguities. In addition, some of the shortcomings of the protocol were knowingly accepted because there seemed no other possible means to satisfy the diametrically opposed positions of the two parties. However, it did bring about the cessation of a tragic war and, despite its deficiencies, it was the only basis for action by the mediatory group.[1]

THE PROTOCOL PROVIDED for the calling of a peace conference by the President of Argentina. The conference, which held its first meeting on July 1, 1935, had three principal functions as defined by the protocol: (1) "to promote the solution of the matters in dispute between Bolivia and Paraguay by direct agreement between the parties"; (2) to settle practical questions arising in the execution of security measures established at the time of the cessation of hostilities; (3) to promote an agreement about the exchange and repatriation of prisoners. If the dispute was not settled by "direct agreement," Bolivia and Paraguay "undertook" to settle it by "juridical arbitration," presumably with the help of the conference.

The problems of prisoner repatriation and security measures caused many anxious moments during the three-year life of the conference. The 17,000 Bolivians held by Paraguay and the 2,500 Paraguayans the Bolivian army had captured were repatriated in July, 1936, on the basis of the protocolary act of January 21, 1936. The security measures involved demobilization of the armies in the Chaco and the establishment by the Neutral Military Commission of lines of separation of the armies in the Chaco. The maximum size of each army, after demobilization was completed on September 30, 1935, was 5,000 men; Bolivia demobilized 140,000 men and Paraguay, 139,826. The lines of separation of the armies remained very close to the battle line at the close of hostilities; the distance between the lines was forty-five miles at the maximum, at the northeast end of the line, while in the southwest near Villa Montes the separation measured less than five miles.

One provision of the protocol remained inoperative. The conference was supposed to establish a commission to give an opinion on "the responsibilities of every order and of every kind arising from the war." Although the conference did its part in drafting a resolution and later a protocol, signed on October 2, 1935, providing for a commission of three judges, one from the highest court of each of the belligerents and one from the United States, the protocol was not ratified by Bolivia or Paraguay, and in the treaty of July 21, 1938, the two countries reciprocally renounced "all actions and claims deriving from responsibilities for the war."

In carrying out these and other duties the conference acted as an administrative body. With regard to its principal function, the bringing of Bolivia and Paraguay to agreement on a boundary in the Chaco and so to a treaty of peace, the conference was several bodies in one. It was a mediator, consoler, pleader, and negotiator; it was also a forum for the belligerents, a center for political intrigue, and an arena for the display of varied ambitions by the peacemakers.[2]

The mediating states were limited to five despite Hull's desire that the other members of the Commission of Neutrals be included.

Hugh Gibson, the Ambassador to Brazil who acted as representative on the mediation group and later as delegate to the conference for the first six months, reported that his Brazilian and Chilean colleagues opposed any increase in the number of conference participants beyond the planned five—Argentina, Brazil, Chile, Peru, and the United States. Gibson added:

The tasks of the Conference and negotiations on matters calling for expeditious decision will be difficult enough under present conditions in view of the erratic character of its chairmanship, lack of organization and the uncontrollable eloquence of some of its members. It is important to restrict to a minimum the amount of time consumed in speech-making and this will, it is contended, be less for a group of six than for double the number.

As a result, Uruguay was the only state added to those originally contemplated as members of the Chaco Peace Conference.

Washington did not accept Gibson's recommendations. Hull noted that at no time had all the American states made a "concerted effort" for peace in the Chaco, because of the lack of "adequate peace machinery" in the Americas; if the past six years' experience was to be valuable, the United States should seize this favorable opportunity and join "with other powers of this Continent in an initiative to suggest the need for the creation of adequate peace machinery."[3] However, Hull's desire was successfully resisted by Saavedra Lamas, who suggested that a general conference be held to discuss peace machinery. The views expressed both by Saavedra Lamas and by the Department of State were influential in the decision to convene the conference at Buenos Aires in 1936.

The attitude of officials in the Department of State toward the approaching negotiations was a workmanlike one. There was a job to be done—the completion of a treaty of peace and the drawing of a boundary line. It was immaterial to the United States government just where the boundary line should be; its interest was in seeing all American states at peace and in trying to find ways to avoid war in the future. Having accepted a responsibility for bringing about a settlement, United States officials demonstrated their willingness to work for a long period and to exercise great perseverance in discharging that responsibility. They were almost entirely without any desire to obtain either personal or national credit for reaching a settlement; it is clear from the course of the negotiations that both Hugh Gibson and his successor, Spruille Braden, were eager to let others obtain any credit that might accrue.

There were certain differences in the attitudes of other countries members of the conference. The Uruguayan and Peruvian governments played relatively small parts in the negotiations; their sympathies had been with Paraguay and Bolivia, respectively, but it does not seem that these sympathies affected the course of the negotiations.[4] They were represented throughout the conference by their ambassadors in Buenos Aires, Eugenio Martínez Thédy and Felipe Barreda Laos.

The government of Brazil maintained an attitude of correct neutrality throughout the war. It was concerned about the possibility that Argentine influence might be extended by an overwhelming victory by Paraguay, but it was less involved with either belligerent than Chile or Argentina. Its delegate at the conference, Ambassador José de Paula Rodrigues Alves, worked closely with the United States delegates and was equally animated by a desire to bring about peace as rapidly as possible.

In the case of Chile, the attitude of its governments and people during the war was pro-Bolivian. Diplomatic relations with Paraguay had been strained and on one occasion had been broken off. Chilean army officers had, until prohibited by law, volunteered for service in the Bolivian army. Outside observers thought that Chile would not have been displeased if, by obtaining a port on the Paraguay River, Bolivia's desires for its own outlet on the Pacific were lessened.

The position of Argentina, and particularly of its foreign minister, was of a special character. Argentina and Chile had permitted the shipment of arms and munitions through their territories to Paraguay and Bolivia, respectively, during the war. It was widely believed that Argentine assistance to Paraguay, both governmental and private, had taken the form of substantial supplies of arms and money. It was known that individual Argentines owned tracts of land in the Chaco and had concessions there from the Paraguayan government, and it was assumed that they had contributed to the Paraguayan cause. Direct evidence on these points is limited, but there are many indirect suggestions that Argentine aid was provided on a large scale.[5] One of the principal indirect evidences is the combination of the inadequacy of the Paraguayan national budget to support a three-year war and the unavailability of any other source of funds except Argentina.

Perhaps the strongest evidence that the Argentine government and Argentine business firms gave financial assistance to Paraguay is offered by Vicente Rivarola, Paraguayan Minister to Argentina. In his memoirs Rivarola states that at various times during the war he secured loans for the Paraguayan government from the Argentine government and from private sources totaling 8 million Argentine pesos.[6] Rivarola reported that in Argentina, President Justo, the Minister of War, General Manuel A. Rodríguez, and the Finance Minister, Federico Pinedo, aided him to secure loans. Pinedo is quoted as saying in August, 1934, that it was to the interest of Argentina that Paraguay should be the victor in the war and prosperous afterward, hence Argentina " 'must provide her now with arms and munitions and make money available without conditions.' "[7] Saavedra Lamas, on the other hand, was said to have written to President Justo in 1934 that he was completely unaware that the Argentine government was furnishing arms to Paraguay.[8] In view of Saavedra Lamas's hopes to gain the Nobel Peace Prize, it would, of course, be advisable for him to have a statement of this kind on the record, although it is difficult to accept his protestation of ignorance of the facts, especially since Justo complained to Rivarola about "indiscretions" of Argentine businessmen about loans to Paraguay.[9]

In a talk with Welles, Brazilian Ambassador Oswaldo Aranha said he "felt that the real crux of the problem from a practical point of view was that Paraguay was enabled to continue the war solely on account of financial assistance she was obtaining from third persons." Welles commented that the Ambassador

obviously referred to, although he did not specify, the financial support which it is alleged Paraguay is receiving from Argentina and in particular from certain Argentine capitalists who were alleged to be financing the Paraguayan offensive in the Chaco war in return for concessions which the Paraguayan Government has promised them when the war is over. The Ambassador maintained that it was impossible to conceive of Paraguay being permitted to make peace unless the territory in the Chaco retained by Paraguay as a peace settlement included the areas for which these concessions were to be granted.

The situation suggested to the Ambassador a possible line for the United States policy to follow:

As a practical solution he believed there was only one way to bring about peace in the Chaco and that was for the more powerful states of the continent to "bail" Paraguay out of her existing financial obligations to the concession seekers by making a loan to Paraguay. He said he was confident that Brazil through an internal loan could participate effectively in such a move and that he thought that Argentina would be willing to do the same.

Welles said that, though this was a practical suggestion, he felt sure the Ambassador knew

the difficulties such a proposal would encounter in the United States. I reminded him of the feeling on the part of American public opinion as to intergovernmental loans and also remarked that I believed it highly unlikely that our Congress would authorize our participation in any such move in view of the economic crisis still existing here.[10]

These considerations gave to Argentina a larger material stake in the war than was possessed by any other nonbelligerent and produced an unwillingness to exert pressure upon Paraguay to accept any solution of the boundary question unpalatable to its government.

Since the conference was held in Buenos Aires, Saavedra Lamas was, by diplomatic protocol, its chairman. As Foreign Minister, he had markedly greater formal prestige than that of any of the other conference delegates, who were no more than permanent ambassadors accredited to the Argentine government or, like Gibson and Braden, were special ambassadors for the purpose of representing the United States at the conference only. Alexander Weddell was the Ambassador of the United States accredited to the Argentine government.[11]

The relations of Saavedra Lamas and President Justo were such that the Argentine President took almost no part in the determination of foreign policy but left Saavedra Lamas a free hand.[12] In his position as chairman, Saavedra Lamas was able to exert a dominant role, particularly in the determination of the pace at which the conference worked. He decided when meetings were to be held, and he decided whether or not subcommittees were to be appointed. Moreover, in his capacity as Foreign Minister he had relationships not only with the Bolivian and Paraguayan representatives at the conference but also with the foreign ministers, which allowed him to exert an influence in La Paz and Asunción that could not be matched by any of his conference colleagues.

Because of the locale and chairmanship of the conference, the secretariat was composed exclusively of officials of the Argentine foreign office. This situation gave the chairman a source of information not equally open to other delegates; it also offered an opportunity to try to write history *à la* Saavedra Lamas by providing inaccurate minutes of the meetings of the conference. Gibson remarked that in the meeting of July 25, 1935,

the chairman's remarks were given in full and our share of the debate completely deleted. . . . There was general indignation among the delegates at the tricky methods of the chairman and at the meeting on the 26th the Brazilian delegate and I took a firm stand that the minutes could not be approved until they were amended to give a true picture of the proceedings. The chairman gave in without argument and blamed the Secretary General [Luis A. Podestá Costa] for what had happened.[13]

Incidents of this sort may have been in the mind of Macedo Soares, the Brazilian Foreign Minister, who told Chargé Gordon that "the substantially all-Argentine set up of the Conference is in his opinion bound to lead to a definite and imminent break down." Gordon reported that "Macedo wished to propose to you that in place of Podestá Costa an American be named secretary of the Conference, preferably [Allan] Dawson, as he is on the spot. Such a selection would, he was certain, command the approval and confidence of all delegations represented at the Conference."

The Department of State replied thanking Macedo for "this further expression of friendly confidence in the Government of the United States and in its representatives," but stating that in view of the fact that Podestá Costa had already been unanimously approved by the mediators,

this Government would be disinclined to make any move for his substitution, particularly owing to the fact that such a move would inevitably be resented in certain quarters, and that the creation of this feeling of resentment might threaten the successful outcome of the negotiations. You may make it quite plain that, even if later on the Conference desired to name some Secretary General other than Dr. Podestá Costa, this Government would not be willing to have one of its own representatives act in that capacity.[14]

Because of his preeminent position, the personality and attitude of Saavedra Lamas were of crucial importance to the work of the conference. At the outset of the conference, according to Gibson:

It is an accepted fact here that the essential immediate difficulty is not the solution of territorial and other problems but the personality of the presiding officer. Saavedra Lamas is on his home ground and he intends that this Conference shall be his. He is openly resentful of any ideas or suggestions put forward by other members and it would appear that if necessary he will drag things out until he has exhausted opposition to his plans.[15]

Three weeks later, he reported:

Saavedra Lamas desires a solution but only on condition that he appear as its sole author. We are continuing in our efforts to convince him that he can have all the credit, that our only interest is in reaching a satisfactory solution and that we will support him in any steps in that direction. We have managed to maintain friendly personal relations with him and feel that our best hope lies in keeping him on the rails as far as this can be done, opposing him only when his trickery is too flagrant. and in urging him on in the right direction.[16]

The difficulties of dealing with Saavedra Lamas did not decrease as the conference wore on. At one point in mid-1935 Gibson reported that Saavedra Lamas "revealed himself as openly pro-Paraguay; said that we must recognize that Paraguay had won the war, that Bolivia must pay reparations. . . . His statements were in the form of peremptory orders in complete disregard of facts and his voice was shrill and at times hysterical." [17]

These difficulties with the chairman of the conference were serious. The difficulties with the delegations of Bolivia and Paraguay were even more serious. The heads of the two delegations during the first year of the conference were Tomás Manuel Elío, and Gerónimo Zubizarreta, respectively, each of whom had ambitions to be president of his country and could not therefore take positions regarded as reasonable by those who, like Gibson and Braden, wanted to settle the controversy. Within the two countries, attitudes in the postwar period were not conducive to compromise.

In Bolivia, President Daniel Salamanca had been seized and forced to resign by a group of army officers when he was visiting the Chaco front on November 28, 1934.[18] He was later released, and he retired to Cochabamba, where he died on July 17, 1935.[19]

Salamanca was succeeded by the Vice-President, José Luis Tejada Sorzano. The term of Salamanca would have ended in

August, 1935, and the presidential elections of November 11, 1934, had given victory to an anti-Salamanca candidate, but Tejada Sorzano was authorized to remain in office for an additional year by special action of the congress. In turn, he was forced to resign by an army coup on May 17, 1936, and Colonel David Toro, who had served in the Chaco, was installed as president by an army junta. A little over a year later, the leader of the 1936 coup, Lt. Col. Germán Busch, led another army move that deposed President Toro. Busch became president on July 13, 1937, and it was his regime that was in power when the Chaco dispute came to an end.

Although it could not be denied in La Paz that the Bolivian armies had been driven out of most of the Chaco, neither would it have been accurate for outside observers to say that the Bolivian army had been routed. Indeed, it seems to have been the capacity of the Bolivians to counterattack in the early months of 1935 that made the Paraguayan government willing to accept the cease-fire lines of the June 12 protocol. The Bolivian army was an organized force holding strong positions in the foothills in front of Villa Montes and other towns. While the Bolivian people and their government were not willing in mid-1935 to make the sacrifices necessary to advance again to the positions held in 1932, it was not impossible that, with the passage of time and the accumulation of additional arms, there might be a renewal of hostilities. No vital portion of the Bolivian economy had been lost to Paraguay; the oil regions were behind Villa Montes and the tin mines were out of reach, high on the Andean plateau. The Paraguayans had been stopped and were not strong enough to threaten Bolivia seriously. There was, therefore, every reason that La Paz should attempt to employ all the resources of diplomacy to obtain the best possible settlement and so to gain by peaceful negotiation some part of the territory from which her soldiers had been driven during the war.

In Paraguay, President Eusebio Ayala, who had successfully conducted the war, was forced to resign on February 17, 1936, after an army coup, and he and Estigarribia spent several months in jail.[20] He was succeeded by Colonel Rafael Franco, one of the Chaco commanders. General Franco survived a revolt by partisans of ex-President Ayala in May, 1936, but he was overthrown on August 13,

1937, by another military group. Franco's successor was Dr. Félix Paiva, and he remained as President until August 15, 1939, when, after national elections, General José Félix Estigarribia, the Chaco's greatest hero, was inaugurated. Paiva's term was a turbulent one, but two attempted revolts were subdued, and his government, greatly aided by Estigarribia, finally made peace with Bolivia.[21]

The situation in Paraguay was rather different from that in Bolivia. The Paraguayans felt that they had literally saved their country from destruction. The prestige of the army was high, and there was grim determination on the part of nearly all Paraguayans to keep the Bolivians as far from Asunción as possible. They had not been able to capture the oil-producing region nor to detach the province of Santa Cruz de la Sierra from Bolivia. What had been gained was space, rather than resources. Space, however, was treasured, not alone because it was the compensation for the sacrifice of forty thousand lives but because it symbolized safety from another Bolivian attack. Since the Chaco was principally space, it was primarily of military value, and partly for this reason the judgment of the Paraguayan army leaders about the Chaco was given great weight. In addition, the army commanders were the proud possessors of great prestige, and the governments of Ayala and Paiva existed by the sufferance of the military. President Ayala told Chargé Thurston in March, 1935, that

he knew that he would be accused of enlarging Paraguay's demands, but that there is no country in the world of similar size that could ignore the claims of a victorious army which includes ten per cent of the total population and which represents an effective majority of all citizens. . . . He observed that when he spoke of the army he did not mean a few officers or a military clique. He stated that the army and the people are one and the same in Paraguay today. . . . He prefers to continue the war rather than risk almost certain internal disturbances or revolution by agreeing to peace terms which would be considered by the Paraguayan people as a surrender of what has been won at great sacrifice during three years of a war which was forced upon them by Bolivia.[22]

Neither in Bolivia nor in Paraguay, of course, were the problems of the Chaco settlement the only important political issues of the years from 1935 to 1938. There were, for example, many questions arising from demobilization such as those of finding work for veterans. To Paraguay the possession of the Chaco was more important than to Bolivia, however, and the final outcome of the negotiations is probably not an inaccurate measure of the relative importance ultimately attached to the Chaco by the two countries.

Failure at Boundary Drawing

In the first three months of its existence, the Chaco peace conference was concerned primarily with security measures: the lines of separation of troops; demobilization; and plans for the organization of a tribunal of war responsibilities. These problems were not all settled in this period, but it was necessary to deal with some of them before the terms of a treaty of peace could be arranged. In addition, there was also reluctance on the part of the delegates to attack the territorial question because of a feeling that the two countries were so far apart on their claims to the Chaco that it would be useless to try to reach an early settlement.

On September 2, 1935, however, Zubizarreta, chairman of the Paraguayan delegation, said he was willing "to consider" a boundary line that would give Bolivia a few miles of river bank along the Paraguay, and that Bolivia might also have a free port on the Paraguay farther south.[23] This apparent concession encouraged the conference delegates and spurred them into proposing a treaty of peace on October 15. The crucial provision of the treaty was the proposed boundary, a straight line running from Fort D'Orbigny on the Pilcomayo northeast to a point on the *thalweg* of the Paraguay River between Bahía Negra and Puerto Caballo. The line was at all points east of the lines of separation of the armies, and, in the interior, it divided into approximately equal parts the territory between the original positions of the troops on June 1, 1932, and the positions on June 12, 1935. At the controversial northeastern, or Paraguay River, end of the line, Bolivia was to receive a few miles of swampland north of Bahía Negra. As Gibson explained the conference plan, it would give to Bolivia at Puerto Caballo a " 'psychological' port without her access to the river being of such a nature as to be dangerous to Paraguay." [24]

In defense of the proposal, Gibson said that the delegates were agreed that

both parties are entirely unreasonable but there is a bare chance that this solution may be accepted and if it is not this will show that the chance would be even less good of continuing negotiations on separate problems. If the plan is accepted we are out of the woods. A refusal by either or both parties would enable us to tackle the next phase which is the elaboration of an arbitral agreement.[25]

The Department of State approved the plan as "reasonable," while noting that it "went a little beyond anything" that Elío had stated Bolivia would accept.[26]

The proposal was a compromise in the classical tradition of conciliation. Neither side was willing to express its serious demands until the conference had produced something specific.

Three days before the conference plan was presented to Bolivia and Paraguay, Gibson cabled that Saavedra Lamas was "in a state of panic lest the present negotiations collapse and affect his personal prestige. His immediate aim, which he has openly pursued during the past few days, is to find a convenient scapegoat." He had suddenly evinced interest in the general conference that had been proposed by the United States, "as something on which the Chaco problem could be unloaded." Gibson thought Saavedra Lamas's idea "savors of going over Niagara Falls in a barrel," although it might later be desirable to arrange the proposed general conference. Gibson concluded: "In the light of the unfortunate experience of this Conference it is clear that any conference entrusted to the guidance of Saavedra Lamas will be handled with a maximum of ineptitude and a minimum of hope." [27]

The Conference chose to prepare its territorial plan in secret and without presenting it to either belligerent before simultaneous and formal delivery on October 15. It was rejected by both Bolivia and Paraguay.[28]

Gibson's interest in the Chaco seems not to have ranked first among his concerns. He was, of course, on leave from his ambassadorship to Brazil; he returned to it in September, and he frequently expressed to Washington his desire to leave Buenos Aires.

His low opinion of the Chaco dispute was summed up in a comment made a week before the presentation of the October 15 proposal:

I am convinced, however, that if it is decided to press this plan we should interpret our role of mediator broadly and exercise a friendly but definite pressure upon both parties to end this conflict on the ground that it is not only senseless as between themselves but a public nuisance for the other countries of America. I believe that such definite and concerted pressure is essential as both Governments are quite prepared to [play?] fast and loose with the problem for their own political ends.[29]

In mid-November Gibson was permitted to return to his beloved Rio de Janeiro, and he was succeeded by Spruille Braden, who served as the American delegate to the conference until its end. Braden had lived in Mexico as a boy and spoke Spanish fluently. He had followed a business career until his appointment as a member of the United States delegation to the Montevideo Conference in 1933. Following the Chaco Conference, he served as Ambassador in Colombia, Cuba, and Argentina, and as Assistant Secretary of State from November, 1945, until June, 1947. Gibson had looked on his own connection with the Chaco dispute as a rather distasteful chore, but Braden regarded the Chaco as a serious international problem worthy of his best efforts as a diplomat. Throughout the conference he displayed high qualities of energy, patience, and tact. He held his colleagues together at times when discouragement threatened to break up the conference; he drove them on through many setbacks to the final treaty, and all the while he maintained an impartiality of demeanor that won the respect of the other representatives. Not the least of his accomplishments was his outmaneuvering of the redoubtable Saavedra Lamas for two and a half years, and then, when the Argentine Foreign Minister went out of office with President Justo, Braden led the last final rush to the long-sought goal of the treaty. If any one individual from a country apart from the belligerents can be said to have been principally responsible for the ultimate settlement in the Chaco, Braden most nearly fits that role.

President Ayala told Minister Findley B. Howard that he appreciated "the disinterested friendship" displayed by the United States and realized its wisdom "in working very quietly and unostentatiously rather than to undertake to dominate or even to appear to attempt to dominate the Conference." [30]

One indication of Braden's attitude toward the problem of the Chaco at this time is found in his remark to Elío denying a rumor that the United States intended to leave the Conference, and asserting that "we regarded this situation as of more importance to us than the Italo-Ethiopian conflict." [31]

Prisoners and Avoidance of Incidents

The territorial question was avoided by the Conference for over a year following the collapse of the October 15 plan. However, the Conference did not adjourn, and later, when it seemed desirable for a time to let special questions be handled by subcommittee, it was said merely that the Conference was in recess.[32] Various subgroups dealt with the two delicate and complicated problems of the return of prisoners and "the security question," that is, the policing of the area between the lines to which the troops had been withdrawn in the Chaco.

The prisoner question was settled in mid-1936, when the Paraguayans retreated from their original position that they would return prisoners only after the final treaty of peace was signed. The reasons for this retreat seem to have been the uselessness of the prisoners as a bargaining counter with Bolivia and the fact that Paraguay began "to find the Bolivian prisoners a burden." The Bolivian government apparently had not been anxious for the prisoners' return because it feared a sharpening of "political and unemployment problems." [33] In the final settlement of maintenance claims, the Bolivian government paid to Paraguay the sum of about 2,400,000 Argentine pesos.

The action of the United States was influential at two points in the early stages of negotiations about the prisoners issue. Braden reported:

The majority of the neutral delegates are worn out and have frayed nerves due to long and trying months of unproductive labor here. . . . The Paraguayan attitude has so incensed some of the neutrals that . . . Nieto [del Rio], the Uruguayans and to some extent Saavedra Lamas urged that the Conference . . . declare direct agreement impossible, summon the two ex-belligerents to draft an arbitrary compromise [*sic*] and, if as anticipated Paraguay refuses to submit the entire territorial question to arbitration, to declare that Paraguay is violating the terms of the Protocol and dissolve the Conference.[34]

Braden added: "I strongly oppose this program with Brazilian and Peruvian support." This was the first of several occasions on which Braden successfully pleaded for a continuation of the Conference's endeavors when others were inclined to give up.

Later in the month, when negotiations on the prisoners were at a standstill, Saavedra Lamas asked that a Paraguayan delegate go to Asunción to explain the situation in Buenos Aires. Countering, the Paraguayans asked that Braden go to Asunción with Vicente Rivarola of their delegation. Braden was reluctant to go, for he did not wish to be later accused of exercising pressure, but he finally did so, in company with Argentine, Brazilian and Chilean representatives, and they gained some significant concessions from Ayala on the prisoner question. Gibson told the Department of State that he was "convinced that the successful outcome is due chiefly to the energy, resourcefulness and incorrigible optimism of Braden."[35]

The security question, unlike the prisoner question, was never really settled during the life of the Conference. There were two main aspects of the security question. The first, which was solved, was that of the physical separation of the armies and demobilization. Despite several anxious periods and one or two minor "frontier" incidents, there was no more fighting. The second aspect was the problem of the precise location of the line of separation of the armies for purposes of the exercise of control over the territory between the troop lines. This problem arose because of the defective drafting of the relevant part of the protocol of June 12, 1935, which referred both to "lines of separation" and "line of separation."

The Neutral Military Commission during the summer of 1935 actually laid down five lines in the Chaco. A central line was called the intermediate line; to the west of it were "a line of fire" and then "a line of separation" for Bolivian troops, and two corresponding lines to the east for the Paraguayans. The whole area between the two outermost lines—the lines of separation—was called the zone of separation; the width of the zone varied from about sixty miles in the far north to five miles in the critical region near Villa Montes where the rival forces were concentrated.

The Conference took the position that it alone possessed authority to establish regulations for the administration of the zone of separation. The Bolivian government was willing to accept this claim, but the Paraguayan government held that its control extended throughout the area between its line of separation and the so-called intermediate line, which was in the middle of the zone of separation. This difference of opinion was not resolved during the Conference, and it was important because, if the Paraguayans controlled the area up to the intermediate line, they could cut off traffic at will on the road between Villa Montes and Boyuibe. This road led northward to Santa Cruz de la Sierra, the principal town in the northern Bolivian lowlands, and southward into Argentina.

In practice, the Paraguayan army did control the road, although it permitted nonmilitary traffic on it according to its own definition of that term. The Conference maintained military observers, supplied by the six mediating countries in rotation, in the zone of separation. These were usually stationed at or near Villa Montes. Their functions were to observe the situation and report to the Conference on such matters as the numbers of troops in the Chaco and the methods of control over the road.

Negotiations about the security question were long and complicated, and they need not be detailed here. Braden's position was that, since "the occurrence of some more or less serious incident along the lines of separation is a definite possibility," [36] the road should be under neutral rather than Paraguayan control. The attitude of the several Paraguayan governments seems to have been based on a desire "to retain control of the Villa Montes Road as a trading element in the final territorial negotiations" and the fear that any concessions on this point might weaken their shaky internal positions.[37]

The influence of internal politics in the ex-belligerent countries took many forms, and it was probably the single most important reason for the prolonged nature of the negotiations. When the October 15 line was proposed, Ayala felt he would be turned out of office by the military if he approved it. Following the revolution in March, 1936, which brought Colonel Franco to power, Minister Howard in Asunción reported that he thought that "because of the internal situation and to justify their own position the present régime finds it difficult or impossible to approve, locally at least, any act of the previous government." [38]

The course of the negotiations was marked by constant efforts by the Conference to assert its right to control the zone of separation and by expressions on the part of Paraguayan delegates both orally and in writing of willingness to accept the proposals of the Conference—expressions which were not accepted in Asunción. Sometimes the complete process of approval and rejection was fully achieved in Buenos Aires, most frequently and successfully by the Paraguayan delegate, J. Isidro Ramírez. On one occasion, Braden reported that Ramírez denied having agreed to Conference control of the Villa Montes road "despite unanimous testimony of ten mediatory delegates and his own colleague." [39] Talks about the security question dragged on until the spring of 1938, when they were set aside, and in the final treaty the Paraguayan withdrawal eastward left the road fully in control of the Bolivian government.

A memorandum summarizing the experience of the Chaco negotiations at the end of 1935 stated:

Events in connection with the Chaco peace negotiations have, on the whole, indicated that the nations of the western hemisphere are not willing to make many more real sacrifices in the interest of peace than is the rest of the world. A great deal of lip service has been paid to peace and to the prevention of war, but immediate national interests of territory, trade and finance remain the dominating factors in formulating policies and influencing actions.

Noting that there had become evident "latent suspicion and distrust between Argentina and Brazil" as well as between Argentina and Chile, the memorandum concluded:

A definitive settlement will remove one of the last boundary disputes from the field of Latin American relations, may have a very helpful influence in a similar settlement of the Ecuadoran-Peruvian boundary question, and might create an atmosphere favorable to the adoption of measures to prevent future wars on the American continents. [40]

Frustration until Retirement of Saavedra Lamas

It was not until the end of 1936 that another effort was made to approach the boundary question—the fundamental question for which the Conference was intended to help to find an answer. Earlier, however, Enrique Finot, the new Bolivian Foreign Minister, said to Braden and others that

"Bolivia has absolutely no practical use for a port on the Paraguay river." He went on to say that "the Chaco is worthless and that the entire question is one of public psychology and sentiment; that cost what it may Bolivia must reach a definite settlement; and that the Protocol provisions for arbitration are of value only insofar as they may be used to force Paraguay to come to a direct agreement within the Conference."[41]

This opinion, so directly contrasting with earlier Bolivian official opinion, may be compared with that of Ayala, when president of Paraguay, who said that "it would benefit Paraguay to grant river port but it was a matter for experts to decide proper place and this must be left to negotiation following peace. In case port was granted he would be satisfied with demobilization of Bolivian army as security against renewal of conflict."[42] The opposite view came later to dominate Paraguayan policy. In 1934, however, Ayala appeared

quite anxious to make arrangements for a Bolivia port. He observed that Bolivia owns many millions of acres of oil lands which are not involved in the Chaco dispute. Pipe lines to a river port would be of advantage to Paraguay, calling for the building of refineries, increasing population and assuring cheaper gasoline for Paraguay.[43]

The Department of State's care in presenting an impartial front in the Chaco dispute is shown in its rejection of a suggestion by Braden that Minister R. Henry Norweb in La Paz be instructed "to point out to President Toro the serious consequences for the conference which Elío's withdrawal might entail." Elío, the chief Bolivian delegate, had resigned after receiving "a discourteous telegram" from Foreign Minister Finot. It was the view of the Department that it would be inadvisable for this Government to appear to intervene in a dispute arising between the Bolivian Foreign Minister and the Bolivian delegate in Buenos Aires . . . the Bolivian Minister for Foreign Affairs would properly resent this Government going over his head in a matter involving relations between himself and another official of the Bolivian Government.

The Argentine government was less cautious, and it despatched Horacio Carrillo to La Paz to try to get the Bolivian government to revoke its decision to send David Alvéstegui as a successor to Elío. Carrillo told Norweb that he had said to Finot that Alvéstegui "was personally antagonistic to several of the neutral mediators" and his appointment would confront the conference with an impossible situation; Finot did not change his mind, however, and Carrillo's intercession with President Toro was without result.[44]

The desire of the Department to avoid seeming to dominate the Conference or to exert pressure of any kind gave rise to a comment by the Chilean delegate, Nieto del Río, who told Braden that the United States was "giving these minor states an inflated opinion of themselves, 'the United States must demonstrate its authority and the fact that a strong hand of control still exists.' " [45]

In a summary of the situation in November, 1936, Braden emphasized the difficulties for the Conference caused by the revolutions in Bolivia and Paraguay, which "meant that for weeks at a time we were without either Paraguayan or Bolivian representatives with whom to deal." [46] Besides, the new governments were weak and uncertain of their popular support.

Following revolutions in each country, groups of political refugees gathered in neighboring Latin American capitals. The deposed Ayala was joined in Buenos Aires by members of his administration. Braden stated that one of the reasons the security question was not settled was "by reason of the violent accusations launched against the present government by representatives of the old régime who claimed Paraguayan interests were being sacrificed by Franco and his supporters." [47] The difficulties for the Conference created by the Paraguayan refugees had reached serious proportions by December. However, the refugee question was given a new twist when ex-President Franco arrived in Buenos Aires as expellee, rather than expeller.

In view of the possibility that he might shortly return to power, Braden reported:

Throwing out an anchor to windward, as it were, I invited Colonel Franco and his brother-in-law Sr. [Marco Antonio] Laconich to lunch with Ambassador Rodrigues Alves and myself on September 28. We apparently impressed the former president with the urgency of reaching an early and complete settlement of the Chaco problem. In fact, both my Brazilian colleague and I feel that we have improved our relations with Colonel Franco to a degree that will prove helpful if he returns to power, an eventuality he expects shortly. Furthermore, he promised that, if we reached a reasonable settlement with the Paiva government, he would approve it publicly and prevent his followers from sharpshooting at it for political motives.[48]

By the end of 1936 the Conference had come to have a kind of life of its own. It continued to carry out certain administrative duties, and it planned a new attack on the territorial question. In addition, the prestige of the mediating nations had become involved, and, more immediately, the prestige of the mediating representatives as individuals was at stake. The success or failure of the Conference would be their own success or failure. The fact that nearly all the individuals serving as representatives were kept in their posts for the duration of the Conference tended to enhance their personal motivation toward reaching a settlement. If there had been many changes in the personnel, the urge to bring Bolivia and Paraguay together might have been less strong, there might not have been a treaty, and the war might have been resumed.

A new approach to the territorial question was begun at the end of 1936. In October, 1935, the Conference had offered a plan without previous negotiations with the ex-belligerents. This had failed completely. The new approach was based on the view that the Conference should not adopt any one frontier as "the Conference line." Instead, the individual members began to talk to both Bolivian and Paraguayan delegations about a number of possible lines. In this way the tenacity of each side on all points in dispute might be judged, if not measured, and, while compromises might not be made on some points, compensations might be found for both sides to offset sacrifices made by each to the other's intransigence. This process, continued for a year and a half, influenced, of course, by many kinds of political pressures, both external and internal, was the one which produced the finally acceptable boundary.

An injection of political realism into thinking about the course of the Conference was offered by Minister Norweb in La Paz, as coming from several sources. In March, 1937, the Bolivian government confiscated the properties of the Standard Oil Company. The Company's wells all lay on the Bolivian side of the intermediary line, although some of the rigs, in the Aguaragua hills, could be seen by the Paraguayan troops. In the later stages of the war, acquisition of part of the oil lands appeared to have become one of Paraguay's war aims, although this was not officially admitted. At the time of the Carrillo mission to La Paz, the Argentine government had expressed an interest in Argentine exploitation or control of the oil resources and offered to support the Bolivian government "in readily reaching a satisfactory solution" in the Chaco. Finot apparently concluded that "the only way the present Government can hope to obtain a sufficiently satisfactory settlement of the Chaco controversy that may save its face with the people of Bolivia is . . . through a rapprochement with the Argentine." [49] and this meant some measure of satisfaction for Argentina's interest in the oil fields. Such satisfaction was provided in subsequent agreements between the two countries, although it does not appear that they had any influence on the final territorial settlement.

Another note of extra-conference politics was struck when the Brazilian Foreign Minister, Macedo Soares, in talking with Braden, suggested that "the United States could not hope to offset the concentrated efforts of Great Britain in Argentina and that we should deal with Argentina, Uruguay and some of the other Latin American nations indirectly through Brazil—" 'let them [Brazil] fight our fight.' " Braden replied that many aspects of United States relations with those states required direct negotiations and that " 'just as Brazil had further cemented her cordial relations with Argentina so we too hope to do the same thing, always preserving the ties of affection and friendship between Brazil and the United States.' " [50]

The balancing of relations between the United States on the one hand and Argentina and Brazil, on the other, was a subject raised more than once by Brazilian diplomats. Welles reported that the

Brazilian Ambassador had showed him a letter from President Vargas saying that

the basis of Brazilian foreign policy should be a complete understanding with the United States on all matters affecting inter-American interests and, even more extensively, world interests—both for the development of inter-American commercial interests and for the promotion of peace and stability on the Continent. President Vargas likewise expressed some concern regarding the closer relations which had developed during the past twelve months between Argentina and the United States and to the peculiarly friendly relations which had been created between the Secretary of State and Dr. Saavedra Lamas during the Montevideo Conference. With reference to this latter point, I said to the Ambassador that he could, of course, well understand that one of the fundamental reasons for the Secretary's visit to Montevideo was his desire to create such close and friendly relations with every government on the Continent and that if this relationship had been established with the Government of Argentina, it was most decidedly desirable from the point of view of this Government. The Ambassador replied that, of course, he understood this, but that I naturally must take into account the susceptibility on the part of the Brazilians concerning anything which implied particularly friendly relations between the United States and Argentina when Brazil had always maintained that relationship with the United States herself.[51]

Through months of negotiations Braden continued unceasingly to seek a settlement, keeping up his hopes while fully recognizing the difficulties of the situation. After almost two years, he summarized the problems:

(*a*) delays occasioned by the ambiguities of the June 12, 1935, Protocol; (*b*) the inherent difficulties of the problem mostly resulting from the fact that the war ended with theoretically neither a victorious nor a vanquished party; (*c*) the revolutions in Bolivia and Paraguay; (*d*) the intractable personalities of some of the mediatory and exbelligerent delegates; (*e*) the Indian suspiciousness especially of the Paraguayans; (*f*) the precautions made necessary in order to avoid any crisis occurring prior to or during the maintenance of Peace Conference. With the exception of (*f*) these considerations still prevail but are not generally appreciated.

He then analyzed the positions of each of the other states concerned and described his interpretation of the position of the United States as desiring to bring about peace; to preserve the inter-American peace system; to prevent a return to reliance on Europe

by the Latin American countries; to avert a loss of prestige for the
mediatory governments and their representatives. This interpretation was not commented on by Washington, and, since it may have
fairly represented the views of the Department of State, it deserves
quotation:

Being entirely free of any direct interest in the dispute our sole objective
is the consummation of a permanent peace between Bolivia and Paraguay,
not alone for reasons of humanity and good neighborliness but still more
to prevent the almost inevitable resumption of war, sooner or later,
following upon a failure of the Conference. Of greater importance than
the Chaco or the pretensions of the two ex-belligerent nations is the
preservation of the laboriously constructed American peace system
recently strengthened at the Maintenance of Peace Conference. Another
war would greatly damage this peace structure and probably throw back
to European influence those discouraged elements of Latin America
which under the recent strong leadership of the United States have been
signally oriented toward pan-American cooperation. So prominent has
been our Latin American policy that a failure of this Conference would
react with especial force on the United States. Also, there would be loss
of prestige for all the mediatory governments and the heaping of re-
proach and ridicule upon the individuals involved.

Finally, Braden stated that "the principal obstacle to a final peace
is the frame of mind of present Paraguayan leaders." Therefore, "all
possible legitimate pressure" must be used "to bring them to
reason." This should include a statement by the conference that, if
this were not achieved in direct negotiations or through an arbitral
settlement, the conference would

adjourn and issue a declaration placing the blame where it belongs—
probably, Paraguayan disinclination to reason. . . . The threat of a
Conference declaration along the above lines might bring Paraguay to
heel. It is even possible that its issuance would upset the Franco régime,
bringing in other politicians who . . . would be willing to compromise
and effect a settlement.

This is the only occasion in the history of the good neighbor policy
when a declaration by a peace conference was proposed to his own
government by a delegate of the United States as a means of ousting
a government of one of the American republics.[52]

   Among pressures that might be exerted on Paraguay, Braden proposed that "perhaps some use might be made of the Trade Agree-

ments holding out a favorable accord as an inducement for Paraguay's making peace with Bolivia." To this drastic measure, however, Welles replied that "the trade agreements program cannot be used in any effective manner to induce favorable action in the Chaco negotiations upon the part of the Paraguayan Government." [53]

At the Conference session on April 28, the chairman announced that no more subcommittees would be appointed but that the Conference would meet once a week, "at which time Dr. Saavedra Lamas would, in all loyalty, report on his negotiations with the parties—he apparently being the one Conference member not subject to the restrictions he attempted to impose on the delegates' extra-Conference activities." Braden regarded this as another maneuver to delay the work of the Conference, and on the following day he read into the record a statement that the United States government had instructed him to express its pleasure that the mediators were agreed that

we are resolved to go to the bottom of the territorial question with energy, wholeheartedness and determination, giving at the same time sufficient publicity to our activities so that the only chance of success lies in our being prepared to meet every day and if necessary, all day, at any time and any place.[54]

This statement apparently had no effect on the chairman, and the situation was regarded so seriously by the representatives of Brazil, Chile, and the United States that they held several meetings to consider how to get around the blockade set up by Saavedra Lamas. Feeling it hopeless to talk directly with him, the group accepted the suggestion of Nieto del Río that they discuss the problem with Julio Roca, Vice President of Argentina, "so that he might carry the result to the knowledge of the President of the Nation." Roca made arrangements for the three representatives to meet with President Justo and Saavedra Lamas at dinner on April 29. Following the meeting with Roca, "the Delegates had a satisfactory impression of the step they had just taken, without discounting the dangers in it, since in the last analysis the conversation with Dr. Roca and that which they would soon have with H. E. the President consisted in very daring diplomacy." [55]

It was daring diplomacy indeed to appeal to the Vice President of

Argentina against the dilatory tactics of Saavedra Lamas and to prepare to discuss the situation with the President himself in the presence of the Foreign Minister.

At the dinner meeting the three delegates concentrated, not on
the personality of Saavedra Lamas nor upon tactics alleged to be
adopted by him, but on one point—their view that it was necessary
to make every effort to obtain the final territorial settlement as
quickly as possible. They employed three principal arguments to
strengthen their case: (1) "if we fail to reach a solution to the territorial problem another war is inevitable"; (2) even more important
than the renewal of war

or the interests of Bolivia and Paraguay is the preservation of the
American peace system developed by President Justo and his Foreign
Minister, together with the other presidents and foreign ministers,
particularly of the mediatory nations. . . . Certainly another Chaco war
would do untold damage to the American peace system and to the
authority and prestige of all our presidents and statesmen and would
bring ridicule upon us delegates who have been directly involved in the
negotiations;

(3) a new element had recently been made available to the
negotiators—

"I may assure you that Bolivia will supply a considerable sum of money,
perhaps two hundred thousand pounds, for a prompt and good arrangement . . . the Conference has at its disposal a most useful element . . . to
convince the Paraguayan government, if we do not allow a long time to
pass, for we must be aware of the price of tin."

The response of Saavedra Lamas to these views was to emphasize
the need for patience and tranquility, and slowness of action. He
noted the political instability in the two ex-belligerents and relied on
the advice of Argentine military men that there was no danger of
the renewal of hostilities in the Chaco, since both were exhausted.
"When the President interrupted him to add the words 'and firmness' to those of tranquility and patience which he had used, the
Foreign Minister did not give any sign of agreeing with the clear
intent of General Justo." [56]

The specific action which the three diplomats asked President
Justo to take was to give "an atmosphere of authority" to the open-

ing of the debate in the Conference on the territorial question by presiding over the first session. Justo neither accepted nor refused this suggestion at the time, but he did not in fact inaugurate the formal "territorial phase" of the Conference discussions.

Among the impressions of the three representatives, as listed by Nieto del Río, were the following:

(1) That the Foreign Minister saw with profound displeasure this meeting for the purpose of showing the President and Vice President that the Conference is taking a wrong course under the policy of Sr. Saavedra Lamas.

(2) That the President got a thorough idea of the object of the meeting and, although he did not exactly indicate what he intended to do, used the word "firmness" in a tone equivalent to an order directed at his Minister for Foreign Relations.

(3) That he got a direct statement that there were no individual interests nor divergent opinions among the mediatory nations, and moreover that they were probably circulated by the Foreign Minister to conspire against the Buenos Aires negotiations. . . .

(7) That Sr. Saavedra Lamas, through wounded *amour propre*, may increase his policy, carrying it into the realm of personalities, and in this case it is incumbent upon the governments to keep together and to seek the support of General Justo who is more disposed to accommodating action.[57]

This "daring diplomacy" failed. There was no solemn ceremony presided over by General Justo, nor was there any change for the better in Saavedra Lamas's obstructionism. Instead, the last impression of the three diplomats was fulfilled.

The Argentine Ambassador in Washington showed to Under Secretary of State Welles part of a cable from Saavedra Lamas, received on July 27, which to Welles,

seemed to indicate that Dr. Saavedra Lamas was once more in one of his customary crises of nervous exaltation. He alleged that Brazil and Chile were trying to remove the seat of the Conference from Buenos Aires to Rio de Janeiro, and that the Chilean and Brazilian delegates to the Conference were undermining his "painful and excessively fatiguing labors" to bring about the submission of the dispute to the World Court. He further alleged that the Paraguayan Government believed that the American delegate, Mr. Braden, was under the influence of the Standard Oil Company, and said that he, Saavedra Lamas, was doing his utmost to persuade the Paraguayan authorities of the falsity of this rumor. He said, however, that Mr. Braden had joined forces with the Chilean and Brazilian delegates to undermine his own authority as Chairman of the Conference, and that, if there was going to be sabotage within the Conference of this character, the Paraguayan Government would withdraw from the Conference and the whole peace efforts which he had undertaken during the past three years would be hopelessly ruined.

Welles defended Braden, and said that he had heard nothing of any plan to shift the Conference to Rio de Janeiro. He added that he would write to Braden asking him to try to obtain "a friendly and harmonious atmosphere" at the Conference, since it appeared to Welles "that nerves were getting very strained and that nothing would be more unfortunate than personal altercations which would jeopardize the ultimate success of the Chaco Conference." [58]

Braden concluded in August that the Conference had failed "to make measurable progress" during 1937. The main reason for this failure, in his opinion, was that

the supreme consideration of Dr. Saavedra Lamas, Conference president, is to preserve his personal reputation as the Great Peacemaker. He fears to face the difficulties which necessarily will arise in the territorial negotiations or the drafting of the arbitral compromise and frequently has admitted of late that his earnest hope is to pass the Chaco question to the World Court for solution. Failing in this, his program will be through procrastination and obstruction to avoid the Conference actively entering the territorial negotiations until he has retired from office, so that the responsibility will fall on his successor as Foreign Minister and Conference president. . . . He would disparage success as an unimportant detail made possible by his own efforts, and ridicule failure as evidence of incompetence by his successor in contrast to the accomplishments attained under his own leadership.[59]

Other contributing factors were mutual recriminations in the press by foreign ministers Finot and Stefanich and "further delays and quibbling over interpretations by the Paraguayans through Dr. Ramírez, head of their delegation." Braden also listed as "a possibility," although he was not prepared to say it was important,

Dr. Saavedra Lamas' desire for Argentine domination—at least economically—over the Chaco and southeastern Bolivia, coupled with a fantastic fear that his country is surrounded by envious neighbors who are forming "blocks" with one another directed against Argentine interests. This reasoning by the Foreign Minister perhaps leads him to believe that the best policy to pursue is either to make the final peace alone, free from the other mediatory powers, or to perpetuate the division between at least two of Argentina's five neighbors—*divide et impera*.[60]

Braden thought the time had come for a fresh start, and new methods were put into effect at two conference sessions on July 30 and August 2. The first, which had been scheduled and then cancelled by Saavedra Lamas, was held in the absence of the chairman because Braden insisted on adhering to schedule. Braden read a statement concluding that "nothing has been done" and expressed the opinion that "the only manner in which we may hope successfully to arrive at a territory-boundary agreement, will be . . . by meeting morning and afternoon and, if necessary, at night." [61]

As early as August 10 Braden reported that "things have taken a decided turn for the better," a result which he attributed to his recently adopted new tactics. President Justo told Saavedra Lamas that he wanted a solution in the Chaco before his administration went out of office in February, 1938, and Saavedra Lamas "for the first time in many months declares his firm belief that the final treaty can be reached by direct negotiations within the Conference." Also, the troops in the Chaco had been withdrawn from the intermediary zone, and everything was "tranquil." [62]

The coming to power of the government of Colonel Busch in Bolivia on July 13 and that of Provisional President Paiva in Paraguay on August 15 opened new possibilities for the mediators, although the immediate effects were to delay negotiations while new delegates were appointed and new foreign ministers gained confidence in their unfamiliar offices.

In Bolivia the change of government, while significant, was of less importance to the Conference than that in Paraguay. In June Chargé John J. Muccio in La Paz had commented on the pacific tone of recent statements by the government and by editorials in the press:

This peaceful attitude of the Bolivian Government may, of course, be interpreted as evidence of its belief that it cannot renew hostilities with much hope of success. Bolivians who served as officers during the war have expressed the opinion that any attempt to conscript men for further fighting would meet with serious resistance because of the disgust of the veterans and of the people as a whole with the way the war was conducted by the Bolivian Command.[63]

The change of government in Bolivia apparently did not represent any significant change in policy, but in Paraguay the disappearance of the Franco regime, which "Paraguayan Liberals are accustomed to refer to . . . as the 'Saavedra Lamas government,' " [64] was thought by Braden to be favorable, since the new government "will enjoy greater authority than the recent one. Also, it would seem to betoken a larger influence in affairs by the old Liberal leaders . . . and should therefore be more amenable to reason." [65]

In connection with the recognition of the Paiva government, the question had been raised whether any attempt should have been made to secure its adherence to resolutions or protocols formulated by the Conference. The view of the Department of State was that it

especially desires to avoid any action that might result in the charge that this Government is endeavoring to force the Conference to take any position with regard to recognition of the new Government in Paraguay which could be construed as tantamount to intervention in their domestic affairs.[66]

Braden apparently had not favored conditional recognition but had brought up the question in a session of the Conference. A week later, he indicated that he favored recognition of the new Paraguayan government without delay because a prolongation of nonrecognition would be interpreted "as undue pressure, not to say, intervention," and, if the Paraguayan government took offense at such prolongation, the hopes of the Conference might not be attained. Also, if the new government was not encouraged, it would be replaced by one that would be less democratic and "surely would drive the country towards dictatorship and Fascism." [67] Recognition was extended to the Paiva government by the United States on August 26, 1937, but the Conference could not recommence its work until mid-October because of the absence of a Paraguayan delegation.

While the Conference marked time, Braden wrote of some of the conflicts of interest among the major powers that complicated the work of peacemaking.

The long standing rivalry of Argentina on the one hand and Brazil and Chile on the other might well have disappeared within the last few years had the direction of the former's foreign relations been in sounder hands than those of Dr. Saavedra Lamas. . . .

Countless incidents indicative of the attitude of the Argentine Foreign Minister . . . have continuously irritated the Brazilian and Chilean delegates to the Chaco Peace Conference and their governments. By using the Conference for other ends than composing ex-belligerent differences, he has confused the issues and thereby created well understandable fear in Bolivia and Paraguay that their interests were not the primary ends sought by the ABC powers in this mediation. Peace negotiations have suffered in consequence.

To illustrate Saavedra Lamas's outlook, Braden cited his

ingenuous admission to me many times during the last four years that the great Rio de La Plata delta with all its affluents constituted a geographical and economical unit. That is, Argentine domination, at least economically, over Uruguay, Paraguay, the Chaco Boreal, Santa Cruz, and even the Beni and Altiplano districts of Bolivia, is a development logically to be expected, towards which his policies must be shaped.

Braden referred to previous reports that Bolivian governments were willing to make arrangements with Argentina for oil concessions and for a railroad to be built from Yacuiba in Argentina through Villa Montes to Santa Cruz de la Sierra, "in return for which they expect Argentina to force through a final boundary sufficiently to the east so that this area will never again be threatened by Paraguayan arms." [68]

The Brazilian government was also interested in the possibilities for developing an eastern outlet for Bolivian trade through Santa Cruz, Roboré, and Puerto Suárez in Bolivia, and Corumbá in Brazil, which was intended to be the western terminus of a Brazilian railway that had been built to within sixty miles of that city. At a meeting with Baldovieso and Alvéstegui at which Ambassador Rodrigues Alves pointed out the possibilities of a Bolivian outlet via Corumbá, Braden supported the Brazilian route, rather than that through Yacuiba in Argentina, on the ground that the former offered more possibilities for the development of railway traffic along the projected route in Bolivian territory.[69]

Of the Argentine-Brazilian rivalry, Braden wrote:

That this jockeying for position or influence by Argentina and Brazil in Paraguay and Bolivia has become a factor in the Chaco Conference is further demonstrated by my Brazilian colleague's conviction that the endless obstructions and delays created by the Conference president [Saavedra Lamas] have been motivated by the latter's desire to postpone any territorial settlement in the Chaco until he has first concluded agreements with the ex-belligerents which will assure Argentina exercising the maximum domination obtainable in both countries, and especially over the Santa Cruz agricultural area and the supposedly rich petroleum fields to the south. This may be a secondary thought in Dr. Saavedra Lamas' mind but I believe the principal objective of the Conference president is to find a face-saving out for himself which will preserve his reputation as the Great Peacemaker.

Nevertheless, so concerned is Ambassador Rodrigues Alves that he has strongly urged upon his own Foreign Minister, Sr. [Mario de] Pimentel Brandão, that Brazil immediately take steps to oppose Argentina's incursions into southeastern Bolivia by herself extending a transportation system to Santa Cruz from Corumbá.[70]

So far as the United States was concerned, Braden felt that it was necessary to dispel Paraguayan suspicion, by demonstrating "my own and my government's complete disinterestedness and neutrality in all directions. Yet, I naturally cannot play a lone hand in these negotiations and collaboration with my Brazilian colleague is especially desirable." He was concerned about the situation because

Self-evidently these rivalries looking to the creation of zones of influence contain the germ which if allowed to grow will inevitably bring on dangerous competition, in armaments and otherwise, which in turn would mean the establishment on this hemisphere of disorder analogous to Europe, leading to war and destruction of the American peace system so laboriously launched by the American government. This situation justifies both careful study and appropriate action in which I believe the United States both can and should play an important, useful part.

It appeared to Braden that the difficulties were largely the creation of Saavedra Lamas's "ambitions to expand Argentine domination to the north," and asserted fears of "a 'Pacific bloc' or of the

'Diagonal' (Brazil-Bolivia-Chile) as combinations directed against Argentina." However, Argentina's recently begun rearmament program was, in Braden's opinion, attributable to deeper causes than the ambitions and fears of Saavedra Lamas. He saw the possibility of a local fascist movement:

In short, Argentina is heading towards at least a species of economic imperialism and a dangerous measure of militarism, abetted by a type of fascist ideology among many who are now influential in directing the nation. The mutual jealousies, suspicions, and fear which have appeared between Argentina and her two largest neighbors may, in due course, bring about the very system of blocs and alignments which as yet exist only as phantasma raised by Dr. Saavedra Lamas. This state of affairs already prejudices the Chaco negotiations and may, if allowed to endure, endanger the American peace system. With the Chaco dispute unsettled Bolivia and Paraguay will inevitably go to war again and those two countries may become the "Balkans of South America." The situation in all its aspects merits, in my opinion, the Department's careful consideration.

What could the United States do about this situation? Braden thought it reasonable that

The United States could effectively help by discreet suggestions and guidance; by frankly drawing attention to the facts and disposing of the unfounded fears, suspicions and bogies; and by serving as intermediary and conciliator. Such a role is possible because developments are still in a process of incubation and our government is thoroughly trusted by Chile and Brazil and most responsible Argentines either now have or are steadily gaining confidence in our integrity, our principles and our disinterestedness.

It is the minorities—Saavedra Lamas, the nationalists or fascists and some of the military—who are nurturing these malignant ideas. If allowed to grow they will become uncontrollable by either their creators or by the mass of sound public opinion here. Hence, the counter-acting efforts of the United States must be concentrated first on Argentina and next on Chile, which is especially sensitive to the fact that it is no longer on a parity with the other two members of the ABC and therefore resents more quickly Argentine displays of superiority. In my opinion, Brazil will cooperate.

Braden did not make any specific recommendations about United States policy, and the reaction of the Department of State was in the most general terms:

Efforts for a successful settlement of the controversy between Bolivia and Paraguay will continue to receive this Government's strong support. As concerns relations among Argentina, Brazil and Chile, no opportunity will be neglected to assist in any appropriate way to lessen the rivalries and friction that you mention. The Department will be glad to receive your comment and suggestions on the situation as it develops.[71]

Braden remained irrepressibly optimistic about a final settlement, even though reporting in October that "the Bolivian and Paraguayan theses are so divergent that if adhered to it would be impossible either to reach a direct agreement or to draft the arbitral compromise in accordance with the Protocols." He had had talks with Alvéstegui and Zubizarreta. The former said that the Toro government had been overthrown "because Colonel Busch and the army felt the Chaco question was being neglected. The government, the army, and the people are unanimous that Bolivia must have a sovereign port on the Paraguay river." In addition, since the Bolivians felt that these terms would be unacceptable to Paraguay and that Paraguay was "preparing for war," Bolivia considered that the Conference could not be successful and was taking steps to prepare for necessary action. Alvéstegui had admitted that Bolivia had made railway concessions to Argentina "in order to get her support in pushing Paraguay eastward." Zubizarreta, on the other hand, had told Braden that Bolivia could not have a sovereign port on the Paraguay River; that Paraguay might relinquish some territory near Villa Montes but would do so only if compensated territorially farther north "along the Parapiti [*sic*] river"; and that Paraguay would not give up any territory for cash.

In summary, Braden reported:

Always providing we are not delayed by more revolutions in the ex-belligerent countries, I believe that while we will have to go through moments of the greatest difficulty and even of despair, nevertheless a solution is possible. We must take first things first, however, and the greatest obstacle of all is Dr. Saavedra Lamas . . . how to circumvent his incompetence and deliberate obstructionism is a problem we must endeavor to solve as we go along. I have, however, told the Brazilian and Bolivian delegates that in my opinion the Conference should not take a recess but should continue earnestly endeavoring to find a solution, always realizing that it may be impossible for us to make genuine progress until the Ortiz administration comes into office and a new Foreign Minister assumes the presidency of the Chaco Peace Conference.[72]

An example of the kind of discussion carried on by Braden with the Paraguayans at this time is given in a despatch written early in the new year. Noting that he felt it was of little use to argue on legal grounds with Zubizarreta, as other mediatory delegates were inclined to do, Braden pointed out:

frequently during the past two and one-half years opportunities to settle the Chaco had been lost by Paraguayan delay and intransigence; fortunately the question had not yet been injected into Bolivian politics, but if it were, there would be little hope for a pacific adjustment; despite the Bolivian government's instructions to its delegate to demand a sovereign port, the mediators were willing to work for a solution such as we had urged during the last few weeks and we felt we would be successful if Paraguay would only give us a starting point; a withdrawal in the west would be more than compensated by the assurance of permanent peace, Paraguayan retention of a major portion of the Chaco and the economic advantages included in our proposal. . . . I maintained that for Paraguay to remain in its present positions, even if Bolivia signed a treaty to that effect, meant that Paraguay would be a continuing threat on Bolivia's doorstep, if not within the door, and would eventually bring war; just as Dr. Zubizarreta called the Paraguay river sacred to his country—so the upper Pilcomayo–Villa Montes–Boyuibe–Parapiti line was sacred to Bolivia; we all recognized Paraguayan bravery during the recent war but also I knew of officers who swore they never would fight in the Chaco again—it wasn't worth it, they would escape over the frontier first; if another war came Paraguay, even though victorious, could gain little, whereas under the handicaps of greater distance from bases, etc., the miracle of the last war might not be repeated; thus, she had everything to lose and nothing to win; the Paraguayan people did not want war, in fact it was only the propaganda of the newspapers and the politicians who kept the dispute alive, and I added one job he could do in Asunción would be to silence those two disturbing elements.

Braden added that Saavedra Lamas had informed the Conference "that President Justo has sent a personal letter to Provisional President Paiva . . . observing that 'while that nation [Paraguay] had many military heroes, its need now was for civilian heroes.' "[73]

Probably this kind of practical, political-military-economic argument had greater weight with the Paraguayans than discussions over the interpretations of the June 12, 1935, protocol or the August 3, 1932, declaration on nonrecognition of territorial aggrandizement by force. On an earlier occasion, Braden felt he "was able to convince the Paraguayan delegates pretty thoroughly that these petroleum fields [near Villa Montes] are commercially unimportant." [74] Braden was in touch with General Estigarribia, who, although still in exile in Argentina, apparently still had

an appreciable backing and influence in the country, probably principally among army officers and ex-combatants. General Estigarribia recognizes the fact that Paraguay could not hold the present line of military occupation as a permanent frontier in the absence of a definitive settlement with Bolivia. [75]

Stimulated, perhaps, by an urge akin to that which accounts for New Year's resolutions, Braden summarized the position of the Conference early in January, 1938. He said that the achievement for 1937 was "zero, except for the intangible credit due it for having prevented the renewal of war." He restated the boundary demands of Bolivia and Paraguay and said that, in view of confidential Bolivian declarations, if Paraguay could be persuaded to agree to withdraw slightly near Villa Montes and accept the intermediary line as the starting point for trading, the following boundary might be approved by both countries: "starting from a point between D'Orbigny and Ballivián on the Pilcomayo—north to latitude 20° South —east to the Paraguay river." However, the Bolivians would probably accept this only "under pressure," and success could be reached only if the Paraguayans "adopt a more conciliatory attitude," if Saavedra Lamas permits negotiations to go on, and if the six mediatory states "are unified on a concrete program which they will support wholeheartedly." He indicated that exiled Paraguayans, including Colonel Franco, General Estigarribia, and ex-president Ayala, had promised to support the above boundary.

Braden requested the views of the Department on the situation. Although he had noted that "there exists some disposition among my mediatory colleagues to threaten Paraguay with a rupture of diplomatic relations if that country's intransigence causes the Conference to fail in reaching a pacific settlement," there appeared no disposition in Washington to take so strong a step. A memorandum to the Under Secratary suggested that the "discouraging" outlook in Buenos Aires might make it "desirable or necessary in the near future to again consider united action in an effort to settle the Chaco matter." The "united action" suggested, however, was no more than the taking of an initiative by the Chaco conference by calling the attention of Bolivia and Paraguay to the Declaration of Principles of Inter-American Solidarity and Cooperation and to the Convention for the Maintenance of Peace, which had been approved at the Buenos Aires Conference. It was noted that these documents were not binding on either Bolivia or Paraguay, and that they "have been ratified by very few of the other American republics. However, the Chaco Peace Conference might well cite the spirit of them in the event that it is decided to attempt to gain the support of the other American republics in bringing the Chaco negotiations to a successful conclusion." [76] It does not appear, however, that Braden was instructed to recommend an initiative of this kind to his colleagues.

A week after his summary despatch, Braden commented on the possibility of new fighting in the Chaco:

The inherent danger of another Chaco war resulting from a failure by the Conference has greatly concerned my Brazilian colleague and me not alone because of the tragedy involved in such a catastrophe, but still more because of our fear that this time, one or more neighboring nations may possibly be sucked into the conflict and, above all, that such a conclusion would be disastrous to the budding American peace system so laboriously erected under the guidance of the United States.[77]

The security question continued to plague the Conference, and it threatened to reach a crisis through Bolivian demands that the Conference put into effect the security regulations accepted on April 23, 1937, but not ratified by Paraguay. Braden remarked:

To avoid the onus of retiring from office with the Chaco negotiations in a critical state the Justo Administration might reasonably be expected to force Paraguay either to reach a final settlement or at least to dispose satisfactorily of the security question. The Brazilian representative and I will work for this but the erratic behavior of the Conference chairman is more likely to make him (*a*) try to break up the Conference so that his successor could get no credit for a final peace or (*b*) capitalize confusion of Conference in order that Ortiz retain him in Cabinet. I believe the Brazilian delegate and I can block (*a*) but (*b*) would be disastrous not only for the Conference but for all America. Therefore, it may be best for the Conference to temporize until after February 20.[78]

In response to these communications, the Department of State advised Braden that it "concurs in your opinion that the best immediate course for the Conference may be to avoid forcing any issues until after February 20." With regard to the fundamental question

the Department, at the present time, reiterates its opinion that the most promising approach may be an effort to delimit definite zones adjudicated *prima facie*, one to Bolivia and one to Paraguay, with an intermediary area comprised between those two zones to be submitted to arbitration.

In view of the many complications attendant upon procedure to submit the Chaco dispute to the World Court, the Department will give attention to means whereby Conference work may be given a new impetus after February 20. It would be desirable for the mediatory delegates, in consultation with their governments, to reach agreement upon a definite program for a final Conference effort to settle the outstanding issues. In this connection, the Department will be prepared to urge directly upon the other mediatory governments the desirability of supporting before the governments of the two disputants in every appropriate way whatever program is agreed upon.[79]

Faced with the dismaying prospect of retirement in three weeks, Saavedra Lamas made a new attempt to hold his positions and find a Chaco settlement. The Conference gave him permission at the end of January to try to secure a boundary settlement through personal negotiations. The Argentine Foreign Minister's final effort included a proposal to shift the intermediary line so as to let Bolivia control the Villa Montes-Boyuibe road, with compensation elsewhere for Paraguay. Further, the boundary was to be studied by a commission of geologists and geographers over a period of several months, during which time the Conference would be in recess.

If Bolivia and Paraguay accepted this proposal, Saavedra Lamas would be able either to retire with a show of success for his personal handling of the situation or to urge strongly that President-elect Ortiz retain him as Foreign Minister so that he might bring about a final peace under purely Argentine auspices.[80]

Neither of these eventualities would have been regarded with pleasure by Braden and his other colleagues, but the situation was saved by the refusal of the Bolivian government to have anything to do with the Saavedra Lamas formula as presented by Horacio Carrillo in La Paz. The new Foreign Minister of Bolivia, Diez de Medina, said that his main objections to the plan were that it would lead to the dissolution of the Conference, that it practically recognized the intermediary line as the boundary, and that it did not provide for a free port for Bolivia on the Paraguay River.[81]

This was Saavedra Lamas's supreme effort at peacemaking. Its failure did not, however, settle the question of whether he would remain as Foreign Minister. Saavedra Lamas had learned that an envoy of one of the South American countries had tried to induce the government of Brazil to bring influence to bear in Buenos Aires to prevent Saavedra Lamas's reappointment. The suggestion had been rejected in Rio de Janeiro, as it would have been in Washington, but Saavedra Lamas gave the news both to President Justo and to President-elect Ortiz, and, in Braden's opinion, he "so effectively capitalized" on the incident "as to practically clinch the position but he lost out this week because of a violent altercation" with one of his cabinet colleagues.[82] It was not until February 18, however, that Braden was able to breathe easily about the situation; on that day he talked with Ortiz, who told him that Saavedra Lamas "with whom both he and Justo had wide differences was out completely." [83]

The leave taking between Saavedra Lamas and the conference delegates was arranged in a formally amicable fashion, although not in the manner desired by Saavedra Lamas. He had, through an intermediary, proposed to the Brazilian and Peruvian delegates that they try to "get approval of plenary session at which each delegation including the ex-belligerents would praise the retiring conference President." Braden hoped that a plenary session would not be held and that the Conference would hold a "luncheon without speeches" as a farewell ceremony.[84] He thought that "a Conference session of homage" might be viewed by Ortiz "as an implicit criticism of his not having reappointed Dr. Saavedra Lamas." Also, at least one of the delegates to the Conference said he would not participate in such a session.[85] Although Saavedra Lamas at first rejected the luncheon proposal, he later accepted it, and the affair was held on

February 19. Braden made a speech largely given to praise of President Justo, and Saavedra Lamas responded.[86] On February 24 the Conference passed a resolution "expressing its appreciation of collaboration of Argentine delegation and ex-Chairman and another resolution emphasizing ex-President Justo's contribution to the Conference and concluding by conferring upon him the title of Honorary President." [87]

After February 20, 1938, Saavedra Lamas was unable any longer in an official capacity to obstruct the work of the Conference of which he had been chairman for thirty-two months, but he continued for an additional month to exert a behind-the-scenes influence. Braden reported on March 15:

Markedly less reasonable attitude today of Paraguayan delegation in committee opinion results from interference by Saavedra Lamas. Zubizarreta admitted former Minister's satellite, Carrillo, described to them day before yesterday the Bolivian anxiety for peace treaty even on basis of this morning's proposal.

Paraguayan delegation has asked for appointment with President of the Argentine Republic "to discuss their mission in the Conference" before Zubizarreta leaves for Asunción next week. This is perhaps also due to Lamas encouraging Paraguayan stalling by assuring them that he will be reappointed Chairman Argentine delegation on arrival Cantilo.[88]

It was not until early in April, with the arrival in Buenos Aires of the new Foreign Minister, José María Cantilo, and the final dashing of Saavedra Lamas's hopes, that the latter's baneful influence was removed from the Conference, except for one unavailing bit of meddling in July.

CHAPTER V

The Chaco Peace Conference—Fulfillment

ON THE RETIREMENT OF SAAVEDRA LAMAS, no progress had been made on the territorial question; Bolivia and Paraguay were both thought to be rearming, and there was serious concern about the possibility of a renewal of hostilities. Braden's opinion, expressed a week before Saavedra Lamas relinquished his position, was that now "for the first time in conference history there can be an intelligent, incisive drive unhampered by Saavedra's intrigue so that fundamental negotiations may be intensified with full Argentine collaboration and a conclusion reached one way or the other in quick order." [1]

Braden's plans for action by the Conference were:

A few weeks of all-day negotiations every day with the parties will ascertain the maximum mutual concessions obtainable from the ex-belligerent delegations in Buenos Aires. As soon as that has been done, the trips to Asunción and La Paz should be made and, within a few weeks thereafter, either a definitive peace treaty should have been agreed upon or we will have established the impossibility of adjusting the Chaco dispute at this time. If this program is successful, all secondary issues will be disposed of automatically; if it is not, the Conference should then decide how it will handle these secondary issues and determine the best course for it to follow.

This program was approved by the Department "provided there is substantial agreement upon it by the mediatory delegations, and no determined opposition to it from either Bolivia or Paraguay." [2]

Braden and Rodrigues Alves tried unsuccessfully to get ex-President Justo to serve as chairman of the Conference, but work was begun quickly under the chairmanship of the acting Foreign Minister, Manuel P. Alvarado, without waiting for the arrival from Italy of Saavedra Lamas's successor, José María Cantilo. On March 8 Braden was named chairman of a committee of the Conference "to pursue intensive territorial boundary negotiations. In my [Braden's] opinion this means that for the first time in over 2 years an intelligent incisive effort can now be made to reach a final solution and very shortly we should know whether or not it is possible of accomplishment at this time." [3]

Not only were the dilatory tactics of Saavedra Lamas no longer a problem, but Alvarado was willing to adopt a strong line to bring about a more "reasonable" attitude by Paraguay; Braden said Alvarado "would be delighted to accomplish during his short tenure of office what S. Lamas failed to do in over 2 years." [4]

Alvarado's opinion was that

(one) the territorial negotiations must now be vigorously pushed to a conclusion; (two) Paraguay must be made to understand that in event of conference failure, (A) that body would make public reasons therefor frankly placing blame on Paraguayan unreasonableness; (B) friendship of mediatory powers for Paraguay would be alienated; (three) at psychological moment the united pressure of mediatory governments would be required and the conference could then count on full support of himself, President Ortiz and Justo.

These views caused concern in Washington, but Welles pointed out that the points in question were the views of the acting Argentine Foreign Minister, and added: "I am inclined to think that unless the Argentine Government is willing to talk vigorously to the Paraguayan along these lines, there isn't the slightest chance that Paraguay will do anything except delay proceedings. For the time being, consequently, I would let things ride." [5]

Welles's decision was a wise one, since it seems clear that the attitudes of Alvarado and Ortiz, and later of Cantilo, were of determining importance in sufficiently reducing the Paraguayan demands. Braden reported that "President of the Argentine Republic [Ortiz] in interview with Zubizarreta with map in hand demanded that a compromise frontier be agreed on as soon as possible." [6] This was a distinctly new experience for the Paraguayan delegate, since former

President Justo had left negotiations entirely in the hands of Saavedra Lamas.

The situation reached no more than a month after Saavedra Lamas's exit was summarized by Braden in a despatch on March 22:

The one decidedly encouraging development is the active collaboration and forthright attitude of the Argentine Minister for Foreign Affairs *ad interim*. Prospects for a final treaty perhaps largely depend on the measure in which he, supported by President Ortiz and General Justo, is able to force Paraguay to accept a frontier approaching Conference proposal No. 1, delivered yesterday, i.e. Ballivián—27 de Noviembre—Ravelo, mouth of the Otuquis [Negro] in the Paraguay River.

That proposal, in the unanimous opinions of the mediatory delegates, should satisfy both parties. While denying a sovereign port to Bolivia it pushes the Paraguayan frontier and military outposts back sufficiently to give ample security. It is distinctly a compromise but in addition to supporting the main pre-war thesis of Paraguay that Bolivia should have no sovereign port, it gives the former country permanent possession with a clear title to approximately 226,000 square kilometers of the Chaco as against some 86,000 square kilometers before the war. Paraguay would thus own an area of the disputed territory considerably larger than: (*a*) the maximum ever contemplated in the various pre-war draft treaties and projects; (*b*) was suggested by the mediatory powers in their October 15, 1935 proposal.

Quite apart from the exclusive interests of the ex-belligerents, Braden noted that

the Brazilian delegate throughout has been adamant that Bolivia must retain a section of territory across the northern Chaco together with the triangle ceded to that country by Brazil. He frankly admits that Brazilian policy in this particular is predicated on the necessity for this Bolivian buffer against a future Argentine aggression. I have told him I thought his fears groundless but they are deep seated and apparently not easily removed.[7]

An amusing side issue arose at this time with one Paraguayan proposal that the western portion of the boundary should run along the Ibibobo hills southeast of Villa Montes. Braden cabled that "great confusion exists as to location exactly of Ibibobo hills. Can the Department help in this respect?" From Washington came word that a 1934 map of Bolivia showed a town called Ibibobo between Villa Montes and Fort D'Orbigny on the Pilcomayo.[8]

The difference in the position of the United States, on the one hand, and that of Argentina and Brazil, on the other, in bringing influence or pressure to bear on Bolivia and Paraguay was illustrated clearly by several incidents at this critical period of the negotiations. The greatest length to which the United States went at this stage was shown in a comment made by Ambassador Weddell to Pablo Max Ynsfrán, Counsellor of the Paraguayan Legation in Washington, who was in Buenos Aires. Weddell said that

only a frontier which the mediators considered satisfactory and as affording complete security for both parties would be complemented, in the final treaty, by the moral guarantee of the mediators. The Ambassador pointed out that the giving of a moral guarantee is a new departure in American diplomatic history. The United States is willing to join with the other mediatory powers in giving it, but if Paraguay insists on a frontier and achieves it—which in his opinion is not sufficient to give security against the renewal of war, he will oppose the United States giving its moral guarantee to the frontier.[9]

The term "moral guarantee" as an obligation of the mediatory nations had been employed in the protocolary act of January 21, 1936, and in the conference resolution of June 8, 1937. The attitude of the office of the legal adviser, sent to Braden, was:

In view of the qualifying word "moral" it is not believed that the guarantee contained in the above quoted agreement [resolution of June 8, 1937] involves an obligation on the part of the United States to exercise force for the purpose of maintaining observance by Bolivia and Paraguay of the agreements already made for reaching a settlement of the boundary between their territories or any agreement which they may make as a result of the conference concerning the boundary. On the other hand, it is believed that the "moral guarantee of the six mediatory nations" means that they are expected to endeavor by peaceful methods to induce Bolivia and Paraguay to abide by the agreements already made.

In the covering instruction sent with the above opinion, the Department asked Braden to "stress the features of cooperation and consultation with the other mediatory powers as essential parts of the policy of this Government." The Department considered, further, "the 'moral guarantee' by the mediatory nations to be an integral part of the obligation of the two Parties to carry out in spirit as well as in letter the provisions of the various agreements reached at the Conference." [10]

In his talks with delegates, Braden seems to have been circumspect about possible influence that the United States might bring to bear. In a talk with the Bolivian delegates and Rodrigues Alves, Alvéstegui had said that "unless Brazil, Chile, and the United States obtained a sovereign port on the river for Bolivia, that country must deliver herself, lock, stock, and barrel, to Argentina." Braden replied that "there was practically nothing the United States could do aside from our participation as a mediator in the Conference, and there was little hope of Bolivia obtaining a sovereign port on the river, since Paraguay was resolutely opposed to that condition above all others." [11]

In contrast, Alvarado, for Argentina, was able to offer material advantages to Bolivia and material threats to Paraguay.

When the mediatory delegates had become convinced that they had secured the maximum concessions possible from the delegates of the ex-belligerents in Buenos Aires, they organized two groups, which visited La Paz and Asunción in the early part of April. Braden, with Manini Ríos, the Uruguayan delegate, and Orlando Leite Ribero, a substitute for Rodrigues Alves, went to La Paz, and the delegates of Argentina, Chile, and Peru, Ambassadors Isidoro Ruiz Moreno, Manuel Bianchi, and Felipe Barreda Laos, respectively, made the trip to the Paraguayan capital.

In La Paz, Braden found that

While the mass of population only desires peace those in control are divided into two groups:
(1) As represented by the President of Bolivia who want peace and probably will accept a line approximating meridian of D'Orbigny but feel must have Bahía Negra in order to justify relinquishing practically all of Chaco.
(2) Group headed by Minister of War uninterested in any settlement confident Bolivia with greater economic and numerical strength having learned lessons of last war can and should look only to a war of revenge.[12]

In a vote in the junta, the Minister of War's faction defeated President Busch and other moderates. However, Braden here, as on other occasions, resorted to informal tactics. With elaborate precautions for secrecy, he met with President Busch and one other person on the night of April 13, 1938, and obtained Busch's personal promise that Busch would accept, and would gain official Bolivian acceptance of, a boundary line in the Chaco that, owing to Busch's promise, was "feasible in Bolivia" and was in Braden's opinion "more than fair to Paraguay." Busch kept his word; Braden and his colleagues pressed their views of "fairness" on the Paraguayan delegation, and this secretly approved line was in all essentials the line as finally drawn.[13] This secret interview was of major importance both as fixing the minimum demands of the Bolivian government and as providing a solid basis for Braden's subsequent dealings with the Paraguayans. Under Braden's consequently confident leadership, the Conference decided on a "showdown"; it would make "with considerable fanfare" its final proposal for the boundary.[14] The proposal would be kept secret until newspaper publicity had been arranged; the "theatricals" successful in the armistice of June, 1935, would be repeated.

Cantilo invited the foreign ministers of the ex-belligerents to attend meetings in Buenos Aires to begin on May 24. Braden felt that Paraguayan acceptance "will depend upon degree of pressure put on Paraguay by Argentina." He urged this view on Cantilo, who was pessimistic and wanted to find a way for the conference "to dissolve gracefully in the event of failure." Braden was more hopeful and said that "the one time a mediator had pounded the table . . . Paraguay promptly backed down and I was convinced united forceful stand by mediators would bring desired result." Braden's reference here was to Rodrigues Alves's telling Zubizarreta that the latter's proposal that the triangle ceded to Bolivia by Brazil in the Treaty of Petropolis should be taken by Paraguay in the final settlement "would 'seriously prejudice friendly relations' between Brazil and Paraguay. Thereupon Zubizarreta replied as follows: They would not make an issue of the triangle." [15]

Braden stated that Cantilo "seemed impressed" and said, significantly, that he would warn the Paraguayans "(1) they must expect totally different attitude from Argentina than in the last war if another conflict occurs; (2) while Paraguayan intransigence will be interpreted as aggression against Bolivia it will be taken as a 'moral aggression' against the mediatory countries." [16]

As a part of the "theatricals" arranged for the meeting of the Conference with the two foreign ministers, Braden addressed the American Club in Buenos Aires, on May 24, with the approval of the other mediators. To those not familiar with the situation in the Conference, the speech might well have appeared to be merely an appeal for peace directed equally at Bolivia and Paraguay. To the insiders, however, and notably to the Paraguayans, the speech was undoubtedly recognized as an expression of dissatisfaction by members of the Conference in general and by the United States in particular with the policy of Paraguay. When Braden said that "two countries, still small in population and who require collaboration of their neighbors, killed over 130,000 of their citizens and maimed countless others to gain possession of an area much of which is, at best, of hypothetical value because of its remoteness and other unfavorable conditions of nature," Paraguayans may have felt that their "victory" was belittled and their unwillingness to compromise sharply attacked.

Paraguayan confidence that the Conference, on the basis of article I, section 3, of the protocol of June 12, 1935, could not "relinquish its functions" until arbitration had been agreed upon, must have been seriously shaken by the lightly veiled threat made by Braden:

By persistence and patience, at long last we have reached the final crucial moment when a permanent frontier, and peace, *must* be established. I say "must" because things cannot continue as they are . . . the two countries have failed to renew official relations; they are rearming and are reported to have military and para-military effectives in excess of the protocol provisions. Of such stuff wars are made. . . .

The parties must remit some rights that they may enjoy others; they must subordinate formal claims to practical necessities; they must make sacrifices of both real and imagined rights. To do these things calls for that rare quality—the courage of a statesman. . . .

For three years, with a patience perhaps unparalleled in history, the representatives of the mediatory nations have worked with those of the ex-belligerents until today the respective claims, policies, and considerations are as well known to the Conference as to the parties themselves. . . . Based on this experience and their knowledge of the subject, and after careful deliberations, the six neutral governments, unbiased by any selfish motives, have unanimously agreed upon a concrete proposal for the settlement, once and for all, of the Chaco dispute.

Linking the Conference's concern to the foreign policy of the United States, Braden said:

There is one common denominator of the foreign relations of all the American republics. By a brilliant rhetorical stroke, it has been called the "Good-Neighbor" policy. That policy is not the unilateral undertaking of a single country: it is a multilateral obligation. Its fundament—its *élan vital*—is that disputes between nations shall be composed by the use of reason and not aggravated by resort to force.[17]

The local reaction to the speech, Braden cabled, was favorable. His colleagues expressed "strong approval . . . Very impressive tone of all Buenos Aires newspapers calling for settlement at this time and most of them urging acceptance of conference proposal." [18]

It is impossible to judge the net effect of this speech, since it was combined with messages from the presidents of the mediatory states and with an Argentine attitude entirely different from that of the previous administration. In any case, it could only have been made by the representative of the United States, and it represented the maximum pressure that the United States at that time was willing to exert. An outline of the speech, but not its text, had been approved by the Department of State, with three suggestions for changes.[19]

President Roosevelt cabled to President Busch and Provisional President Paiva his hopes that the Conference formula would be accepted, and he "strongly urged" this course on both governments. Roosevelt called the plan an equitable one, offering "every possibility for lasting peace, security and the national interests of the two parties." To La Paz, the President's words were that the United States government "has a vital interest, in common with its sister republics of the Americas, in preserving peace in our hemisphere." [20]

The new boundary proposed by the Conference was not greatly different from Conference proposal No. 1, of March 22, mentioned above (p. 139), except that the southern end was now slightly farther west on the Pilcomayo and, in order to try to secure Puerto Caballo at the mouth of the Negro River in the Paraguay River north of Bahía Negra for Bolivia, the Conference assured Paraguay of the payment by Bolivia of "monetary consideration." [21]

The Bolivian Foreign Minister accepted the Conference plan on May 31; on the next day the Paraguayan delegation rejected it, stating that they could not accept cession to Bolivia of any territory on the Paraguay River or on the Negro River south of the mouth of the Otuquis River. Zubizarreta said that Paraguay's position was due "to need of military security, Paraguayan settlements and interests near Bahía Negra and sentimental reasons." Braden's response was that "Paraguay would have complete security against any possible aggression . . . while respecting Paraguayan sentimental valuation these are outweighed by peace; furthermore opinion of America would be scandalized to know when the time came that negotiations had failed on account of 6 kilometres of swamps." [22]

Zubizarreta's refusal to discuss any Paraguay River littoral for Bolivia was regarded by Braden as "the essence of intransigence." An explanation of Zubizarreta's defiance of the Conference was given to President Ortiz by Foreign Minister Cecilio Báez, who said Zubizarreta "was building in the Conference his political platform for the Presidency" of Paraguay.[23]

At the first meeting of the Conference when Báez and Diez de Medina were both present, Báez made a remark to the effect that " 'one nation at Habana inter-American Conference [1928] asserted the policy of intervention but that 20 Latin American republics rose up and defeated that policy.' " Braden thought this obviously hostile reference to the United States resulted from the combination of his speech on May 24 and President Roosevelt's telegram to President Paiva.[24]

President Roosevelt's letter to Paiva was used by a Conservative newspaper in Asunción, *Patria*, for a political attack on the Liberal régime. The paper stated editorially on May 27 that for the United States to "urge strongly" the acceptance of the Conference plan was an "insolent and inexcusable impertinence," which was the result of the "servile diplomacy" of the Liberal Party. A second editorial on May 28 stated that Paraguay should adopt a firm attitude toward the effrontery of governments which violated the respect due to the Paraguayan people who had "sacrificed 40,000 of its best citizens" to suppress Bolivian aggression and so had rendered a service to continental peace, which is a thousand times more sure and effective than the ambiguous and deceitful diplomacy of the "great power of the North."

Seeking to find a way around Zubizarreta's firmness, Braden suggested to the Department that it inform Estigarribia, then Paraguayan Minister in Washington, that Zubizarreta's stand would mean eventual war if it were not modified, and also that President Ortiz and other officials had told the Paraguayan delegates "that in the event of another conflict they must count on no help from Argentina." [25] Laurence Duggan talked with Estigarribia, who said he thought that Paraguay was being asked to give up too much territory and that Paraguay would not favor accepting money for land that it had lost lives to acquire. He was unimpressed by Ortiz's statement and protested "vigorously that no Argentine support had been received during the last war." [26]

Exploring other means of circumventing Zubizarreta, some of the mediators "suggested Argentina might exert decisive influence either by sending an army officer as confidential agent to Asunción or having President of the Argentine Republic telephone President of Paraguay but Argentine Minister for Foreign Affairs opposed the steps as excessive pressure." [27]

Another suggestion was also made along this line. Braden commented that the Paraguayan delegation had "not fully informed the authorities in Asunción of the negotiations here including important phases of the Conference proposal." He wondered, consequently, whether "an airplane visit to Asunción by the Brazilian delegate, myself and one other preferably Argentine, might turn the trick if the trip were made at Paraguayan invitation." This idea was given up, however, since "no invitation was elicited from Paraguay and I do not wish to press the matter as it might be interpreted as undue pressure on Paraguay by the delegate of the United States." [28]

After further negotiations, a "final" counteroffer was made by Paraguay on June 24—D'Orbigny-Capirenda-Carandaity-Matico-

Ravelo to the mouth of the Otuquis. This was considered "totally unacceptable" by the Conference, but the Paraguayans were told that the Conference would try for two or three days to get concessions from Bolivia, and then a final offer would be made to Paraguay "making clear to Paraguayans no further negotiations are possible and if it is rejected direct negotiations will be declared terminated." At this stage Braden reported that "aside from Paraguayan intransigence principal handicap is timidity of the Argentine Minister for Foreign Affairs [Cantilo] vis-à-vis Paraguayans, the fact that he is poor negotiator and his main concern to get rid of the Chaco." The Paraguayans were apparently still bargaining at this late hour, a tactic which was due, in Braden's view, to "the peculiar Paraguayan psychology." Cantilo said that the junior Paraguayan delegate, Efraím Cardozo, had told him that the counterproposal "was made to give an opening to negotiations; that civilians in Asunción were disposed to accept Conference proposal in the interior but that military insisted a fight should be made for a better line before accepting." [29]

During this phase of the Paraguayan resistance the Bolivians became restive. Diez de Medina said that he would withdraw Bolivian acceptance of the Conference line in a few days and would leave Buenos Aires if no progress was made. The Chilean delegate informed the Conference of Chilean army reports confirming information from Bolivian sources "that pro-war party in that country is growing rapidly," and unusually large arms shipments through Arica to Bolivia were reported in April, 1938. [30]

The statement of the Conference's intention to terminate direct negotiations "visibly moved" the Paraguayan delegation. Even before this, however, Zubizarreta had shown signs of climbing down to a position that would make agreement possible. He said that the differences between Bolivia and Paraguay were over a small area only and that "if Bolivia does not insist on littoral [on the Paraguay River] south of Otuquis an agreement on balance of the line appears feasible; if Bolivia will not, then nothing remains but to end direct negotiations." He suggested that a committee of the Conference go to Asunción, prepared to spend a month if necessary, to negotiate directly with civilian and military leaders. Then, "if a gentleman's agreement resulted respecting the frontier the Paraguayan Government which now has all of its electoral system organized could submit it to an informal plebiscite including women." A plebiscite was necessary because the Paraguayan government would "fall immediately" if it accepted a settlement unsatisfactory to the people and the army.[31]

Spurred by Bolivian threats to publish a memorandum attacking Paraguay and the Conference, the mediators asked Paraguay in writing if it "would accept Conference line in west and north if Bolivia gave up littoral for a free port and money were omitted from settlement." Braden personally promised Cardozo that, if this was accepted in principle, "the Conference would then be willing to send a committee of delegates to help put over the plebiscite." [32]

The reply to this inquiry, received on July 1, was in the negative, although additional negotiations were requested, but by that time it had been superseded by a new proposal.

At Braden's request, Sumner Welles pointed out to the Bolivian Minister in Washington the "inadvisability of publication of the Bolivian memorandum at this time," and the minister said he would so inform his government.[33]

The situation at this moment was critical, with war, so far staved off by the Conference, more likely than ever. Chargé Walter Thomas Prendergast reported that on June 24 the Bolivian constitutional convention had passed a law "authorizing the Bolivian Government to raise the sum of £1,000,000 sterling, largely for the purchase of arms, in view of the possible failure of the Chaco peace negotiations." Prendergast added that Bolivians were not being allowed to leave the country without special permission "in view of the precarious international situation. There is a very evident feeling in La Paz that the peace negotiations at Buenos Aires have, to all intents and purposes, broken down." [34]

Zubizarreta suggested for the first time on June 26 that "war will be the outcome." This conclusion he reached as a result of his conviction that "the Argentine Minister for Foreign Affairs and Government including President are uninterested in a solution and only desire to be rid of the question and the Conference"; and because he expected a negative reply from Asunción on the question by the Conference that had been sent off that day. He had no hope that an agreement could be reached on the terms for an arbitral settlement. Zubizarreta urged that Braden go to Asunción with Rodrigues Alves to press for the Conference solution and a plebiscite.[35]

In consequence of this conversation, Braden stated:

> It is apparent that neither the Paraguayan Government nor delegation dare assume the responsibility of accepting any line materially divergent from their counter-proposal. I am satisfied of their good faith in proposing plebiscite and visit to Asunción by committee of mediatory delegates.

Braden favored this procedure, on the basis of a boundary line that, as it turned out, was almost identical to the final solution, and that the Bolivian delegation thought could be approved by La Paz. However, opposition to visits to Asunción and a plebiscite was expressed by the Argentine and Peruvian delegates, and Braden admitted that the problem was difficult if the Paraguayan delegates and government were "to avoid committing themselves in advance." [36]

Finally, out of these frenzied negotiations, Braden and Cardozo, with the knowledge of Zubizarreta, developed a plan that solved the problem of procedure and within ten days resulted in the signature of the treaty. They were greatly assisted by word from La Paz that Bolivia would accept a line that did not include any territory on the Paraguay River "for the sake of peace," but it would insist on the retention of the rest of the boundary proposed by the Conference on May 27 (see pp. 144–45).

The plan, as reported to the Department of State, was that President Roosevelt would instruct Braden to make a proposal in a plenary session of the Conference. The proposal would suggest that there was only a narrow zone between the Conference offer of May 27 and the Paraguayan counterproposal of June 24 and that the frontier should be fixed within this zone by "an arbitration *ex aequo et bono*." [37] The arbitrator or arbitrators would be a president or presidents of the mediatory countries; Bolivia and Paraguay would immediately sign an agreement for this arbitration, which would be ratified in Bolivia by the constitutional convention and in

Paraguay "by a plebiscite possibly including women to be held within 20 days, the arbitral award to be given 10 days thereafter." Braden added in the final paragraph of this important telegram:

During the 30 days after signing the *compromis* the Conference and parties would be ostensibly informing the arbitrator. It will be understood hitherto [*sic*] between the Conference and the Bolivian and Paraguayan delegations that the award will be the line described in the fourth paragraph my telegram No. 164, June 24, 9 p.m., on which, as I reported yesterday, there is already virtual agreement.

The line to which Braden referred was: "D'Orbigny; 27 November; a point approximately 20 [*sic*; i.e., 19] degrees 45 south 61 degrees 10 west; a point midway between Ravelo and intermediary line; to approximately 19 degrees 15 south 59 degrees 9 west passing close to Galpón and Patria; to mouth of Otuquis." [38]

In reply, the Department of State said it was "delighted" at the encouraging prospect for a settlement, but it believed that "the proposal should come from the Conference rather than from President Roosevelt." However, Braden might inform "the other mediatory delegates that your Government has instructed you to strongly support the presentation and adoption of such a Conference plan." The Department thought that all six mediatory presidents should serve as arbitrators, but otherwise had no changes in the Braden-Cardozo suggestion.

The remarkable proposition that the final line to be determined "ostensibly" by "an arbitration *ex aequo et bono*" would actually be known and accepted in advance by Bolivia and Paraguay and promised by the Conference was not questioned in any way by the Department of State. Hull's cable simply stated that "the Department assumes that there will be a clear understanding concerning the award as set forth in the final paragraph of your telegram." [39]

This gem of diplomatic finesse, perhaps outsparkling any other in the history of arbitration, appears to have been called the "Roosevelt formula," at the Conference, and this term was used in a speech by Braden on January 5, 1939, at The Johns Hopkins University. Braden later stated that

Dr. Cardozo and I drafted and baptized this formula; it was a concrete written formula—not merely our conversations; the expression "Roosevelt

Formula" was generally used by Paraguayan authorities, including the Minister for Foreign Affairs *ad interim;* the Bolivians also employed it and all the other mediatory delegates, excepting only Barreda recognized that it emanated from the American Delegation and was the basis of the July 21 Peace Treaty. . . . This formula originated with the delegation of the United States, who also obtained its acceptance by the parties and by President Ortiz; it was the "break" or turning point in the Conference which resulted from our plans and strategy; it is historically important and we may well be proud of it.[40]

Braden's account of the origin of the "formula" is contested by Cardozo, who writes that the formula originated with him in a memorandum, a copy of which exists in his own archives. This formula, he adds, "was accepted by Braden who presented it as his own in the Peace Conference." [41]

The formula had many facets. Under the protocol arbitration was an alternative to direct negotiations. This proposal combined two two-in-one solutions. The plan overcame the irresolution of the Paraguayan delegation and government, since neither would now have to take public responsibility for precise, debatable places on either side of the boundary; the mediatory presidents would determine the exact line somewhere between the Conference proposal and the Paraguayan counterproposal, which was regarded in Asunción as the worst frontier the government could suggest and still avoid a revolution. In addition, the Paraguayan government and delegation were protected by the plebiscite, since the Paraguayan people, including the women who did not vote in regular elections, would have accepted the possibility that the full Paraguayan claims might not be secured. Finally, since the Paraguayan government, but not the Paraguayan people, would know beforehand exactly what the arbitral award would be, it was assured of gaining what it regarded as essential for its security and for its sentiments of patriotism. The Bolivians, having decided that access to the Paraguay River was not a vital matter, were assured by the advance understanding about the arbitral award that the boundary in the southwest would be satisfactorily far from the Villa Montes–Boyuibe road, and the Busch government felt sufficiently secure so that a direct appeal to its people was not necessary. President Busch's views at this time were reported by Chargé Prendergast:

A Bolivian owned port on the Paraguay River was, after all, merely a question of national pride and would have little utilitarian value. As he expressed it, six months of the year the port would be under water, and the other six months the river would be too low for practical navigation. Furthermore, in his [Busch's] opinion, a free port would avoid the necessity of large expenditures on Bolivia's part for its maintenance and upkeep.

The President . . . wanted at all costs to avoid a renewal of the Chaco conflict. There was, he said, no heart in the Bolivian people for a further war, and he, who had taken part in the last one, did not wish to have to fight in another.[42]

Since the mediatory governments were weary of the whole dispute, and none of them was willing to use effective pressure to induce Paraguay to make further concessions, this plan offered a settlement reasonably close to the line proposed by the Conference on May 27, and that was sufficient.

The way to peace had been traced from afar, but the path had still to be traveled, and the way was found devious. The incorrigible Saavedra Lamas once more breathed chilling words against the flickering warmth of agreement; he told Zubizarreta that Bolivia would accept the boundary demanded by Paraguay. Zubizarreta then tried to obtain changes in the Braden-Cardozo formula, which he had accepted a day earlier and which had been approved by President Ortiz. This effort was beaten down by the mediators, whose patience was further tried by the discovery that Cardozo "had made flatly contradictory statements" to both Cantilo and Braden.

Difficulties were also created by the Bolivians.

Before the session this morning Bolivian Minister for Foreign Affairs confirmed to the Peruvian delegate and me that he would accept the arbitration under discussion including as the award the line [of the Braden-Cardozo formula]. This afternoon Bolivian Minister for Foreign Affairs [Diez de Medina] and delegate [Finot] in Finotesque manner denied to us both separately that he had ever mentioned or heard of it. The Bolivians realize Paraguay is yielding a little and want to take advantage of this to get a more favorable line.[43]

A later incident of this kind caused Braden to remark that "my colleague [Rodrigues Alves] and I are satisfied recent difficulties have been provoked by personal ambition of Finot who, while at outs with Bolivian Minister for Foreign Affairs, nevertheless cows him." [44]

Braden's hopes were dashed also by the action taken by Cantilo, who, without consulting other mediators, told Zubizarreta that the Braden-Cardozo plan "was no longer under consideration" and demanded that Paraguay present a new proposal the next day. Braden commented that "we know Paraguay can make no proposal which would be acceptable and must persuade Argentine Minister for Foreign Affairs to desist from his idea." [45] This specific notion was abandoned, but on July 4, according to Braden, the Conference agreed "to allow Argentine Minister for Foreign Affairs 48 hours in which to try personally to bring about full agreement between the ex-belligerent delegations. I do not like this procedure but can do nothing about it." [46] Braden does not tell anything about the activities of Cantilo in the next two days, but, when they were over, simultaneous agreement by the Bolivians and Paraguayans was reached. The jockeying of the previous week, which had seen the two delegations agree to the same plan, but on different days, was ended,[47] but what Cantilo may have said to Zubizarreta and to Estigarribia, who had just arrived from Washington, is not known.

Finally, on the evening of July 5 the two delegations accepted the Conference formula in the presence of the mediatory delegates, and arrangements were made to hasten the signing of the treaty so that it could occur on the Argentine national holiday, July 9. Approval by the two governments was given without further difficulties, and a draft treaty was initialed at three o'clock in the morning of July 9; the final treaty was signed on July 21. The treaty was, of course, an agreement between Bolivia and Paraguay, but it was also signed by Braden and nine other representatives of the six mediatory countries under whose "auspices and moral guaranty" the treaty was concluded, in the words of the preamble.

The treaty was a treaty of peace and friendship and also an arbitral *compromis*.[48] Paraguay granted to Bolivia "the amplest free transit through its territory, and especially through the zone of Puerto Casado," of Bolivian imports and exports, and direct negotiations were to be undertaken for economic and commercial conventions. The two countries renounced "all actions and claims deriving from responsibilities for the war" and "solemnly bind themselves not to make war on each other or to use force" to settle future differences. It was provided that ratification should be by the Bolivian constitutional convention and "by a national plebiscite in Paraguay," both within twenty days after July 21.

On the great question of the boundary, the treaty stated that the line should be determined by the six mediatory presidents "in their capacity as arbitrators in equity, who, acting *ex aequo et bono*" would fix the line in the north between the Conference line of May 27 and the Paraguayan counterproposal, "excluding the littoral on the Paraguay River south of the mouth of the River Otuquis or Negro." The western line would begin not farther east than Pozo Hondo, near Fort Guachalla, nor farther west than Fort D'Orbigny. The award would be given within two months after ratification of the treaty. Finally, the arbitrators, which meant in fact their deputies, "shall render the decision after having heard the parties and according to their true knowledge and understanding, taking into consideration the experience acquired by the Peace Conference and the suggestions of the military advisers to that organization." There was no provision for a money payment to Paraguay by Bolivia, presumably since that had been contemplated only if it induced Paraguay to permit Bolivia to obtain a sovereign port on the Paraguay River.

The principal "experience acquired by the Peace Conference" was that it had been impossible to arrange for the arbitration at all until agreement had been secretly reached, before the treaty was signed, on six crucial places on the boundary line that the arbitrators would be bound to make in their award. Braden described the terms of this agreement explicitly as follows:

Both parties have agreed secretly with mediators individually that the line of award in the arbitration under consideration shall be Esmeralda, 27 of November, Captain Ustares, Palmar de las Islas, Chovoreca, mouth of Otuquis. Forts Galpón and Patria would probably be destroyed or quietly moved westward a short distance to allow Bolivian access to the triangle.[49]

Braden added the depressing observation that the Bolivians insisted that the western line from Esmeralda to Captain Ustares "must be written into the arbitral *compromis*," because "they did not trust the arbitrators to award it." In fact, however, this line had not been included in the part of the treaty containing the *compromis* because it was unacceptable to the Paraguayans. Nevertheless, adequate satisfaction was given the Bolivians by the secret arrangements with the mediators that this line would be part of the arbitral award. This procedure resulted in an arbitration that was not an arbitration at all, *ex aequo et bono* or otherwise. It was simply a ratification of secret negotiations; its justification was that no settlement could have been reached without it.

To the Bolivians the secretly arranged line was the uttermost limit of retreat in defense of their national interests; to the Paraguayans, as was admitted by Braden and others, public knowledge of the acceptance of this line would have meant the fall of the government. The Bolivians could not place their trust in arbitration as a procedure, and the Paraguayans had to insist on arbitration as a procedure. It was necessary, therefore, to make arbitration appear to be the mode of settlement. It was equally necessary that arbitration play absolutely no role, in fact, in the settlement. The Conference performed feats of prestidigitation, in the open and behind the scenes, to meet the apparently incompatible demands upon it.

Paraguay, the gainer in the war, was able to have its "vital" interest at Bahía Negra protected openly in the public treaty. At the western end of the line where Paraguayan troops would have to be withdrawn, the arbitrators provided an essential service in taking public responsibility for a decision the Paraguayan government could accept only in secret. Bolivia, the loser, accepted publicly the possibility of an arbitral decision that would have inadmissibly endangered the Villa Montes–Boyuibe road. Privately, however, Bolivia received from the Conference delegates, who were in fact the arbitrators, satisfactory assurances that no such arbitral award would be handed down. The exact nature of these assurances is not known. The Bolivians did not get a written pledge in the *compromis* that the limit of their admissible concessions in the area of the Villa Montes—Boyuibe road would not be surpassed. In view of their cynicism about the good faith of any arbitrators, however, it may be confidently asserted that they received written assurances from the mediators on this essential point.

To the mediators, this arrangement appeared to be the only way to complete their task. Braden had told the Department that he did not like the idea of a secret agreement proposed early in June by the Brazilian delegate, and the Department agreed that "no attempt should be made to keep secret the terms of any agreement accepted by the two parties." [50] In July, however, Bolivian mistrust of any and all arbitrators made necessary a resort to secrecy, which was maintained as long as politically necessary.

The Department of States does not appear to have issued any instructions to Braden nor to have commented upon the secret agreements between the parties, on the one hand, and the individual mediators, on the other. It seems probable that in Washington it was assumed that no other solution was politically feasible and that, given the time and effort already expended on the Chaco and the opportunity for making a settlement in this way, it would be quixotic to insist at this moment that the arbitrators should actually have some significant element of free judgment that they might exercise. In any case, the presidents were expected to delegate their authority to their mediatory representatives in Buenos Aires, and those representatives had already determined that the line secretly agreed upon was the only line acceptable to both governments. In addition, the zone within which the arbitrators were formally given an area of discretion under the treaty was narrowly circumscribed in the treaty itself.

Rarely indeed have the positive advantages of the existence of an international body been so clearly demonstrated. The Conference, guided by principles of amity to which neither contending government could subscribe, was able to provide a practical solution that was beyond the capabilities of Bolivia and Paraguay alone. The Conference was able to relieve the Paraguayan government of political responsibility by apparently shifting the burden of decision to the eminent agency of the distinguished arbitrators, while at the same time guaranteeing in advance to Paraguay and to Bolivia that their irreducible boundary demands would be satisfied. Since the Paraguayan counterproposal was written into the treaty as one limit of the arbitral award, deviation from that limit could both be blamed on the arbitrators and defended in Paraguay as a virtuous sacrifice made in the cause of peace. With these solid advantages to both sides, it is understandable that no difficulties were raised about this tortuous and perhaps unique application of what was made to look like the technique of arbitral settlement.

Between the initialing of the treaty and its signature a number of minor changes were made in the text. Estigarribia and Cardozo flew to Asunción and successfully obtained governmental approval for the treaty. Zubizarreta resigned on July 14 as chief delegate, and Estigarribia replaced him. Owing largely to the latter's influence, the army did not oppose the treaty, nor did the Liberal Party, of which Zubizarreta was then president.[51]

With pardonable if long-deferred satisfaction, Braden cabled to the Department of State that "we may justifiably point to the practicability of the American peace machinery, both in its operation and its results." He was warmly congratulated by Secretary Hull, and others, and authorized to say in his speech to the Argentine Congress that the settlement was "a vindication of the possibility of the pacific settlement of international differences and of the effectiveness of the inter-American system of consultation and cooperation." [52]

The signing of the treaty was received with pleasure throughout the continent, except in Bolivia, where there was expressed neither satisfaction nor opposition. *El Diario* (La Paz), July 22, stated:

This peace, resulting from an unfortunate war, has been received in Bolivia with a serene feeling of dignity which is far from conducive to manifestations of satisfaction and gaiety. Of the celebrated event in Buenos Aires the Bolivian people has been an indifferent spectator, or, more properly, the usual and traditional "Juan Pueblo," largely accustomed to sacrifices and mutilations.[53]

In Brazil July 21 was declared a national holiday. In Paraguay, where until the afternoon of July 13, there was still serious question about the acceptance of the treaty, the signature was greeted with "relief and happiness." There were spontaneous and unofficial demonstrations of pleasure, and the treaty was given the approval of the Archbishop of Asunción.[54]

Although Braden expressed some concern about the securing of ratification in Paraguay, the process in both countries was completed successfully. In Bolivia the constitutional convention ratified the treaty on August 10 by a vote of 102 to 9, and in Paraguay, on the same date, the plebiscite ratified the treaty by 135,385 votes to 13,204.[55]

The Conference sent an Advisory Military Commission to survey certain of the boundary areas, and the so-called arbitral college, acting in accordance with the terms of the secret arrangements, gave its foreordained award on October 10, 1938, with minor changes as recommended by the report of the Commission, exactly two months after the ratification of the treaty. The proceedings of the arbitral college, appropriately enough, were secret; its members were the six representatives of the states that were members of the Conference. The award was accepted by the two governments within three days, and the arbitral college was dissolved. On January 23, 1939, the Conference itself declared its functions ended and thanked President Ortiz for his country's hospitality, the presidents of the mediatory countries for "their valued collaboration," and the governments of Bolivia and Paraguay "for the lofty spirit shown during the negotiations." The work of setting up the boundary markers was carried out later by a mixed commission, composed of two members each from Bolivia and Paraguay, with an Argentine colonel as chairman.

On the occasion of the arbitral award, *La Prensa*, of Buenos Aires, printed an editorial entitled: "A Fair American Example," the theme of which was:

We can celebrate this occasion with double satisfaction, since, if it is the result of the primacy of reason over force, it represents also an exclusively American achievement. It demonstrates our capability for understanding that allows us to dispense with foreign interventions in a case where an amicable settlement is to be reached after differences have arisen.

This indirect reference to satisfaction that European participation in the solution of the Chaco dispute had been avoided was also the theme of an earlier (July 11) editorial in the Santiago daily *El Imparcial*, which noted that the young nations of America

have invariably looked toward Europe as if only from the Old World could emerge formulas that could solve our differences, and it was thus that we adhered for a long time to anachronistic mechanisms like the

League of Nations, which has revealed its absolute incapacity either to prevent armed conflicts or to find for them equitable and just solutions.

The paper added that it might be permitted to record something that gave it cause for pride:

We have constantly pleaded in these columns that for American problems should be found American solutions, because we, the members of this great family, are the most capable to judge our issues and to take part in their solution with the most elevated spirit of true brotherhood. . . . We can and we must settle our disputes within this great home that is our America.

In a similar vein, although without such clear references to outsiders, Sumner Welles issued a statement to the press on October 10:

The success of the effort of two American republics, with the help of six other friendly American nations, to solve peacefully a dispute which had at one time resulted in actual war and which had cost the lives of many thousands of people is heartening and encouraging. It justifies the faith of the American peoples in the efficacy of pacific negotiations. It shows the value of disinterested and impartial mediation. It translates into fact the unanimous will for peace of the American democracies.

After its ratification in the ex-belligerent countries, the treaty was accepted, and there seems to have been little disposition to call it into question again. The treaty was approved unanimously by the Paraguayan Senate, and a speech by the president of that body expressed views that were perhaps representative of civilian politicians in Paraguay in February, 1939. Dr. Justo Pastor Prieto said that the treaty did not satisfy "our traditional aspiration, neither as to territory nor as to economic advantages." He placed the blame for this situation on the revolt and subsequent policies of Colonel Franco and said that, in 1938, Paraguay "was a country convulsed by internal struggles, a country which did not demonstrate in peace the greatness which it had shown during the war." He complained that the conference had not provided an arbitration "by right" but only one of equity, "which is always dangerous for the side which has the soundest legal position and therefore does not have the duty to be generous." In addition, he apparently voiced the feeling of many Paraguayans in saying that the conference had done little or nothing to carry out the parts of the June 21, 1935, protocol referring to the economic development of the ex-belligerents. Nevertheless, Dr. Prieto recommended that the treaty be approved, feeling that no other solution was possible in the situation.[56]

In the course of the final negotiations, there seems to have been no reference to the declaration of August 3, 1932, concerning the nonrecognition of territorial conquest, based on the Pact of Paris. The treaty itself makes no mention of this declaration, despite the importance that had been attached to it in several statements by representatives of the government of the United States. How is its use to be regarded in the case of the Chaco?

The declaration of August 3, 1932, stated: "The American nations further declare that they will not recognize any territorial arrangement of this controversy which has not been obtained by peaceful means nor the validity of territorial acquisitions which may be obtained through occupation or conquest by force of arms."

The purpose of the declaration had been to prevent the Chaco War. In this sense it was a failure. It was referred to in article IV of the protocol of June 12, 1935, as follows: "The declaration of the third of August 1932, regarding territorial acquisitions, is recognized by the belligerents." The declaration seems to have had no influence upon the work of the conference nor upon the final treaty. No reference to it was made in the Conference's proposed treaty of peace of October 15, 1935, which "offers to both an honorable means of settling by compromise the conflict which for long years has separated the two countries."

The final boundary line was realistically and correctly described by Dr. Prieto when he said that "our victorious army" achieved an advance "which more or less determined what was later awarded to us by the Treaty." Bolivia was unable to drive the Paraguayan army farther eastward, and none of the mediators would use force to bring about a Paraguayan withdrawal. The final boundary was, therefore, essentially achieved by Bolivian acceptance of the military situation. With Bolivia's giving up any claim to a port on the Paraguay River, the Paraguayans gave up any attempt to reach the oil district beyond Villa Montes and agreed to relinquish enough territory in that area to assure Bolivian control of the Villa Montes–Boyuibe international route.

The official report of the United States delegation to the Chaco conference included, without comment, the above quoted portion of the text of the August 3, 1932, declaration. Was the treaty line a recognition of a territorial acquisition by Paraguayan occupation or conquest? It was much farther west than any of the lines in the Chaco established by the unratified treaties of 1879, 1887, or 1894, and it gave to Paraguay some 50,000 square kilometers more than it would have had if the Pinilla-Soler line of 1907, establishing limits of military advance, had been accepted as the territorial frontier. It did not, however, at any point touch the extreme claims described by Paraguay's own definition of the Chaco Boreal.

In 1932, it will be recalled, the declaration was looked upon by its originator, Francis White, as of fundamental importance. He had taken the position, later approved by the Commission of Neutrals, that an armistice could only be made on the basis of a return of the troops of Bolivia and Paraguay to the lines occupied on June 1, 1932, and he and his colleagues therefore rejected an offer by Bolivia, which was supported by Argentina, to accept an armistice on the lines occupied on August 3, 1932. This action was thought "intransigent" by some of the neighboring countries, but White stuck by it, saying that "we should do nothing which would impair or invalidate the doctrine of August 3." [57] A year later, President Salamanca in a public address, said that, if the Neutrals had consulted Paraguay when Bolivia offered to accept an armistice on the basis of positions occupied in August, 1932, the war would have ended in its early stages. [58]

The declaration, in this way, became associated with the line of June 1, 1932, for purposes of obtaining an armistice, although it was never stated officially that gains beyond that line would be the same as "occupation" or "conquest" for either side. Neither in 1935 nor in 1938, with Paraguayan troops 160 miles west of the June 1, 1932, line, does it seem to have occurred to the mediators in Buenos Aires that the moral value attributed to the declaration by White and Carr should outweigh the practical necessities involved in securing Paraguayan acceptance of either an armistice or of the final boundary.

It is at least doubtful that the boundary of October 10, 1938, was a "territorial acquisition" for Paraguay, since no previous legal line had been established. At one point, on the Pilcomayo, the final line was about forty miles east of the conference compromise line of October 15, 1935, but this point seems to have been determined by Bolivian insistence, and not by the concern of the mediators to have their original line recognized to some degree nor by any feeling that this point was necessary to establish as a way of making a bow toward the declaration of August 3 as the embodiment of the Stimson doctrine. In these circumstances, it is possible that the omission from the United States delegation's report of comment on the declaration, with the exception of Laurence Duggan's remarks quoted below, may be attributed either to forgetfulness of the importance once attached to it or to a silent admission of the ineffectiveness of the Stimson doctrine in this case.

No more than a few references to the declaration were made in the diplomatic correspondence after 1932. At the end of 1934, the minister in Uruguay reported that "there exists in Uruguay a feeling in favor of Paraguay which perhaps may be best defined as a romantic interest. . . . Uruguayan sentiment is reflected at present in a belief that Paraguay should retain the territory conquered by its army." Although Uruguay adhered to the declaration, "when reference is now made to this declaration, as applied to the hostilities in the Chaco, the universal feeling among Uruguayans is that it would be an injustice to deprive the Paraguayans of the fruits of their military successes." [59]

President Ayala, toward the end of the conflict, told Minister Nicholson: "Our object in the war is to recover what belongs to us and to obtain the satisfaction that corresponds to the victim of a crime. The declaration of the 3rd of August will always be on our altar. Paraguay does not propose conquest. Its ambitions are just and reasonable." [60] A little later, in a circular published by the Bolivian Foreign Minister, Dr. Alvéstegui, it was stated: "The Government of Bolivia has the conviction that the peace with Paraguay must be juridical in accordance with the American declaration of August 3, 1932, and it is sure that the best procedure to reach this result is that established in the recommendations of the League of Nations." [61] This statement, coming within two months of the end of the war, may be regarded as an attempt to use the declaration as a means of limiting the Paraguayan victory rather than as evidence of previous Bolivian attachment to its principles. It does not appear that the Bolivians placed any reliance on the declaration in later negotiations nor that they complained that the mediators were acting inconsistently with the declaration in approving the treaty of peace.

In the light of the role of the August 3 declaration in the Chaco dispute, it is curious not only that Laurence Duggan, Chief of the Division of the American Republics of the Department of State, should have made the following statements in an address on August 27, 1938, but also that it should have been printed in the report of the United States delegation to the Chaco conference:

It is a particular pleasure today, upon the tenth anniversary of the signature at Paris of the treaty providing for the renunciation of war as an instrument of national policy, to pay tribute to two nations of this hemisphere which recently have given a striking proof of good faith in adhering to the principle of pacific settlement of international disputes. We rejoice today that the Governments and peoples of Bolivia and Paraguay translated their peace-loving words and promises into acts by signing and ratifying the treaty of peace, friendship and boundaries of July 21, 1938. . . . The treaty . . . is a fair test of the effectiveness of the pacific settlement of international disputes because major and vital interests were involved. The peace effected rests upon agreement, upon mutual concessions, upon the expressed will of the people and of their representatives. It is not a peace imposed by force of arms upon a weaker adversary but was made possible by constructive leadership, overwhelmingly supported by a public opinion throughout the Americas, desirous of peace. . . .

It would be difficult to cite any one event of greater significance in inter-American relations today than the pacific settlement of the Chaco dispute. One of the potentially most serious problems of the Americas has ceased to threaten the gathering momentum of the movement for real cooperation and friendly relations among the American Republics. Proof has been given of the effectiveness of our peace machinery and of our system of consultation and cooperation in solving our problems.[62]

It is quite possible that a renewal of the war may have been prevented by the efforts of the mediators, and for this achievement they are entitled to due credit. However, there had been a fierce and bloody war, carried on to the very limits of the capacity of the combatants. After those limits had been reached, war as an instrument of national policy had then been "renounced." This was hardly the kind of renunciation intended by the authors of the Kellogg-Briand Pact. If Duggan intended his fulsome praise for the effectiveness of American peace machinery to apply to the avoidance of a renewal of the conflict, his comments possessed a color of justification. His remarks, however, seem strangely unreal when it is recalled that the declaration of August 3, 1932, did not delay or halt the fighting, had no effect on the course of the war, and was utterly ignored by the mediators in arranging the terms of settlement. At best, it was a renunciation of the renewal of war in 1938 and not a renunciation in 1932—a secondary but not a primary renunciation —for which the erstwhile combatants might be praised.

Other spokesmen for the United States Government also expressed pleasure over the outcome in the Chaco. President Roosevelt cabled President Ortiz that the treaty "offers concrete evidence of the existence of a very real and lasting inter-American solidarity and of the ever-increasing insistence on the part of public opinion in all of our nations that war be abolished from this hemisphere." Secretary Hull said:

The peaceful determination of the complicated Chaco differences is an outstanding triumph for the spirit of peace and the principles of order based on law over the doctrine of force and aggression. The happy outcome of the negotiations . . . offers a powerful demonstration of the practicability and effectiveness of methods of cooperation in the settlement of international disputes. The fidelity of the Governments of Bolivia and Paraguay to those basic principles which alone can assure conditions of peace and orderly progress offers an inspiring example to the friends of order based on law in every part of the world.

Summer Welles stated in a radio broadcast that "there has been no inter-American dispute which has been more bitter than this one, and yet it has been solved because of the determination of the parties to the controversy to find an equitable and peaceful settlement, and because of the efficacy of the inter-American system of consultation and cooperation." [63]

The authors of these statements, except Laurence Duggan, made no reference to the fact that a war had actually been fought, and they might be regarded as having given grounds for charges that they were hypocritical. To critics bringing such charges, however, the answer may be made that these statesmen were fulfilling some of the essential and most praiseworthy of diplomatic functions.

Diplomacy in the broad sense has a civilizing mission as well as one of serving the interests of individual states. The ceremonial aspect of this mission is an important one that should not be under-estimated, for it serves in a conspicuous way to reaffirm the highest ideals of the diplomat's profession. True, pledges may be broken and ideals may not be attained; it is true also that victory in war receives a respect that through time may acquire laurels no less green than those freely granted to peaceful achievements. In conflicts where the physical or legal existence of a nation is at stake it may be impossible for diplomats to mediate if their intention is to do no more than that, and this was the situation in the early stages of the Chaco war. If the issues are less vital, mediation may be difficult and even hazardous, for failure may mean a loss of prestige; success, however, is deserving of honor. In terms appropriate to their era, therefore, Roosevelt and Hull, Welles and Duggan were carrying out a statesmanlike function by praising those who had striven for peace in the Chaco, by commending them on a hard-won victory, and by exhorting others to follow an inspiring example. To criticize them for ignoring some aspects of the history of the Chaco conflict would be to misinterpret their roles at the time; they were speakers at a graduation ceremony and not investigators of educational techniques.

The Chaco experience was an educational one for American diplomats. Failure to prevent war in the Chaco was one of the principal reasons for the convocation of the Buenos Aires peace conference of 1936. The acceptance of the principle of consultation at that conference was in part a result of the realization of lessons learned from the Chaco negotiations. Although the principle of consultation was not applied to the conflict between Ecuador and Peru in 1941, it was energetically developed afterward at the initiative of the United States with regard to inter-American solidarity toward

World War II, and its application played an important part in the creation of attitudes favorable to the postwar establishment of the Organization of American States.

Between Bolivia and Paraguay peace has reigned. There are no triumphal arches in Asunción, and there are no battlegrounds preserved as monuments in the Chaco; it would be difficult now to find any vestiges of Fort Senator Long. In the plaza on which the Paraguayan presidential palace faces there is on a grassy knoll a light tank that once belonged to a unit of the army of Bolivia. On the tank is a plaque bearing this generous inscription: "Homage to the valor and heroism of two peoples of the same family, who fought each other through human mistakes and injustices." [64]

PART TWO

The Leticia Dispute

CHAPTER VI

Background and Outbreak

THE LETICIA DISPUTE arose over a Peruvian attempt to repudiate a valid treaty and to regain by violence territory ceded to Colombia. The government of the United States, to its later embarrassment, exerted influence from 1923 to 1928 to secure the treaty's ratification. Therefore, when the dispute broke out, the Department of State felt a strong sense of responsibility for trying to prevent an armed conflict between Colombia and Peru, and from 1932 to 1935 it played the role of an anxious and admonitory, if unsuccessful, peacemaker.

After many years of controversy over the boundary, Alberto Salomón Osorio and Fabio Lozano Torrijos signed for the governments of Peru and Colombia, respectively, the Salomón-Lozano treaty on March 24, 1922.[1] One feature of the treaty was Peruvian agreement to Colombian sovereignty over some 4,000 square miles in the Leticia quadrilateral, which, at its southernmost side, gave to Colombia about sixty-five miles of river frontage on the northern bank of the Amazon. Leticia, at the southeastern corner of the quadrilateral, was a small village on a low plateau in the midst of a vast marshy jungle. It had no communication by road with any other town in Colombia; it was occasionally visited from southwestern Colombia by river launches motoring eastward on the Putumayo to the Amazon, about 150 miles below Leticia, and thence westward. It might be considered, like Bahía Negra to Bolivia, a psychological port, since, although it opened no route for the export or import of goods to Colombia, it provided to that state a cartographical point on the continent's greatest river and so gave to Colombia, however tenuously, the coveted status of an Amazonian power. Bahía Negra had neither a hinterland nor a navigable channel in the Paraguay River, but Leticia was reached by ocean-going vessels, which could continue some two hundred miles farther upriver to Iquitos, Peru's chief city in the province of Loreto.

Another feature of the treaty was the fixing of the boundary between Colombia and Peru at the Putumayo River westward from the northwestern corner of the Leticia trapezium to Güepi. This meant that Colombia ceded to Peru territory north of the watershed between the Napo and Putumayo rivers (see Map II), although that watershed had been established as the Colombia-Ecuador boundary in the Muñoz Vernaza–Suárez treaty of 1916 between those two countries. Thus the boundary agreed upon in 1916 between Colombia and Ecuador became in 1922 the southern limit of territory recognized as Peruvian by Colombia in the secretly negotiated Salomón-Lozano treaty. Furthermore, cession to Peru of this strip of territory more than three hundred miles long and about forty miles wide removed Colombia from direct contact with any possible Ecuadoran Oriente and so not only withdrew any support the 1916 treaty gave to Ecuadoran territorial claims but made illusory any Ecuadoran hopes for Colombian military or other backing in its dispute with Peru. This outstanding advantage gained by Peru from the Salomón-Lozano treaty has been largely neglected by the treaty's critics in Peru, who have concentrated attention almost exclusively on the loss of Leticia to Colombia. To the Colombian government the cession of the strip south of the Putumayo was the price for Leticia, and a reasonable one, in its view, for the coveted Amazonian port.

The Ecuadoran government regarded the Salomón-Lozano treaty as a violation by Colombia of the terms of the treaty of 1916, and Quito broke off diplomatic relations with Bogotá when the former treaty's terms became known in 1925. The Ecuadorans were brusquely confronted by a three hundred mile boundary with their enemy, Peru, instead of the same line with Colombia, a country they had formerly regarded as a friend.

This series of events may well be regarded as an extraordinary diplomatic achievement by the Colombian government, if, indeed, it was the result of long-range calculation. A confident judgment on this point must await further research and the availability of documents in still jealously guarded archives. To the Peruvian government, whatever the irritations that might derive from Colombia's possession of Leticia, it had secured a geopolitical position from which it could deal with Ecuador on its own terms and at leisure. The position of the Ecuadorans was, of course, seriously weakened by these maneuvers. Ecuadorans were reported as saying: "In time of crisis the weakest is sacrificed, since this is the easiest way out." [2]

In 1923, at the request of President Pedro Nel Ospina of Colombia for the good offices of President Calvin Coolidge, Ambassador Miles Poindexter in Lima was instructed to say to President Augusto B. Leguía of Peru that the United States government "would be highly gratified if he could arrange for submission of the treaty to the Peruvian Congress." [3] The keynote of the Department of State's interest in the affair over the next decade was sounded at this time: "The Department wishes its action kept within the limits of that of a friendly power earnestly interested in the welfare of both Peru and Colombia, an interest to be expressed whenever favorable opportunities may arise." [4] However, the Department did "not desire to appear as the agency suggesting or initiating measures which, if brought to the attention of the other party, might incline it to view further informal action with disfavor." [5] This was a desire that the Department found it impossible to fulfill.

When, toward the end of 1924, Leguía submitted the treaty to the Peruvian Congress, the government of Brazil objected to the cession of the Leticia quadrilateral as not having been contemplated by it in the treaty of October 23, 1851, which had fixed the boundary between Peru and Brazil in this area.

Shortly afterward, Secretary of State Charles Evans Hughes showed signs of wishing to crown his accomplishments in office by settling this tripartite dispute. He telegraphed to Ambassador Edwin Vernon Morgan in Brazil:

You will please say to the Minister for Foreign Affairs, and if necessary to the President, that as I am leaving office on March 4, [1925] it would be very gratifying to me should it be possible to settle the boundary question with Colombia before that time. While this Government is acting as a means of communication between interested parties, it is a medium of communication which is also profoundly interested in a just and prompt settlement. Please endeavor to have the matter given prompt consideration.[6]

This peremptory desire on the part of Secretary Hughes to be a peacemaker resulted in speedy and slap-dash diplomacy ending in the signing on March 4, 1925, Hughes's last day in office, of an agreement between Brazil, Colombia, and Peru that resolved all difficulties and cleared the road for Peruvian ratification of the treaty in 1928.[7] Throughout the previous month and a half the cables from the Department to the three South American capitals revealed Hughes's desire for negotiatory haste with their exhortations to the United States diplomats to obtain "prompt" replies and to "expedite" conversations.

These pricks of pressure in the cause of peace were, of course, both felt and remembered by Latin Americans, and seven years later a bitterly anti-Leguía regime in Peru charged that the then hated Salomón-Lozano treaty had been imposed on Peru by a Secretary of State seeking one more laurel. In 1932, before any Peruvian comments had been heard by the embassy in Lima, Ambassador Fred Morris Dearing asked the Department for

the reasons for our Government's insistence upon the signing of the *procès verbal* in Secretary Hughes' office in 1924 [*sic*] . . . the Embassy's records . . . seem to show such evident urging on the part of our Government that the treaty should be made, that it arouses a number of questions as to the degree to which we are responsible for it. The old records seem to indicate that neither Leguía nor Salomón desired the treaty and were brought, by our representations, to sign it against their will.[8]

The Department replied, a bit stiffly, that the United States had acted

in harmony with the traditional policy of this Government of assisting wherever it appropriately can in the peaceful solution of international difficulties and conflicts. It is probable that what you term this Government's insistence on the settlement of this question was due to the natural desire of the outgoing Secretary of State [Hughes] to conclude a matter of such importance and in which he had taken a great interest, prior to the relinquishment of his office.[9]

There is no question that Hughes's pressure was directed most strongly at Peru. Pressure in Bogotá was unnecessary since the Colombian government greatly desired the treaty, and the influential Lozano family regarded its signature as a personal triumph. For example, in a telegram sent at eleven o'clock at night on February 28, 1925, Hughes informed Poindexter that the Colombian minister rejected one of the remaining Peruvian modifications in the formula that Hughes had developed. Hughes instructed Poindexter to

call upon President Leguía and point out to him that of the three countries concerned Peru is asked to do the least. . . . The insistence of the Peruvian Government on the modifications will make it necessary to reopen negotiations with Bogotá and Rio thus making it impossible to sign the Procès Verbal by March 3. You will please explain to him again the desire if possible to bring about this amicable settlement before I leave office on March 4, which means the Procès Verbal must be signed not later than Tuesday afternoon, March 3. . . . You will please state to President Leguía that the Department is making this last effort to bring about a friendly agreement between the three countries concerned and that it would very much regret to have to inform Brazil and Colombia that the Department's good offices had been unfruitful because of the apparent disinclination of Peru to accept the friendly suggestions proposed.[10]

Leguía refused at first to change his position, despite Poindexter's best efforts, but finally came around to the acceptance of a new text, which was hastily cleared with the Brazilian and Colombian representatives in Washington, Chargé Samuel de Souza Leão Gracie and Minister Enrique Olaya Herrera. The last cable from Lima, sent at 2:00 A.M. and received in Washington at 7:01 A.M. on March 4, carried news of a rejection of a Colombian textual change. However, Hughes settled this problem with Olaya, and, at five o'clock in the afternoon, the agreement was signed by Hughes, Olaya, Peruvian Minister Hernán Velarde, and Souza Leão. Brazil withdrew its "observations"; Colombia and Peru agreed to ratify the treaty; and Colombia and Brazil agreed to accept the 1851 boundary as the eastern edge of the Leticia quadrilateral, the so-called Tabatinga-

Apoporis line. All three governments stated that they accepted this "friendly suggestion" of the Secretary of State.[11]

Having barely met his schedule, Hughes, with this small triumph, finally left the desk that his successor, Frank B. Kellogg, had been entitled to occupy several hours previously. In retiring, he left on that desk the problem of how strongly to urge Peruvian ratification of the Salomón-Lozano treaty, with which Kellogg was to be concerned occasionally during the subsequent three years. During 1926 Poindexter prodded Leguía "to urge favorable action" on the treaty by the Peruvian Congress. Leguía said he would do everything possible, but he was not sure that he could persuade the congress, in which there was powerful opposition, particularly by deputies from Loreto province. In January, 1927, Kellogg asked Poindexter to renew his efforts, stating that "there is real danger that Colombia may sever diplomatic relations if the treaty is not ratified after repeated promises of President Leguía. Such action would naturally cause serious embarrassment to the Government of the United States which sponsored the protocol." [12]

No action was taken by Leguía until the end of the year, however. Chargé Pierre Boal reported from Lima in November:

The treaty appears to be on the eve of being presented to Congress where there is much opposition to it and much agitation regarding it. With the general public the treaty is without doubt unpopular. I have been reliably informed that the president of the House of Deputies in his attempt to convince vacillating members has told them that the Government of the United States has been bringing pressure to bear upon Peru to ratify the treaty.[13]

In December the Peruvian Congress finally approved the treaty by a vote of 102 to 7, and the exchange of ratifications on January 23, 1928, appeared to have settled the matter.[14] This was the case so far as the existing governments were concerned. However, President Leguía, who had been elected for a fourth term in 1929, was forced to resign by a revolution in 1930. Following a chaotic year in Peruvian politics, Colonel Luis M. Sánchez Cerro, who had led the revolt against Leguía, was elected president. His regime was supported by the army and by several groups of conservatives, notably the Civilista Party. The Civilistas had bitterly opposed Leguía's policies as destructive of the traditional social and economic order in the country. The Salomón-Lozano treaty was one of Leguía's achievements that the Civilistas wished to nullify; in this effort they found allies among the rough and ready frontiersmen of Loreto, who held that the Amazon should be a wholly Peruvian stream from its source to the Brazilian border.[15]

The immediate origins of the Leticia dispute are difficult to interpret with assurance. During the night of August 31, 1932, a group of armed Peruvians forcibly, but without bloodshed, took control of the hamlet of Leticia. Ambassador Dearing reported immediately that "Apristas captured an *intendente*, four employees and only one gendarme." The action took the government in Lima completely by surprise, according to its own account. Communications with Iquitos were poor, and President Sánchez Cerro's statement to Dearing was that it was "a political plot intended to embarrass the Government, distract attention and prepare the way for an Apri-Communist outbreak in Lima." He was said to have "convinced the Colombian Minister he will cooperate with him in every possible way to prevent the incident from becoming serious." [16]

This assertion by Sánchez Cerro was supported by the account given to Dearing by Solon Polo, Under Secretary for Foreign Affairs, who stated that on September 4 the President and Cabinet had met and decided "to maintain the boundary treaty with Colombia . . . to dominate the present situation in Iquitos . . . to put no obstacle whatever in the way of the Colombian Government's expelling the Peruvians who seized Leticia." [17]

As the news came filtering in from various sources, however, it appeared that it was at least probable that Sánchez Cerro had known that plans were being laid for the Leticia expedition.[18]

Although his reactions as expressed to Dearing convinced the Ambassador at first that Sánchez Cerro was both surprised by the news and persuaded that the affair was a plot by "Apri-Communists," it is not improbable that the President's course was a carefully planned one. This is not meant to suggest, however, that at that time he intended to hold Leticia at the risk of war with Colombia, for he does not appear to have made preparations for war. It is possible, however, that, if he knew of the Loretanos plans, he may have calculated that he could turn the situation to his own political advantage in Peru and that there was a real chance that Colombia, confronted with a situation in Leticia requiring a major national effort to reestablish its position, would prefer to renegotiate the Salomón-Lozano treaty. This interpretation would seem to account for a situation in which the Peruvians, initially much stronger than Colombia at Leticia, did not make serious preparations for war before the outbreak and then showed surprise at the determination of Bogotá as manifested by the despatch of an expedition to retake Leticia.[19]

From the view that the captors of Leticia were "Apri-Communists" and that the government must oppose them, the President glided into the position that the Leticia affair had aroused patriotic demands that he was unable to resist if his government were to remain in power. While Solon Polo continued to assure Dearing and Lozano that the Peruvian government would secure the withdrawal of the invaders, Sánchez Cerro refused to disavow the capture publicly or to make a satisfactory written statement to Bogotá.

The Department of State was concerned about Peru's internal stability, and it raised the question with Dearing, at the same time asking him to talk with Foreign Minister Carlos Zavala Loaiza, "in an entirely informal and very friendly manner" and without putting anything in writing, to "urge in behalf of Peru's own best interests, that the boundary treaty be upheld" and that the incident be prevented from becoming an international question.[20] Dearing was properly circumspect in dealing with Zavala, saying to him: "I would be happy to know precisely how Peru felt about the situation and the extent of the internal menace, and the problem confronting the nation, but that I did not wish to appear unduly curious about Peru's internal affairs and merely desired to promote peaceful solutions and good relations." [21]

Dearing's own view of the situation, as given in this despatch, was that the government was still master of the situation:

At first there was complaint that there would be overwhelming reaction throughout the country, but the people have been somewhat apathetic. Next, it was said that the Loretanos would rebel and now it is beginning to appear that neither of these reactions in any exaggerated sense is a certainty, that the character of the reaction will depend a good deal upon what the Government does. . . . At first all was deference, reasonableness and assurances towards Colombia, next no concessions were to be made to Colombia, and at present a latent opposition is fast developing and is being fanned into a flame of opposition and aggressiveness.

A quite different opinion was, however, urged upon Dearing by a former Foreign Minister of Peru, who said that Sánchez Cerro was the only man in the country who could "hold it together and give the nation a strong administration." A new twist to the pervasive Latin American "fall-of-the-government" argument was offered by the statement that, if the Colombian government should fall because of an acceptance of Peruvian demands for revision of the treaty, the result would not be serious, since another political party would come to power. However, the ex-Foreign Minister said: "The dislodgment of the Sánchez Cerro Administration would mean the advent of Communism in its worst and most terrifying form." [22] The implied suggestion that the United States should choose, on the basis of these alleged alternatives, to support Peru does not appear to have been given serious consideration in Washington.

A concrete indication, either of Foreign Minister Zavala's real judgment of the internal situation or of the way he thought best to affect Washington's attitude, was given by him in a talk with Dearing. The Ambassador had suggested that Peru should not use the occupation of Leticia to coerce Colombia into a revision of the treaty but should plan to raise the question of revision after Colombia had reoccupied Leticia, meanwhile getting the Peruvians there to return to Iquitos and promising them that revision would be discussed later with Colombia. Zavala replied that "if he made such suggestions without something concrete from Colombia beforehand he would be hanged." [23]

In Colombia, President Olaya was also concerned about the fate of his government, although less gruesomely about his own. He remarked to Ambassador Jefferson Caffery, after rejecting a Peruvian proposal for the appointment of a conciliation commission:

"No Government in Colombia could last an hour that would agree to participating in such a commission at this time. . . . We cannot allow any commission to discuss our right to recover territory which has been taken from us illegally by force. As I see the matter now, it seems that either I must fall or Sánchez Cerro must fall. I certainly would not wait to be put out. If things go badly and a clamor arises for a change of Government . . . I shall step out." [24]

In other talks with Caffery, Olaya had dwelt on the folly of a war, the unarmed condition of Colombia, the probability that service of the Colombian foreign debt would be discontinued because of the cost of war preparations, and his hope that the United States would act to preserve peace. On this last point, he remarked: " 'Anything else means that every Latin American country must stay armed to the teeth in order to guard its legitimate rights.' " [25]

Besides his official position, Olaya had at stake a certain matter of personal prestige that may have affected his attitude. He had been Foreign Minister in 1911, when a Colombian force of some seventy men had been defeated by a larger force of Peruvian troops under Major Oscar Benavides in the battle of La Pedrera on the Caquetá River, a well-remembered engagement in the century-long boundary dispute. Fabio Lozano y Lozano, Colombian minister in Peru, told Dearing that the Leticia situation was a serious personal affair for Olaya, who had been held responsible for the "fiasco" in 1911.[26]

The Colombian government mounted a strong propaganda campaign in Europe and the Americas that included the publication of opinions favoring its position by foreign statesmen and international lawyers.[27]

Six weeks after the incident, Dearing reported that "the capture of Leticia is now believed by many to have been due to the desire of the Administration to secure support from the various sections of Peru and from the armed forces, and thereby stave off the waning of its influence," and the Ambassador had so far revised his own impression of the sources of the affair as to say that "the President has conjured the first stage of this new situation with Colombia." [28]

It does not appear that the capture of Leticia was part of a revolutionary movement, but it is possible that, if the government in Lima had not supported the action, a revolt in Loreto would have occurred. Minister Jefferson Caffery in Bogotá quoted a British source as stating that a Junta Patriótica had been organized in Iquitos and that troops and arms were shipped to Leticia from that city on September 2. The Junta had ousted the prefect, and at its request Lima had flown in his successor, Oswaldo Hoyos Osores, who arrived in Iquitos on September 6 with word that Lima was fully backing the Loretanos.[29]

The formation of the Junta Patriótica was apparently the work of a few Peruvians whose economic interests had been damaged by the transfer of Leticia to Colombia. They were able to gain popular support in Loreto for the expedition to Leticia because of resentment against Colombia's access to the Amazon as provided in the Salomón-Lozano treaty. Peruvians had been accustomed to move freely in this region since the days of the rubber boom in the early 1900s, and the people of Loreto felt strongly that the Amazon above Tabatinga, the Brazilian town on the frontier, should be wholly Peruvian. The Colombian authorities at Leticia were accused of imposing excessive charges against Peruvian ships stopping for supplies; Loretanos also resented having to pay Colombian duties in Leticia on their exports going to Colombian towns far up the Putumayo. In addition, several influential Loretanos had owned property in the quadrilateral before the cession to Colombia; it was these men, principally Julio C. Araña and Enrique A. Vigil, who were the activators of the seizure of Leticia. Vigil published a letter in *El Oriente*, of Iquitos, February 13, 1933, describing how he helped to organize the expedition to Leticia and justifying his part in it. He said that, having been encouraged to establish a sugar plantation in Leticia by President Leguía, he later had to leave the place and move his sugar-milling equipment to Peruvian territory, since he could not sell sugar in Iquitos because of Peruvian tariffs, there was no market in accessible Colombian territory, and the Colombian government had refused to buy his holdings for the 80,000 Colombian pesos (about $40,000) he had demanded.[30]

The expedition to Leticia was said to have been led by Vigil's ranch foreman, Jorge Giles, other employees, and additional Peruvians from near Leticia and was aided by some of the Peruvians in the village itself.[31] Vigil's attitude is expressed in his letter:

I was the propitiatory victim of the Lozano-Salomón treaty. . . . We have not taken an inch of Colombian territory, not one Colombian, but Colombia took advantage of an insane dictator and a shameful government of Peru, to jump from the Caquetá to the doors of Iquitos, without firing a shot, but by maneuvers of her obscure diplomacy and megalomaniac audacity.[32]

Making this filibuster possible were the frontier conditions and corresponding political attitudes in Loreto: the weakness of the Colombian government in Leticia itself, where there were stationed only a prefect, three or four clerks, and a half-dozen "guards," and the initial passivity of the Peruvian army officers in Iquitos, which changed literally overnight into support for the expedition, with the despatch to Leticia on September 2 of the gunboat *América*, carrying supplies for Vigil's adventurous band.[33]

For both countries Leticia was a remote area. Trans-Andean communications were extraordinarily difficult, and the only way either could bring heavy military equipment to the region was by way of the Amazon. Leticia was 1,700 miles from Pará at the mouth of the river, and from Pará to Barranquilla, the nearest port in Colombia, the distance was about 2,200 miles. From Callao, the port of Lima, the voyage via the Panama Canal to Leticia covered almost 5,500 miles. Overland, from Lima to Iquitos, it was possible to send lightly armed soldiers successively by train, automobile, muleback, canoe, and launch in a minimum of seventeen days, while the few available light planes made the trip in two days. Colombia had no way of reaching Leticia except by way of the Amazon or by seaplane, since Peruvian forts controlled stretches of the upper Putumayo and there were no Colombian airfields in the region. Peru had some five hundred soldiers in and near Iquitos and two armed river vessels, while Colombian forces were nonexistent after the fall of Leticia.

CHAPTER VII

Fighting and Mediation

THESE WERE SOME of the elements in the situation which confronted the Department of State. ("Confronted" is an appropriate term, because some form of influence on the course of the affair by the United States was expected by all parties concerned.) The United States had taken a prominent part in the settlement of the Tacna-Arica dispute between Chile and Peru, and it was at the moment not only closely engaged in efforts to stop the fighting in the Chaco, which had broken out two months previously, but was also assisting in the settlement of two other Latin American boundary controversies. In addition, since Secretary Hughes, for the United States government, had (to use Secretary Kellogg's word) "sponsored" the agreement that made possible the ratification of the Salomón-Lozano treaty, the Department of State took as lively an interest in the Leticia dispute as it had shown in promoting the ratification of the treaty.

The Department is much concerned over the situation the obvious danger of which lies in the very difficult internal situation in Peru and the possibility that the movement "to regain lost territory" may become too popular in Peru to be withstood. . . . The procès verbal relative to the boundary settlements between Brazil and Colombia and Colombia and Peru was signed at the Department under the good offices of Secretary Hughes in March 1925, and . . . consequently this Government has a direct interest in the matter.[1]

Although the Department might have acted without a request from either Colombia or Peru, its first move followed an expression of hope from President Olaya Herrera of Colombia that the United States use its good offices. The United States did not go so far as to offer its good offices to Peru, but the day after news of the taking of Leticia was received, Ambassador Dearing was instructed to call on President Sánchez Cerro and say "very discreetly" that it was hoped the situation would not become serious and that it was "highly important for the Peruvian Government immediately to disavow the attack on Leticia and to take energetic measures to see that no arms or other assistance are sent from Peru to those occupying the town." [2] Dearing did so and reported:

There is no such thing as using discretion with Sánchez Cerro. At the very first mention of our friendly hope the President became stubborn, defiant and uncommunicative and but little information was to be got out of him. He insisted the matter was purely domestic although he had stated the moment before that the Government knew but little about it and was investigating. He inquired testily whether our Government was "mixing into this matter," to which I replied that our sincere friendship for Peru and Colombia warranted an expression of the hope that no serious international consequences would flow from the incident and that of course we wish to prevent any possibility of a conflict. . . . I told him his word "mixing-in" did not seem friendly to me and carried disagreeable implications and told him he had not comprehended what I was saying to him. Whereupon he denied intending any unfriendliness but his manner belied his words. . . . He assured me Peru was a serious Government, that it knew its duty and would perform it . . . that I could say that Peru was doing everything the situation required.[3]

This suspicious truculence in Lima contrasted with Olaya's statements in Bogotá that he relied on the United States and that " 'the only moral force in America which can preserve peace in this case is the United States.' " [4] Olaya had been Colombia's minister to the United States on March 4, 1925, and as President he had shown an amicable spirit in both political and economic dealings.

For its part, the United States government adopted what it viewed as a position of impartiality toward Colombia and Peru; it certainly had no other interest than that of keeping the peace. However, Dearing's discreet inquiry was a unilateral action by the United States, and it had been made without any indication from Peru that assistance from outsiders was desired. It was no doubt difficult for Washington to conceive that the government in Lima could actually plan to support a band of private citizens in a raid of this kind that violated an international treaty, and Secretary of State Henry L. Stimson's first moves were less cautiously made than if he had anticipated that a serious international dispute might arise. Consequently, neither he nor Dearing was prepared for the intensity of the resentment toward the United States that marked the reaction of Sánchez Cerro and other Peruvians.

In the classic manner of those who wish to exploit an opportunity to gain an advantage by the use of force, Sánchez Cerro complained of "undue interference" [5] by third parties, in this case the United States. In the classic manner of those who seek to avoid or terminate a trial by battle, Olaya appealed for assistance from an outsider. In practice, in conflicts between states in Latin America in the first half of the twentieth century, the positions adopted by disputants in this regard are a nearly infallible test either of the identity of an attacker or, as in the Chaco, of the combatants' own estimates of the ebb and flow of conflict. The attacker, or confident government, wanted to be left alone by "outsiders," and the attacked, or weaker state, welcomed third party assistance.

To an immediate request from Olaya for the sale of two hydroplanes, the Department of State replied that the U.S. Navy could not sell the planes, although it referred Olaya to manufacturers in the United States who might provide them. To Ambassador Caffery the Department stated that, even if amphibians were under construction for the Navy, "the possible international aspects of the situation might make the diversion of such planes to Colombia somewhat embarrassing." [6] In an interview with the Colombian minister, Fabio Lozano y Torrijos, Secretary Stimson said he thought "it would be consistent with our policy" for him to convey the Colombian desire for speedy procurement of planes to the Department of Commerce. His response, however, was based on his opinion that "fortunately this incident did not appear to have taken on any international aspect, and he sincerely hoped that it would not do so, but he felt that we must not lose sight of the possibility of this." [7]

The presence of a United States naval mission in Peru caused some concern in Washington, although the Colombian government does not appear to have raised any questions about it. The principal purpose of the mission had been to improve the training of Peruvian naval personnel, and its contract would have been terminated automatically in case of war. However, the mission had, at the request of the Peruvian government but apparently without Washington's knowledge, taken part in the preparation of Peruvian war plans, one of which had envisaged the possibility of war with Colombia. On learning of this unwelcome news from Dearing, the Department immediately cabled that "it is essential that members of Mission refrain from participating in any way whatsoever in formulation of war plans directed against Colombia." Dearing suggested that Washington might soon receive a protest from Colombia and reported that the Naval Mission was merely doing "what they were brought to Peru to do . . . . they must in logic give their advice, but as a practical matter this may be injurious from the Colombian point of view but it is certainly extremely valuable to the Peruvian Government at this moment when it has no central coordinating office or facilities for making war plans, and if it were not for the War College and the knowledge of our two naval officers on the Naval Mission, the situation for Peru would certainly be much worse than it is now." Officers in the Department of State placed question marks in the margins of this despatch.[8]

However, the international aspect of the dispute almost immediately became apparent. While Sánchez Cerro privately stated that his government disavowed the filibusterers, he refused to say it publicly or put it in writing. On September 7, Dearing reported that, while "so far I have believed in Sánchez Cerro's good faith," "persistent rumors" now credit him with saying that "he would support the seizure of Leticia and ask the Constituent Assembly to seek a revision of the Salomón-Lozano Treaty." [9] The Peruvian Foreign Minister was reported to have said that, if Sánchez Cerro stood by the treaty, "his Government will fall, if the contrary Peru will be shamed before the world and be in conflict with Colombia." [10]

As early as September 8 Caffery reported that Olaya thought that Peru was helping the Leticia captors and that a war was possible.[11] To a request by Lozano y Torrijos that Secretary Stimson talk with Peruvian Ambassador Manuel de Freyre y Santander, however,

Assistant Secretary of State Francis White said: "I did not think he could count on our doing anything else for them in Peru. We have made our position clear and we are glad to do this. However, our action in the matter had at first been considerably resented by President Sánchez Cerro." [12]

A few days later, however, Secretary Stimson invited Freyre to call. The Department was aware by this time that Colombia was planning to send an expedition to reoccupy Leticia. Edwin C. Wilson, Chief of the Division of Latin American Affairs, with whose opinion Francis White concurred, suggested to Stimson that he tell Freyre

that the essential thing in this case is to see that the validity of existing treaties is upheld. With the troubled condition of the world today and the conflict in the Chaco at a serious stage, it is essential that the American states show that they intend to honor their treaty obligations and not allow any incidents which occur to lead to a serious situation. . . . It would be inexcusable to upset this treaty now. I doubt the wisdom of again making the specific suggestion to the Peruvians that they publicly disavow the Leticia incident. . . . Sánchez Cerro is undoubtedly under great pressure to support a movement to revise the treaty. Any such suggestion from us at this time might cause resentment and bring about the opposite of what we are hoping for. Probably a general statement that we are confident that the Peruvian Government will take all steps appropriate to keep this incident from becoming serious and threatening the validity of the treaty will be the wisest thing. [13]

In his talk with Freyre, Stimson emphasized the desirability of treaty observance and said "that there could be no excuse for capturing a town in the territory of another friendly country" but that Peru was "condoning" such action in this case. "If this sort of thing were to be indulged in, there would be no telling where the end would be." Freyre explained some of the problems of controlling the people in Iquitos, and Stimson said he realized the difficulties "but thought the situation would be aggravated if the Peruvian Government did not express its disapproval. It could at least do that." On this last point the Secretary apparently thought his advisers too cautious. Stimson also said he regarded the present Peruvian position inconsistent with its adherence to the declaration of August 3, 1932, that reaffirmed the Kellogg-Briand Pact and applied it to the Chaco war. Freyre said he would take the matter up with Lima "and urge the respect of international agreements." [14]

An account of this talk was given the same day by White to the Colombian minister who had called to ask that the Department of State do everything it could to help avoid an apparently inevitable conflict with Peru. White said, however, "that it is not the function of the United States alone to take action in these matters"; although "we were of course willing to do our part." He suggested that Colombia might ask some other signatories of the declaration of August 3 to "say something in Lima." [15] This advice was acted on by Bogotá, but it met with a negative response.

Along this same line, White expressed his views informally to Dr. Leo S. Rowe, Director General of the Pan American Union, who had asked the Secretary to make a public statement on Leticia. White said: "I did not feel that the United States alone should make any declaration in the matter; we are not the sole guardian of peace in South America, and there is no reason why we should always jump in and assume such a role. Such action on our part might well be resented in other parts of South America." For the moment he did not see anything more that the United States could do.[16]

Stimson's admonitions to Freyre had no visible effect on Lima's policy. Foreign Minister Zavala complained to Dearing, who had talked to him about respect for treaties, that Dearing "was dealing in Aristotelian logic, whereas he [Zavala] is undertaking to deal with immediate practical necessities." [17] Earlier Zavala had neatly summarized the Peruvian view in a statement to Dearing that he

recognized logic and technical correctness of the Colombian position but declared that the treaty was iniquitous in essence, that he as a judge knew the fair thing was to consider the equity in a situation, that the Peruvian people were opposed to the treaty and that it had been secured by pressure and the betrayal of the country by Leguía and Salomón.[18]

Against the principle of the observance of treaties, Peruvians placed three principal arguments. The legal one was that there also existed in international law the principle that changes in conditions might make treaties inapplicable, and the situation in Leticia proved the inapplicability of the Salomón-Lozano treaty.[19]

The second argument, a political one, was that Leguía had been a tyrannical dictator who had betrayed his country by ramming the treaty through congress in secret session and concentrating troops in Loreto to prevent demonstrations or a revolt. Leguía was pictured as having been duped by Fabio Lozano Torrijos, then Colombian minister in Peru. General Oscar Benavides, the victor at La Pedrera, had written an earlier protest against the treaty, which was published in *La Crónica* (Lima), November 10, 1932. He stated:

The Colombian minister in Peru should be proud of his work! Cleverly exploiting in his public speeches the exaggerated egotism, the immeasurable vanity of Augusto Leguía . . . he was able to present to his country the welcome surprise of extending its territorial domain over areas it never had claimed even in its most exaggerated demands.

He alleged that the Peruvian congress, behind closed doors and without a single public session, had approved the treaty.

Thus, Augusto Leguía, in the shadows, gagging this victim [the Peruvian people] so that it could not voice its grief, tying it so that it could not defend itself, with all the brutality of his tyrannical power, plunged his murderous dagger into its heart.

Benavides claimed that the treaty surrendered to Colombia at Leticia "the keys of our military security and of our commercial life east of the Andes, and received nothing in exchange. . . . For Americanism, for the love of peace, sacrifices should always be made, but not when they involve an assault on the vital interests of the nation—not when they mean suicide." [20] These, in 1928, were the views of the man who, five years later, became President of Peru and who brought about the peaceful settlement of the Leticia dispute without gaining a revision of the treaty.

Benavides's opinions were shared by others. Victor Andrés Belaunde, later President of the General Assembly of the United Nations, considered that the Salomón-Lozano treaty was an " 'inconceivable concession' " by Peru.[21] Similarly, Luis Alayza y Paz Soldán records that he told Alberto Salomón in 1951 that he found "frankly inexplicable" the Salomón-Lozano treaty.[22] Alberto Ulloa, a distinguished Peruvian lawyer, called the Leticia triangle "absurd," "unnatural," and an "unjustifiable concession." [23] There is in these comments a suggestion that Leguía had been responsible for a mysteriously un-Peruvian action in relinquishing exclusive Peruvian control over the Amazon-Marañón above Tabatinga.

The third argument was directed against the alleged pressure by the United States exerted, first, by Secretary Hughes in 1925 to get the procès verbal signed and, second, by President Coolidge to induce Leguía to bring about approval of the treaty by Congress. This pressure, the argument ran, was an error of United States policy and imposed on the Department of State the duty to help eliminate the unhappy results of the treaty. *El Comercio* (Lima) argued that, in view of the Hughes episode, "no people is more obligated than that of the United States, not only to carry its impartiality to the greatest degree in the Leticia dispute, but also to remove every obstacle which might disturb a flexible and understanding mediation which could really lead to peace through justice and international equity." [24]

It was even suggested that Secretary Hughes had desired "to remove Colombian resentment over Roosevelt's seizure of Panama, by giving Colombia a greatly desired outlet on the Amazon." [25]

Three weeks after the "act of piracy" at Leticia, as the Colombians called it, the danger of war became apparent. About September 20, Peru despatched a military mission to Japan to purchase arms, and an internal loan of 20 million soles was authorized by the Constituent Assembly. On September 22 the Colombian government was authorized to float a loan of 10 million pesos for war supplies, and, in answer to an appeal from Bogotá, gifts of large quantities of money, jewelry, and even wedding rings were made by the Colombian people.[26]

Ambassador Dearing became concerned when he learned from "the most trustworthy authority that Peru is determined upon having war with Colombia over the Leticia incident, or having her way," and he asked whether he should "make any new representations" to Peru.[27] The Department, however, felt that "we should avoid the appearance of taking any initiative in the matter of representations to Peru or of attempting to mobilize Latin American opinion against Peru. If such an impression were to be gained the effect might be contrary to the Department's desires that the incident be kept within proper bounds." [28]

The first formal proposal from Peru for the settlement of the situation arising from the Leticia incident was a note of September 30 to Colombia, stating the Peruvian case for revision of the treaty and suggesting the appointment of a conciliation commission under the Gondra Treaty, one of six treaties for pacific settlement to which both states were parties. Ambassador Freyre explained this proposal in an interview with White and said that the Salomón-Lozano treaty was most unpopular in Peru and should be revised. White replied that he "personally thought the Peruvian point of view, as expressed by him, was astounding, and that on the basis he set forth, namely that his Government could not control its people there, any international agreement might be overthrown." Freyre said that Lima, in the present state of opinion in Peru, could not put their citizens out of Leticia, and White noted he was not asking that, but he "certainly felt" that Peru should not oppose Colombia's reestablishing "her own authority in her own territory. . . . There was only one solid basis—respect for international obligations. I told him quite frankly that I was astounded at any other doctrine he had set forth." Freyre said the matter should be handled in "a practical way," and White said "that of course it is a matter for Colombia to decide; the United States has no part in it whatsoever." [29]

Two days later, in a talk with Lozano Torrijos, White suggested that Colombia might give thought to the possibility that Peru "may be looking to the Conciliation Committee to make a recommendation so that it can back out gracefully from the position it is in at Leticia"; if so, the Committee might be able to help settle the affair by "making it easier for the Peruvian Government to withdraw from the position it is now in." [30] Olaya did not take this advice but in mid-October rejected Peru's proposal, although he sent at the same time a good-will mission to Lima. The mission was not instructed to take the initiative in negotiations with Sánchez Cerro, but it was intended by Olaya to offer an extra-diplomatic means of negotiation, if Lima wished to change its policy. White told Freyre that he "personally thought that the Colombians were fully justified in rejecting the Peruvian request as long as the Peruvians remained in Leticia or at least their presence there was not disavowed by the Peruvian Government." [31] Freyre's answer was that "no Peruvian

Government could possibly last" if it acted as White suggested. Earlier White had refused to take seriously Freyre's suggestion that "the Colombians should discuss the matter with the Loretanos in Lima, the Peruvian Government keeping out of the matter and just watching developments from the sideline." White's temper may have been tried by Freyre's remark that "the Colombians ought to be able to readily understand the difficulty Peru had in controlling the inhabitants of the Oriente as the Colombians thirty years ago had had the same difficulty with the Panamanians," but he only commented that he "thought the Colombians might rightly feel that it was up to the Peruvians to deal with their own inhabitants." [32]

In another review of the situation a week later, when asked by Freyre for his suggestions, White replied:

we do not want to butt into this matter in any way whatsoever or to seem to take any preponderant role, but that if his Government wanted us to make any inquiries and asked us to do so we naturally, in our desire to be helpful to two countries with which we have the most friendly relations, would be glad to do anything we properly could with the understanding, of course, that such action would be agreeable to both parties. [33]

While Washington was doing no more than making cautious suggestions, Dr. Rowe of the Pan American Union again tried to stimulate a stronger line of action to prevent "a bad situation." He told White "the United States ought to take the leadership and have another continental statement made such as that of August 3 last." White stuck to his view that "the United States is not the policeman of South America"; he felt that some other country, either Argentina or Brazil, should take the initiative. Rowe said that

he did not think anybody would take the leadership but the United States. Our leadership is the only one that would be respected in Peru. He thought that despite my reluctance to have us play a predominant role that it was one of the prices this country has to pay for its great power. We are the only one who can take the lead and we would be respected for doing so. We may well be criticized afterwards, but he thought we could be callous to that. I told him that I had not yet given up hope that something would be worked out and that I hoped that next week the Peruvian Ambassador might have more encouraging news. [34]

Rowe's recommendations raised issues of fundamental importance, but they do not seem to have been persuasive; at this time and throughout the next decade, Washington's policies were marked by evidences of sensitivity to criticism, rather than by callousness. An equally unsuccessful suggestion for leadership by the United States came from quite another source in the person of the Foreign Minister of Ecuador, who said to Minister William Dawson that "he feared that the incident would eventually result in war between Colombia and Peru unless the United States took steps to bring the two countries together." [35]

A Peruvian bid for the support of the United States in a move to solve the situation was also rejected by White. Victor M. Maúrtua, Peruvian special envoy, proposed that White aid in getting Colombian agreement to the following plan:

Peru would agree to help Colombia to reestablish by peaceful means her authority in Leticia and in return Colombia would agree that when this is done she will negotiate with Peru through a conciliation commission regarding the situation produced by the Treaty of 1922, commercially and otherwise, but with the understanding that there would be no territorial diminution of Colombia. Peru would merely ask for some boundary rectifications.

White said that he would transmit this to Bogotá, if Maúrtua asked him to do so, but he would not endorse the plan since the United States would then appear "to take sides regarding the Treaty of 1922 and to support the Peruvian thesis that the treaty had been negotiated unfairly and for that reason should not be respected but should be modified." [36]

This United States position was summarized by White in a talk with the Brazilian Ambassador, Rinaldo de Lima e Silva, in which White said he thought Brazil was the neutral country "having the greatest interest in the peaceful solution of this question" and suggested that Brazil might take some initiative in the Leticia affair. Rio de Janeiro, however, declined to take any initiative—alone, with Argentina and Chile, or even with all the American states together.[37]

The Peruvians continued to try to get the Department's support for their position, and Freyre was reduced to such a dubious argu-

ment as his statement to White that, "whatever the juridical position may be, we must get down to facts and the facts are that unless
the two countries can get together and discuss this matter there will
be war and that we should not run the risk of a war just to save a
juridical principle." White said that more than "a mere juridical
principle" was involved. What assurance would the Colombians have
that some future Peruvian government would not repudiate any
new agreement that might be reached about Leticia? White could
not support any proposal "unless I thought it was fair and equitable. . . . Respect for treaties is the foundation of all international
dealings and . . . unless this were maintained we were opening a
situation of chaos." He added that unless Peru got out of Leticia,

Peru would have forcibly seized territory and refused to give it up unless Colombia agreed to certain conditions. . . . This would be contrary
to the Kellogg-Briand Pact . . . and the matter would therefore affect
not only Peru and Colombia, but would be of very great concern to
sixty other nations of the world as well. I told him I thought it well to
consider that aspect of the problem.[38]

Faced by the assertion that the Peruvian government would fall if
it accepted White's suggestions about a settlement, the Department
turned to Colombia and proposed that it "call Peru before an investigation commission," to settle the Leticia problem.[39] This idea met
in Bogotá the same kind of "absolute" argument put up by Freyre.
Caffery reported that Olaya "feels that if he attempted to do anything of the kind he might be turned out of Office." He must first
recover Leticia. In return, Olaya had some suggestions for action
the United States might take: (1) it might "publicly reprimand
Peru"; (2) it might "mobilize the American nations against Peru"
for violating the Kellogg Pact; (3) it might notify Lima that it
should publicly disavow the capture of Leticia; (4) it might make a
"public declaration that we will permit no fighting on the Pacific
coast of Colombia or Peru."[40] These proposals were clearly unin-
viting to Washington, which desired to maintain an impartial public
posture and had no wish to serve as a "policeman" in South America. Caffery had earlier reported that Olaya felt that the United
States should have been willing to assist Colombia in the Leticia
dispute in return for what Olaya considered to have been his

friendly cooperation on issues such as the Colombian oil law, the Barco concession, and problems of the United Fruit Company in Colombia.[41] A further report by Caffery stated that he had noted a "changed attitude on the part of many prominent Colombians who formerly were exceedingly hostile to any intervention on the part of the United States in the affairs of Latin American countries." He said that "former President Abadía Méndez remarked to me (in effect) that only the intervention of the United States could prevent war between Colombia and Peru, and he intimated that he very much hoped that the United States would take action in that sense." [42]

Olaya's feelings were demonstrated to Caffery by his remark that

the Department of State could settle the Leticia controversy, if it so desired, in forty-eight hours. I, of course, attempted to explain to him that he is in error on this. However, I believe that he persists in his theory, for I heard yesterday that his brother-in-law . . . had remarked that the United States could settle the Leticia controversy in twenty-four hours.[43]

Following up these remarks, White told the Colombian special envoy, Pomponio Guzmán, that he had heard that Colombians felt that

the United States could settle the Leticia matter in forty-eight hours if it wanted to and that we were criticized for not jumping in and doing so. I told him that the Colombians should remember that for our action to be effective it must be evident that we are acting in an impartial manner and that we would have to have either definite proof or acknowledgment by Peru that Peruvian troops were in Leticia. I said that I had made this charge in conversation with Maúrtua and he had admitted it but of course we had nothing in writing. . . . I said that . . . we just are not convinced as yet that the time for the United States to make any public declaration has arrived.[44]

Mediation: First Phase

At this time White felt that an impasse had been reached and that "conditions are drifting more and more toward war." He hoped that it might be possible to make a fresh start by trying to get "informal conversations" going between Colombian and Peruvian representatives in Washington.[45] New possibilities were opened up by a burst of activity on the part of the governments of Chile and Brazil. As early as September 17, Foreign Minister Carlos Saavedra Lamas of Argentina had suggested to the Colombian minister in Buenos Aires that a Pan American conference might be called to examine continental conflicts, including Leticia, but Olaya had rather sharply rejected this proposal on the ground that Colombia had no international problem to be settled at such a conference; the Leticia incident had been created for Colombia only by "a group of pirates," and the only problem raised was Colombia's reestablishment of its authority in Leticia.[46]

The Chilean Ambassador to the United States, and later Foreign Minister, Miguel Cruchaga Tocornal, offered to both countries a proposal for the establishment of a commission in Santiago, composed of two Colombians, two Peruvians, and himself, to study the reestablishment of Colombian authority in Leticia and changes that would be made in the 1922 treaty, but this suggestion was accepted neither in Bogotá nor Lima.[47]

An ultimately more fruitful line was followed by the Brazilian government at the end of the year. During the last three months of 1932 military preparations had been going on in both Colombia and Peru, and, just before Christmas, the Colombian expedition to retake Leticia, consisting of some one thousand men in five ships under the command of General Alfredo Vásquez Cobo, arrived at Pará at the mouth of the Amazon River. On December 27 Caffery reported that the Brazilian government had agreed to permit the Colombian flotilla freedom of navigation on the Amazon in accordance with the treaty of November 15, 1928. On December 30 Afranio de Mello Franco, Brazilian Foreign Minister, proposed to Colombia a plan for Peruvian delivery of Leticia to Brazil and the restoration of Leticia to Colombia by Brazil, on the understanding that Colombia and Peru would "settle the territorial dispute" by talks in Rio with Brazil as mediator.[48] The Department of State welcomed this initiative, and White advised Lozano Torrijos that he hoped that Colombia would "examine any proposal with greatest care, to see whether it offered a satisfactory way out." [49]

For its part, the United States immediately ended some tortuous negotiations with Maúrtua that had been proceeding during the previous ten days. Maúrtua had proposed, orally, a solution for the dispute that seemed so reasonable to White that it was immediately sent to Bogotá, and Olaya found it satisfactory. Maúrtua, however, who had promised White to support the plan in Lima, sent quite a different proposal to his Foreign Minister, a fact that came to light in Dearing's reports. White, somewhat embarrassed at having sent to Olaya a "plan" that Maúrtua himself said White had misinterpreted, gave Maúrtua a bad quarter of an hour in an interview and asked him to put his "plan" in writing "so there would be no misunderstanding whatsoever exactly what he would stand by." [50] White was perhaps a bit incautious in falling a victim to Maúrtua's deception, but he appears to have acted only out of a sincere desire to be helpful. He should first have made sure Maúrtua was speaking for Lima; his hasty action may have been due to the fact that this was the first suggestion in four months that looked like a real chance for peace.

White personally sympathized strongly with the Colombian position. To Alfonso López, Colombian minister to London, who passed through Washington, he said that he was "absolutely convinced of the justice of Colombia's cause and had sustained it so vigorously with the Peruvian representatives . . . that for over six weeks they had not come to see me or discussed the matter further until the day before yesterday." López had said in this talk that "Colombia does not want war; that his Party [Liberal] especially had fought the military clique in Colombia and had broken down the military caste." Caffery had mentioned on more than one occasion Olaya's fear that one result of having to prepare for war might bring about a renewal of the power of the military in Colombia.[51] The day before, White had told López that he thought "Colombia was sitting back expecting somebody else to do the work for her and had not herself developed her case to the point where some effective aid could be given her. For instance, I said that it had not been brought out officially yet that Peruvians are in Leticia." In this talk, the conscious, accepted futility of the position of the government of the United States was clearly delineated. White asked López to suggest what the United States might do. López replied that "we could tell the Peruvians that they should get out of Leticia. I told him that we had said that; that I had said this in no uncertain terms to both Freyre and Maúrtua but Peru had not gotten out." López had no other suggestions.[52]

The Brazilian proposal of December 30 touched off a series of rapid-fire diplomatic exchanges. Colombia accepted it; Peru rejected it unless changed so that the talks with Colombia were held before Brazil would return Leticia to Colombia. Colombia refused this change. In response to a request for backing from Brazil, a request that went to all American states, the United States on January 10, 1933, having previously asked Colombia to take no action pending the explorations by Brazil, sent a note to the new Peruvian Minister of Foreign Affairs, José Matías Manzanilla, stating its understanding of the Brazilian proposal and supporting it in the following terms:

The United States Government has noted that the Peruvian Government recognizes that the Treaty of 1922 is valid and in effect. In view of this the United States Government is confident that the Peruvian Government will welcome the honorable and decorous way suggested and offered by the Brazilian Government by which this matter may be settled. The United States Government feels that it expresses the sentiment of public opinion in the hemisphere when it states that it would learn with the greatest satisfaction that the Peruvian Government has accepted the proposal of the Brazilian Government.[53]

This note was reported to have "made both Foreign Minister and President furious." [54] Manzanilla's reply said that, in the Peruvian government's examination of the Brazilian proposals, "the desires and opinion of the Government of the United States . . . will be given consideration in all their high significance." [55]

The nature of the contempt in Lima for the United States representations became clear a few days later, when the Peruvian rejection of the Brazilian formula became known, and Caffery reported from Bogotá that "Mello Franco admits completely unsatisfactory nature of Peruvian reply." [56] It did not matter that Mello Franco's formula as presented to Lima was slightly different than the one the United States and Colombia understood he was offering.[57] Mello Franco was actually taking some liberties in his role as mediator and holding out to Peru a little more than he knew Colombia would concede, at the same time telling Lima that Colombia had accepted his proposal. The Colombians, when they learned the text of the Mello Franco plan as presented to Lima, were disturbed, because they recognized they would find it difficult to reject it, but Manzanilla saved them from this embarrassment by rejecting it himself.[58]

The fact that Peru rejected this favorable proposal only made the tone of Manzanilla's reply to Stimson the more offensive. Although there is no direct evidence to this effect, it appears likely that the impudent style of Manzanilla's note may have been one of the factors bringing about a quick and vigorous reaction on the part of the Secretary of State, manifested on January 25. The other, and more important, factors were the receipt of a Colombian note addressed to signatories of the Kellogg Pact and the desire of Secretary Stimson, in view of the advance by Vásquez Cobo toward Leticia, to act as promptly as possible. He would probably not have been deterred even had he received in time Dearing's advice that Peru

will make no concession of any kind unless forced to do so. The indications are that the force will have to be physical, as there are no signs that the pressure coming from Brazil, our country, the Pope, the Permanent Commission of Conciliation, the British Government, the Spanish Government, the Chilean Government, and the Italian Government, and very likely from other quarters is having any effect upon Sánchez Cerro and his advisers.[59]

The Application of the Kellogg-Briand Pact

From the beginning, the applicability of the Kellogg-Briand Pact to Leticia had been in the minds of United States officials, who, in the declaration of August 3, 1932, had taken a leading part in developing the principles of the Pact into a doctrine of the nonrecognition of territory acquired by conquest in the Chaco. In Leticia it was for a long time unclear whether Lima was supporting the Loretanos or not, so the United States did not refer to the Pact. In a talk with White, Maúrtua had taken the offensive and charged that Colombia was violating the Kellogg Pact by refusing to accept Peru's offer of consultation, which had been made twice. White noted that the Gondra treaty, under which one of these offers was made, was not binding on Colombia, since its ratification had not been legally completed by that country. White recounted that Maúrtua claimed that, if Peru could not get the dispute discussed in Washington,

they would take the matter to the League of Nations. I told him that if he was trying to upset me by any such a statement he was wrong because I thought that might be a sensible thing to do. He said that if the two countries went to war that would be the end of the Kellogg Pact and that the Kellogg Pact was being violated by Colombia in not discussing the matter peacefully.

White then quizzed Maúrtua about the situation in Leticia and concluded by saying that

it seemed to simmer down then to the fact that Peruvians, by force of arms, had seized Colombian territory and refuse to evacuate it unless Colombia will consent to revise a valid treaty between the two countries. I told him that it seemed to me that this constituted the use of force as an instrument of national policy and, as such, was clearly contrary to the terms of the Kellogg Pact and the declaration of August 3, last, and that it would therefore seem to be Peru, rather than Colombia, which was violating the Kellogg Pact. Colombia certainly has the right of self defense against invasion. Doctor Maúrtua said the invasion was over.[60]

A month later, White was informed of a cable from Olaya stating that Olaya proposed drawing up a memorandum charging Peru with violating the Kellogg Pact, among other treaties. The purpose of the memorandum would have been to give the United States an opportunity to take a public initiative to try to avoid a war and to announce its support of the principle of the sanctity of treaties. Olaya wished to know what action the United States might be prepared to take if the memorandum was sent and asked for White's advice as to whether it should go to the United States alone, to all American states, or to all the countries of the world.[61] White's response was to recommend that Colombia should first bring out Peru's responsibility for supporting the Peruvians in Leticia. If Peru admitted that its troops were in Leticia, "we might be able, under the Kellogg Pact, to ask the other signatories to join us in demanding that Peru withdraw." If Peru did not reply to a Colombian inquiry, "we might then have to smoke her out by saying that silence on the charges would be tantamount to admission" and take the same sort of action. If Peru denied that troops were in Leticia, "the Kellogg Pact signatories might ask that a commission of investigation be sent to Leticia." [62]

With this encouragement, Olaya made plans to appeal to all signatories of the Kellogg Pact. He deferred action, first, because of the false hopes aroused by White's transmission of Maúrtua's deceptive "plan" and, then, in order to see whether the Brazilian formula might bring about an agreement. In the meantime Vásquez Cobo was slowly but steadily moving up the Amazon. Resting at Pará until Maúrtua's balloon had been popped, he advanced to Manaus and lay over there until it was evident that Peru had rejected the Brazilian proposal. On January 17 he left Manaus for Teffe at the mouth of the Caquetá River, arriving there on January 21, where he was within three days steaming from Leticia.

Meanwhile Olaya had been relieved of the necessity of clarifying Lima's position on supporting the filibusterers. On January 6 General Victor Ramos, commander of the Peruvian fifth division in Iquitos, cabled the Colombian Consul in Pará that the entry of the Colombian flotilla into the Amazon meant the outbreak of hostilities and that he had ordered military measures to prevent Vásquez Cobo from arriving at Leticia. [63]

The Ramos telegram was cited by Olaya in his note to signatories of the Kellogg Pact on January 23; he claimed that Peru had violated the Pact and was "employing force in support of unlawful and inexcusable acts of aggression in the territory of a friendly nation." Olaya asked the signatories to deny Peru "the benefits furnished by that treaty," to call the attention of Peru to its obligations under the Pact, and "to urge that Government that it do not violate that treaty." [64]

The response of Washington to this note was immediate and important. Stimson asked the ambassadors of France, Germany, Great Britain, and Japan to meet with him at his home at six o'clock on January 24. He explained that his view was

that there is no question regarding the title of Colombia over Leticia and that Peru has recognized Leticia as Colombian but now wants Leticia to be transferred to Peru and states that she will forcibly oppose the legitimate efforts of Colombia to reestablish her authority in her own territory and will only go to a conference to discuss the matter provided that Colombia agrees, in advance, to turn over Leticia to Peru. The Secretary said that this is a clear cut violation of the Kellogg Pact.

Stimson said:

he thought it would be very unfortunate if the first time one of the Pact signatories invokes the support of the other signatories to prevent a violation thereof the call should go unheeded. The French and British Ambassadors said that they agreed and the German and Italian Ambassadors assented. The Japanese Ambassador made no comment throughout the meeting.[65]

Without waiting for action by the ambassadors' governments, Stimson sent a note, dated January 25, addressed to Manzanilla. The note reviewed the Leticia incident and the claims of Colombia and Peru. The United States government, said Stimson, saw no alternative to the conclusion that, "if it were conceivable that Peru was seeking to obtain her desire to modify the Treaty of 1922, not by pacific means, but by a forcible and armed support of the illegal occupation of Leticia," such a position would be "entirely contrary to the provisions of Article 2 of the Kellogg-Briand Pact." [66]

The Department of State informed American missions in all Latin American countries that this note had been sent, and also despatched a copy to Consul Prentiss Gilbert in Geneva for informal transmission to the Secretary General of the League of Nations. The Council of the League had been officially asked on January 24 to act in the Leticia dispute by a Peruvian request that it "order" Colombia to cease "aggressive measures," in the form of the movements of Vásquez Cobo's flotilla. On January 26 the Council sent a telegram to Peru, stating that it "feels bound" to point out that it was Peru's duty to avoid "any intervention by force on Colombian territory" and "should not hinder" Colombian authorities from exercising full sovereignty in Colombian territory. At the same time, the cable to Bogotá declared that it "trusts that in the exercise of their legitimate rights" the Colombians would not violate Peruvian territory, and would make it clear they had no intention to do so.[67]

The Peruvian government replied to Stimson's note on January 27, by a note from Manzanilla that, both in tone and substance, was a source of no satisfaction to Washington. Manzanilla stated that, since Colombia was sending an expedition to Leticia, "it was an act of unavoidable prudence for the authorities of Loreto to take measures which have been only of a purely defensive character in prevision of unexpected emergencies." Although the Peruvian government "had absolutely nothing to do with the events of September 1, 1932 at Leticia," it cannot be indifferent to the lot of the Peruvians who are occupying Leticia.

The true significance of my Government's declarations, [Manzanilla stated], is that it cannot view with indifference the aggression against the Peruvians at Leticia, gathered there to demand that their rights be respected. . . . We are not violating the Briand-Kellogg Pact, because Peru is the very country that is seeking a peaceful settlement of the conflict that has arisen. It is Colombia that prefers to impose her will by violence and that has mobilized considerable forces for that purpose, while on our part not a soldier nor a vessel has left our territory and we have not acquired a single vessel more.

He went on to accuse Colombia of purchasing ships and arms abroad and of enlisting "legions of adventurers in European and American ports in order to make use of the perverse inclinations of those people in the execution of its purpose of drowning in blood the patriotic aspirations of the Peruvians in Leticia." [68] He noted that Colombia had refused to negotiate through the conciliation commission in Washington, as proposed by Peru, and that Peru had accepted the Brazilian peace proposal in part. He concluded by stating that "Peru will comply strictly with the international pacts which it has signed, and particularly, those guaranteeing peace between the nations of the American continent. She has not forgotten the Pact of Paris and will comply with it." [69]

Stimson's reply to Manzanilla was brief and did not try to deal with any of the Foreign Minister's contentions. He noted Manzanilla's statement that Peru had not forgotten the Pact and would abide by it and hoped that Peru would accept the Brazilian proposal "without modification so that bloodshed may be avoided and this situation may be definitely and peacefully settled." [70]

In return, Manzanilla stated that he had accepted the Brazilian formula in such form that Colombia, as well as Peru, would request the transfer of Leticia to Brazil pending negotiations; "with this and the proposal for general arbitration, my Government believes it has given new proof of its love for peace and its friendship toward Colombia and the mediating Government." [71]

It is not clear why Stimson did not react more strongly to Manzanilla's rejection of his contentions in the note of January 25. It is possible that he may have thought that the case that Peru had violated the Kellogg Pact would not be fully made unless Peruvian troops actually took part in opposing a Colombian attempt to retake Leticia. Although he had told the ambassadors that the existing Peruvian position was a violation of the Pact, his note to Peru was carefully drawn so as to suggest no more than that any aid by Lima to the Leticia adventurers would be contrary to the Pact. The note did not charge that a violation had occurred. Such aid as had been given so far might be withdrawn before shots were fired, and in that case the violation would presumably not take place. Stimson may have been hopeful that Mello Franco would soon be successful in his mediation. He may also have wished to await the response of other American governments to his request of February 1 that they appeal to Peru as the United States had done. [72]

On this occasion Stimson exhibited a certain degree of boldness as that quality is measured with respect to the application of the Kellogg Pact. On the three previous occasions when Washington initiated diplomatic correspondence on behalf of the Pact—the Sino-Russian fighting in 1929, the Sino-Japanese conflict in 1931, and the Chaco dispute in 1932—notes had been addressed in each case to both parties. In the Leticia affair, however, the appeal for peace was sent only to Peru, and Peru alone was warned that a continuation of its apparent policy would violate the Pact. Stimson was not so bold as to assert that Peru was or might become an aggressor, but the fact that Peru was the sole recipient of the note clearly implied that the United States government would regard Peru as responsible for any conflict that might ensue. Manzanilla did not refer to his country's being singled out for all the world's attention, perhaps because such reference would only have underscored the fact, but there can be little question that Stimson's action was fully appreciated and hotly resented in Lima.

Stimson's effort to mobilize the signatories of the Pact met, on the whole, with a substantial response. Guatemala had appealed to Peru about January 25, recalling the obligations of the Pact. Following the publication of Stimson's note and his request for support, Ecuador, Honduras, and Panama sent notes to Peru referring to the Pact. Eight states—Chile, Costa Rica, Cuba, Dominican Republic, Haiti, Nicaragua, Paraguay, and Venezuela—immediately sent notes to Peru, urging it to accept the Mello Franco formula. This action, however, did not satisfy Stimson, who requested United States representatives in those countries to ask that they also appeal on the basis of the Kellogg Pact. For example, a cable to the Dominican Republic on February 4 inquired: "Has Government made representations to Peru on basis of Kellogg Pact as requested by Colombia? I consider this important." [73] In response to this request, seven of the above states sent new appeals, referring to the Pact. Chile alone refused to do so, stating in response to the circular of January 23 from Olaya, that, as reported by Ambassador William S. Culbertson, "no basis for action under the Pact has arisen since Peru has not rejected the proposal of Brazil and therefore Peru may be considered still to be seeking a settlement by 'pacific means.' " [74] However, Cruchaga and Saavedra Lamas, then meeting at Mendoza, cabled to Lima urging the acceptance of the Brazilian formula. Mexico sent no note because it had at the time no diplomatic relations with Peru. Japan sent no note to Peru but the governments of France, Germany, Great Britain, and Italy joined their voices with that of the United States. The British government's action was taken only after it had learned that Peruvian troops, as distinguished from Peruvian private citizens, were in Leticia.[75] The French government, informing Washington of its note to Peru, suggested that the various peace efforts should be coordinated, particularly those based on the Covenant and the Pact. In reply, the Department described its activities and the support by other countries, and stated:

It is hoped that this action will prove effective in maintaining peace and in bringing about a settlement of this question. Should it appear later, however, that further action is necessary, the American Government will be prepared, of course, to take appropriate action and to consult with the other interested Powers.[76]

During the first week of February there were four distinct moves under way to avoid fighting in Leticia. The setting in motion of a fifth was proposed by the Director General of the Pan American Union, but this was headed off by the Department of State when it refused to take the initiative in calling a meeting of the chiefs of Latin American diplomatic missions in Washington to "consider the attitude that should be taken by the respective Governments in the Brazilian proposal." [77]

The Council of the League of Nations was giving attention to the question. Mello Franco was acting with all diplomatic speed, making several changes in his formula. The United States was activating world opinion to appeal to Peru not to violate the Kellogg Pact. Finally, the British government entered the lists with a plan of its own, which was withdrawn within a few days because of strong objections by Secretary Stimson. The British plan was that Leticia would be administered by Brazil for four months; if after two months Peru and Colombia could not agree on a solution, the dispute should be submitted to a commission, made up of representatives of Brazil, the United States, and Great Britain, which would decide "whether Leticia shall be handed over to Colombia or to Peru."

Stimson pointed out that the British plan was based on a mistaken understanding of Mello Franco's proposal. More importantly, however, since Leticia had become part of Colombia by the 1922 treaty, letting a commission decide its status would "put a premium on the forceful seizure of territory and would be a derogation of the all important principle of the sanctity of treaties." In addition, the plan overlooked Colombia's vital interests in the dispute, and its application would conflict with the negotiations already commenced by Mello Franco. In an instruction to London, Stimson asked Ambassador Andrew Mellon to

discuss the matter at once with Sir John Simon and point out the reasons why I feel this proposal is thoroughly unsound and urge him to make representations in Lima to the Peruvian Government to abide by its commitments under the Kellogg Pact and to support the real Brazilian proposal. Otherwise there will be great confusion.[78]

Mellon reported that Sir John had sent word to Washington that
" 'In view of the attitude of the United States Government I shall
proceed no further in the matter and can only hope that serious
conflict will not ensue.' " [79]

Even though Stimson's campaign to get American and other nations to mention the Kellogg Pact in their notes to Lima had been
successful, it cannot be said that the effect on the people or government of Peru was significant. The people in Peru were kept in ignorance of the world opinion about Leticia that Stimson had been
able to muster. Dearing reported:

> The Peruvians have not yet dared to publish here Mr. Stimson's note of
> January 25th, and somewhat astutely are referring to the rejoinder to
> Manzanilla's reply to the note of the 25th as being the American note,
> and have published Manzanilla's reply to this second note as being Peru's
> reply. The public at large is, therefore, completely in the dark and merely
> takes the last two notes exchanged as being the whole correspondence.[80]

El Comercio (Lima) published an editorial on February 2, attacking the position of the United States government, although without
referring to the note of January 25; it stated that the spirit of the
Kellogg Pact had been changed, since it was being used "to impose
rigid solutions which are in disaccord with equity among nations,
and which serve to consecrate international injustice."

Concerning the government, Dearing reported that, in his opinion, Sánchez Cerro "means to fight because he thinks he will win
and will continue diplomatic maneuver as long as he thinks anything
can be gained by doing so." Dearing judged that the "Department
may, I believe, abandon all hope of effecting a change in this attitude unless powerful continuous pressure can be brought to bear directly on this Government which continues to disregard the opinion
of the world." [81] Dearing also reported that the Peruvian Foreign
Minister, whom he called "the wily Manzanilla," had talked with
the British minister who had "pointed to adverse opinion of world
and Peru's opportunity under Brazilian Plan to save her face. Manzanilla stated world opinion would have to be ignored if it meant
abandoning captors or Loreto and that Peru had been trying to save
Colombia's face." [82]

Mediation: Second Phase

While the peace efforts were reaching a climax, Vásquez Cobo made another move in his carefully timed journey westward. He left Teffe on January 26 and halted again at Santo Antônio do Iça. Which way would he go? This was at last a vital question, since he could go either northwestward up the Putumayo (Iça) to Tarapacá, at the northeastern corner of the Leticia quadrilateral, or southwestward to Leticia itself. If he took the latter course, he could not turn aside but must attack Leticia or retreat. If he ascended the Putumayo, he would move on Tarapacá, a place that was weakly held by the Loretanos, and then later he might be able to join forces on the upper Putumayo with Colombian gunboats that had so far been blocked from moving down the river by Peruvian forts. When Vásquez Cobo's departure from Teffe was reported from Lima, Dearing cabled: "Peru inquires of Brazilian Minister what would be attitude of Brazil if Colombia uses gas or Colombian boats return to Brazilian waters. . . . Conscription continues. . . . Foreign consuls Iquitos express alarm over possible air bombing that place." [83]

Vásquez Cobo was in close touch with Bogotá, where Olaya was weighing his moves with great care. When speeches by the opposition or critical editorials seriously weakened his internal position or when he felt Colombia's dignity could bear inaction no longer, he would redress the balance by adding a few more miles of Amazon traversed by Vásquez Cobo. When the pressure of Stimson or Mello Franco to hold up the force on the Amazon until the peace negotiations could be further explored became irresistible or when his own sincere desire to avoid fighting was allowed to express itself freely, he would level the balance by putting in a few days or even two weeks of delay in the flotilla's advance. This precarious equilibrium was maintained for over a month after Caffery had reported that "the breaking point has about been reached" by Colombian public opinion. [84]

Meanwhile the negotiations of Mello Franco had been going badly, but they were kept going, despite constant difficulties, by the energy and patience of the Brazilian Foreign Minister. One serious problem had arisen with the Peruvian minister in Rio de Janeiro, Ventura García Calderón. Caffery reported that Olaya had heard from his minister in Brazil that

Mello Franco "is completely disheartened" and "has lost all hope" of negotiations succeeding; Peruvian Minister at Rio has just told him that instead of transmitting actual Brazilian formula to his Government he through a misunderstanding informed it that formula provided for delivery of Leticia to Brazil for 90 days, attempts at agreement during this period and return of territory to attackers should attempts fail, and that if he now altered it his Government would think him "crazy." [85]

Previously, according to Dearing, Garcia Calderón had reported to Lima that the Colombian minister in Brazil "had accepted Peruvian modifications [of the] Brazilian plan. This erroneous report was widely disseminated here as great Peruvian diplomatic victory and a settlement of the dispute." [86] Within two days García Calderón sent another report to Lima, which was inaccurate, probably deliberately so: he cabled that Colombia had withdrawn from the mediation sponsored by Mello Franco. This second "inaccuracy" was one too many for Mello Franco, who apparently brought such pressure on García Calderón that he cabled to Lima admitting that both his reports were erroneous.[87] Dearing, who in this telegram had referred to García Calderón only as "a thoroughly mischievous and dangerous adviser to the Lima Government," later revised his opinion and said that he "was not so much the informer and adviser of his Government as a conniver with it in trying to distort and falsify the Brazilian Plan." This view was based on the observation that Manzanilla's note of January 16, replying to the Brazilian formula, "virtually supports the confessedly incorrect reports of the Peruvian Minister at Rio and virtually incorporates them in the note." [88]

Mello Franco had replied to Manzanilla's note by maintaining that his formula was unchanged and hoping that Peru would find it possible to accept it. When the Department of State had ended its brief and unsatisfactory exchange with Manzanilla about the Pact, Stimson proposed to Mello Franco that, if he found that Peru did not agree to his formula of January 13, Brazil might ask that Peru avoid interfering with the Colombian forces advancing toward Leticia and propose further negotiations.[89] Mello Franco said he would adopt this suggestion if circumstances permitted, which, as it turned out, they did not. However, with the Council of the League of Nations inactive and the appeal to Peru on the basis of the Kellogg Pact rejected by Lima, on February 6 White tried to breathe new life into the Mello Franco formula by persuading Olaya to accept a modification of the formula as rejected by Peru. That formula had also been unsatisfactory to Colombia, as mentioned above, because it contained changes in the original formula that Olaya had approved. Olaya at first accepted the new proposal and then almost immediately rejected it on the advice of his Foreign Affairs Advisory Committee. The new formula provided that "Peru would turn over Leticia at once to Brazil; conference would start at once Rio de Janeiro and no matter what result of conference Brazil would deliver Leticia to Colombia at expiration of 60 days." [90]

Stimson cabled Caffery that "Department is extremely disappointed that Olaya has withdrawn his acceptance," and, on February 7, Caffery reported that "Olaya agrees to renew acceptance." [91] This last shift by Olaya was a difficult decision. Caffery cabled: "I hope that the Department realizes grave responsibility Olaya is assuming by going counter to advice of his advisers and that he runs risk thereby. The two principal leaders of the Liberal Party and a Conservative candidate for the presidency in 1930 are in agreement on insistence on original Brazilian formula. Their advice is not capricious, going as it does against their personal interests (they stand to lose politically if Vásquez [Cobo] becomes military hero)." [92]

Although the Department had said on February 6 that it hoped Caffery "would be able to persuade Olaya that in case proposal is accepted ships would be withdrawn to Manaus or at least to Teffe," Caffery replied in his cable of February 7 that Olaya "insists that he must bring boats except *Mosquera*" into the Putumayo and Caquetá rivers and added that Olaya "said he would not last 48 hours if he left all boats in Brazil." This decision, however, was one of the less belligerent of the alternatives before Olaya, since it meant that he did not intend that Vásquez Cobo should attack Leticia immediately. The Putumayo led only to Tarapacá, where Vásquez Cobo could reoccupy a Colombian town, reassert Colombian authority in the quadrilateral, and so enable Olaya to mollify Colombian opinion while deferring a battle at Leticia and providing more time for the testing of the possibilities for peace. Stimson, in the meanwhile, speeding arrangements in Rio by telephone so that the new proposal to Peru would be made in exactly the terms that Olaya had accepted, cabled Caffery: "Please endeavor to have advance of boats delayed as much as possible." Caffery replied:

Olaya today told me his position was more serious than he ever imagined it could be. Military have become restless; conservative opposition potentially dangerous; he received yesterday violent telegram from Santos attacking him for accepting 60 days suggestion. . . . Olaya declares he puts himself "in the hands of the Department" but not in those of Brazil whose attitude he terms ambiguous and uncertain. Pressure for advance of Amazon expedition has become overwhelming; he has held it at Tonantins for almost 2 weeks but can no longer do so; the main force is now proceeding very slowly up Putumayo. I consider the question of the boats moving to be a critical one for Olaya. If he is overthrown no matter who comes into office our interests here will certainly suffer.[93]

Olaya's reference to the Brazilian attitude was appreciated in Washington, where Mello Franco's response to its repeated inquiries about the text of the new proposal were both less clear and less swift than was desired. After several baffling exchanges of telegrams, Stimson cabled to Ambassador Morgan that "Brazilian Government apparently does not realize urgency of situation." [94] On the same day, however, Mello Franco sent a telegram to Colombia and Peru, proposing a change in his formula, but stating only that "in the shortest period possible," rather than in sixty days, Brazil would reinstate Colombian officials in Leticia.[95] The sending of this telegram demonstrated Mello Franco's appreciation of the urgency of the situation, but not his agreement with Stimson as to what should be done about it. News of the sending of the Brazilian note prompted Stimson to respond immediately that "Department finds it difficult to understand why Brazilian note does not definitely state that if after 60 days negotiations there is no agreement between the parties Brazil will return Leticia to Colombia." This cable stated:

[Vásquez Cobo] has been ordered not to reach Tarapacá until Sunday [February 12]. This is a considerable delay which Olaya has brought about at the earnest request of this Government. In view of the internal political situation in Colombia . . . Department will not make any further representations to Olaya to hold up expedition. There is therefore little over 24 hours for Brazil to clear this matter up and get an answer from Peru.[96]

By one final effort, the seventh urgent telegram within the week, Morgan was informed that "Department must emphasize again the urgent need for quick action if the Brazilian proposal is not to arrive too late." After commenting on what it viewed as inadequacies of the Brazilian note of February 10, Stimson stated: "Important thing however is to have Brazilian Government clear up these points regarding its proposal and make the proposal promptly. There is no time to be lost and you should impress this clearly on Brazilian Government." [97]

The tone of these cables, verging on the peremptory, may well have made Morgan's task a difficult one, although it is not known in what terms he spoke with the Brazilian Foreign Minister. Mello Franco's position, which was not made known to Washington until February 13, was that a sixty-day time limit "would make the situation more difficult for the Peruvian Government without corresponding advantage." [98]

The Battle of Tarapacá

Olaya could wait no longer. Vásquez Cobo was ordered to restore Colombian authority in Tarapacá. Before advancing, he called on the Peruvian commander to allow him to occupy Tarapacá peacefully. The request was refused, and on February 14 his three gunboats moved toward Tarapacá. While still in Brazilian waters, the ships were bombed, but not hit, by Peruvian planes, which soon were driven off by Colombian planes. The Peruvian bombing appears to have been the first "shot" fired in the engagement. Vásquez Cobo pressed the attack on Tarapacá with bombs and naval gunfire, and on February 15 he reported the capture of the place, along with six mountain guns and other supplies. Apart from the aerial and naval bombardment, there seems to have been little, if any, fighting, and there were no Peruvians taken prisoner.[99] Casualties were light.

On April 8 the Colombian government published the news that, since the commencement of the fighting, 8 Colombians had been killed in action or died of wounds and 19 had died from other causes.[100] On the Peruvian side, it was reported at the end of the year that 25 men had been killed in action, and that 800 had died of disease.[101]

Just after the Tarapacá engagement, the Department of State had another occasion to defend its impartiality in the dispute. Olaya asked if a United States observer could be sent to Leticia "to verify that it is the Peruvians and not the Colombians who start the fighting." White had previously suggested to Olaya that "they ought to have a Brazilian boat present, if possible, to verify exactly what happens." He thought such an observer could obviously not go on a Colombian ship; it would be "embarrassing for us to suggest to the Brazilians that an American observer was necessary to give an impartial report." [102]

Olaya also desired observers from Brazil and from the League of Nations. Replying to a cable from Caffery on this subject, Stimson stated:

To send an official observer with Colombian forces might well be considered as a sign of partiality. . . . While this Government considers . . . that Colombia is justified in this matter, nevertheless the dispute is not between this Government and Peru and this Government can not take action which might be considered as partial or unneutral as regards the prosecution of the conflict. You should be careful not to let Olaya get the idea that this Government can perform services for Colombia which it is clearly the function of Colombian Government to perform for itself.[103]

Although White, in talking with George Rublee, considered that an observer might be sent if an invitation came from Brazil, it was apparently decided that this observance of Brazilian susceptibilities could be overlooked in view of the utter lack of a United States source of information nearer Leticia than Lima, Bogotá, or Manaus. Consequently, Ambassador Morgan was asked to secure facilities from the Government in Rio de Janeiro for an officer of the United States Army to proceed to the "scene of operations," and the Brazilian government generously provided transportation and other assistance to Major William Sackville for this purpose.[104]

CHAPTER VIII

Pacification

ON THE DIPLOMATIC FRONT, Mello Franco quit the field temporarily, formally withdrawing his mediation of February 15, and almost nothing more was heard of the Kellogg-Briand Pact initiative of the United States. One significant attitude within the Department of State at the time was expressed by Edwin C. Wilson. Commenting on the news of the Peruvian bombing of the Colombian flotilla near Tarapacá, he said:

It would be difficult to find a clearer case of the use of force [by Peru] as an instrument of national policy, resulting in a violation of the Briand-Kellogg Pact. In view of this it is worth considering what action we can take in support of the Pact and in order to make effective the statement in the preamble thereof that a violation of the Pact would entail a denial of its benefits to the signatory power which violated it.

In the absence of legislative authority to put an embargo on shipments of munitions to Peru, presumably our market remains open for the Peruvians to obtain munitions in this country. Or could it be held that, in view of Peru's violation of the Kellogg-Briand Pact to which we are a party, we would be justified in depriving Peru of access to our market? Perhaps Mr. Rogers [James Grafton Rogers, Assistant Secretary of State] and Mr. Hackworth [Green H. Hackworth, Legal Adviser] might be interested in considering this. Of course, to be effective, agreement would have to be reached with other powers parties to the Kellogg Pact to take similar action.[1]

No action seems to have been taken by the Department along these lines. Similarly, there appears to have been no attempt by the Department to employ the Pact, when so requested by Colombia, to prevent munitions for Peru from being shipped through the Panama Canal.[2] Stimson's note of January 25 was finally published in Peru on February 27 in English, but not in Spanish, in the *West Coast Leader* (Lima), at a time, presumably, when the government considered its publication no longer dangerous. The Department gave no attention to a suggestion by former Acting President Dr. Alberto Guerrero Martínez of Ecuador that the United States should take "a more energetic stand" in the Leticia affair. Guerrero said that "in 1910 when Eucador and Peru were on the verge of hostilities the United States had virtually told the two countries that they could not go to war," and he thought that similar action should now be taken, particularly since the other American states were not in so strong a position as to exert economic pressure. Minister William Dawson said that "the United States had been subjected to no little criticism on account of their alleged intervention in Latin American affairs." To this, Guerrero replied that, although the United States "had been criticized for intervening in the domestic affairs of various countries," its "interposition to maintain international peace had never been and never would be resented." [3]

Colombia broke off diplomatic relations with Peru on February 15, because of the "attack by Peruvian planes on Colombian vessels in Brazilian and Colombian waters." [4] In Bogotá, the news of the victory at Tarapacá had been greeted with patriotic demonstrations; the government had stationed a small police guard before the Peruvian legation, but the crowds made no attack upon it. In Peru, however, a mob looted and partly burned the Colombian legation, and Minister Lozano y Lozano barely escaped being killed. Thirty years later this event may hardly seem noteworthy, since observance of the inviolability of diplomatic premises has recently declined. At the time, however, and especially in Latin America where the general rules protecting legations and embassies were reenforced by the frequent and acute needs of heads of state and others for asylum, this incident was regarded as an extraordinary departure from civilized patterns of international behavior. Dearing blamed the Peruvian government for "dilatoriness and inaction" in failing to protect the legation.[5] He added: "Foreign representatives thoroughly aroused and fearful for their safety," and he asked the Department of State "to consider most seriously whether a war vessel should not be despatched to Callao immediately from the nearest point possible on a declared friendly visit but to remain here during period of uncertainty. Vessel and equipment should be adequate for dealing with hostile mobs of considerable size." [6]

The Department of State took a cooler view of the situation. In reply to Dearing, it noted that the Peruvian government had given assurances of future protection; "in view of this, and as it does not appear from your reports that American lives are at present in any actual danger, the Department, as at present advised, believes that the despatch of a war vessel to Peruvian waters would not be warranted." [7]

This brief exchange was supplemented by a longer despatch from Dearing, which, with comments by Department officials, illustrates policy attitudes in Washington on the advisability of making a show of force in Latin America. Justifying his request for a "war vessel," Dearing wrote:

> In this general connection my concrete suggestion would be that our Government begin from now on a series of friendly visits every little while so that the ports of South America will become accustomed to the sight of our war vessels engaged in friendly missions, and they can come with more and more frequency, and thus not stir up resentment and excitement. [Marginal comment: "I disagree: I believe they are usually misunderstood and cause friction." H. F. M(atthews). Comment on Matthews comment: "I agree." E. C. W(ilson).] Moreover, they will then be within closer call when needed. The vessels of other countries come and go, notably the British, French, Germans and Italians, and unless some very great expense is involved, it seems to me our vessels should make far more frequent visits also. [Marginal comment: "As a general rule, they should not make any to L.A." E.C.W(ilson).] The policy of making very few results in a situation in which any visit now made is immediately interpreted as having ulterior purposes and being in a sense admonitory. We can accomplish all the practical purposes needed, the experience will probably be good for our vessels, and at the same time, I believe, allay rather than excite general feeling throughout South America by having our vessels come more often and by emphasizing the social and friendly character of the visit.
>
> If such a general policy were adopted, I believe that in situations such as the one existing at present in Peru Americans and their interests would be far safer and certainly the feeling among our citizens here, who are

entitled to every respect and every measure of protection that can be given them, would be much more confident and happy. It will then be unnecessary to wait until some tragedy occurs to supply the justification for the despatch of a ship. It is only common sense to take preventative measures and to take them in time. The Embassy realizes, however, that certain preventative measures arouse great suspicion and under the present circumstances would create the actual state of danger I have outlined above. For that reason I suggest again that this general policy of friendly visits be given careful consideration in order to assure the protection of our citizens in future years. They can be made without upsetting the general South American psychology, they can be made without involving us in any local or domestic disputes, and they can be made in such a manner as to leave full and complete responsibility for the protection of American interests with the various Governments down here. At the same time their frequent appearance in South American waters will, I believe, create an atmosphere which will be helpful for American interests, add to our general prestige, and be impresssive in an unobjectionable way not only in South American countries but for European and Asiatic Governments as well.

As I stated in my telegram, I have no wish to alarm the Department or to be embarking upon large matters of policy which it belongs to our Government at home to deal with, nevertheless, I have a duty to perform in protecting our people here; this duty involves some comment upon our policies and such suggestions as I am able to offer, and we are confronted by a practical and actual situation which requires action every little while. In view of this I trust the Department will consider this despatch with indulgence as well as with close attention.[8]

From this time forward, the United States took a less prominent part in the Leticia negotiations, although the Department of State maintained a constant interest in their course and occasionally exerted some influence on it. Several reasons may have combined to affect this withdrawal from the spotlight. The inauguration of Franklin D. Roosevelt was at hand. As Edwin C. Wilson's memorandum had shown, uncertainty existed as to a next step that the United States might take. The rainy season on the upper Amazon was expected to limit further fighting until July. The resources of the League of Nations were beginning to be explored by the disputants, now that American initiatives had failed. Finally, there was open expression of strong feeling in Peru against the United States.

Manzanilla, in a note to "friendly governments," after Tarapacá, restated the Peruvian claims to Leticia, charged Colombia with opening "a dangerous and menacing perspective in its relations with Peru," and, for his government, declined all responsibility for the Colombian "aggression." He stated that the Brazilian government had "presented some observations" on the Salomón-Lozano treaty, "which were only withdrawn 3 years afterwards due to the intervention of the Government of the United States of America." [9]

To this note, Stimson merely replied: "I find nothing therein to change the views which I frankly and fully expressed to you in my cable of January 25th." He regretted that Peru had not accepted "the very equitable proposal suggested by the Brazilian Government" and hoped that it would be able to accept a formula presented to Peru by the Council of the League of Nations on February 23.[10]

Evidence of the feeling in government circles in Peru at this time was given in an editorial in *El Comercio* (Lima), on March 3, 1933. This paper was the preeminent newspaper in Peru; its owners, the Miró Quesada family, strongly upheld the Sánchez Cerro government and were opposed to all the works of the Leguía regime. Its editorials had approved the government's policy on Leticia, and Dearing reported in February: "*Comercio* editorials all almost certainly prepared by Manzanilla." [11]

The editorial of March 3 expressed the hope that the Roosevelt administration would follow a different line of policy from that so far taken by the United States. Its criticism of the Department of State was outspoken:

> The policy of the Department on Leticia has been most unwelcome to Peru. It not only justifies our resentment, but we may venture to say that the determined support given in Washington to the Colombian thesis has greatly contributed to the force of Colombian intransigence, leading it down the path of hostilities, instead of along the road to conciliation.
>
> The attitude of Colombia would have been quite different if, instead of making its declaration on the intangible sanctity of treaties, and instead of peremptorily recommending to Peru the acceptance of Brazilian mediation without changes, the Department of State had, from the White House, made Colombia understand that the peace of America stands above all other considerations, and that the keeping of the peace should never be sacrificed to the text of a diplomatic agreement which, while negotiated to promote harmony among peoples, was converted into an instrument of hatred and a cause of war.

The United States, more than any other country, should have done this service to the cause of American peace, not alone because of its great moral authority in the continent, but also because its own intervention in the making of the Salomón-Lozano treaty, should have readily enabled it to advise Colombia to be flexible and to compromise. If the voice of the United States had been heard to recommend that the treaty of 1922 should not be made into a yoke which would eternally subjugate the Peruvians in Leticia, but into an effective means of consolidating peace and Peruvian-Colombian friendship, the angry conflict in the Amazon would have taken on an entirely different character. . . .

Unhappily, the United States has revealed disturbing prejudices in this affair which have not harmonized well with the sense of high impartiality which it should have demonstrated as a neutral and a friend of the two peoples in conflict. . . .

Leticia has been and will continue to desire to be Peruvian; despite this conventional respect for treaties, however unjust, which now is invoked by the League of Nations, there has been forgotten the sacred principle of self-determination which belongs to the population of any territory, and which was the founding principle, the reason for the existence of the international organization which sprang from the lofty spirit of President Wilson. . .

We cherish the hope that the new administration in the United States will look on the Peruvian-Colombian problem with a more understanding and practical spirit, and will reach the heart of the dispute without wasting time in sterile technicalities nor in dead texts which are unreal and are discordant with the fundamental objective of maintaining, above all, peace on American soil.

It would be a painful disappointment for us if the change in administrations . . . did not change the policy of the White House on Leticia, a policy which has been so rigidly opposed to our national interests and to our conception of justice and humanity as the unchanging foundation of a just law of nations.

An alleged expression of popular feeling in Loreto, which may well have been officially or semi-officially inspired, was published on April 7, 1933, by *La Crónica* (Lima). An article gave the purported text of a declaration by the people in the town of Leticia, which stated in part:

"We must defend our rights and nationality that is menaced by the warlike aspect of Colombia and by the moral pressure of the League of Nations and of Secretary Stimson of the United States.

"It was resolved: to burn in effigy in the public square of Leticia, Alberto Salomón and Fabio Lozano, the signers of the treaty, and also the Yankee Secretary Stimson, who encouraged our annihilation in order to compensate Colombia for the Panama Canal Zone and obscure petroleum deals." [12]

El Comercio's appeal went unheeded in Washington, as did another, from the American Society of Peru. The Society, composed largely of United States business men in Lima, cabled to President Roosevelt that it desired to "invoke your interest in situation and request continuance [of] good offices [by] our Government whenever requested seeking a just and lasting understanding between our mutual friends, Peru and Colombia, when consistent with high principles universally recognized essential to amicable intercourse between nations." [13]

The Department of State sent a noncommittal reply to this message. It had been previously informed by Dearing that Manzanilla had told the lawyers of United States firms that the sending of such a cable "would be a desirable thing." Manzanilla had suggested that the cable should "express the hope that some basis—more satisfactory than the League plan—would be found" for the Leticia dispute and had asked that the lawyers not disclose that he had suggested the idea.[14]

President-elect Roosevelt had in January issued a statement supporting Stimson's policy of the nonrecognition of territorial conquests. Stimson and Roosevelt, in discussing the statement, were thinking primarily of Manchuria, but it was made in terms general enough to apply both to the Chaco and to Leticia.[15] A measure of continuity of policy was provided by the retention of Francis White as Assistant Secretary of State until his appointment in June as Minister to Czechoslovakia, and Edwin C. Wilson remained as Chief of the Division of Latin American Affairs. In any case, the attention of the President and Secretary of State Cordell Hull was centered on other matters, and they seem personally to have taken little interest in Leticia. The United States public appears also to have been little concerned by the possibility of war over Leticia. The Department of State was certainly under no significant pressure to follow any other policy than that which it had independently determined. During the Leticia negotiations, it received a few letters from peace groups praising its attitude, and a few communications that were critical, but nothing approaching a public controversy blew up.[16]

In contrast to the attitude of *El Comercio* in Lima, fulsome praise for Secretary Stimson and his policy was offered on the eve of his leaving office by L. E. Nieto Caballero in an article in *El Tiempo* of Bogotá, on February 6, which Ambassador Caffery said "expresses the general feeling of gratitude to the Secretary prevailing in Colombia." [17] Nieto hoped that President Hoover's policies toward Latin America would be continued by the new President, and said of Stimson:

To him his party owes the transformation of a resistance, muffled or clamorous, in our America, into a smile which augurs well for rapprochement. Other men as well intentioned as he failed to obtain comparable results. Even Wilson, with all his moral elevation, could not avoid bitter interventions. . . .

Secretary Hughes . . . with his famous theories which he explained as potential intervention in white gloves, which, however, in reality are of iron, left in Havana the impression of a shadow of an equivocation. . . .

Colonel Stimson knows us better, understands more deeply the Latin-American psychology with its caprices and its foolishnesses [*necedades*]; its fears and its strength, its guile and its subtlety; above all that part of it which is affable, cordial, hospitable, like a playful child made defiant by a frown, or smiling by cordiality of manners. . . .

In the case of Leticia, Stimson comprehended the situation quickly and clearly. He played with the sophistries of Peru, crumbled them in his fingers, threw the pieces to the ground and wrote some formidable notes. It was he who was first in the United States to denounce the miserable practice of inventing international problems in order to develop support for a government otherwise lacking in prestige, and he condemned it appropriately.

In like vein, Pomponio Guzmán on his return to Colombia stated in a newspaper interview that United States public opinion favored Colombia's stand on Leticia, and added:

"It is natural that justice should be recognized in a country with the democratic traditions of the United States. That democracy, which in less than a century has reached the apex of culture, has a great number of virtues; among them stands out the feeling of justice, which has become almost a habit, caused by its moral sense, although the psychology of the race has sometimes hidden this." [18]

After the failure of the first phase of the Brazilian mediation and Peru's disregard of the consequences of a violation of the Kellogg-

Briand Pact, Washington does not appear to have regarded the entry of the League of Nations into the Leticia question as other than a natural development. In the Chaco dispute, the Department of State had resisted the League's entry into negotiations so long as there appeared any chance for the success of the Commission of Neutrals. However, no such joint effort was under way concerning Leticia, and there was no stand-in for Mello Franco's role; it seemed preferable to let a new company go on with the play.

The League's work in bringing about a settlement of the dispute was supported in several ways by Secretaries Stimson and Hull. Endorsing the first League proposal, made on February 25, Stimson cabled to Bogotá and Lima his opinion that it was "a most straight-forward, helpful one, which, if accepted by both parties, should make possible a peaceful solution of the present controversy, honorable to both Governments. In giving my fullest support to this proposal I have the honor to express the hope that your Government will see its way clear to accepting it." [19] Olaya accepted the proposal without conditions, but Manzanilla would not agree to the reoccupation of Leticia by Colombian troops, even though they were to be "placed at the disposition of the commission of the League of Nations," as provided in the Council's plan.

A subsequent report and resolution, adopted unanimously by the Council on March 18, was also accepted by Colombia and rejected by Peru. In response to an invitation to the United States, along with Brazil, to cooperate with an Advisory Committee of the Council, which was to assist the members of the League in their future action concerning Leticia, Secretary Hull authorized Minister Hugh R. Wilson to attend the meetings of the Committee but not to take part as a member.[20] Brazil accepted cooperation on similar terms.

This measure of collaboration with the Council did not mean that the United States necessarily approved its policies. Its support of the first plan was based on its own judgment that the proposal was a fair one. A problem soon arose, as reported by Wilson:

It is obvious that League members, especially the more ardent protagonists of the integral application of the Covenant, including article 16, are anxious to establish a precedent based on the case of Leticia, which can be invoked in considering the much more serious Manchurian matter or future eventualities elsewhere. The case against Peru is so clearcut that to the doctrinaire mind it is almost welcomed in order to put into motion the machinery established by the Covenant and create a precedent for the further and more important use of this machinery. Futhermore, I believe that the thought uppermost in the minds of these League members is the punitive aspect of an embargo and their desire to take action against an aggressor.[21]

The Department did not favor the application of an arms or other embargo. Authority was lacking in United States legislation, and it was doubted that an arms embargo would be desirable in the Leticia dispute.[22] In Latin America, there was no evidence of any sentiment favoring the application of sanctions to encourage policies of peace. With the exception of Venezuela, which had come forward briefly with a proposal for peaceful settlement shortly before the battle of Tarapacá, the South American countries appeared determined to remain entirely neutral. This policy, Eduardo Santos was quoted as saying, "constitutes a complete absence in the continent of a spirit of intervention which the European powers might have harbored." Santos reported that there was no knowledge in Geneva of "possible action by Washington, which would be the only decisive factor." [23]

For three weeks after Peru's rejection of its proposal, there was no formal action on the League's part, although the Advisory Committee held several meetings. During this period, and following the battle of Tarapacá, preparations for war had been going forward swiftly in Colombia and Peru. The battle had been used in Lima to generate popular sentiment favorable to the policy of the government. A "monster patriotic demonstration" was held on February 20.[24] The campaign was continued with energy:

The internal propaganda system in Peru is now on a war basis. Every obscure orator and editor is finding work in getting out patriotic exhortations. *El Comercio* leads in its attacks on Colombia and is devoting every energy at this time toward exciting public opinion and gaining public support for the Government's policy. The patriotic slogan has become: Leticia will always be Peruvian.[25]

In Colombia the situation was similar; the people were urging the government to act. The press, with the notable exception of *El Tiempo*, had unanimously opposed the League plan accepted by the

Colombian government. "The general public has had its fill of procrastination and formulas and wishes complete and unconditional recovery of Leticia as soon as possible." The public was demanding military action to regain Leticia, and Olaya was barely able to contain it. Caffery's own judgment was that both Olaya and the Colombian people had shown "patience and restraint." [26]

Both governments recognized that, as Olaya put it, " 'it is control of the air which will decide the fate of Leticia,' " [27] and both governments made every attempt to obtain planes and pilots from abroad, in addition to other types of arms.

The influence of the United States during this period was exerted to restrain Colombia from a further military action—the capture of two Peruvian forts on the Putumayo River, at Güepi and Puerto Arturo. When the Department had been informed of such plans, immediately after the battle of Tarapacá, Stimson had suggested that there were "possibilities of Colombia's position before world opinion being adversely affected in case she took the initiative on attacking these Peruvian positions." [28] Caffery took a similar line in talking with Olaya, who immediately gave orders to call off the planned attack, and instead cabled Eduardo Santos in Geneva to appeal for League action under Article 16.[29] The Colombians, however, became concerned about the possibility that their long supply line via the Amazon might be cut off by Brazilian restrictions and wished to open communications for Vásquez Cobo with Colombia by way of the Putumayo. On March 8 Caffery again counseled that "an unprovoked attack by the Colombian military forces on the Peruvian garrisons on the Putumayo might have certain unfavorable repercussions abroad," and later he told Olaya that it would be "a serious mistake." [30]

After the Peruvian rejection of the Council's resolution of March 18, Olaya apparently decided he must act, both for the safety of the expedition and to show Colombian opinion that he was continuing an active policy, and on March 27 Güepi was captured, assuring an open supply route from Pasto to Caucaya, about a third of the way down the Putumayo to Tarapacá. The Güepi engagement was the final encounter in the Leticia conflict. The Colombian government admitted that four of its soldiers were killed and claimed that twenty-four Peruvians were captured and ten killed; the remainder of a garrison estimated at five hundred escaped. The Peruvian government asserted that Colombia was now clearly the aggressor, since Güepi was a Peruvian outpost in uncontested territory. Lima's announcement of the recapture of Güepi on April 17 was no more than a false statement issued for domestic political purposes; Bogotá calmly denied that there was any enemy activity at Güepi, and in May the falsity of the Peruvian claim became evident when the Peruvian delegate in Geneva said his government "attached great importance" to the inclusion in the armistice agreement of the statement that "Leticia and Güepi should be evacuated simultaneously" because "the mention of Güepi would counterbalance that of Leticia." [31]

The action at Güepi was reported to the League Council by Peru, and it may have been of some influence in contributing to the Advisory Committee's adoption of a third plan for settlement in Leticia, known as the "Lester modifications," presented to both countries on April 7.[32] The most important part of the Lester modifications was the elimination from the March 18 plan of the provision that Leticia was to be returned to Colombian authority; they proposed that a League commission would "take charge" of Leticia, during further negotiations but said nothing whatever about the resumption of Colombian sovereignty. This represented a real concession to the Peruvian contentions maintained during and since the Mello Franco mediation, and Lima promptly accepted the proposal.

It is possible that the Lester modifications originated in Lima; *Peru Ilustrado* of April 10, 1933, stated that this "appeared" to have been the case and that the British and Italian ministers in Lima took part in the formulation of the proposal.[33] At any rate, London exerted strong pressure in Bogotá. Caffery reported that

the Colombian authorities are much intrigued to know why the British Government continues to insist on its accepting the Lester modifications . . . the British Government has been able to persuade the French, German and Italian Governments to renew their recommendations here that the Colombian Government accept the Lester modifications.[34]

Acting immediately on the receipt of the Lester modifications, the Department of State sent them to Caffery, stating that "as this appears to offer a reasonable solution of the difficulty, you are authorized to discuss it with President Olaya and to say that the Department very much hopes that he will find it possible to accept." [35]

Olaya, however, reminded Caffery "of the many times he has supported unpopular proposals in the face of a hostile public opinion when he believed in the justice of the cause . . . but this time he says he can not fight the public. . . . Santos at Geneva is strongly opposed to Lester's modifications as are all political leaders here." [36]

Two days later, Ambassador Freyre gave a memorandum to Under Secretary William Phillips, announcing Peru's acceptance of the Lester modifications and stating that "any friendly suggestion to the Colombian Government, tending to advise them also to accept these proposals, would be appreciated." Freyre said that "President Olaya would need some friendly council [sic], in order to overcome the political drive which might be made against him if he should decide to accept the League proposal." Freyre mentioned President Roosevelt's "use of the term 'good neighbor,' the Secretary's reference to 'good neighbor' yesterday, and said that he hoped the United States would now use its influence as a good neighbor in an appeal to Colombia." [37] In his memorandum of this talk, Phillips did not record that he made any statements whatever to Freyre in response to this early interpretation of the good neighbor policy, one of the first to be made by a Latin American diplomat. It may be presumed, however, that he did not mention that the United States government had already done precisely what Peru desired nor that Olaya had not found it possible to accept the Department's counsel. Had Freyre called on Phillips two days earlier, he might have been given word that the Department thought the Lester modifications "a reasonable solution" and had so advised Olaya; Freyre might have been pleased to learn of this first instance in the Leticia affair when Lima and Washington were in accord; Phillips might have been gratified to be able to demonstrate to Peru in unimpeachable fashion that the United States was impartial in the dispute, and the opportunity might have been seized to give the good neighbor policy a specific application in the Leticia affair.

There is at least one good reason for reflecting, however, that it was just as well that Freyre had not called on Phillips earlier. This was the nature of the plans Manzanilla was reported to have had in mind for the delivery of Leticia to a League Commission under the' terms of the Lester modifications. Dearing received word "from a most trustworthy source" at the end of April that the Peruvian civilians would not evacuate Leticia and that "the International Commission will receive Leticia from the hands of the Chief of the Peruvian troops upon the express condition of returning Leticia to this Chief the moment the settlement has been reached no matter in what form." Colombian troops in the area would "fall back" from the borders of Leticia "and may not advance unless the Commission so orders." "A plebiscite, a revision of historical documents, the sole will of all the inhabitants, and the former boundaries shall serve as the principal basis for the Commission's investigation." Under this stipulation, since Peruvian troops would reoccupy Leticia whatever the outcome of the work of the League Commission, Peruvian acceptance of the Lester modifications was no more than a temporizing measure, if the report was accurate. For the moment, however, it served to make it appear to Geneva that the onus for rejecting an internationally sponsored settlement was placed on Colombia.[38]

The great difference between Manzanilla's plans at this time and the arrangement reached at the end of May was due entirely to the change of government in Peru that occurred in the first week of that month.

In Lima, *El Comercio* made good use of President Roosevelt's Pan American Day speech on April 12. An editorial on April 16 noted Roosevelt's concern about existing conflicts in Latin America and stated that, in order to carry on a good neighbor policy, it was necessary to remove obstacles that prevent international amity, such as treaties that were not in harmony with "legitimate aspirations of men for liberty and freedom." The Leticia conflict offered an opportunity to apply the Roosevelt formula. "Peru desires to live as a good neighbor with Colombia but cannot do so because of the insuperable obstacle of the errors" of the treaty of 1922, a treaty which Colombia refuses to modify, as shown by its rejection of the most recent proposals from Geneva.

Feeling now in a strong diplomatic position, Solon Polo, a high official of the Peruvian foreign ministry, told Dearing that "something similar to Secretary Stimson's note of January 25th might now very appropriately be sent to Colombia." [39] The Department of State held off and did not declare itself further on the Lester modifications until after receiving Olaya's counterproposal that the League Commission should receive Leticia from Peruvian forces "in the name and representation of the Government of Colombia." [40] Six days later, the Department cabled to London and Geneva that "this new Colombian proposal modifying the Lester Formula offers an eminently fair and reasonable solution." [41]

Whereas the Lester modifications themselves were "reasonable," the Colombian plan was "eminently fair and reasonable"—a distinction that may have reflected the Department's judgment of their respective merits, as well as its views of the degree of emphasis required by its relations with Bogotá and with London and Geneva. From London came word that "the Foreign Office 'deplored these Colombian proposals' since in its opinion Colombia was amply protected under the Lester formula." However, the Foreign Office agreed to support the Colombian position except on the fundamental point demanded in Olaya's counterproposal above. The Department upheld Olaya and on May 2 cabled to London that it "very much hopes, therefore, that the British Government will support this latest proposal in its original form and urge its acceptance at Geneva." [42]

The Foreign Office, however, maintained its position that it would not support Olaya's counterproposal "in its present form," but it was willing to keep on working toward a peaceful solution, and it was continuing talks with Eduardo Santos. The British attitude as expressed by Robert Leslie Craigie, Counselor at the Foreign Office, was that "if an attempt were made to settle the dispute on purely academic and legal viewpoints it might lead to no settlement at all but rather a resort to force. This he felt should be avoided and could be avoided if some way were sought for the Peruvians to withdraw without loss of too much *amour propre*." [43]

In Bogotá, Olaya was deeply concerned. The situation of the expedition on the Putumayo was deteriorating. "In addition to bad weather conditions, the troops are now contending with disease and

I believe that a great many of them are ill. Mosquitoes and other insects exist by the millions, making life for the soldiers far from agreeable; also I believe that their food supply is not very satisfactory." [44] By the end of the month, General Vásquez Cobo, who had been staying for some weeks in the mountains apart from his troops, left Colombia for France without visiting Bogotá.[45]

In addition, a new and menacing move had been made by Peru. A new naval odyssey had commenced, strangely paralleling that of Vásquez Cobo's fleet. Peru, the fourth naval power of Latin America, had finally mobilized its naval forces, which were greatly superior in firepower to those of Colombia. At the end of April a cruiser, the *Almirante Grau*, and two submarines left Callao for an unknown destination, feared in Colombia to be a Colombian port but later shown to be the upper Amazon. They passed through the Panama Canal by May 4 and continued their trip, as the Colombian fleet had ascended the river, by slow stages. The *Grau* could reach Tarapacá during the rainy season and presumably could force the Colombian ships to retire up the Putumayo.[46]

It is not clear why Sánchez Cerro had delayed so long in making use of his navy. However, the cruisers were old, and it may have taken eight months to ready one of them for the long ocean voyage, with the limited facilities available in Peru. In January the Department learned that the cruiser *Bolognesi* had left Callao for Balboa to obtain repairs in the drydock at the Canal. The trip had been arranged with the authorities in Panama by the chief of the United States naval mission in Peru, rather than through the Peruvian Ambassador in Washington, as had been the custom. Although the ship was already en route and actually arrived at Balboa, the Peruvian government was told that drydocking would be refused at the Canal, because "in the case of possible armed conflict between two American states it is the policy of this Government to refrain from facilitating in any way the preparations of either party." [47] The refusal of governmental facilities did not, of course, mean that either Peru or Colombia was prohibited from purchasing vessels or arms from private firms in the United States, and both governments made such purchases. It is possible that the *Bolognesi* would have proceeded to Iquitos when refitted. In the case of the *Grau*, however, no drydocking was requested. The cruiser was capable of making the trip, and the Department of State took the position that the *Grau* might obtain fuel, water, and provisions from private sources in Panama and would be allowed to pass through the Canal.[48]

Finally, Olaya was resisting pressure from European countries to accept the Lester modifications, now accepted by Peru, and he was not hopeful that he would be able to get them changed.[49] About May 1 he cabled to his Special Financial Adviser in the United States, George Rublee, expressing his feeling that the United States "should make some supreme effort to end the conflict between Colombia and Peru, and that if such an effort were made at this time it would succeed." Edwin C. Wilson commented that "this seems simply another instance of Olaya's almost pathetic conviction that this Government is omnipotent and can settle anything if it so desires." [50]

Suddenly, however, the whole situation was transformed. President Sánchez Cerro was assassinated on April 30.[51] The new president named by the Constituent Assembly was General Oscar Benavides, the hero of La Pedrera and a former president. After the battle of Tarapacá, it was reported that he had insisted on returning home and had finally been permitted to do so by Sánchez Cerro on March 25. Benavides was a member of the Civilista Party.[52] He was a close personal friend of Alfonso López, a leader of the Liberal Party in Colombia, a fact that soon became of vital importance in the peace negotiations.[53]

Benavides's assumption of the presidency did not cause the *Grau* to halt. It refueled at Curaçao on May 8 and steamed toward the Amazon.[54]

An imminent crisis developing from the advance of the *Grau* was one of the considerations before the Council's Advisory Committee when it met on May 10 and adopted a new proposal on Leticia to be "presented as the final views of the Committee and not open to amendment." [55] This proposal met Colombian desires in stating that the League's Commission "in the name of the Government of Colombia will take charge of the territory." It also provided for a private communication to go only to Bogotá, stating that the Commission "will call solely on Colombian military and police forces" to maintain order in Leticia. The plan as made public stated merely that the Commission "shall call upon the military forces of its choice" for this purpose.

The Department of State, as in the case of every other League of Nations proposal on Leticia, including the Lester modifications, also gave its support to this proposal, stating in cables to Bogotá and Lima that it was "happy" to say that "in its judgment the recommendations of the Advisory Committee offer a peaceful and honorable means of terminating this unfortunate controversy," and it hoped both governments would accept them.[56]

In Lima this note was not presented immediately to the Foreign Minister because of a new development. Two days after the death of Sánchez Cerro, direct negotiations on Leticia were commenced by Alfonso López and President Benavides. Manzanilla, who had stayed on as Foreign Minister, informed Dearing that López was coming to Lima for talks with the President and that "bases for peaceful settlement will be laid within a week." The Peruvian government did not wish to accept the League proposal of May 10 "and expects to do better in the direct conversations." In this situation, Dearing proposed to Washington that "developments be awaited," but the Department instructed him to deliver immediately its note of May 11.[57] Colombia accepted the League plan, including the private understanding, on May 12.

The *Grau* and the two submarines arrived at Trinidad on May 12 where they "were fueled and given facilities," and they left for the Amazon the next day, probably intending to stop again in the Guianas.[58]

Lopez arrived in Lima on May 15, and left on May 21, after talks in which Benavides agreed to accept the League plan of May 10. Benavides was unable to persuade his cabinet, still composed largely of appointees of Sánchez Cerro, to endorse his agreement with López, but he obtained the approval of a majority of the members of the congress. When López on May 6 had cabled his congratulations on Benavides's becoming President of Peru, Benavides had replied immediately, inviting Lopez to visit him in Lima.[59] López's visit was a risky one for his own political fortunes, since Benavides had announced his intention to carry on the policies of the late

President. At this moment, before the presentation of the League's "final" plan of May 10, Benavides may have hoped to persuade Colombia to accept the Lester modifications, but the final plan was presented before López's arrival.

The decision in Lima to make a sharp turn in policy and accept the League plan may have been due in part to financial problems encountered in preparing for war. In addition, Benavides was reported as stating to the congress:

Peru is not in a position to carry on a war with Colombia with any hope of a satisfactory conclusion. We will probably not be able to withstand the Colombian drive now being made on Puerto Arturo. We are isolated among the countries of the world and our diplomatic position is even worse than our military one. The ships that we have just sent to Pará have had a most unfortunate trip, owing to the united action of the countries at whose ports these ships stop for provisions and fuel. This shows that these countries are united against Peru. I fear that all the countries belonging to the League will shortly withdraw their diplomatic representatives from Lima as a sign of protest; that there may likewise be an embargo on arms and possibly an economic boycott.[60]

There remained details to arrange, but peace had come to Leticia, and, while a renewal of fighting appeared possible more than once in the next year, the two countries, through what Benavides called a " 'humane and serene discussion [of the] Leticia incident for definite and honorable settlement,' "[61] finally reached an amicable understanding.

The details, settled by an agreement signed on May 25, consisted of ways of saving face for Peru and of handling the actual transfer of control of Leticia from the Peruvian forces to the League Commission of three members. Although Lima had been informed of the intention of the Commission to make use only of Colombian troops in Leticia, the Peruvian request that a copy of the Advisory Committee's letter to Bogotá not be officially communicated to Lima had been granted.[62] It was also agreed that the words " 'legitimate interests of Peru' " should appear in identic letters to the two countries from the Committee, together with the statement that Güepi was to be returned to Peru simultaneously with the Commission's assuming the administration of the town of Leticia.[63]

Leticia was evacuated by Peruvian troops, and peacefully delivered to the League commission on June 25.

> The Peruvians have derived considerable satisfaction over the way in which the Peruvian flag was removed from Leticia. A great deal had been made in that country over promises never to haul down the Peruvian flag at that port. . . . The flag was not hauled down but . . . the flag pole with the flag attached was taken up and carried across the river to Peruvian territory, where it was replaced in the ground with the flag still flying.[64]

For the Peruvian flag and flagpole were substituted two flagpoles and two flags: Colombia's red, blue and yellow standard and the blue and white banner of the League of Nations.

President Roosevelt, acting on the advice of Secretary Hull that, "inasmuch as we have cooperated fully with the League in order to bring about a peaceful settlement of this conflict, thus carrying forward your policy of the 'good neighbor,' I earnestly recommend that we should informally advise the League that there would be no objection to an American army officer serving on the Commission," [65] nominated Colonel Arthur W. Brown for appointment by the Council to the Leticia Commission.

The League Commission was to administer the town of Leticia for a maximum period of one year; it had no jurisdiction over the Leticia quadrilateral as a whole. The Commission was to withdraw at the end of a year; the agreement did not provide for the return of Leticia to Colombia at that time. Within the year ending June 19, 1934, Colombia and Peru had agreed to carry on negotiations and the League Council was to stand by, ready to provide good offices if so requested. The agreement of May 25, 1933, therefore, was an armistice; it was not yet clear that peace terms acceptable to both parties could be found, and there had been no arrangement made for what might happen when the Commission left the territory. At the time of the armistice, however, general satisfaction was expressed in both countries. In Peru, "the country is strongly with Benavides on the peace plan, regardless of the reversal of the Sánchez Cerro policy. . . . The attitude of the Army regarding peace is not yet clear. The Army, of course, holds the key to the situation, but most of the officers who have been in Loreto are not anxious for war." [66]

In Colombia, "the reaction of Colombians of all classes" was one of "sincere satisfaction." However, *El País* (Bogotá) and other Conservative papers soon began a campaign against the government for "weakness" in accepting the League's proposal. Although these papers were said to have tried to obtain the support of the army, Chargé Allan Dawson dryly commented: "It will hardly be successful; conditions on the Putumayo have not been such as to lead those actually engaged in military operations in that region to desire their continuation." [67]

Evidence of the good faith and statesmanlike qualities of Olaya is provided in the statement of his position he asked Chargé Dawson to transmit to the Department of State, following the departure of the League Commission and the reoccupation of Leticia by Colombian forces. He spoke of the disastrous consequences of a renewal of hostilities and said it is "incumbent upon him and other men of good will in positions of authority in the two nations to attempt to avoid it if humanly possible." The national honor of Colombia had been satisfied by the return of Leticia, and it might be possible to seek an "equitable and practical" solution of the dispute without "undue insistence" on the provisions of the Salomón-Lozano treaty since sovereignty over Leticia and a portion of the left bank of the Amazon "is not in itself absolutely essential to Colombia."

Olaya recognized that "the Department of Loreto, and perhaps Peru as a whole, has the feeling that possession of Leticia and both banks of the Amazon as far as the Brazilian boundary is vital to its interests." He was willing to consider the possibility that Colombia might cede to Peru the southern part of Leticia in return for sufficient Peruvian territory along the southern bank of the Putumayo to make the Putumayo a Colombian stream until it reached Brazilian territory. Such an arrangement, however, would be dependent on a tactful attitude by Peru at the coming conference at Rio de Janeiro, in which attacks on the Salomón-Lozano treaty would be avoided, and on a new Colombian-Brazilian treaty ensuring freedom of transit of the Amazon for Colombian ships of all types in war and peace. In addition, Olaya hoped that Peru would agree to permit an Ecuadoran delegation to participate in the conference; if so, he thought a settlement might be arranged between those countries that would give Ecuador some territory along the upper Putumayo and allow Peru to have full jurisdiction along the lower Napo River. This suggestion for a settlement of these two disputes was based in part on Olaya's judgment that " 'past experience has shown that a river is a bad boundary between neighbors of comparable strength.' " [68] At the conference, it was not found advisable to make such a compromise settlement, and, in view of the strength that Lozano was subsequently able to muster against the protocol, it is highly doubtful that such settlement could have received the consent of the Colombian congress.

The amassing of war materials continued in both countries despite the armistice, and a lively difference of view came to light, with the publication in *La Prensa* (New York), on May 27, of a letter by Lozano Torrijos. Minister Lozano, as the Colombian negotiator of the Salomón-Lozano treaty, was watchfully jealous of his creation, and quick to resist any hint, however wispy, that it might be changed. His letter, written in answer to a news despatch to the effect that the forthcoming negotiations would aim at a settlement of the "territorial dispute," asserted that the negotiations would have nothing to do with territorial matters but would deal only with commercial and navigation matters. In a reply of June 5 in the same daily, Ambassador Freyre referred to the phrase in the agreement of May 25, stating that the "legitimate interests of Peru" should be considered in the negotiations, as grounds for asserting that there could be no exclusion of the territorial question from the agenda. This interchange did not affect the policies of the two governments, and negotiations were begun in Rio de Janeiro early in October, 1933.

Mediation: Third Phase

The talks went very slowly depite the best efforts of Mello Franco, who, after his resignation as Foreign Minister of Brazil, agreed to continue to assist the two delegations. By the end of the year, Olaya was reported by Minister Sheldon Whitehouse as evidently considering that war was "not only possible but probable." [69] Shortly afterward, Minister Lozano asked that the United States government send an aviation mission to Colombia to help improve Colombian military aviation. Edwin C. Wilson told Lozano that this could not be done: "We must of course be careful to be absolutely impartial in this question . . . the apprehension which the Colombians felt regarding future developments in the matter were an added reason for us to be scrupulous." [70]

During the first few months, the United States took no part in the negotiations at Rio de Janeiro, officially or unofficially. After the turn of the year, prompted perhaps by reports of preparations for war, the Department of State bestirred itself to give the impression that it was again willing to be helpful if asked. Secretary Hull, recently returned from his trip up the west coast of South America on the way home from the Montevideo conference, told Ambassador Freyre "very delicately" that some journalists who were impartial on the question,

suggested to me the fear, if not the belief, on their part that those two countries [Colombia and Peru] were unduly suspicious of each other's purpose and attitude and that both were secretly arming, whereas if either should cease doing so the other would be glad to do so. I said that of course I was a warm friend alike of both countries and that I earnestly hoped this rumor or report was inaccurate. I said that it would break the hearts of all the friends of peace in this Hemisphere if two outstanding nations like Peru and Colombia could not avoid hostilities, but should allow themselves to be dragged into war. I inquired whether the land in the Leticia controversy was of any value, and he [Freyre] said, "None." I said, "Then it is a task for statesmen which they unquestionably should be able to meet by preventing hostilities." . . . I stated that if contrary to our anxious desire there should occur any complications in the future that might be solved by a simple remark here or there by wholly disinterested friends of the two countries and anxious friends of peace, that I hoped he would let me know. [71]

The meetings in Rio de Janeiro were stalled. There was "dissension" in the Peruvian delegation, and little work was possible during the conference at Montevideo. [72] Ambassador Hugh Gibson was asked to discover whether active negotiations might be resumed, and he reported in mid-February that Mello Franco was getting the delegates together to recommence the talks. Mello Franco was not pessimistic, although he feared press campaigns might develop in

Colombia and Peru. "He is informed that both Governments are purchasing arms and is unofficially urging upon the two delegations that if they hope to maintain the ascendency of the civil authorities over the military they must come to a [prompt?] and reasonable agreement." [73]

The *Almirante Grau* had returned to Peru in August without going up the Amazon, but Peru purchased two destroyers in Esthonia, and in February, 1934, one of these was stationed at Ramón Castilla, across the river from Leticia. Colombia countered by buying two destroyers that a British firm had nearly completed for Portugal. Both countries were purchasing airplanes from manufacturers in the United States. The Colombian government apparently hoped that it might secure planes with the aid of a loan from the "new organization for the financing of American foreign trade," which was the subject of a bill in the United States Congress, but Edwin C. Wilson marginally commented on the despatch containing this suggestion: "This Govt. shld. not assist." [74]

After making a trip to the area early in February, Allan Dawson concluded: "The general feeling of everyone in the region, Colombians, Peruvians, Brazilians, and others, seems to be that a resumption of hostilities after the expiration of the League Commission's term of office is certain." [75] This opinion was buttressed by the view of Minister Sheldon Whitehouse that "an impasse at Rio is almost certain to lead to hostilities." He wrote to Hull that "four million dollars in foreign exchange have just been thrown away by the Colombian Government for the purchase of two British-built Portuguese destroyers, and further large expenditures for military aircraft are in prospect." He suggested that the United States initiate talks "with the other American Powers" in the near future about the policy to be followed when the League Commission left Leticia in June. Hull replied that, in view of Mello Franco's work and the vigilance of the League of Nations agencies, it appeared better to wait until June 19, and then, if necessary, "urge upon both Governments the desirability of extending the League's mandate. . . . As you know, we are deeply interested in this situation and it is of course our policy to do everything that we can appropriately to use our moral influence on behalf of peace." [76]

As a result of the vagueness of the agreement of May 26, 1933, about what would happen when the Commission left Leticia, this question became acute in the spring of 1934. Whitehouse informed Washington that the members of the Commission "expect to turn that territory over to the Colombian authorities at the expiration of their year's mandate." [77] This was also the view of League officials in Geneva, who were concerned, however, about the possibility that, if Colombia sent a new body of troops to occupy Leticia on the departure of the Commission, hostilities with Peruvian forces might be provoked. [78]

Minister Wilson reported that on these and other points League officials "would be very grateful for our confidential advice. It has been my experience that the small committees have usually come to us for confidential advice and any views which we might express would be given due weight and would, I believe, be appreciated." Offering advice in Geneva, however, was a responsibility the Department decided to avoid, and it replied that, since Mello Franco remained optimistic and because "for the moment at least we do not feel sufficiently informed of all developments and details of this matter," the Department did not wish "to venture an expression of views." [79]

At this moment, it seemed that the time had come for the utterance of what Secretary Hull in his talk with Freyre had called "a simple remark here or there by wholly disinterested friends of the two countries and anxious friends of peace." Freyre himself called on Assistant Secretary Sumner Welles to inquire about the negotiations at Rio. Welles gave him some information and said that

it would be a sad commentary upon the progress of civilization in this continent if, after the twelve months period had elapsed, two of the great powers of the American hemisphere were not able in a fair and just manner to solve this dispute without resorting once more to armed hostilities. . . . I asked the Ambassador, in reply to his Government, to state our deep interest and our frank concern as well as our hope that negotiations might be expedited in a friendly and frank manner either at Rio or in any other way upon which the two governments might determine which would render it possible when the month of June came for the continent not to be faced with the possibility of another war.

On parting from Welles, "the Ambassador stated, significantly, in my judgment, that frequently a government which found itself in the position in which Peru now found herself needed leadership to extricate her from that difficulty, and in what better place, he remarked, could such leadership be found than the Department of State in Washington."

To this open appeal, Welles recorded that "I told the Ambassador before he left that I would be very grateful to him for any information which he might receive which would throw light upon the existing situation and upon the manner in which the discussions between Peru and Colombia are progressing." [80]

Welles viewed the situation with greater equanimity than Whitehouse, who cabled that the news from Rio was bad, that the Peruvian delegates had tried to question the validity of the Salomón-Lozano treaty, and that the Colombian government "had decided that the only course to take was to prepare for war in the hope that if Colombia showed herself sufficiently prepared Peru might hesitate to begin hostilities." Whitehouse's policy recommendation was: "If the disastrous expenditures are to be stopped pressure must be brought on Peru to take immediate concrete steps to prove that her pacific assurances have some meaning. Colombian Government is also acting in haste from fear that the Amazon might be closed which would be more disadvantageous to them than to the Peruvians." [81]

A few days later came word from Colombia that Alfonso López hoped that Secretary Hull "would use all your influence at Lima to make the Peruvian Government see common sense." [82]

Confronted with alarming reports of preparations for war, with requests from both parties for "leadership" and "influence," and with news from Geneva that the Advisory Committee was meeting on April 12, coupled with the suggestion from Wilson that "if we hold strong views on any of the points mentioned it would be well for me to have them as soon as possible since a good deal of work can be done quietly in anticipation of the meeting," [83] the Department decided that the time for action had at last arrived. However, its action did not go further than to suggest to Mello Franco that he take action. A cable was sent to Wilson stating that the Department had no desire to express any opinion on the points he had raised. A cable was also sent to Gibson in Brazil, asking him to suggest to Mello

Franco that, since the parties seemed deadlocked, he might now come forward with a proposal of his own.

If a reasonable proposal were made by Mello Franco, who is so widely known for his high sense of impartiality and justice, it might conceivably meet with the approval of the two Governments, which could satisfy their public opinion by explaining that while they had invariably declined every proposal made by the opposing side, they did not feel that they could afford to disapprove an equitable solution proposed by such an outstanding personality as Mello Franco, representing the fervent desire and appeal of the American countries for a peaceful solution of this difficulty.

Gibson was to tell Mello Franco "that it would be a matter of deep gratification and relief to your Government to hear that he had proposed on his own initiative to both delegations a fair and just solution giving hope of a peaceful and lasting settlement of this difficult question."

At the same time, Gibson was to

make it abundantly clear to him that the last thing we have in mind is any attempt to interfere with his handling of the situation; and that our views as set out above arise from our anxiety over the situation between the two countries and our desire to be of any assistance we appropriately can to him in his work for a peaceful settlement.[84]

Mello Franco's response to this idea was a counterproposal. As Gibson reported it, he

raised the question whether as being a perfectly excellent solution, you would feel disposed to have a talk with the Peruvian Ambassador and ask him as of your own motion why the whole matter could not be simplified by Peru taking the initiative in expressing regrets for the incidents of September 1st (which she has maintained were caused by rebellious frontiersmen) and furthermore for the burning of the Colombian Legation in Lima. . . . He particularly stressed the fact that if you decide to broach this idea it should be as one which occurred to you without reference to any suggestions from Rio de Janeiro. . . . It seems clear to me that he felt there was greater hope of the matter being entertained sympathetically by both sides if the suggestion should come from you in informal conversation.[85]

There was no indication in this cable that Mello Franco had any plan of his own to propose, although he expressed appreciation for the Secretary's suggestions. Gibson reported that Mello Franco's counterproposal was based on his knowledge that two of the junior delegates, Victor Andrés Belaunde of Peru and Luis Cano of Colombia, "have been working very privately and without the knowledge of the chief delegates" on a plan for Peru's expressing regret for the occupation of Leticia, acknowledging the validity of the treaty of 1922, and "proposing arbitration." [86] If the suggestion for this solution could come from Washington, Mello Franco felt that it might be helpful; he could not suggest it himself without the risk of compromising the two delegates who had been in contact with him.

Another complication in Rio de Janeiro was caused by a characteristically false report given to Mello Franco by Maúrtua, then in the city as one of the principal Peruvian delegates, that "the Department supported the Peruvian stand in regard to the prolongation of the mandate" of the Leticia Commission.[87] Gibson said that Mello Franco "did not seem to take this too seriously," but the Department took it seriously enough to reply: "We of course have made no statement to the Peruvian Ambassador which would warrant such an impression." [88]

The Department replied to Mello Franco's counterproposal that "while we are somewhat [inclined?] [*sic*] to doubt the wisdom of our making the suggestion to the Peruvian Ambassador mentioned by Mello Franco, we will give careful consideration to the idea and will advise you later." [89] This advice, however, does not seem to have been sent, and it became unnecessary after Mello Franco on April 24 presented a protocol that, after considerable revision, became the text of an agreement signed on May 24 and, after a year and a half, with the exchange of ratifications, was turned into the document marking the settlement of the Leticia dispute.

The settlement became possible as the result of a change in the position of the government of Peru. The reasons for this change are not fully known, but some of the considerations involved may be suggested, after a brief review of the situation in Lima and of Peruvian attitudes toward the United States. As late as May 8, Dearing's opinion was that "it is impossible to predict what course this Government may pursue." [90] In his talks with Solon Polo, who had replaced Manzanilla as Foreign Minister, and with President Benavides, he had not been able to find any indication that the government was ready to compromise. Polo had "sought again to impress upon me the disturbance that would result within Peru, declaring that the people would be simply *'incontenible'* (uncontrollable) in case the League should withdraw and Colombia should take possession of Leticia prior to an accord being reached at Rio de Janeiro." [91]

President Benavides, in a talk with Dearing, "definitely voiced the desire of his Government for the return of Leticia to Peruvian sovereignty and the intention to work the problem out along that line if possible." He also spoke of the "adverse reaction" in Loreto that the return of Leticia would provoke and dwelt on the view that "the Leticia doorway was useless for Colombia," since a land approach was "practically impossible" and Colombia could reach the Amazon by way of the Putumayo. Dearing did not encourage Benavides in any of these suggestions. "I endeavored to get him to see some of the results of drifting into war, but he gave no very tangible evidence that they made much impression upon him, bothered him or changed his point of view." [92]

The drift toward war was continuing. Colombia was readying a new expedition to occupy Leticia on the withdrawal of the League Commission; the 150 Colombian troops which the Commission had utilized in Leticia to aid its administration would then be substantially reinforced. Peruvian naval personnel left in mid-April for the United States, where new river gunboats were nearing completion at a private shipyard. Colombia was recruiting airplane pilots in the United States, and the Peruvians made another attempt to get one of their cruisers, the *Bolognesi*, repaired at the Panama Canal. Repairs at the Canal had been permitted for the *Almirante Grau* in August, 1933, on its return trip to Peru. Acting Secretary of State William Phillips had considered that, while the general policy that had prevented the *Grau's* being repaired on her outward journey would continue to be followed, it now seemed that the circumstances of the acceptance of the League's recommendations by both countries warranted such repairs and provisioning as would be provided under normal conditions.[93]

These last two moves caused considerable resentment in official circles in Lima, which Washington attempted to allay with no more than partial success. The recruiting of pilots for service in the Colombian forces was stopped by the Department of State, which pointed out to Lozano that such action was "in violation of the spirit, if not the strict letter of the law." [94]

The Department stated publicly that "the Government of the United States disapproves of American citizens taking service in the armed forces of any foreign Government and if Americans do so it is on their sole responsibility and risk and they cannot look to their own Government for protection while in such service." [95] The Department refused to issue passports to Americans signing contracts to serve in the Colombian forces, but it did issue passports to Americans who signed contracts to serve as instructors for the Colombian air force, and several American pilots left for Colombia on April 12 under this arrangement. [96]

Concerning the *Bolognesi*, in which it was desired to have new boilers installed and which arrived suddenly and unexpectedly at Balboa on April 10, the Department maintained the position it had taken the previous year; it allowed the cruiser to take aboard the boilers that had been shipped from Great Britain but would not permit their installation. President Benavides told Dearing that he had prevented the publication of "a flood of messages" on the Department's decision, "as they were of so incendiary a character that for them to be published would undoubtedly arouse resentment against the members of the American colony and he was anxious for that not to happen." [97] The Department was not turned aside from its policy of impartiality in the refusal of United States governmental facilities to either country, by the threat implied in Benavides's remark. Although it was not uncommon for United States diplomats to express to the Department their fears for the safety of United States nationals in Latin American countries, this remark by Benavides is unusual in hinting that he had it within his power to treat the members of the American colony as hostages to try to force a change in the policy of the United States. [98]

These incidents gave rise anew to the feeling in Lima that the

United States was "partial to Colombia." Dearing stated that "the fact that Colombia happens to be quite justified in her attitude towards Peru's ruthless seizure of Leticia does not much change the Peruvian point of view, and it will be inevitable that expressions of this resentment at what is considered to be our favoritism, will appear from time to time." [99]

Resentment of what Lima called partiality toward Colombia did not mean that Peruvians would have been satisfied with what they would have admitted to be impartiality on the part of the United States. The President of the Council of Ministers, José de la Riva Agüero y Osma, complained to Dearing about Colombian "dilatoriness" at Rio de Janeiro and said that "a friendly word from our Government to Colombia to cease obstruction would effect a satisfactory arrangement and dissipate the fast growing menace of an unfortunate incident, hostilities, and war, long drawn and disastrous." Dearing thought this "meant, if it meant anything, that we should frankly espouse the Peruvian point of view." Riva Agüero said that "in spite of our good neighbor policy we are not as disinterested as we assert, and do and can exert direct influence in political situations in this part of the world." This remark gave Dearing a chance to expound the good neighbor policy:

I told him that it was fine, of course, for our Government to interfere with advice in political situations in South America so long as the nations concerned happened to like it, but that if they did not, we were immediately accused of a number of crimes and of being a sort of monster endeavoring in some subtle way to implant our ideas and make them prevail. I stressed it to him that our Government's present policy of the good neighbor was completely and absolutely sincere, and there could be no doubt about it whatever, that it was a cardinal point with us that our South American friends should be left alone to work out their salvation in their own ways, and that particularly when questions become difficult, they should energetically and self-sacrificingly search within their own capacities the means for just and reasonable settlements. I pointed out moreover that except on the basis of an absolute impartiality and a complete friendliness for both sides, and that possibly even then, indications from our Government as to what should be done involved a very great responsibility and one which having been assumed could not casually be laid aside, and that later developments in the exercise of such a responsibility might not prove to be acceptable even to the nation so earnestly invoking good offices in immediate circumstances.[100]

The position of the United States, Peru, and Colombia was discussed at this time by *El País* (Bogotá) in an article of May 11, 1934; *El Mundo Gráfico* (Lima) was quoted as saying that with United States money Colombia was able to buy war materials and hire foreign military men and that in this situation Peru was forced to proceed with

"prudence and calmness, to develop a friendly arrangement with Colombia on the basis of respect for the Salomón-Lozano treaty, knowing that behind Colombia is the protecting hand of the United States, an imperialist and acquisitive [*absorbente*] country that is the real arbiter of the nations of this continent, who, instead of engaging in mutual alienation, ought to move toward unification in order to withstand the common danger which menaces them."

El País denied that the United States had given any aid to Colombia, but it used the occasion to attack President Olaya for his pro-United States policy, asserting that to his Calvinist temperament

success and money are the only possible virtues of man. . . . The true American danger is not in North America but in the docile instruments that Anglo-Saxon capitalism employs in our countries to solidify its imperialist power. Only fortifying ourselves resolutely in the soil of our ancestors can we liberate ourselves from the forceful influences of other races.

The views of *El Mundo Gráfico* are of interest as showing the difficulty the United States found in divesting itself of its influence and presumed interests, even when it attempted to act with greatest impartiality. This statement also demonstrates that the attribution to the United States of power to dominate a situation in South America may provide a useful means of escape—a lightning rod—for a state that for other reasons decides to adopt a line of action that, but for the opportunity to attack the United States, might cause it to be diplomatically embarrassed. This same function, of course, is also one of the principal services provided by international political organizations, as was well illustrated by the participation of the League of Nations in the Leticia dispute. What better reasons could be alleged for Peru's final willingness to accept Mello Franco's formula than the official one that the action was being taken as a contribution to American unity and friendship and the unofficial one that there was no other course because of the concentration of the power of influence of the United States on the side of Colombia?

The effective reasons, as distinct from the formal justifications, for Peru's acceptance of the Mello Franco proposal, were undoubtedly more complex than the available evidence suggests. One of them appears to have been the lamentable unreadiness of the Peruvian navy, as evidenced by the *Bolognesi*'s need for new boilers, compared with the capacity of Colombia shown by the arrival at Trinidad on May 22 of Colombia's reoccupation expedition consisting of two transports bound for Leticia with 1,650 troops.[101]

A second reason appears to have been a financial one. Dearing reported on April 12 that the Peruvian Secretary of the Treasury was opposed to the continuation of the war,[102] and it appeared that the government was having serious difficulty in financing its existing scale of preparations. Connected with this consideration may have been the realization that no financial return could be expected from regaining control over Leticia. Profitable rubber operations in the region had ceased with the development of plantation production in Southeast Asia, and the principal remaining export was timber, largely mahogany. Even if the whole of the quadrilateral were secured by Peru, the prospects that either the economic or the strategic value of the place would be significant in the visible future were remote. It was the opinion of one of the Colombian delegates at the Rio de Janeiro mediation meeting that the fact that "General Benavides knew the Amazon territory so well had been a factor of great importance in reaching a peaceful settlement; that centuries would pass before the region would be of any value to mankind; and that the area in dispute was not worth the lives of 'ten Colombians or ten Peruvians.' "[103]

In the third place, President Benavides was apparently seriously concerned about the attitude and possible reactions of other countries in case of war. Dearing's view was that "the approaching embargo on the shipment of arms and munitions of war to the Chaco, which could so easily have been extended to the Leticia conflict, has tremendously aided and speeded up the decisions reached in Rio de Janeiro." [104]

In addition, there is some evidence that Lima was worried about the possible entry of Ecuador on the side of Colombia if war should come. Early in the course of the Leticia dispute, Quito had declared in a note to all American governments that "Ecuador is and will be an Amazonian nation." [105] Dearing reported that

the present opportunity would seem to be the most favorable one Ecuador has had since 1830 to obtain the recognition by both its neighbors of its rights to part of the Amazon. . . . It is clear that the sudden realization that Ecuador could seize the opportunity of hostilities between Peru and Colombia to assert its claim to half the Department of Loreto, has tempered the ardor of the directors of Peruvian foreign policy. This attitude of Ecuador may conceivably be the factor which will decide Peru to retreat from its position regarding Leticia. [106]

A possible alliance of Ecuador with Colombia apparently did not strongly influence Sánchez Cerro, but it may have been important in the thinking of Benavides, a more cautious man. The dispute with Ecuador involved territories far larger than Leticia, and it may well have seemed prudent to Benavides to relinquish dubious claims to Leticia in order to avoid any risk whatever that Peru's position with respect to Ecuador might later be weakened.

Finally, Benavides had by this time strengthened his internal political position. Gradually the Sánchez Cerro supporters had been removed from positions of power, and on May 15 the resignation of Riva Agüero took from the Cabinet one of the strongest advocates of the retention of Leticia. Benavides's survival of the ensuing Cabinet crisis was evidence of his political strength. If the President was strong, he must have made satisfactory arrangements with the Peruvian army, and this meant that the army was satisfied that the Mello Franco formula provided a solution satisfactory for itself and for the nation. The acquiescence of the army may also have involved other considerations; it may at least be speculated that it received promises that it would be strengthened in the future. It is possible that a lesson had been learned in Leticia; communications overland with Iquitos were so difficult that Peru could not quickly exert military power in Loreto, and the country's lack of an air force had been demonstrated as an element of weakness even in comparison with Colombia, which was in the same position at the start of the Leticia incident.

Once the Peruvian decision was taken, about the middle of May, agreement was only ten days away. The part of the United States in the final arrangements appears to have been a small one. On May 17, identic telegrams were sent to the missions at Bogotá and Lima requesting them to advise the foreign ministers orally that the United States government regarded the Mello Franco formula "as equitable and as offering an honorable and peaceful method of reaching a permanent solution of this serious controversy" and hoped that it would be accepted by both countries.[107] In commenting on this action, Dearing noted that until May 10 there was still intransigence on both sides. "Happily, almost simultaneous Cabinet changes in both countries assisted the issue, and the kindly intervention of our own Government served to induce both Peru and Colombia to make the necessary concessions, rendering a peaceful solution possible." [108] This appears, however, to have been an overstatement of the situation, since the Peruvian government's determination to accept the general lines of Mello Franco's proposal had been reached three days earlier, and the views of the Colombian government were already close to the terms of the current revision of the Mello Franco formula.

In the Protocol of Peace, Friendship and Cooperation and Additional Act of May 24, 1934, the mediatory ability of Mello Franco, coupled with the forbearance of the Colombian delegation, achieved the agreement that settled the Leticia dispute without any mention whatever of the territory or town of Leticia or of the regaining of sovereign authority over Leticia by Colombian forces.[109] The nearest reference to Leticia was the statement in the first article that "Peru sincerely deplores, as she has previously declared, the events which have taken place since September 1, 1932, which have disturbed her relations with Colombia." The protocol managed also to avoid any reference to the League of Nations, whose officials might have been entitled to feel that that organization had been rather ungraciously treated. Not only did the preamble of the Protocol state simply that Colombia and Peru were in the process of "executing the agreement adopted by them in Geneva on May 25, 1933," but it went on blandly to point out that both countries

assert as a fundamental duty of States the proscription of war . . . That this duty is the more agreeable for the States which compose the American community, among which exist historical, social, and sentimental ties, which cannot be weakened by divergencies or events that must always be considered in a spirit of reciprocal understanding and good will.

In substance, the two countries agreed to renew diplomatic relations, and they stated that the treaty of 1922 was a "juridical tie" that "may not be modified or affected except by mutual consent of the parties or by a decision of International Justice within the terms below established in Article 7." This article provided for recourse to the Permanent Court of International Justice under Article 36 of the Court's statute. Colombia and Peru obligated themselves not to make war or employ force for the solution of any problems whatever arising between them, and they agreed to continue negotiations "in order that all pending problems may receive a just, lasting, and satisfactory solution." A commission was established to demilitarize the frontier between the two countries, and in the Additional Act there was made a series of agreements about matters of transit, navigation, and customs. The apparently incomplete nature of the agreement was made possible by the fact that with the retirement of the League Commission, the Colombian troops there would simply remain in possession and Colombia's sovereignty over Leticia would be reestablished.

President Roosevelt sent his "heartiest" congratulations to Olaya, and his "warmest" congratulations to Benavides on the signing of the Leticia protocol. Dearing commented from Lima:

Such congratulations are of great significance and effect in Latin American countries, as can be readily appreciated by a glance at the local newspapers which carry a long list of messages of felicitation exchanged between the President and the Minister for Foreign Affairs, the heads and foreign ministers of various Governments, and other prominent personages. It is one of the best ways in the world in which to assure the local Administration of its worth and identity and to give it the moral courage and support needed to persevere in the laudable and proper course which has at last and with so much difficulty been decided upon.[110]

The news was greeted with acclaim in both countries. In Lima "a solemn Te Deum was held in the Cathedral on May 26th, and on the 28th a parade of unequalled proportions took place to manifest the satisfaction of the people and their gratitude to the Administation which had accepted the settlement and saved the country from a needless and disastrous war."[111] In Loreto also there was general acceptance of the agreement, and none of the forecasts of forcible protests were fulfilled. When the League Commission withdrew from Leticia, the town was "turned over to the Colombian Government . . . without incident."[112]

The United States and the Protocol of Rio de Janeiro

There remained only the exchange of ratifications of the protocol, which had provided for the completion of this action by December 31, 1934. The Peruvian constituent assembly approved the protocol by a vote of 61 to 11 on November 2, 1934.

In Colombia, ratification was dragged out over many months and the United States took one more part in the drama's long run. President Olaya's term of office ended shortly after the signature of the protocol, and he was succeeded by Alfonso López. The members of the Conservative Party in the Senate, led by Laureano Gómez, the owner of *El País*, decided to make ratification a partisan issue, and, when they were joined by Lozano Torrijos, the proud author of what he called the Lozano-Salomón treaty and a nominal Liberal, the fate of the protocol appeared to be in doubt. Lozano was not satisfied with the outcome of the Leticia dispute, even though in effect "his" treaty had been upheld. He took the position that the protocol should be rejected because there existed the possibility that the treaty of 1922 might be brought into question before the Permanent Court of International Justice.[113]

In Lima these developments were regarded with concern, and the Foreign Minister again raised the bugaboo of possible adverse reactions in Loreto if ratification was not completed by the end of the year. Polo "definitely inquired whether our Government would be willing in the interest of peace and good understanding to send some appropriate message to López or at least make an inquiry which would make the Colombian Government aware of our interest and concern." [114]

The Secretary of State, acting on these appeals, authorized Chargé Samuel W. Washington to say to the Colombian Foreign Minister that "we wish to express our interest in the maintenance of friendly relations among the American states and our confident hope" that the protocol "may receive ratification in Colombia" before December 21.[115]

The sending of this message was appreciated in Lima, but it caused an uproar in a secret session of the Colombian senate on December 26. The acting Foreign Minister informed the senate of the receipt of messages from the United States and Brazil, hoping this news might help bring about ratification. However, it was reported that, on the contrary, Laureano Gómez was inspired to make a patriotic speech, "declaring that the matter of ratifying the treaty is to be determined by the Colombian Congress, and it alone, and that it would stand no interference from foreign imperialistic powers." [116] Although the Colombian house of representatives approved the treaty, with most of the Conservatives absent, the situation in the senate was so delicate that on December 29 President López extended the extraordinary session of congress "to enable it to finish its study of the Rio pact." [117]

The strength of the Conservative Party in the senate was shown in January when Lozano Torrijos was elected President for that month by a vote of 29 to 26; the majority included 27 Conservatives, Lozano, and one other Liberal.[118] Chargé Washington reported that Olaya said President López was thinking of getting the time for ratification extended so that it might be completed after election of a hopefully Liberal congress in May, 1935. One of the Conservatives stated that he and some other senators "would now willingly allow the pact to pass if there were some way by which they could save their faces." On the question of the expression by the United States of hope for ratification, made on December 15, Olaya said he thought this and other messages from abroad "did a lot of good," which was useful even though the opposition tried to capitalize them in a secret session of the senate. "I believe that if an appeal is made by any foreign countries now it should be done publicly so as to affect Colombian public opinion and I strongly urge that nothing be done to make it appear that the appeal is led or promoted principally by the United States." [119]

Although a request was made of the Department of State by the Peruvian Ambassador on January 24 to "send a message to our Minister in Bogotá urging that the Protocol be disposed of and not shelved," Under Secretary Phillips, acting on the advice of Edwin C. Wilson, decided to take no action at the time.[120]

The reluctance of the Department of State to be criticized a second time in Colombia apparently caused it to make no further attempt to influence the course of the debate in the Colombian Congress. When the question arose in Bogotá whether Mello Franco had been accurately quoted on an interpretation of one of the articles of the protocol, Olaya, who became Foreign Minister on February 5, asked whether the Department of State would indicate to Mello Franco the concern of Bogotá in the matter. Secretary Hull replied that "we cannot escape the feeling that it would be unwise and open to misinterpretation if we should now seek to intervene in a highly confidential matter which has already been the subject of discussion between the Colombian Minister at Rio de Janeiro and Dr. Mello Franco." [121]

This same degree of delicacy was not exhibited by the ministers of France, Great Britain, and Italy in Bogotá, who, at the end of January, expressed the hopes of their governments that the protocol would be ratified. The Advisory Committee of the Council of the League of Nations had reconvened in mid-January, and these governments were presumably expressing the views of the Committee. However, Chargé Washington advised the Department that the situation in the Colombian senate was not within the control of the administration and that "unless the United States Government very much desires to associate itself with the other friendly nations in this gesture in favor of international peace I believe that little can be accomplished by representations to the Colombian Government at this moment." [122]

On February 6 the Colombian senate failed to approve ratification by a vote of 28 to 28; President López immediately brought an end to the session of the congress. In Lima this action was regretted, but Dearing cabled that the news was "received with a remarkable absence of excitement, even the *Comercio* being calm, fair and dignified. It is realized that Lozano's pride and partisan politics are responsible and López, Santos and Olaya are rather confidently expected to be able to control situation eventually and accomplish ratification." [123]

This expectation was realized, with the help of an accommodating attitude in Lima that permitted the extension of the ratification period initially to September 30 and finally to November 30, 1935.[124]

The Colombian senate approved the protocol on August 21, and this action was followed by the house on September 17. Ratifications were exchanged on September 27, 1935, and the Leticia dispute was officially closed. Unofficially, the people in Loreto accepted the settlement.

Relations between Colombians and Peruvians in the border region are reported by Colombian members of the mixed commission to be cordial and peaceful, especially since the ratification of the Rio de Janeiro Protocol. It is interesting to note that a football game was recently played at Leticia between the Colombian garrison team and a Peruvian team from a garrison across the border, a silver cup having been donated by the Colombian Ministry of War.[125]

This happy state of affairs was maintained after 1935, and the boundary question has not since been a source of difficulty between Colombia and Peru. Indeed, this is one of the most secure boundaries in Latin America, for Peru will hardly question Colombia's title to Leticia so long as Ecuador seeks to undermine the validity of the Protocol of Rio de Janeiro of January 29, 1942.

PART THREE

The Marañón Conflict

CHAPTER IX

Origins

IN THE CHACO WAR and in the Leticia dispute the victorious countries enjoyed widespread sympathy in the American states, and both the military decisions and the peace treaties were accepted by the losers. These circumstances made mediation look successful, and diplomatic overstatement about the effectiveness of pacific settlements by American states could be given a gloss of justification.

In the conflict between Ecuador and Peru, however, the military victor had the sympathy of few, and the loser, even after ratifying the treaty, still protests its terms. Consequently, however correct the legal formalities were, the mediation appears to have been unsuccessful. The American states were baffled in this dispute, for they were not at the time prepared to deal with a quick, decisive victory, after which the victor occupied part of the loser's territory until the peace settlement was negotiated. But this was what happened in the conflict between Ecuador and Peru, which will here be called the Marañón dispute, since the principal issue at stake was, and still is, whether Ecuador should possess territory at any point on the northern bank of the Marañón River, the name given the Amazon above Iquitos.

Ecuador and Peru began to dispute the limits of their territorial inheritances from Spain as early as 1829. The dispute concerned a small area on the Pacific Ocean, and some 120,000 square miles in the Oriente lying between the equator and the Javarý River, and between the Andes and Leticia.

The dispute was carried on for a century on three levels—military, diplomatic, and demographic. In the west, between the mountains and the sea, the boundary became fairly well recognized along a series of river courses in the areas of Jaén and Tumbes, where it corresponded roughly to lines of civilian as well as military occupation. In the Oriente, however, the frontier was a fluid one, and throughout the nineteenth and early twentieth centuries there were sporadic, minor clashes of troops in isolated outposts in the region the Peruvians called Mainas.

In diplomatic transactions no decision had been reached at the end of the first hundred years. In 1887 an arbitration convention submitted the whole question to the decision of the King of Spain. The arbitral decision was delayed, pending direct negotiations, and in 1910 the King declined to hand down a verdict. This action was due to a partial and premature disclosure of the terms of the award and to indications by the Ecuadoran government that it would reject the anticipated terms.[1]

There was a war scare in 1910, but it died down after strong representations made at the initiative of the United States and supported by Argentina and Brazil. These three countries firmly declared:

It is unthinkable that Ecuador and Peru should go to war over a boundary dispute which both, by solemn agreement, submitted to arbitration. Neither would it be conscionable to sanction the repudiation of the award in advance by either party, for such sanction would dishonor the enlightened institution of arbitration, to which institution of an advanced civilization the American Republics are committed.[2]

The three states also offered to act as mediators between Ecuador and Peru, and, although the offer was accepted, the mediation did not produce an agreement. At one moment, when Washington thought Ecuador recalcitrant, Minister William C. Fox was instructed to protest in terms considerably stronger than those customary in the more polite days of the good neighbor policy. He was directed "discreetly but forcibly to impress upon the President" the views of the United States that Ecuador's failure to be conciliatory "can only be regarded by this Government as an evidence of (1) a disinclination to reach a peaceful and honorable solution of the boundary difficulty or (2) lack of confidence in the mediating powers." [3] The Ecuadorans opted for peace, honor, and faith and thereafter saw the relative military power of the two countries develop in favor of Peru.

As to the demographic situation, Peruvian settlers, traders, and soldiers gradually extended their occupation of the Oriente region. The Ecuadorans, while maintaining a few troops at outposts like Rocafuerte on the Napo River and a few missionaries at several places, did not establish any civilian population in the Oriente, except in the extreme southwest and northern portions, and did not found any town remotely comparable to Iquitos to serve as a base for economic or political development or for military operations. As late as 1936 it was noted in Washington: "The fact is that there are several thousand Peruvians in the disputed area and relatively few Ecuadorans." [4]

The interest of the government of the United States was engaged in the dispute again in 1924, when Ecuador and Peru, by the Ponce–Castro Oyanguren protocol, agreed that, with the consent of the United States, they would negotiate in Washington about the boundary to determine the questions that they would later submit to arbitration by the President of the United States. The meeting in Washington was delayed for twelve years, and in the meantime attention was drawn to Ecuadoran claims in the Oriente as a result of the Leticia affair. In October, 1932, there was a border incident at the western end of the frontier, caused by disputes over islands formed by changes in the course of the Zarumilla River. The incident itself was settled satisfactorily, but, in conjunction with the possibility of war between Colombia and Peru over Leticia, it was probably influential in the development of what was reported to be "an increasing sentiment on the part of the Ecuadoran public that the Ecuadoran Government should not stand idly by while events which may affect her territorial rights are taking place." [5]

Ecuador did take the occasion to assert its claims in the Oriente through a declaration made to all the American Governments by Foreign Minister Gonzalo Zaldumbide on November 12, 1932:

America is not unaware of the fact that Ecuador is and will be an Amazonian nation. Her geographic location, her numerous juridical rights, the imperative demands of her economic life and the requirements of her normal biological development, the right that every people has to a proportionate territory, and the indisputable fact that the Amazon forms the inland sea and the common outlet toward the East for the countries of this part of the New World make Ecuador's right to be an Amazonian State, as she is and always has been, since the first colonial centuries, irrefutable and indisputable.[6]

At this time Peru was so far from admitting that Ecuador might be an Amazonian nation that, as Ambassador Dearing reported from Lima:

All Peruvian maps for the past twenty-five years have shown the Eastern Ecuadorian frontier to be about twenty kilometers East of Riobamba and Latacunga and only forty kilometers East of Quito. The Peruvian public in general has been so accustomed to this boundary line that they have assumed that it is a definite and uncontested one, and the realization that Ecuador claims immense territory on the Paute, Pastaza, and Napo comes as a shock to almost all the people of Peru.[7]

Ecuador made repeated requests to be invited to take part in the negotiations at Rio de Janeiro over Leticia, but it was excluded because of Peruvian objections.[8] The Department of State took the position that it could not urge Lima to change its attitude.

Beyond making these diplomatic moves, Ecuador was unable to gain any advantage from the involvement of Peru in the Leticia dispute. It is possible, however, that the assertion of Ecuadoran claims to be an "Amazonian nation" may have influenced later Peruvian policy; the impression may have been gained in Peru that a favorable diplomatic settlement was out of the question. If this impression existed, it was probably reinforced when later negotiations failed to find an acceptable basis for a legal decision.[9]

Direct negotiations were reopened in Lima in 1933, and early in 1934 the two governments requested permission to send delegations to Washington for discussions that Ecuadorans hoped would lead to arbitration by President Roosevelt. Assistant Secretary of State Sumner Welles recommended to the President that the United States should "offer to these two Governments our friendly assistance in the manner requested in order that they may arrive at a peaceful solution of their long-standing controversy." [10] This recommendation was approved, both as to the holding of the talks in Washington, and as to the acceptance of the responsibility for giving an arbitral award if the negotiations should succeed.

The conference between the two delegations began in September, 1936, at Washington, on the basis of an agreement signed in Lima on July 6, 1936.[11] One of the important features of this agreement was the provision that the two countries "shall maintain the *status quo* of their present territorial position" in the disputed areas until the termination of the discussions in Washington. The "line of the *status quo* of 1936" was frequently referred to in later discussions. (For an approximation of this line, estimated on the basis of several sources, see Map IV.) [12]

The Peruvian version of the *status quo* line of 1936 was described in a note from Lima to the American states in September, 1936, and it claimed, apparently correctly, that Ecuador then held no positions on the Marañón River. It has been admitted by Julio Tobar Donoso, Foreign Minister of Ecuador during the conflict, that "unfortunately at this time [1936] we had no military post or other sign of possession at the mouth of any of the rivers that enter the Marañón. Our garrisons were far away in the upper parts of these rivers." [13]

The negotiations in Washington were fruitless and were broken off in 1938. Throughout, the government of the United States maintained a position of impartiality and refused to take the initiative in matters such as the suggestion of a compromise boundary line.[14] At one stage the Ecuadoran government appeared to be ready to resort to force, and Under Secretary of State Welles, "seriously preoccupied" by this possibility, asked Ecuadoran Ambassador Colón Eloy Alfaro

how it would be possible for the Government of Ecuador, after the peace treaties which it had signed at the Buenos Aires Conference and in view of the unanimous desire on the part of all of the American Republics there expressed always to resort to peaceful means of adjudicating disputes, now to contemplate hostilities when no act of aggression had been committed against Ecuador by Peru.[15]

The government in Quito did not resort to violence, and it shortly afterward proposed arbitration of the whole controversy by the President of the United States. This suggestion was accompanied by an outline of Ecuador's position as to the boundary line itself and by another reference to the risks of war. President Federico Páez's proposal was reported as follows:

If Peru refused arbitration by President Roosevelt, an agreement be made on the line of the García-Herrera Treaty [1890], submitting to the arbitration of President Roosevelt the zone comprised between the Pastaza and Morona Rivers . . . the Ecuadoran Congress had ratified that line, and the Peruvian Congress had also ratified it with the exception of the zone between the two rivers mentioned. The Minister expressed the belief that this is the most reasonable offer that can possibly be made by his Government. He added, parenthetically, that he would probably be stoned by his own people for such a maximum concession.

The Foreign Minister then expressed the pessimism he feels that Peru will not agree to either proposal. At that moment he became especially agitated and remarked "it would seem that war is our only recourse." [16]

The role played by the Department of State is illustrated by Welles's response to the statement of the Ecuadoran Ambassador that his delegation would accept a prior arbitration of certain points by the World Court if the proposal was first made by the Peruvians. Welles replied that

while this Government was acting as host to the two delegations, it did not possess the functions of mediator nor of intermediary and that, while I was prepared and had been prepared to do everything I could to facilitate the successful termination of the negotiations, I did not feel authorized by either of the two Governments involved to suggest specific solutions or methods of procedure.

However, if he found that the Peruvian delegation favored such a procedure, Welles said he would be willing to state that he thought it would be acceptable to Ecuador. [17]

In a talk with Ambassador Manuel de Freyre y Santander and Francisco Tudela, head of the Peruvian delegation, Welles was told that the principal difficulty between the delegations was whether Ecuador should secure any territory on the north bank of the Marañón or Amazon rivers. Tudela said that "Peru could not possibly agree to relinquish her existing control of these rivers." Welles said he thought this might mean the breakdown of the negotiations and the possible refusal of Ecuador to attend the eighth conference of American states at Lima. Welles then said that "perhaps a way out of the difficulty was to revert to the Peruvian suggestion *re* prior arbitration" and asked for Tudela's opinion about such an arbitration on the points mentioned by the Ecuadoran Ambassador without, of course, mentioning the source of the suggestion. Tudela promised to convey Welles's remarks to Foreign Minister Carlos Concha.[18]

Ambassador Freyre reported to Welles at the end of March that "the Peruvian Government was prepared to accept the suggestions I [Welles] had proffered as a basis for the definitive settlement of the boundary dispute with Ecuador." [19]

However, before the two delegations could work out this hopeful development into an agreement, a frontier clash occurred at Rocafuerte that took on serious proportions when both sides reinforced certain boundary positions. Welles telegraphed both governments, stating that the incident "appears to give ground for concern" but that the United States government was confident that the incident would be adjusted so that the negotiations might proceed "to the successful outcome that is the hope of all." [20] Both governments replied with protestations of pacific intentions, and the dispute's flare-up gradually burned down to its chronic smoky glow.

At this time, and at others in the course of the Marañón dispute, Welles seemed reluctant to exert pressure on the Peruvian government. He appeared to retain a keen appreciation of the resentment by Peruvian officials of Secretary Stimson's denunciation of their government's position in the Leticia affair and, therefore, desired to avoid stirring up comparable resentment in the present case. He does not seem, for example, to have talked to any Peruvian at this time in the terms he used with the Ecuadoran Ambassador on June 10, 1937.

The settlement of the Rocafuerte incident did not bring agreement in Washington, and on August 31, 1938, Ecuador took the venturesome step of sending an announcement to the American states, and to the League of Nations, that Ecuador was proposing to Peru the immediate submission of the entire dispute to President Roosevelt for a "juridical arbitration." [21]

The United States government did not indicate whether it approved or disapproved of the proposal, presumably because this announcement was a request by only one of the two parties.[22]

This move may have been intended by Quito to embarrass Peru, since it had been the Peruvian contention that any arbitral settlement should be based on legal claims only, and not on considerations of equity. It may have been hoped also that the publication of the proposal would either induce a more conciliatory attitude by Peru or place on Peru the responsibility for the anticipated failure of the Washington negotiations.

The Peruvian reaction showed no inclination to make any concessions on the substance of the dispute. On September 29 Concha broke off the Washington talks, giving as a reason the claim that the Ecuadoran proposal for arbitration of the entire question was not contemplated in the Ponce–Castro Oyanguren protocol of 1924. In addition, however, he shocked the new Ecuadoran government headed by Provisional President Manuel María Borrero, by making public an exchange of letters in the spring of 1938 between President Alberto Enríquez Gallo of Ecuador and President Oscar Benavides of Peru in which Enríquez had proposed that, in case the talks in Washington were not successful, they should be continued in Lima. Benavides had accepted this proposal on May 20. Concha was able in this way to turn the tables on the Ecuadoran foreign office and state that, of course, Peru "accedes to the suggestion received, disposed as always to exhaust every pacific effort to settle juridically its boundary dispute." [23]

It later appeared that the existence of President Enríquez's letter was known only to three Ecuadorans—the President himself, his Foreign Minister, and the Minister in Lima—and that it had been sent without consultation with the Cabinet or the Advisory Council. It is hardly likely that the declaration of August 31 would have been made had the new Foreign Minister, Tobar Donoso, known of this correspondence. It is possible that the Enríquez letter may have been prompted by the Ecuadoran Minister in Lima, who felt that a diplomatic, rather than a legal solution, was necessary and who persuaded President Enríquez that he would be able to work out a satisfactory direct settlement with Concha.

The new Ecuadoran government, however, did not wish to go

alone to Lima for further discussion of the dispute. Knowing themselves to be weaker than Peru, they continued the tactics that had brought about the talks in Washington, where they had hoped, unavailingly, to strengthen their position. Quito took the occasion of the announcement of the arbitration award in the Chaco War to request on October 10, 1938, that the states (other than Peru) participating in that arbitration agree to mediate its controversy with Lima; it may have hoped that Washington, freed from the impartial imperatives of a potential arbitrator, might as mediator exert more pressure on Peruvian policy than it had in the recent past.

Before replying, the Department of State sent a memorandum to all its co-mediators in the Chaco dispute, except Peru, that noted that "within the existing peace machinery of this hemisphere there exist procedures believed adequate and effective for bringing about peaceful settlement of disputes between nations" and stated as its view that, if Ecuador wished to go "outside of the peace mechanism established by treaty" to call on the mediators, "such a procedure must also meet with the approval and have the support of the Government of Peru." [24] The other four mediators approved of this position, but on October 12 the Peruvian government stated publicly that no diplomatic action that was not bilateral would be justified, and it followed this immediately with word to Rio de Janeiro and Santiago that it would not accept the Ecuadoran proposal. [25]

Although the United States memorandum had proposed an "exchange of views" among the mediators and had stated that the United States "will await the outcome of the present consultation and any others that may seem necessary in order to bring about this unified approach prior to replying to the message from the President of Ecuador," the Chilean government, without any consultation, sent on October 14 a reply to the Ecuadoran request for mediation, stating that Chile would be pleased to accept if a similar request were also made by Lima. In a memorandum informing Ambassador Norman Armour of this action, the foreign office stated that it would have been pleased to assist the two countries but, " 'due to the existence of negotiations, in the customary diplomatic channels, Peru has declared that it does not accept any intervention in its dispute with Ecuador, which makes impossible at this time, a démarche promising real results.'" [26] The Chileans thus brusquely killed whatever chances this United States initiative may have had.

In these circumstances the Department of State saw no alternative but to inform Quito that the United States would be happy to participate in a mediation if Ecuador and Peru should both desire such action.[27] Since it was known in Washington that Peru opposed mediation and that Chile had previously replied in the same sense, this telegram was an empty gesture. However, there seemed to be no other course open, particularly since the formula had been prepared originally in the Department of State.

Secretary Hull was apparently annoyed at what he called "the precipitancy of Chile." He also stated:

I myself in conversation with the Peruvian Ambassador here have expressed our very earnest hope that Peru would not shut the door to the possibility of permitting other disinterested and friendly American Governments to try and cooperate in assisting Peru and Ecuador to find a satisfactory method for the solution of their dispute.[28]

This is a significant statement, because Hull here placed on Peru the responsibility for "shutting the door" on a mediatory effort. However, the Peruvian government did not feel called upon to take further official action on the Ecuadoran request; its position had been fully safeguarded by the Chilean government, which had both rejected Quito's proposal and broken up any possible move toward the formation of a group of mediating countries. An editorial that appeared on October 20 in *La Prensa* (Lima) may be taken to represent the views of the Peruvian foreign office. It stated that the responses of the five states to Ecuador's unilateral request could not have been different without "causing irreparable damage to the delicate mechanism of conciliation." Peru considered that there was no danger that diplomatic relations with Ecuador would be broken and that direct negotiations would now supersede those undertaken in accord with the 1924 protocol. "A mediation requested by only one party would have been impertinent."

Thus, the American states feebly let slip the last favorable opportunity to end the boundary dispute in peaceful fashion. Despite the spirit and the terms of the conventions of the Buenos Aires Conference and despite the experience gained in the Chaco conflict, long-range mediation by means of diplomatic correspondence was tried once more, and once more found wanting. No attempt was made to breathe life into the principle of consultation or to hold a meeting of the American republics. As had happened so often in the past, the interests of one country had prevented the unity that alone could have produced effective pressure. That the country here in question was Chile was not necessarily cause for censure; other countries had been similarly responsible in other cases. The failure to arrange for consultation or mediation was the result of a lack of single-minded concern for the maintenance of peace coupled with the continued inability to bring rapidly into existence a consultative meeting. The lack of such "machinery" had been deplored, at least in Washington, through the preceding decade. The strength of Peruvian resistance to peace moves by other states was an ominous sign; it was allowed to pass almost unheeded by statesmen who at the time were more deeply concerned with the Munich crisis in Europe.

CHAPTER X

Hostilities

THE DIPLOMATIC FIASCO of the Washington efforts ended for more than two years any attempt by outside states to settle the dispute. The attention of the Department of State was, of course, centered on the great events in Europe and the Far East, and the Latin American states showed no inclination to take an initiative that would be resented by Peru. Negotiations were not renewed on the part of the two disputants.

During the eighth conference of American states, held at Lima in December, 1938, several unofficial attempts were made to gain a settlement of the controversy. Afranio de Mello Franco of Brazil continued talks initiated before the conference; Tobar Donoso vainly proposed several procedures to Concha; and Hull brought his concern to the attention of Concha, whose support in securing the adoption of the conference's declarations of solidarity and American principles Cordell Hull said was "very helpful." Hull reported to Welles:

I have told him that the world situation requires that the peace of the Americas be maintained; that public sentiment in the Americas is unanimous in its insistence that there be peace on this hemisphere; that the Ecuador-Peru boundary dispute is the only major blight on the peace of the Americas; that because of its resources, strength and experience Peru should take the initiative although Ecuador of course should do its full part; and after complimenting Dr. Concha for his handling of the Conference, appealed to him to take upon his shoulders the responsibility for removing the last major obstacle towards peace in the Americas. Dr. Concha has assured me that the President [Manuel Prado] is genuinely desirous of a settlement of the dispute and I believe that Dr. Concha was impressed by my personal appeal to him to take the initiative and endeavor to find a solution. . . . Under the circumstances, I believe I have done all that I possibly can.[1]

The declaration of American principles approved by the conference included, among others, the following:

1. The intervention of any State in the internal or external affairs of another is inadmissible.
2. All differences of an international character should be settled by peaceful means.
3. The use of force as an instrument of national or international policy is proscribed.[2]

These principles, along with many other similar declarations of American states, are cited by defenders of the Ecuadoran position in the Marañón dispute as having been violated by the Peruvian invasion in 1941.[3]

However, the Ecuadoran delegation left Lima without reaching an agreement on further talks, and none were held on the dispute as a whole before hostilities broke out in the summer of 1941. The core of the diplomatic aspect of the dispute at this time was Peruvian insistence on bilateral negotiations with Ecuador in Lima and Ecuadoran efforts to arrange mediatory action, preferably involving Brazil and the United States. During 1939 and 1940 there were border incidents, resulting in charges by Lima and Quito that troops of the other country had committed a "bloody attack."[4]

The relations between the two countries were steadily growing worse, and toward the end of 1940 there were rumors emanating from Quito, and in early 1941 from Lima, of movements of Peruvian troops toward Ecuadoran positions both in the Zarumilla sector in the west and in areas east of the Andes. In 1940 the Ecuadoran government began to build a road from Cuenca to Loja, which, as Tobar notes, would allow Ecuador for the first time to "carry war material to the southern provinces with relative speed."[5] In addition, Ecuador began to establish military posts at certain points in the Zarumilla sector that had previously been occupied only by Ecuadoran civilians, and Peruvian protests were quickly forthcoming.

The policy of the United States toward the dispute was the subject of press and official comment at this time as the result of an article by John Lear of the Associated Press, which appeared in *El Telégrafo* (Guayaquil) on January 20, 1941. Lear stated that an arrangement was under consideration by which the United States would receive from Ecuador the right to establish naval and air bases in the Galápagos Islands and, in return, the United States would support Ecuador in its demand for arbitration of the boundary dispute. Lear reported that United States officials in Ecuador denied that their government had taken any initiative in this regard. President Carlos Alberto Arroyo del Río and Foreign Minister Tobar Donoso issued statements to the effect that there was no basis for the allegations in Lear's article. However, the subject was taken up in Lima by Alberto Ulloa in an article in *El Comercio* on February 10, 1941. Ulloa gave credence to the report, asserted Peru's great interest in the question, and raised the possibility that any such arrangement would threaten continental solidarity. No statement was issued in Washington at this time concerning the incident, but the Department of State was, of course, informed about it.

In Ecuador the danger of war with Peru was fully recognized by December, 1940. Tobar reports that the army urged breaking diplomatic relations with Peru; he first offered his resignation because of the army's interference in foreign policy, and, on its being refused, he warned the Advisory Council that Ecuadoran diplomacy could not be effective without military strength. He urged that Ecuador seek time to arm itself: " 'When we are strong . . . the word of the Foreign Minister will possess the power of the word of a man who can defend justice because he has the support of force.' " [6]

At the same time, Tobar asked Ecuadoran diplomats to explain the situation to the foreign ministers of other American states. Foreign Minister Oswaldo Aranha of Brazil, who had communicated with President Prado of Peru about the desirability of a peaceful settlement of the dispute, reported that Prado suggested that Ecuador be " 'prudent and serene.' " Aranha had responded that he could not advise Ecuador to be prudent " 'when Peru's forces were moving up rivers and invading Ecuadoran territory.' " However,

Aranha also referred to the " 'indecisiveness of Washington' " as creating difficulties in the formation of a firm position on the part of Brazil,[7] despite his desire expressed on one occasion to use "vigorous good offices" on the Peruvians.

In Washington, Welles recognized that the dispute "was the most serious element of danger today in the entire Western Hemisphere. . . . It seemed to us that it was in the highest degree necessary for the sake of the peace of the continent that the dispute be settled in an equitable manner by pacific means as soon as possible." These statements were made to Peruvian Ambassador Freyre, who had assured Welles that "Peru believes only in the pacific adjustment of this dispute and in no event will resort to force unless attacked by Ecuador." [8]

Desperately alarmed by reports from Ecuadoran diplomats of Peruvian military preparations near the boundary in the west,[9] Tobar, on April 6, 1941, sent a telegram addressed to the foreign offices of the American states stating his willingness to enter into direct negotiations with Peru, " 'if given guarantees of good faith,' " or to agree to arbitration or mediation, and asked for " 'sympathy' " on the part of other governments, since Ecuador's attitude demonstrated " 'confidence in the community of the American nations.' "[10]

The principal effect of the Ecuadoran declaration was to exacerbate feelings in Lima, where Dr. Alfredo Solf y Muro, the new Foreign Minister who had come into office after the election of President Manuel Prado in 1939, replied in a note protesting the statement that Ecuador would enter negotiations only if given guarantees of "good faith" by Peru.[11] Tobar retorted that he considered that the Peruvian reply gave evidence of the " 'excessive sensitivity' " of the Peruvian foreign office; but this did nothing to allay resentment in Lima. These exchanges were published, and the press in each country supported its government.[12]

This diplomatic exchange may be regarded as marking the end of one phase in the dispute and the opening of another—the last and most important endeavor by third parties to arrange a peaceful settlement. The Brazilian peace moves were at an end. The new phase appears to have been opened by reports to Buenos Aires from Carlos

Quintana, Argentine Ambassador in Lima, about alarming concentrations of Peruvian troops in the Zarumilla sector near the Pacific Ocean. The acting Argentine Foreign Minister Guillermo Rothe suggested to Rio de Janeiro and Washington that the three governments consider some form of action that might bring about a friendly settlement of the visibly looming conflict. This initiative, after consultations among the three governments, resulted on May 8, 1941, in the sending by each of notes to Lima and Quito that expressed their deep concern at the continuation of the boundary dispute and their desire to terminate it. The three governments made the following proposal:

"Impressed by the necessity, in this critical hour, of the American Republics drawing ever closer together in an unshakeable determination to maintain unimpaired their peace, territorial integrity, and security, the Governments of Argentina, Brazil and the United States tender their friendly services in furthering the prompt, equitable and final settlement of the dispute to the Governments of Ecuador and Peru, together with the services of such other governments as they are both desirous of inviting, in such manner as may be deemed appropriate and advantageous." [13]

This offer of "friendly services" was favorably received in Quito and immediately accepted without reservations. Not only did it represent the kind of action constantly sought by Ecuador since the breakup of the Washington talks in 1938, but, in referring to an "equitable" settlement, it held out hope for a solution that might allow Ecuador to become an "Amazonian nation," whatever might have been the prospects for a decision by an arbitral tribunal. Outside Ecuador as well, the tripartite offer was regarded as at least a temporary diplomatic victory for Ecuador.

In Lima the reaction was quite different. The Peruvian reply of May 13, 1941, is noteworthy in several respects. It declared that in 1910 a similar offer by the same three powers had been rejected by Ecuador and that Peru was therefore not responsible for the prolongation of the dispute. It stated that Peru could not admit that its sovereign rights over the provinces of Tumbes, Mainas, and Jaén could be brought into question. Peru was disposed to settle the dispute over frontiers but not to admit as "a matter of argument" any question about the sovereign rights of Peru over the three provinces. The note concluded with the slightly insulting declaration that

"in consonance with the principles stated, which Your Excellency will properly appreciate, the Government of Peru accepts the good offices offered by the governments of Argentina, Brazil and the United States, to the end that the atmosphere of cordiality and sincere collaboration between the two countries may be restored." [14]

What Peru accepted were "good offices" to restore amicable relations with Ecuador. What the three governments offered were "friendly services" to reach a final settlement without delay. These were very different arrangements, both in method and in purpose. Lima had in mind no more than the reopening of bilateral negotiations with Quito. The three powers wished to participate in the negotiations and to make suggestions not only about methods of settlement but also about the course of the boundary itself. Good offices constituted the established form of minimal diplomatic help to disputants and did not necessarily involve mediation. "Friendly services" was not a technical term of traditional usage; it suggested an unlimited and flexible kind of assistance, and the Peruvians feared with some reason that most of the assistance would be received by Ecuador. In view of the importance attached in Lima to the rejection of friendly services, it is possible that Peruvian protests would have been silenced had it been recalled that the government of Peru had signed an agreement in concert with Argentina, Brazil, and Chile in 1932, in which all four governments offered their "friendly services" to Bolivia and Paraguay in the hope of reaching a peaceful settlement of the Chaco dispute.[15]

Had Peru accepted the mediators' offer in view of Solf's calculated substitution of "good offices" for "friendly services" and in view of the express reservations as to the limits on the proffered aid? This was a live question. By accepting "good offices" but not "friendly services" the Peruvian government considered that it had not accepted "mediation" by Argentina, Brazil, and the United States. This point is made perfectly clear by Alberto Ulloa, a former acting Foreign Minister of Peru, whose pronouncements in a series of articles in *La Prensa* (Lima) in 1941 may be taken as expressive of official Peruvian opinion.[16]

The response of the Peruvian government was not regarded as satisfactory by the governments of Argentina, Brazil, and the United States, but they decided to accept it as a basis for further initiatives.[17] However, their unity was shaken, as was indicated by differences in their notes to Ecuador and Peru of May 20, 1941. The United States maintained its offer of "friendly services," but the Argentine and Brazilian notes mentioned only the intention of offering no more than "good offices." The Peruvian reply had succeeded in dividing those who offered help in a situation where the Peruvian government wanted no help.[18] That the Argentine note omitted the word "prompt" was probably noted with grim pleasure in Lima, where a storm of anti-United States feeling had quickly whirled up.

Although unofficially, the Peruvian newspapers outspokenly attacked the mediation offer, and the United States in particular. *El Universal* (Lima) on May 13, 1941, criticized the failure to give Peru advance notice of the notes of May 8 and said that "this hour of anguish seems the least appropriate for solving a problem . . . that the most able men of Peru and Ecuador had not been able to settle in the course of 120 years." The editorial remarked, in an obvious attempt to single out the United States among the three states concerned, that the rapid acceptance by Ecuador and the unusual form of the proposed "good offices" "could only awake, and have in fact awakened, in Peruvian public opinion righteous misgivings and suspicions, which, of course, do not damage nor diminish our constant friendship toward the nations to which we are united by the bonds of common blood and a common historical tradition."

In response to reports from Peru that the United States was showing partiality to Ecuador in the dispute by providing Ecuador with coast guard vessels and airplanes, Secretary Hull stated publicly that: "this Government was motivated in offering to Ecuador and Peru its *friendly offices* solely by the most friendly desire to assist in settling, once and for all, the long-standing boundary dispute between those two neighboring countries." Hull added that the United States government has not, in any way, discussed with Ecuador the question of bases on the Galápagos Islands. Moreover, the willingness of this Government to consider making available to Ecuador two coastal patrol vessels and military supplies has absolutely no relation to the offer of *friendly good offices* but derives solely from a general policy of this Government made known to each and every one of the American Republics, to cooperate insofar as possible in military and naval matters for the purpose of strengthening the defense of the Western Hemisphere. [Italics supplied.] [19]

The italicized phrases in the above statements by Secretary Hull must have been heartening to Peruvian officials, for they were presumably employed instead of "friendly services" as used in the note of May 8, and in the Peruvian foreign office they were probably interpreted, and rightly as events demonstrated, that the United States did not intend to take any measures against Peru that were more threatening than the mild measures traditionally understood when the expression "good offices" was used. Therefore, "friendly services," with its possible overtones of external pressures to bring about a settlement, appeared to have been relinquished by the United States, and President Prado was probably emboldened to continue his military preparations toward a settlement of the boundary dispute with Ecuador.

Nevertheless, the reaction to Hull's statement by *El Comercio* (Lima), Peru's most influential newspaper, was to maintain that it was inadequate. An editorial on May 17 pointedly noted that public statements by Oswaldo Aranha about the mediation "had been received in Peru with real sympathy, because they were inspired by the same sentiments of cordiality which our country has always felt toward Brazil." It suggested that Hull's denial of negotiations about the Galápagos Islands was not sufficient to still all suspicions that the matter was under discussion. Concerning the coast guard vessels to be delivered to Ecuador, the tone of the editorial was harsh:

The defense of the high interests of our country impels us to declare that we do not find satisfactory the form in which Mr. Cordell Hull explains an act of his government that is harmful to Peru. If there is really no relationship between the supplying of warships to Ecuador and the offer of "friendly services," it must be agreed that this is a case of an inopportune coincidence that should have been avoided. It is clear that, when one interferes in a boundary dispute that might be, as has been said, "the origin of dangerous developments," it is inadmissible that whoever fears this result and tries to prevent it, in a friendly way, should provide materials of war to one of the possible contenders. It is still less admissible that such materials should be given to the weaker of the two, since this tends to equalize the forces of the two countries and to stimulate and make possible the struggle.

El Comercio thought the policy of the United States was a strange one if it was aimed at strengthening the defense of the Hemisphere, "since, as we know, the United States has given naval vessels to no other nation of the American Continent, except Ecuador, and certainly Ecuador is not the most obviously qualified country for beginning the task of building up Western Hemisphere defenses." The editorial concluded:

We have believed it necessary to speak with entire frankness, so that there may be no mistake about the future attitude of Peru. We see with natural displeasure that the United States, a country to which we have given clear and constant proofs of friendship, supplies arms to our presumptive opponent. We regret that foreign offices that always have shown respect for the sovereignty and original establishment of the republics of the continent should have offered "friendly services" without warning and therefore in an unwelcome fashion. We had not requested them and, in fact, they signify a form of pressure that affects our sovereignty and endangers our territorial integrity. But, if the nations making this offer do not wish their action to fail, they must accept, as Peru has proposed, that they limit their proposal to "good offices" with the sole aim of reestablishing the atmosphere of friendship, which ceased to exist some time ago, particularly in our neighboring country to the north.[20]

The Peruvian concern over the terms used by Lima and the "friendly" powers was not a quibble. The Peruvian government profoundly feared that the United States was interested in promoting an "equitable" settlement, and what leading Peruvians wanted was not equity but "justice." As Ulloa said, when "only one of the parties, as in this case, has justice on its side, equity would result in a diminution of its rights."[21]

After receiving the three slightly, but significantly, different notes of May 20, Solf cabled to Hull on May 23 that Peru had accepted "good offices" in his note of May 12, but it deems that joint conversations of the representatives of the interested countries and of the friendly countries making the offer are not in harmony with the institution of good offices, a form which would be characteristic of a mediation, which Peru has not accepted. The Government of Peru thinks that the immediate discussion of the boundary difference would heighten the tension between the two countries, producing, precisely, the contrary effect to that which the friendly Governments propose to secure.

He restated Peru's position on the boundary dispute and said that Peru "is disposed to subscribe to a juridical instrument guaranteeing peace between the two countries and establishing a regime of effective cooperation until an opportunity arises to obtain a settlement of the difference." This action, in his opinion, would satisfy the "noble purpose" of the friendly countries to prevent a situation which "may diminish or undermine the strength of continental solidarity." [22]

Such diplomatic language was no more than a pale reflection of intense sentiments expressed in influential circles in Peru. The Miró Quesada family, through the editorial columns of *El Comercio*, carried on a bitter campaign against the United States. Whatever might have been the real aims of Prado and his advisers, the President would have met powerful opposition from civilians and military alike if he had shown any sign of accepting proposals from the mediators that would have risked Peruvian withdrawals from the 1936 *status quo* line. That the United States was being made the target of attacks in Peru was in itself noteworthy; it was apparently felt that there was less risk to Peru in singling out the United States than in assailing Brazil or Argentina, despite the fact that it was known in Peru that Argentina had initiated the mediation. Peruvians may also have thought that this tactic might split the mediatory powers, and Peruvians may have appeared bolder in their own eyes by publicly defying the most powerful state in the hemisphere. Beyond this, they may have calculated that Washington would feel that it had more to lose than the other mediators if Peru refrained from cooperation in measures for the defense of the Western Hemisphere in World War II. If this was the case, they played cleverly upon the sensitivity of the powerful, and they rightly gauged Washington's anxiety to avoid any breach in the solidarity of defensive cooperation or any possibility that Prado's regime might be overthrown if it were forced to change its policy on the Ecuadoran dispute.

Peruvian "resentment" at the offer of "friendly services" apparently was intensified by the use of the term "prompt" (*pronto* in Spanish) in the note of May 8. The welling up of resentment in Lima that accompanied Stimson's effort to prevent war over Leticia in 1932–33 and its recurrence against the United States in 1941 suggest that Peruvian leaders had found that diplomatic ferocity, artificial or real, was a rewarding technique. Secretary Hull's public statement of May 16 was an uncertain retreat, and subsequent diplomatic moves by the United States government demonstrated great reluctance to exert any pressure on Lima to change the course of Peruvian policy.

The basic motivation of the United States in trying to bring about a pacific settlement of the dispute was expressed about this time by Under Secretary Sumner Welles in an interview with Ambassador Freyre of Peru as follows:

In accordance with the spirit and letter of existing inter-American agreements, the United States respects in practice and in theory the complete sovereignty of every one of the other American nations and for that reason has refrained from exercising any kind of pressure upon the parties to the dispute. However, in accordance with accepted tenets of international law and of inter-American relationships, the United States, together with Argentina and Brazil, has offered its friendly services to both Peru and Ecuador to try and prevent the tension arising from the boundary dispute from becoming more acute, in the hope that both sides would reach a final and friendly settlement of the dispute. The United States has joined in this friendly offer all the more readily at this moment because of the increasingly critical world situation and because of the self-evident fact that if hostilities actually did break out between two neighboring American republics, that would be an opportunity which would be gladly availed of by Germany and her Axis partners as a means of fomenting trouble and discord in the new world and as a means of disrupting inter-American solidarity.[23]

With the replies of Ecuador and Peru to the note of the three mediatory powers of May 20, 1941, the first phase of the mediation ended, for hostilities began before the mediators took any further action. Tobar attributes what he regarded as a regrettable diplomatic hiatus to an internal crisis within the mediation. He suggests that "the irritation manifested by Peru against the Argentine foreign office created some concern in Buenos Aires; the fear of further embroilment with Peru weakened the force of the first generous impulse." [24]

There were new border incidents in June, and Washington was informed by both sides about the circumstances and their significance. The charges made by the Ecuadoran press about Peruvian troop concentrations along the coast, at the western end of the boundary, may have been exaggerated so far as numbers of men were concerned, but there was no question that a Peruvian military buildup was taking place there. Washington had been receiving official reports of Peruvian deployments since mid-April, and these troop movements had originally inspired the mediators' first note of May 8, 1941.

One alarmist report in the Ecuadoran press was that Japanese officers and technicians were aiding Peruvian military preparations. There seems to be no foundation for these reports, except perhaps a desire on the part of Ecuadoran journalists to excite opinion in the United States and elsewhere. It is of interest to note that this same charge had been made by Colombian newspapers against Peru in the Leticia dispute, and it was then equally inaccurate. The Department of State did not take these rumors seriously.

The diplomatic tension was broken on July 5, 1941, with the opening of large-scale and continuous fighting on the western front at Huaquillas and Chacras. Tobar informed the other American states that the Peruvian forces were employing artillery and that Peruvian planes were bombing Ecuadoran positions; he asserted that these actions proved that the fighting was not an incident, but that it was " 'the aggression that has been evidently prepared since last February.' " [25]

Tobar stated that on July 5 some Peruvian agricultural workers, accompanied by civil guards, entered Ecuadoran territory along the Zarumilla River. An Ecuadoran patrol came upon them, the Peruvian guards opened fire, and fighting extended to several frontier posts. The affair might have ended only as an incident, in his view, but in the two following days the Peruvian forces continued to attack, and the villages of Chacras and Huaquillas were bombed by the Peruvian air force.[26]

In Peru the foreign ministry issued a statement declaring that Ecuadoran soldiers had attacked Peruvian positions and had been beaten off.

The Department of State regarded the fighting as serious and immediately initiated talks with the Argentine and Brazilian representatives in Washington. Within two days the three countries instructed their missions in Lima and Quito to request joint interviews with the foreign ministers for the purpose of recalling to them the acceptance by both governments of the "good offices" offered on May 8, expressing their concern about "the present hostilities" and making the following proposal:

It would seem that the only sure way of preventing an aggravation of the present hostilities and a recurrence of these incidents would be for the withdrawal by each Government of its forces a distance of 15 kilometers from the line of the so-called *status quo* tacitly recognized previously by both Governments.

If this proposal was accepted, it was to be urged on both Ecuador and Peru that they sign immediately a declaration of friendship and agree to keep their troops behind the proposed lines of separation.

Moreover, for the purpose of assuring the effective and prompt withdrawal of the military forces of each country from the line of the so-called *status quo*, military attachés of the American countries in the two capitals or other military experts will be instructed to collaborate with the authorities designated by the Governments of Ecuador and Peru.[27]

In addition to joining in the above proposal to the combatants, the United States government, together with those of Argentina and Brazil, instructed its missions in all other American states to call upon the foreign ministers and say that the present incident between Peru and Ecuador explained the quickness with which the three mediators acted on May 8 in offering their friendly services to Ecuador and Peru. However, the new outbreak of fighting had demonstrated the need for "an even more ample, common and solidary action on the part of all of the Americas" to terminate an affair that endangered continental peace, unity and safety. The three countries therefore suggested a joint effort by all American states to reestablish peace, and as a first step they made available to them the text of their note of July 8.[28]

Ecuador and Peru promptly accepted the proposal for the withdrawal of troops. Peru's acceptance at first was "in principle," since Solf said Peru could not withdraw its forces until an alleged incident concerning affronts to the Peruvian Consulate in Guayaquil had been settled. Quito quickly gave satisfaction for this incident, and the Peruvian foreign office then indicated it was willing to await further suggestions from the mediators.[29]

However, the mediators were meeting difficulties in trying to get common action by all American states. The difficulties arose from the all but unanimously favorable response from the other American states for representations in support of the note of July 8 to Lima and Quito from the three mediators. Chile alone had not joined the American chorus.

The Chilean government resented its not being included in the offer of "friendly services" on May 8 and was intensely disappointed that, now that fighting had commenced, it was still not one of the mediators. It held that, as one of the principal South American states on the Pacific Coast, it should have been associated in efforts to keep the peace.[30] The three mediators tried to arrange new joint interviews in Lima and Quito to present the view that they would welcome the participation of Chile and of Colombia as mediators. These interviews did not take place, however, because of Peruvian opposition to the inclusion of Chile.

On July 12 Foreign Minister Juan Bautista Rossetti of Chile stated publicly that at the present time it was not necessary to utilize in the dispute any other procedures than those already available in the form of existing inter-American agreements. Without directly saying so, this statement demonstrated that Chile would not support the proposal of the mediatory powers, and it thereby prevented the appeal of the mediators from gaining unanimous support from the American states. It was hardly to Peru's interest to bring about such unanimity by agreeing to Chile's participation as a mediator, so that Solf's action in rejecting in advance a proposal he knew was coming was quite understandable.

This affair rounds out an interesting and possibly instructive episode in inter-American diplomacy. In 1938, it will be recalled, Chile had prevented the commencement of a mediatory effort after the collapse of the Washington conversations. When the new mediatory group was formed on May 8, 1941, at the initiative of Argentina, Chile was not included. The reasons for this action are not known, but it is possible that Chile's noncooperative role in 1938 may have been partially responsible. Although in May, 1941, Chile could have been included without the permission of Ecuador and Peru, the three mediators felt that once their "good offices" had been accepted, the agreement of the disputants was necessary to enlarge the number of mediators in July. Then, however, Peru was undoubtedly happy to be in a position to insure the continuation of the lack of continental solidarity disclosed when Chile refused to support the proposal of July 8.

These considerations redirect attention to the origin of the mediatory effort in May. There are some plausible, if purely speculative, reasons for thinking that that effort may have been inspired by the Peruvian government. It may be assumed that Lima would not have failed to calculate the inter-American reverberations of an outbreak of hostilities with Ecuador in the summer of 1941. By 1941 most of the American states, but not Argentina or Peru, had ratified the Convention for the Maintenance, Preservation and Reestablishment of Peace signed by all of them at the Buenos Aires Conference. This Convention provided that, if intra-American peace were menaced, any one American government might consult with the others, "which, in such event, shall consult together for the purpose of finding and adopting methods of peaceful cooperation."

Furthermore, it may be assumed that Peruvian diplomats were aware of the great importance attached by the government of the United States to this Convention. Sumner Welles had stated publicly:

If experience has taught us anything, it has taught us that the way to avert war is not to wait until the storm is breaking, but to seek the pacific solution when the cloud of controversy no bigger than the palm of a man's hand first appears upon the horizon. The world has also learned that the staunchest safeguard against war which mankind today possesses is the force of public opinion freely expressed. What this convention provides is something which has never before existed on this Continent. It provides that whenever there is any threat to the maintenance of peace in the Americas, however remote that threat may be, any American state shall possess the right to bring about consultation between all of the American Governments in order to avert the danger.[31]

If it be assumed that Lima wished to avert, not the danger of war, but the dangers to its enterprise of consultative unanimity and of freely expressed public opinion, it would seek a way of heading them off. What better way could be found, using the model of the Chaco dispute, than that of initiating a partial consultation that would have little chance of success in keeping the peace by its own efforts and would also forestall the consultation of all American states? If, in addition, Chile were excluded from the partial consultation, assurance of the frustration of the efforts of the mediators would be nearly complete.

Carrying this speculation a little farther, it may be asked whether it was fortuitous that the initiator of the tripartite mediation was the government of Argentina. The Peruvian Ambassador in Buenos Aires was no less a person than General Oscar Benavides, ex-President of Peru. Of the three mediating powers, Argentina was, as a non-ratifier, least likely to be concerned with the provisions of the Buenos Aires Convention and, also, least insistent on the inclusion of Chile in the mediating group. Without knowing anything of what actually went on in Buenos Aires, it may be said that the results of the "Argentine initiative" could not have been more in accord with the interests of Peru than if the Peruvians had themselves made the plans. It may not be irrelevant to recall that, following the presentation of the first note of the mediators, the ire of the Peruvian press, notably that of the well-informed *El Comercio*, was expressed, not against Argentina, but against the United States as the government allegedly responsible for the mediation.

While the mediators were failing to unify the potential peacemakers, they were also making no progress on the fundamental question of stopping the fighting. Both disputants had sent special emissaries to Washington. Carlos Concha, ex-Foreign Minister of Peru, and Homero Viteri Lafronte, Ecuador's representative at the

Washington talks in 1938, arrived on the same airplane on July 11, 1941, and immediately called, separately, on Welles. These and subsequent talks in Washington did not result in any concrete actions toward settlement of the dispute, and on July 16 the Peruvian government formally tested the mettle of the mediators by a note replying to that of July 8. The Peruvian government accepted the suggested plan for a withdrawal of troops, but limited it to the extreme western sector of the boundary, and proposed that the withdrawal be supervised by a commission of civilians and military officers of Ecuador and Peru, thus rejecting the mediators' proposal of the appointment of neutral military observers.[32]

During the next week the mediators were not able to reach agreement on any action, and on July 23 hostilities were renewed along a front of about fifty kilometers in the western sector. Peruvian troops began an advance that carried them several miles into Ecuadoran territory and routed the Ecuadoran forces in three days. In his account of the conflict, Tobar asserts that, whereas what he called the "trial aggression" of July 5–7 had its origin in an incident, the "second aggression" of July 23 was initiated by Peru without any preliminary incident.[33] It appears that the Peruvian government, having tested the reaction of the mediators and found it weak and knowing the Ecuadoran army had become no stronger, was confident that it could safely impose a settlement on Ecuador by force of arms.

The news of the renewed fighting stimulated Enrique Ruiz Guiñazú, Argentine Foreign Minister, to make on July 23 what he called a "supreme appeal" to the two governments to cease fighting and refrain from new hostile acts. This appeal was made by the Argentine government alone, and not as a joint declaration by the three mediators, but it was immediately supported by the United States government.

The appeal evidently had an upsetting effect in Lima, for on July 25 Solf made one of the very few tactical errors attributable to Peru in the whole course of the mediation. He told the ambassadors of the mediating powers that Peru would accept the fixing by the mediators of a definite date and hour for the stopping of fighting and that Peru would agree to withdraw its troops according to the terms of the mediators' note of July 8.[34]

Solf's statement was of great significance, for it gave the mediators an opening, which Sumner Welles immediately seized. Within a few hours, after consultation with his Argentine and Brazilian colleagues, he informed Lima and Quito that the mediators understood that Peru had agreed to cease fire at a time to be determined by the mediators and that the mediators had set 6:00 P.M. on July 26 as the hour. Viteri Lafronte, in Washington, accepted this proposal immediately on behalf of Ecuador and so advised Tobar late in the afternoon of July 26.[35]

The Ecuadoran government responded immediately, and Ecuadoran troops received orders to stop fighting before midnight of July 26.

Why did Quito act so precipitately on a matter of such importance without first confirming the report received by radio or waiting for assurance that Peru would also accept the armistice? Tobar's own account gives two reasons: (1) to present to Peru's determination to advance at least the obstacle of Ecuador's immediate acceptance of the armistice proposed by the mediators, and (2) "to preserve the honor of our armed forces, protecting them by heeding a request from the mediators." Tobar declares that on July 25 the disorganization of the army was such that, of its 1,200 men, facing some 13,000 Peruvians in the west, only 350 remained subject to discipline. Beginning on July 26, desertion by the soldiers was uncontrollable and even the officers were demoralized by the Peruvian planes and heavy artillery. By that date the Ecuadoran army had been destroyed as an organized force.[36]

Despite Tobar's protective action, the defeat of the Ecuadoran army was fully recognized in America. Aranha later asked an Ecuadoran in Rio de Janeiro if, by chance, " 'there was not one man in Ecuador capable of buckling on a sword.' " Tobar thought the question less than just, but he admitted that Ecuador should not try to defend its honor with self-deceptions; the army had demonstrated its heroism, but its heroism had been fruitless in the face of Peruvian superiority in numbers, discipline, and equipment.[37]

Solf's incautious acceptance of the mediators' judgment as to the hour of suspension of hostilities was not ratified by the Peruvian army, which, under General Eloy Ureta, continued its invasion of Ecuadoran territory. Further, Solf's action was not supported by the Peruvian government, presumably on the orders of President Prado himself, for the government set as a condition for Peruvian cessation of fighting that Ecuador should annul a mobilization decree issued on July 24, immediately following the Peruvian invasion of July 23.[38] The annulment of the decree was announced on July 31 over the Quito radio, and only at 6:00 P.M. on that day did Peruvian troops in the western sector finally end their advance, five days after the Ecuadorans had ceased to resist, after General Ureta had attained what he regarded as minimal strategic objectives, and five days after the time set for the cease-fire by the mediators, who had relied on Solf's statement of July 25.[39]

The Peruvian position on the termination of hostilities was expressed in an official communiqué, published in *El Comercio*, August 1, 1941:

Having won the battle of Zarumilla, provoked by the insistent aggression of Ecuador, having recovered the areas invaded by Ecuador, and having punished that country for its provocations and offenses, Peru accepted in principle on the evening of July 25 the friendly invitation of the Argentine foreign minister Ruiz Guiñazú to cease hostilities on the western front.

Shortly afterward, on August 4, *El Comercio* published a commentary on an Ecuadoran communiqué in which it stated that "all America knows, and especially the mediatory powers, that Peru demanded as a prior condition to the cessation of hostilities that Ecuador annul the mobilization decree it had issued." This "prior condition" had, however, been made only after Solf's statement of July 25.

The full story of this incident cannot be reconstructed from the available documents, but some speculations may be hazarded. There seems to be no reason to question that Solf declared that Peru would accept the mediators' determination of a time for an armistice and that his statement was unconditional. His subsequent unavailability to the mediators' ambassadors in Lima was probably due to a purely diplomatic illness, brought on by acute domestic embarrassment. Welles presumably talked with the Argentine and Brazilian ambassadors in Washington before setting the time for the armistice, but it is not clear, in view of the time factor, that Aranha and Ruiz

Guiñazú formally approved the action. Welles may have thought that a speedy move was necessary to create a *fait accompli*, making it difficult either for his mediatory colleagues to propose less drastic measures or for Solf to back out of his declaration. Welles probably did not expect that Solf's commitment would be repudiated by President Prado, whose hand may well have been forced by the field commander, General Ureta, and, when the Peruvian government later set conditions for the armistice, Welles found nothing better to do than strongly advise Ecuador to accept the conditions as soon as possible.

Welles probably was embarrassed by the reception of a cable from Tobar on July 29, stating that, while Ecuadoran troops had ceased firing on July 26 at the request of the mediators, Peru had continued hostilities and had even bombed "open cities where there were no military targets." [40] Such actions, he added, were proscribed by international law, and he noted that the Panama conference of American foreign ministers had appealed to the belligerents in World War II to refrain from " 'bombarding open cities, objects, and places without military value.' " [41] Such actions, added Tobar, "should with all the more reason be repudiated in America, the continent which had offered itself as a model of justice and of Christian civilization."

However, no specific reply seems to have been given by the mediators to this appeal; their effective response was to maintain pressure on Ecuador to annul the mobilization decree of July 24, and this pressure was successful, as has been noted, on July 31. This date Tobar later called "the most terrible day of my civic life, even more bitter than that of January 29, 1942," which was when he signed the protocol of Rio de Janeiro, since the earlier action was a "destruction of Ecuadoran sovereignty," whereas the signing of the protocol was an act of sovereignty by the Ecuadoran government. [42]

Embarrassment may well have been caused in Washington by this cable, by the continued Peruvian advances into Ecuadoran territory, and by publicity in Peru that attributed to the United States the leading part in efforts of the mediation to limit Peruvian military moves.

In Ecuador, where hopes had long been cherished for assistance from the United States, the press expressed strong feelings, occasioned by the cease-fire that was not observed by the Peruvian army and by withdrawal of the mobilization decree on terms imposed by Peru. An editorial in *El Telégrafo* (Guayaquil) of July 30, 1941, declared:

We would never have believed that the United States and all the other American republics would look on impassively at this horrible aggression by Peru that destroys continental harmony, favoring the growth of totalitarian policies.

The echoes are still heard from the sonorous speeches in the Pan American conferences, and the ink is still fresh on the signatures of American diplomats to the lyrical conventions and the optimistic treaties that were to guarantee peace and concord in the Continent. . . .

None of this has remained after the shock with bleak reality. Neither initiatives nor agreements have retained value because they were made of lies and deceptions. Like a house of cards it has collapsed, this structure of falsehoods and mirages that continental diplomacy erected under the perfidious name of the Pan American Union.

In the same paper on the following day there appeared another editorial, inspired, it stated, by the favorable response to the previous article. It asserted that

the principles of the good neighbor policy of President Roosevelt have had absolutely no value; they have not served as guarantees for the maintenance of peace or the prevention of aggression. . . . They have all been deceptions, as has also been the belief that the United States would guard inter-American concord and protect the weak countries of the continent.

All the American nations would now have to arm themselves, since they no longer could "confide in the pseudo-leaders of the continent, and since there now existed the fear that in each neighbor there was a Brutus who might plunge the traitorous dagger into one's back."

The editorial regretted that the United States did not understand the full implications of the Peruvian "attack":

This atrocious aggression not only has harmed our little country, it has destroyed the diplomatic work of half a century and weakened the feelings of mutual confidence and the hopes for cooperation among the

American peoples. The nations of America will not fear the United States, nor can they hope for its aid or intervention in a grave crisis, and each country will seek in some strong or rich state of other continents the armed protection or the economic help that may be needed.

President Roosevelt sent hearty messages to Presidents Arroyo del Río of Ecuador and Prado of Peru on August 1, 1941, expressing his approval of the "agreement" reached by the two governments to cease hostilities "in the frontier region between the two countries" and congratulating them on "this auspicious occasion." [43]

The mediatory powers immediately (August 2) proposed to Ecuador and Peru that each country should withdraw its troops fifteen kilometers behind the *status quo* line of 1936 and that military observers named by the mediators should be enabled to observe the retirement. This proposal was accepted by the Ecuadoran government, but no reply was forthcoming from Lima, which in practice rejected it, and the Peruvian forces remained in the positions they had conquered in the Ecuadoran province of El Oro. These positions were maintained by General Ureta's army for about six months, until after the Ecuadoran government had signed the boundary agreement negotiated at the Rio de Janeiro conference in January, 1942.

Quito agreed immediately to the appointment of military observers by the mediatory powers, but in Lima there was delay and reluctance to accept neutral observers at the advanced Peruvian positions. Finally these observers were admitted to Peruvian positions in the western sector, but the observers never were allowed to visit the Peruvian positions along the boundary in the area east of the Andes, where Peruvian military units continued to advance throughout the month of August, 1941.[44]

The continued Peruvian advances in the eastern sector were known in Washington, and Secretary Hull apparently considered that the Peruvian forces were violating the "agreement" of July 31, which President Roosevelt had regarded as marking the cessation of hostilities. Hull is reported to have

felt obliged to speak firmly to the former Peruvian Foreign Minister [Carlos Concha], who happened to be visiting Washington. Pointing out the parlous state of the world situation, Mr. Hull observed that, without reference to the merits of the boundary dispute, he knew that it should not exist "in this period of crisis when the fate of civilization is hanging by a thread." The two countries, he continued, simply could not afford the risk of starting a conflagration in the heart of South America at a time when the flames of war from east and west were already so clearly discernible.[45]

It is significant that Hull spoke "firmly" to a Peruvian, and not to an Ecuadoran. Hull was acquainted with the fact that the Peruvian army was continuing to advance beyond the 1936 *status quo* line and was continuing to reject the mediators' proposal to withdraw fifteen kilometers behind that line. Nevertheless, however outrageous the Peruvian actions may have been regarded in Washington, the Department of State did not at this time exert any pressure stronger than Hull's remarks to Carlos Concha, and these remarks were no more effective in changing the course of Peruvian policy than were those that Hull addressed to Concha during the Lima conference in 1938.

The Peruvian government had no intention at this time of withdrawing its troops even from El Oro province, which was indisputably Ecuadoran territory. The occupation of El Oro provided not only assurance of Ecuador's acceptance of Peruvian gains in the Oriente but, if necessary, a military position for further advances in the west, toward Guayaquil or elsewhere. The Peruvian frontier claims were not officially known at this time, although there existed rumors that they included the major portions if not all of the provinces of Tumbes, Jaén, and Mainas. The first of these was considered in Ecuador to be part of its province of El Oro. The second was known by the same name in Ecuador and Peru. The third was a Peruvian name that corresponded roughly to the Ecuadoran province of Napo-Pastaza and part of the province of Santiago-Zamora.[46]

The neutral military observers who had gone from Quito to the front after conferring with their colleagues from Lima reported that the Peruvian military objective

"is to remain in the area so far occupied until Ecuador has accepted Peruvian demands for the boundary. Should Ecuador not accept, Peru would be able to continue its advance. The Peruvian commander-in-chief, fully supported by the army, is the principal protagonist of this objective which symbolizes an old Peruvian national goal, and he would strive to attain it even if his government should give him orders incompatible with it." [47]

The mediatory powers could do little more for the moment than maintain the observers in the western military zone as reporters of developments in the situation and, perhaps, as one form of restraint on further moves by the army of General Ureta. That restraint had resulted from the action of the mediators was asserted by the military observers from Lima, who reported the view that emerged from their interviews with General Ureta and other Peruvian officers:

"The mediation of Argentina, Brazil and the United States prevented the carrying out of victorious operations by the Peruvian army, which could have brought peace with Ecuador quickly by means of a decisive military action, thus ending the boundary dispute. The acceptance by the army of the armistice imposed on it by the government of Peru, despoiled the army of the fruits of a military victory of great political importance. Therefore, the resentment of the military forces against the mediatory countries is regarded as perfectly justified. . . .

"The necessity is evident that the mediatory powers define their attitude by making concrete proposals for the termination of the conflict, without any demands for previous retirement of Peruvian troops. Such demands would not lead to a solution, and, besides, the Peruvian army is not disposed to accept them, in defense of the rights and the sovereignty of Peru." [48]

Although the front in the west was quiet for the time being, it was feared that General Ureta was planning to advance and take Guayaquil, and his ability to do so was not doubted, as it had become clear that Ecuador was incapable of offering further resistance to the ably led and well-equipped Peruvian troops. General Ureta had found scope for the successful employment of tanks, and in at least one engagement Peruvian parachute troops had helped to gain a victory.[49]

This was the first conflict between American states in which parachute troops were used. In their use of modern methods of fighting, the Peruvians also tried psychological warfare; they dropped leaflets from planes over Guayaquil on July 29. The leaflets apparently aimed at lowering enemy morale by urging Ecuadorans to be suspicious of their political leaders, who the Peruvians said were bringing on the horrors of war for personal advantage.

The Peruvian army had advanced about twenty-five miles north and northeast of the Zarumilla River on a front of about fifty miles, and it was in complete control of the Ecuadoran province of El Oro. It was quite impossible for Ecuador to dislodge the Peruvian forces. The government of Peru apparently thought that it could afford to disregard the pleas of the mediators, and there was little expectation in Washington that further diplomatic appeals to Peru could be effective.

In the Oriente, where there were no observers, Peruvian advances continued. Quito reported that Rocafuerte had been taken by Peruvian forces on August 11 as one of many alleged cases of Peruvian advances since the truce of July 31.[50]

In view of the inactivity of the mediators, Tobar sent a note to all the American governments on September 15, asserting that the Peruvian army was still advancing in the eastern sector and that even in the western sector, in Ecuadoran territory that had never been claimed by Peru, Peruvian forces had made continued "incursions." [51]

Some messages of sympathy were received by Tobar, but the most important response to his appeal for assistance was made by Ezequiel Padilla, Foreign Minister of Mexico, in a note of September 18, 1941, addressed to the governments of the three mediatory powers. Padilla asked the mediators, in order to maintain inter-American solidarity and to conserve continental peace," to "extend a general invitation to the other American governments to undertake a collective action" to bring about peace between Ecuador and Peru.[52]

The Mexican invitation was not accepted by the mediators, who turned it aside with soft words. They continued their futile efforts to induce Prado to withdraw his army behind the *status quo* line of 1936 and, failing that, to limit Peruvian advances by the mediators' maintenance of military observers on the western front.

The Mexican note was the occasion for an exposition in *El Comercio* (Lima), October 4, 1941, of the Peruvian view that equated joint efforts by the American nations to help solve the dispute with an acceptance by them of the Ecuadoran thesis about the boundary. The editorial stated that Padilla's initiative

contains the original sin of partiality, like that of the "friendly services" offered by Argentina, Brazil, and the United States. The reason is simple. Peru in its boundary dispute with Ecuador has both law and possession in its favor and therefore openly seeks a direct, juridical understanding. Ecuador, however, without title or effective possession, hopes for a solution of equity. Since in order to get something, it is necessary to claim a great deal, Ecuador carries its audacity so far as to question the nationality of the utterly Peruvian provinces of Tumbes, Mainas, and Jaén. Therefore, the mediators took the part of the absurd Ecuadoran thesis in offering their "friendly services to promote the prompt, equitable, and final solution of the dispute."

Hence, the Mexican action in proposing to reinforce the disinterested action of the mediators "means that there is being exerted a pressure that we regard as inadmissible. . . . The proof of the truth of what we say is found in the jubilant demonstrations in Ecuador that have greeted the Mexican initiative." Here, as elsewhere, *El Comercio* repeatedly made references to the term "friendly services" as being diplomatically unconventional and therefore justificatory in itself of Peru's rejection.

The Mexican memorandum of September 18, 1941, although it was not accepted by the mediators, probably made the Peruvian foreign office more keenly aware that it was better able to deal with three mediators than with a conclave of all the American states. There were many resolutions of inter-American conferences that had proscribed the use of force as a means of settling disputes among American states, and Lima preferred to avoid a formal confrontation, since favorable compromises would be easier with the mediators than in a meeting of all the states of the continent. Thus, when "official circles" in Lima reportedly commented that the joint action proposed by Mexico "would interfere with the success of the good offices of the United States, Brazil and Argentina," they, of course, meant that such "success" was so favorable to their cause that they would not wish to see it diminished by a collective move that would more effectively restrain Peru.[53]

The stand taken by the Peruvian government following its

military victory was made clear in mid-September by the presentation to the mediators of a memorandum containing Lima's conditions for the retirement of Peruvian forces from the province of El Oro. This document, dated September 13, is of such importance as to justify its being quoted in full:

1. Recognition by Ecuador of Peruvian territorial sovereignty bounded by the line running from the Pacific Ocean to the Chínchipe River and the Quebrada [ravine] de San Francisco, according to the attached description, in accordance with the traditional dominion of Peru.

2. Direct negotiations between the two countries concerning the territory extending between the line described in the foregoing paragraph and the line of Peru's claim, which was made before the Spanish arbitrator.

3. Recognition by Ecuador of Peruvian sovereignty in the eastern region as far as Peru's present jurisdiction extends, which is comprised within the extent of its legitimate domain, according to the attached description.

4. Direct negotiations between the two countries concerning the territory extending between the line described in the foregoing paragraph and the line of Peru's claim, which was made before the Spanish arbitrator.

5. Once the foregoing points have been accepted by Ecuador and their fulfillment guaranteed by the friendly countries, the territory of the province of El Oro beyond the line designated in paragraph no. 1, will be evacuated by Peru, remaining demilitarized under the supervision of the observers from the countries mentioned.

6. If, after the points of this agreement have been accepted by Ecuador, the agreement is not made into a treaty, within a period of six months, Peru shall take such steps as it may deem advisable.

7. The reimbursement of Peru for expenses incident to its occupation of the province of El Oro shall also be the subject of the negotiation referred to in paragraph no. 2.[54]

The "attached description" mentioned in the first and third paragraphs of this document is not printed in *Foreign Relations of the United States*, but it is of vital importance to an understanding of the extent of territory demanded by the Peruvian government in September, 1941, when Ecuador's incapacity to resist had been fully demonstrated. The text of the "attached description" is as follows:

I. Line of Peruvian territorial sovereignty in the western zone of the frontier with Ecuador, from the Pacific Ocean to the Chínchipe River and the Quebrada de San Francisco, in accordance with the traditional possession of Peru.

1. From the mouth of the Chupaderos in the Pacific Ocean, follow the canal that separates the islands of Tembleque y Pengal to the outlet of the old bed of the Zarumilla River by the inlet of Huaquillas near the village or port of Hualtaco, leaving within Peruvian territory the islands of Tembleque, Delicias, Payana or Salinas, Callejones, Bellavista, Corea, and Matapalo.

2. The Zarumilla River and its tributary Las Lajas or Balsamal, to its most remote origins in the Cordillera de Taguín, it being understood that on the lower part of this river, where its course divides, the line follows the old bed, called "Rio Viejo" or "Callancas."

3. From the principal origin [*formador*] of the Las Lajas River in the Cordillera de Taguín, the line down the Tumbes or Puyango River, following the meridian of this course.

4. The course of the Tumbes or Puyango River until the outlet of the Quebrada de Casaderos.

5. The course of the Quebrada de Casaderos to its origin.

6. A straight line that will unite this point with the point El Salto in the Quebrada de Pilares.

7. The Quebrada de Pilares to its outlet in the Alamor River.

8. The course of the Alamor River to its outlet in the Chira River.

9. The rivers Chira, Macará, Calvas, and Espíndola to their sources in the Nudo de Sabanillas.

10. From this point, continue along the Cordillera until the Quebrada Gramalotal, which has its outlet in the Canchis River, leaving within the limits of Peru the lands of Chicuate which are the property of the Indian community [*comunidad indígena*] of Segunda.

11. The course of the Canchis River to its outlet in the Chínchipe River.

12. The course of the Chínchipe River to the Quebrada de San Francisco.

13. The Quebrada de San Francisco to its origin in the Cordillera del Condor.

[Through this point the line is nearly the same as the 1936 *status quo* line. B.W.]

II. From the origin of the Quebrada de San Francisco, in the Cordillera del Condor, the existing jurisdiction of Peru in the Amazonian Northeast, will be established by the following points:

1. On the Nangueisa or Nangartiza, the sources of its tributary, the Minza or Miasse.

2. On the Santiago River, a point situated about 10 kilometers from the confluence of its sources, the Rivers Paute and Zamora, and another point at the mouth of the Yaupi River in the Santiago River.

3. In the system of the Morona River, a point situated at 10 kilometers from the confluence of the Miazal and Mangosisa Rivers and another at the confluence of the Macuma and Cangaine Rivers.

4. On the Pastaza River, a point halfway between the Peruvian settlement of Andoas and the outlet of the Bobonaza River.

5. On the Tigre River, the confluence of the Cunambo and Pintoyacu Rivers.

6. On the Curaray River, the point called Mascota at the mouth of the Villano River.

7. On the Napo River, the mouth of the Coca River.

8. On the Aguarico, the mouth of the Cuyabeno River.

9. On the San Miguel or Sucumbios River, the boundary with Colombia.[55]

From this document one can sense the attitude of a conquerer dictating terms, rather than the disposition of a state which had accepted good offices, if not friendly services, of other American states. The proposed boundary line in the Oriente was almost identical to the most advanced posts occupied by Peruvian troops. The consignment of the mediators by Peru to the role of guarantors of terms such as these could hardly have made other than a painful impression in Washington. This impression was deepened by reports of an incident created by Peruvian forces in El Oro province that had involved the destruction of property of United States citizens. In August Peruvian soldiers, who had been reported as looting at Puerto Bolivar and elsewhere, had seized some property belonging to the South American Development Company, an American mining corporation in El Oro.

The following month a more serious incident took place. On September 15 at Tenguel two Peruvian planes in separate attacks had machine-gunned a workers' camp, killing a woman and a child, and had dropped about ten bombs, killing one man and damaging buildings of the United Fruit Company. The United States flag was flying over the plantation, and it was reported that the flag itself had been hit.[56]

Fifteen years earlier an affair of this kind would probably have occasioned intervention by United States naval forces for the protection of the lives and property of its citizens. Instead, the formal reaction by Washington was limited to a mild protest in Lima. The protest took the form of a suggestion that the Peruvian airmen knew the Tenguel property belonged to a United States company and a request that the Peruvian government investigate the circumstances. Lima's response was far from apologetic; the foreign office declared that Peruvian planes had bombed the Tenguel property because "Ecuadoran troops were being concentrated there in preparation 'for aggression against Peru' " and added that not only were " 'war elements' " of Ecuador being carried on ships belonging to a "United States banana company" but that the planes had not dropped their bombs at Tenguel until fired on by "Ecuadoran antiaircraft guns." [57]

Certain aspects of the internal situation in Peru were appreciated in Washington as standing in the way of a settlement. It was common knowledge that the Peruvian President's personal background was one of these factors. Prado was the son of a former president of Peru, Mariano Ignacio Prado, who, while in office, had fled the country eight months after the outbreak of war with Chile in 1879. He had left his post, ostensibly to visit "the United States, and perhaps Europe, in the interest of Peru." However, it was reported at the time that "the general belief . . . among all classes seems to be that it was a desertion, a flight from the government, which, under an accumulation of calamities, he felt he could no longer hold with advantage to himself or to the country." [58] It was a safe presumption that Manuel Prado as President of Peru in 1941 would try to comport himself so that the blackened reputation of his family might be redeemed.

Another element in the internal situation, an important and baffling one, was the relationship between Prado and the army. General Ureta and his brother officers had the military, and therefore the political, power to insist that the war be ended on terms that would assure a due meed of glory to the victory-starved Peruvian armed forces. On the one hand, at this stage it would have been a blunder of the first magnitude if General Ureta had been ordered to capture Guayaquil, and, on the other hand, the army could not permanently remain in El Oro province, which was unquestionably Ecuadoran territory. General Ureta's function in El Oro was to maintain pressure on Ecuador and indirectly on the mediators until the Peruvian territorial demands in the Amazon basin and on the eastern slopes of the Andes were satisfied. Peru's demands had to be sufficiently extensive to give satisfaction to its army leaders, to resuscitate the family pride of the Prados, and to appease other Peruvian politicians; they had also to be sufficiently moderate to be accepted, however despairingly, by Ecuador and to fall just short of outraging the rather elastic conscience of America as represented by the mediatory powers. The order given above may well have been the order of priority attached to these considerations by President Prado. The political settlement could not be negotiated until he felt fairly sure of the acquiescence of the army, for the army in Peru, as in certain other countries, could not automatically be counted as politically neutral.[59]

At the same time, Prado's position with respect to the army may have been such as to impel him to strive for a negotiated settlement within a reasonably short time. It may be assumed that he wished to avoid the creation of a situation that would give General Ureta a chance to return to Lima as a conquering hero before the government could gain credit for a Peruvian victory through diplomatic channels. This consideration may have been an impelling one, both for the subsequent negotiations of an armistice in El Oro and for the nature of the terms of the settlement at the Rio de Janeiro conference.

From the point of view of the United States it was desirable that a stable political regime be maintained in Peru and that control of the government should not be secured by the Peruvian army, since it appeared to Washington that the army would be less likely than the civilian authorities to make a speedy and moderate settlement with Ecuador.

With considerations such as these in the minds of men in the foreign offices in Washington, Rio de Janeiro, and Buenos Aires, efforts were made to draft a mutually satisfactory response to the Peruvian memorandum of September 13. These efforts were complicated by the fact that some Peruvians had been struck by sober second thoughts about the appropriateness of their memorandum. Ex-President Oscar Benavides, Peruvian Ambassador in Buenos Aires, made strenuous endeavors to dissuade the mediators from making a written reply to the Peruvian note, and there is some evidence of hesitation and differences of opinion among the mediators about the firmness of their reply.[60] Nevertheless, on October 4, 1941, the mediators presented their response to the Peruvian foreign office. This important note was less censorious than Washington would have desired, but it remained a message strongly denunciatory of Peruvian policy. It left no doubt that Peru had agreed to withdraw its armed forces fifteen kilometers behind the 1936 *status quo* line, that Peru had not fulfilled this pledge, and that the mediators regarded such withdrawal as "essential to the establishment of an atmosphere favorable to the negotiation of a friendly settlement." It was noted that on July 25 the Peruvian Foreign Minister, Solf y Muro, had "formally agreed that the representatives of the mediators should establish a definitive day and hour for the cessation of hostilities." Both countries had finally agreed to an armistice to be effective on July 31, and Peru had at that time agreed to retire its armed forces fifteen kilometers behind the 1936 *status quo* line. However, the memorandum stated that the Peruvian foreign office, in its memorandum of September 13, 1941, had presented "new demands" on Ecuador "as a condition previous to the retirement of its armed forces."

The mediatory powers expressed the hope that Peru would reconsider its attitude, and " 'would facilitate the necessary solution on a basis that would be more harmonious with the irrevocable principles by which the American Republics had repudiated territorial conquests by means of force.' " The mediators suggested to the Peruvian and Ecuadoran governments that, concurrently with the withdrawal of troops, " 'they name plenipotentiaries who would go immediately to Buenos Aires to discuss there all the phases of the boundary dispute,' " with representatives of the three mediatory powers. The note ended with a request for a " 'prompt reply' " from the Peruvian government, so that the mediators " 'may give the fullest possible satisfaction to the right of all the American republics to be fully informed and to be consulted in regard to any question affecting the maintenance of the peace and the security of the continent.' " [61]

The presentation of the mediators' reply to the Peruvian note of September 13 created dismay in Lima, and intense efforts were made by Peruvian diplomats to induce the mediators to withdraw their note.[62] These efforts, vigorously countered by Ecuadoran representations, were in vain, and the mediators' reply was maintained as having been formally presented, to the enduring satisfaction of the Ecuadoran government and the embarrassment of that of Peru. Tobar regarded this reply as "the brand on the forehead of the aggressor." It remains, officially, however, only an Ecuadoran brand, since the mediators themselves have not released an authenticated text in Spanish, Portuguese, or English.[63]

CHAPTER XI

Truce and Treaty

TWO DAYS BEFORE the presentation of the mediators' memorandum, the military commanders of Ecuador and Peru made an agreement, known as the Talara truce, that established a neutral zone between two lines in the provinces of Guayas, El Oro, and Loja. The Talara truce did not in any way affect the situation in the Oriente. The zone varied in width from about twenty to about thirty miles. In general, the Peruvian army maintained most of its advanced positions in Ecuadoran territory, and the Ecuadoran army retired the distance necessary to create the neutral zone. The armed forces of both states withdrew completely from the neutral zone, and observers of the mediatory powers were to exercise supervision and ascertain that soldiers of neither side entered the zone. It should be noted that the creation of this zone had no relationship to the Peruvian agreement to withdraw behind the 1936 *status quo* line, an agreement that Peru did not fulfill.[1] (The lines are shown in Map III.)

An influential role in bringing about the Talara truce was played by the mediators' ambassadors in Lima and by the military observers. General Ureta had been authorized by Lima to discuss with the observers a suspension of military action, and the Department of State had authorized Norweb to permit the United States observers to serve as transmitting agents between the two armies.

The Department of State was pleased with the negotiation of the Talara truce, but it regarded the truce as a strictly military arrangement made by Ecuadoran and Peruvian officers, with which the mediators had no connection or responsibility. Otherwise the Department of State would have in some measure recognized the advances made by the Peruvian army beyond the 1936 *status quo* line, behind which the mediators' memorandum of October 4 had demanded that those forces retire. The Talara truce had been signed by the mediators' military observers as witnesses only, and the truce was not submitted to their governments for approval. The ambassadors of the mediators had apparently encouraged the making of the truce as the best way to bring an end to military operations after it had become clear that the Peruvian troops would not be withdrawn until a settlement of the boundary had been reached.

Although the Talara truce arranged an armistice between Ecuador and Peru on the basis of the existing Peruvian military dispositions, the mediators did not regard the truce as weakening their demand that Peruvian troops should withdraw behind the 1936 *status quo* line. Despite some wavering on the part of Rio de Janeiro and Buneos Aires, the Department of State did not change its position. The mediators' memorandum of October 4 was never withdrawn. Neither, however, were the Peruvian troops withdrawn; they remained on Ecuadoran soil, and the Peruvian government never replied to the mediators' note of October 4. The military control of the situation by the Peruvian forces was therefore maintained.

In Peru there seems to have been a serious difference of opinion at this time between General Ureta at the front and President Prado and Foreign Minister Solf y Muro in Lima. General Ureta was not disposed to reduce the pressure that his army's presence in Ecuador created, and he may even have proposed to advance to Guayaquil. Prado and Solf, more sensitive to the reactions of the other American states, may have wished to secure the maximum advantage from their existing position, rather than to risk their anticipated gains by grasping more territory or exercising more forceful pressure on Ecuador. There does not appear to have been any official support in Lima for the views of Peruvian superpatriots who hinted at the annexation of all Ecuador and who talked about the reincorporation of the Inca Empire. The Peruvian government made certain moves toward a settlement, based on the recognition by Ecuador of the

1936 *status quo* line in the western sector and a line in the Oriente with certain modifications in favor of Peru's claims.[2] These proposals were opposed by Quito, and no important change occurred in the situation before the Japanese attack on Pearl Harbor on December 7, 1941, and the entry of the United States into World War II.

Faced by the silence and noncompliance of the Peruvian government with respect to their strong memorandum of October 4, 1941, and by the evident refusal of Peru to withdraw its army from the Ecuadoran province of El Oro, the mediatory powers began to show signs of disunity and even of a disorderly tendency to request a change of attitude on the part of the government of Ecuador.[3] They had begun to recognize the consequences of the powerful position and evident determination of the Peruvian government, and they turned from attempts to persuade Peru to withdraw its troops and fulfill its promises, as set forth in their memorandum of October 4, to trying to find ways of moderating Peruvian territorial demands.[4]

The Japanese attack on Pearl Harbor, however, created a new atmosphere around the Marañón dispute. Washington's drive for hemispheric unity was accelerated, and renewed urgency was felt in its desire for a permanent settlement of the controversy. The third conference of foreign ministers of the American states, called to meet at Rio de Janeiro on January 15, 1942, was primarily concerned with continental defense. Peru was not anxious to have the boundary dispute discussed, but Ecuador wished the conference to arrange a formula in advance. Quito no doubt had little desire to be left utterly alone at the mercy of Peru, as might well be the case if the attention of the United States were concentrated more single-mindedly than ever on the world conflict.

At the same time, the Peruvians were not in an entirely happy position. The Brazilian Ambassador in Lima received instructions "to impress strongly upon his Peruvian friends the importance of reaching a settlement with Ecuador on the basis of the 1936 line and the unfortunate circumstances of having the boundary question raised at the Rio de Janeiro meeting on the grounds that Peru is occupying Ecuadoran territory by force." [5]

The Ecuadoran government recognized the unfavorable climate created by the involvement of the United States in World War II, and it attempted to defer the proposed meeting of foreign ministers of the American states requested by Washington.[6] This effort did not succeed, but on December 23, 1941, the mediatory powers again proposed to Ecuador and Peru that they accept as the basis for a final settlement the 1936 *status quo* line, that they withdraw their troops behind this line, and that they agree that a conference be held in Buenos Aires to arrange a final boundary.[7]

Ecuador accepted this proposal, but Peru refused it. President Prado

was unyielding in his refusal to accept the 1936 line as the basis for negotiations in the Oriente and insisted that Ecuador recognize that line in the Oriente as its maximum aspirations and the zone between would be the subject of negotiations. . . . I think that Peru may feel that it will have a good case if there is a definitive settlement and withdrawal of troops in the west, since it can claim that advances in the Oriente have been made by both parties and that Peruvian advances are into territory in dispute and not into Ecuadoran territory.[8]

Despite Tobar's best efforts, the boundary dispute with Peru was not given a place on the agenda of the conference of foreign ministers at Rio de Janeiro.[9] Consequently, when the conference opened, the relations between the two countries and between them and the mediators, was undefined, although both Ecuador and Peru finally agreed to participate by sending formal delegations, headed by their respective foreign ministers. It should be noted, however, that the mediators, in notes of December 26, 1941, informed the other American states of their proposal of December 23 to Ecuador and Peru.[10] They did not go so far, however, as to say that they knew Peru would not accept this proposal, nor were they so bold as to suggest that the controversy be placed on the agenda of the meeting of foreign ministers, scheduled to be held in three weeks.

As the delegates converged on Rio de Janeiro, three proposals had been made for settlement of the Marañón dispute, each one supported by a different mediatory power.[11] The proposals of Argentina and Brazil were regarded by Tobar as forecasting a fundamental and unfortunate change in the position of the mediators. "Was

America going to accept accomplished facts in order to achieve an apparent, artificial solidarity?" [12] If so, the situation would be regarded with complacency by Peru and with dismay by Ecuador. However, each side had its champion. Foreign Minister Solf left Lima for Buenos Aires and accompanied Ruiz Guiñazú by ship to Rio de Janeiro. Foreign Minister Tobar left Quito for Washington and traveled in an airplane with Welles to the Brazilian capital.

Tobar relates that, when in Washington, Welles informed him that Aranha had stated in a recent letter that his Ambassador in Peru, Pedro de Moraes Barros, " 'had succeeded in getting the Peruvian government to accept' " a line, which, as it turned out, was the line later written into the Protocol of Rio de Janeiro. This line was at all but one point (on the Pastaza River) east of the Peruvian line of September 13, 1941, and so may be regarded as offering to Ecuador a more favorable territorial position than would have been achieved if Peruvian desires had been uninhibited by the efforts of Brazil and the other mediators, although it did not, of course, offer Ecuadoran access to the Marañón. Further, Aranha had stated to Welles:

"We recognize that this situation would mean a certain material sacrifice [by Ecuador]; however, *we do not see that there is any other solution capable of re-establishing harmony between the two countries*, and, consequently, of permitting America to take, in a general atmosphere of confidence and solidarity, decisions which are necessary for each and every one of the nations of the continent." [13]

In thus supporting the essence of the Peruvian claims, Aranha provided what Peruvians have since praised and Ecuadorans denounced as the "Aranha line." The Argentine formula for the boundary was considerably more favorable to Peru than the Aranha line, and it was also made known to Tobar in Washington at this time.[14]

During their trip to Rio de Janeiro, Tobar gave Welles a memorandum intended to convince him that, "in order to preserve the prestige of continental institutions" Peru should first withdraw from the Ecuadoran province of El Oro. The Argentine and Brazilian proposals were said to be "absolutely contrary to American Law" because they implied the approval of the results of the use of force by Peru. Tobar reported that Welles was "deeply impressed" by the memorandum and said that it would be a basis for the talks he would have with Aranha, "who was, by virtue of his qualities of intelligence and character, the man who would be called upon to settle the controversy." [15]

Tobar soon found that Aranha wanted to settle the conflict during the Rio de Janeiro conference, rather than to arrange a preliminary settlement in accordance with the mediators' proposals of December 26, a procedure that Ecuador greatly preferred. Tobar pleaded in vain for a delay on the ground that the mediators had asked Peru to withdraw its troops from El Oro and that the mediators' note of December 23 had proposed a withdrawal of all troops behind the 1936 *status quo* line and a conference in Buenos Aires for a final settlement. Aranha was determined that a settlement be reached with or without a Peruvian withdrawal, and that the final settlement should not be postponed by referring negotiations to a later conference in Buenos Aires. He told Tobar that the mediators could not give their attention to the Marañón dispute after the conference because of "the grave questions that they were called upon to consider at this time." [16]

At the conference, the Peruvian delegation had a strong position. Peruvian troops were still occupying Ecuadoran territory, with the evident threat that they might advance from El Oro to Guayaquil. Brazil was committed to support a boundary that would give Peru Andoas and Rocafuerte beyond the 1936 line, with some intervening territory. As had become evident from the maps attached to the proposal of December 3 made by Ruiz Guiñazú, Argentina was even more generous to Peru, and undoubtedly the principal aim of Solf's roundabout itinerary was to assure himself of Argentine support of the Brazilian proposal, at the very least. Whereas Colombian sympathies were expected to favor Ecuador, as were those of Mexico, the Peruvians probably believed that they had only the United States to consider as a serious obstacle to securing approval of their demands. Their willingness to exercise what pressure they could on the United States is suggested by a remark made by Solf and reported in the Lima press on January 7. Solf said that Peru did not regard the United States as a belligerent in World War II and, when asked if Peru intended to offer military assistance to the United States, he replied: " 'I do not believe that the United States needs our military aid.' "

The only advantage that Ecuador had in the negotiations was its capacity to refuse to sign the final act of the Rio de Janeiro conference. Tobar used the threat of such a refusal, but only as a means of postponing for twenty-four hours the closing of the conference.

During the entire period of the conference (January 15-29), the mediators informally negotiated with Tobar and Solf. Aranha took the lead in the negotiations, during which the Ecuadorans and Peruvians held no meetings together. Since the dispute was not on the agenda, it was officially ignored by the conference, and not only did the American states other than the four mediators—Chile was added to the group at Rio de Janeiro—take no part whatever in the talks, but their diplomats avoided all efforts of the Ecuadoran delegates to interest them in the dispute.

Sumner Welles had little time to give to the boundary dispute in view of his other negotiations. Preoccupied by threats to the United States from Germany and Japan, Welles appears to have done little more at Rio de Janeiro than follow the lead of Aranha in the Marañón dispute.[17] This lead was inconsistent with two general principles of Brazilian foreign policy: (1) to aid weak states in Latin America against the stronger states and (2) to secure the participation of as many Latin American states as possible in arrangements for control of the Amazon River system.[18]

The principal source of information about the negotiations at Rio de Janeiro on the boundary dispute is Tobar's book, which, since it is a defense of his action, should be used with some caution. However, the tone of Tobar's account, together with the accuracy of his documentation on other aspects of the dispute, provides a reasonable assurance that, in its general lines at least, his story may be given credence.[19]

Washington and other American capitals had advised Ecuador to attend the conference at Rio de Janeiro. The Ecuadoran government finally decided to send a delegation, accepting Viteri's opinion that, since Ecuador was weak, it was essential to go to Rio de Janeiro in order to strengthen the principles that Ecuador must use for its defense.[20]

When Tobar had arrived in Washington, he had talked with Welles about the proposals of Aranha and Ruiz Guiñazú and had said that both of them "implied the consecration of the injustice committed against Ecuador, and the recognition of the accomplishments of violence, in spite of Ecuador's having given no reason for aggression." Nevertheless, he relates, Welles "stated categorically that 'it was impossible to fail to take account of certain facts.' A delicate allusion, no doubt, to the unhappy circumstance that Ecuador had been defeated." [21]

However, Welles probably had in mind a number of other "facts" that he was taking into account. These were provided by the "Report of the Commission of Military Observers in Ecuador Visiting the Peruvian Zone," made in August, 1941.[22]

The Commission of Military Observers visited General Ureta and other officers in the Peruvian positions in El Oro province, and they recorded the following "impressions," which are given here in full, in view of their importance to an understanding of many aspects of the Marañón conflict:

The impressions obtained personally by the Commission following several conversations with Peruvian officers allow of the following conclusions:

a. The political objective of the Peruvian military action is to resolve the frontier dispute with Ecuador, placing the Peruvian army in a threatening position so that Ecuador will accept without delay or qualification the boundary that Peru has always claimed: The whole of the Oriente, with the possible exception of a single route to the Amazon region, and the provinces of Jaén and Tumbes.

b. As security, the Peruvian army will continue to occupy the province of El Oro, as well as all parts of the Oriente presently occupied by Peruvian troops.

c. If Ecuador refuses to accept the terms to be proposed by Peru, the occupation of El Oro will be completed, and an advance will be made on Loja, Cuenca, and Guayaquil. Such action would also be undertaken if Ecuador should delay the signing of the treaty for settlement of the frontier problem.

d. The government of Peru has so far prevented General Ureta from advancing on Guayaquil, Cuenca, and Loja.

e. General Ureta did not agree to stop hostilities on July 26, since he had not yet secured control of El Oro, and his progress toward Pasaje had been delayed because he had had to consolidate a position at Machala instead of continuing his advance farther toward the east.

When the Peruvian government accepted the cease-fire, General Ureta advanced only to obtain secure, advanced positions; so that the army had turned to the right [eastward from Machala on the coast] to enable it to obtain positions menacing Loja and Cuenca, and to oblige the dispersion of Ecuadoran forces to defend those towns.

f. Peru has desired to satisfy the long-standing national aspiration to define, once and for all, its frontier in the north, in accordance with its claims that, it is contended, are adequately justified by its legal titles. Peru desires to achieve this aim now, so as to avoid the possibility that Ecuador might impose its will on Peru as a result of an unfavorable domestic political situation in Peru, an Ecuadoran advantage in military forces, or support for Ecuadoran claims by foreign countries. The possibility of such a situation is envisaged because Ecuador has had earlier opportunities of which it has not been able to take advantage, such as during the War of the Pacific and Peru's affray with Colombia over Leticia, as a result of incapable governments in Quito, discontinuity in Ecuador's foreign and domestic policies, and lack of sufficient resources.

g. Although Peru has not fostered an aggressive propaganda campaign, or a preparation of the spirit of its people antagonistic to Ecuador, the insults and indignities and the continued campaign of hatred that Ecuador had carried on against Peru and the Peruvian soldier had finally produced a profound resentment in Peru.

h. The Peruvian campaign is intimately related to a popular aspiration of all Peruvians, and it has no relationship whatever to any foreign influence, German, Japanese or other.

i. The Peruvian army is an effective force, well equipped with the arms necessary to deal with Ecuador. It has the greatest confidence in General Ureta.

j. Peru does not desire the intervention of the mediatory powers in its dispute with Ecuador; it wants to settle this dispute by itself. The mediation was accepted only because of the weakness of its political leaders, but Peru will not accept the mediators' intervention as arbitrators.[23]

The report of the Commission of Military Observers continued by stating that "Ecuador has not had, does not have, nor can it obtain within a relatively long time, an army that could undertake an offensive or even defend the country despite the extraordinarily excellent topography available for such defense. Ecuador lacks capable officers, trained troops, organization, and equipment."

However, the Peruvian army could at any moment begin an attack even though such action would violate the cease-fire.[24]

As an appendix (No. 2) to the above document (Annex No. 4 to the Report of the Commission of Military Observers), there appears a document entitled "Analytical Commentary on the Views of Peruvian Military Officers: A Faithful Copy of the Information Provided by the Military Observers of the Mediatory Powers in Lima." The salient portions of this document are also quoted here in view of their official provenance, as well as their significance and uniqueness.[25]

The "Commentary" stated that the views of Peruvian officers could be summarized as follows:

"The mediation of Argentina, Brazil, and the United States of America had prevented the completion of victorious operations by the Peruvian army, which otherwise could have quickly secured peace with Ecuador and, by means of a decisive military action, settled the frontier dispute.

"The Peruvian government's acceptance of the cease-fire of July 26, 1941, had deprived the Peruvian army of the fruits of a victory of great potential political importance. Hence, the resentment of the army against the mediatory powers, which brought about this unjust situation, is entirely justified.

"The Peruvian army, having stopped its advance on July 31, is in no way disposed to retire, and much less is it inclined to accept a retirement of fifteen kilometers behind the 1936 *status quo* line, which is presently obsolete in view of new conditions. The Peruvian army considers that, taking advantage of surprise and the complete demoralization of the Ecuadorans, it would have been easy to occupy within fifteen or twenty days the vital centers of Ecuador and impose upon it a definitive treaty of peace and amity, in which Ecuador would recognize for once and for all the sovereignty of Peru over its ancient provinces of Tumbes, Jaén, and Maynas.

"After such a treaty, since Peru has no territorial claims on foreign soil and had no desire to continue occupation of territory that had always belonged to Ecuador, there would be no difficulty about the withdrawal of Peruvian troops behind the frontier, leaving the zones of Machala and Santa Rosa and other Ecuadoran areas that did not form part of the above mentioned provinces of Peru. . . .

"In such fashion, had it not been for the inopportune intervention of the mediatory countries, the conflict would have ended, and American peace would have been obtained, which was the asserted aim of this intervention. Further, the uncertain situation resulting from the cease-fire has resulted in difficult problems of supply and sanitation for the Peruvian army and for Peruvian and Ecuadoran civilians in the occupied zones. The mediators should therefore act quickly to bring about a settlement, without requiring troop withdrawals that would not lead to any solution and that the Peruvian army would not accept. . . .

"The impetuous personality of General Ureta is manifest, and his authority and prestige has the unanimous support of the important army group under his orders. His army feels and thinks as does its leader, and it is clear that it will follow him blindly wherever he may choose to lead it. The support of the remainder of the Peruvian army may be assumed; it sympathizes in its great majority with General Ureta, especially after the victories he has obtained. The authoritarian character of General Ureta is well known, and recently he has been credited with political ambitions. If to this it is added that the campaign in the north was not an improvisation, but that it is a product of a plan directed by General Ureta; that the campaign has been curtailed by the cease-fire; that the Peruvian army's plans had been carefully worked out by the Escuela Superior de Guerra whose director was General Ureta, who is now surrounded by his students who are members of his staff, it can readily be understood that the army leaders are unhappy about the present situation, which has stopped them from gaining the victory over Ecuador that they had planned and toward which they were successfully marching when halted by diplomatic maneuvering. The popularity of General Ureta is therefore growing, and there are possibilities of his having domestic political objectives in view of the existing situation." [26]

Other "facts" that Welles may be presumed to have had in mind when talking to Tobar had been reported to the Department of State following an interview in September with the Minister of Defense of Ecuador by members of the Commission of Military Observers.[27]

The Minister of Defense thought that a Peruvian advance on Guayaquil was quite practicable and that Ecuador would prefer to create a neutralized zone than to run the risk of a renewal of hostilities, even though such a zone would be based on the present military positions. Ecuador did not wish in any case to be left alone to deal with Peru directly but desired the participation of the mediatory powers. Ecuador, however, was entirely agreeable to cede to Peru the frontier of the *status quo* line of 1936 and even the rivers of the Oriente up to the limit of their navigability. The Minister of Defense ended by saying that "the Oriente was practically lost to Ecuador, and it would have been possible to retain it only if Ecuador had continued to form part of "Gran Colombia,' a possibility which even at present should not be entirely discounted." The

Minister expressed his thanks to the mediatory powers and to their military observers, since, he said, without them "Guayaquil would be in the hands of Peru." [28]

It was clear to Welles, when he had talked to Tobar, not only that Ecuador had been defeated but also that the Peruvian army under General Ureta would not withdraw from Ecuadoran territory until a treaty had been made that would give Peru a boundary not much different from that which the Peruvian government had outlined in its note of September 13, 1941. Only superior force on the ground, in Ecuador, would make Ureta retreat. At the time, in late December, 1941, there was no possibility that the United States would divert any armed force from its military effort against Japan and Germany in order to drive the Peruvian army out of Ecuador. If any effective pressure was to be brought against Peru, it would have to be done by the Brazilian government.

From this time forward Welles appears to have been an infrequent participant in the negotiations at Rio de Janeiro. Tobar had learned as early as October that the United States wished to give to Brazil the "preëminent and decisive role in the dispute," and Welles was apparently happy to have Aranha take the lead not only to avoid further resentment against the United States but also because Welles desired to give his whole attention to the gaining of continental solidarity against the Axis powers.

Although Tobar and his colleagues on the delegation tried to win support from the mediators for a preliminary agreement with Peru on procedures for a final settlement that would be arranged later, as proposed in the mediators' note of December 23, Aranha said that such a procedure was out of the question. If the dispute were not settled at the conference, said Aranha, Ecuador would then be at the mercy not only of the civil government in Lima but also of General Ureta and the commander in the Oriente.[29] The present moment, he continued, was a unique opportunity, perhaps the last, for Ecuador to hope for a peaceful solution. " 'You must have a skin,' " Aranha added. " 'A country without frontiers is the same as a man without a skin. You need peace rather than land.' "

In an interview with Welles, Tobar heard the same opinion in different words. Welles said that Peru had rejected the proposal of

December 23 for a provisional arrangement; consequently, the best procedure was for the disputants to accept a boundary line adopted by the mediators.[30] It may have been this interview that has given rise to the opinion held by some Ecuadorans that it was the United States that was primarily responsible for the "imposition" of the terms of the Protocol on Ecuador. This opinion may be developing into a myth, but, if so, the claims to participatory responsibility of Oswaldo Aranha and Enrique Ruiz Guiñazú should not be forgotten. However, in his book on Ecuadoran culture, Pio Jaramillo Alvarado asserts that at the Rio de Janeiro conference, "the United States favored strong Peru against weak Ecuador"; and in a pro-Ecuadoran work by the late Colombian international lawyer, Jesús María Yepes, it is stated that, at the conference, Sumner Welles "coldly notified" Tobar in a secret session, "revealed by the indiscretion of one of the participants," that, if Ecuador did not accept the mediators' proposal, "Peru would invade Ecuador within a short time and that the United States . . . would do nothing to prevent Peru's action." [31]

The Ecuadorans did not give up on this point until after they met with Aranha and Welles together on January 15, when the two mediators declared emphatically that the mediation was at an end and that a final solution must be found at the conference. Tobar said there was not enough time, but Welles claimed there was time and declared that he would stay long enough in Rio de Janeiro to see the settlement through. It was now clear that the Ruiz Guiñazú formula was discarded, since it proposed later negotiations; consideration settled on the Brazilian proposal, which the Ecuadorans and Peruvians, for different reasons, preferred to call "the Aranha line"; by using this name Ecuadorans mean that the line was imposed by the mediators and Peruvians mean it had their approval.

In writing about the opening session of the conference, Tobar states that

none of the speakers alluded to the existence of a case of aggression in America; all of them talked only of the attack by Japan on the United States. . . . The luster of the Conference was not going to be dimmed by even one reference to our situation, despite the fact that it was putting to the test the sincerity and effectiveness of continental institutions.[32]

The Ecuadoran delegation decided, under the circumstances, to refrain from attending any further sessions of the conference and explained its intention in a note to Aranha. The Brazilian Foreign Minister's response was to say that he would then declare the mediation at an end and at the same time release the Ecuadoran note to the other states. Faced with this threat, Tobar gave in, agreed to attend the conference sessions, and in effect placed the settlement of the boundary problem in the hands of the mediators who carried on negotiations separately with the Peruvians. His position was approved by the government in Quito, which suggested three changes in the Aranha line. The change that Quito asked Tobar to try to do everything possible to obtain was that Ecuador should have access to the Marañón from the mouth of the Santiago to the mouth of the Morona.[33]

Tobar told Aranha of Quito's position, and Aranha said that his desire to support Ecuador had been blocked by the insistence of Peru that Ecuador should obtain no outlet on the Marañón, even at the mouth of the Santiago, which, because of the Manseriche Rapids, lower on the Marañón, would be useless in any case as navigable access to the Amazon system. It is reported that about this time Aranha said that President Vargas vainly urged Solf y Muro " 'the man of granite,' " to accept a conciliatory settlement.[34]

The next several days of the conference saw no progress, mainly because the mediators were concerned with resolving the difference with Argentina about the resolution on breaking relations with the Axis powers. When this matter was settled, and Ecuador and Peru had signed the resolution, the mediators bent every effort to get a boundary document completed. Tobar and his delegation decided on the morning of January 27 that, since the demands of Peru could not be accepted, Tobar would speak at the last plenary session of the conference scheduled for that afternoon, explaining Ecuador's position and announcing that it would not sign the final act of the conference. Aranha, however, postponed the session as he and the other mediators plunged into a series of continuous meetings with the Ecuadorans and the Peruvians, alternately. At one o'clock on the morning of January 28 Tobar was given a description of the boundary line that had been drawn up by the Brazilian foreign office and that was represented as being the maximum concession obtainable from Peru.

The Peruvian "minimum" demand was a serious blow to the hopes of the Ecuadorans, who protested on several points. They were given a second blow by the news that the scheduled plenary session of the conference, postponed from January 27 to January 28, would not be held at all; the final session would be that of formal speechmaking only. Tobar asserts that "in this way the Foreign Minister of Ecuador was deprived of the last appropriate opportunity . . . to express to America his calm, dignified, and measured protest against the Peruvian aggression." [35]

After further consultation with Solf, the mediators called in Dr. Arroyo Delgado of the Ecuadoran delegation at one o'clock in the afternoon on January 28 and presented the Peruvian "last word," which the mediators transmitted to Ecuador for consideration and a reply by four o'clock of the same day. Arroyo reported that, in effect, Ecuador was to be definitely excluded from the Marañón and that the dispositions in the northern Oriente were vague and gave Ecuador no compensation for Peru's advantages in the south. Arroyo reported to Tobar that he had said that

even giving full credit to the proffered guarantee of the mediators, the proposed solution did not offer adequate prospects for Ecuador, since documents signed by Peru were without value in international dealings, and the guarantors could only assure Ecuador that they would exhaust their efforts with a country against whose position their influence and prestige had already had little effect. Mr. Welles said: "The Ecuadoran Minister is right." [36]

Arroyo said he would not even transmit the Peruvian proposal to Tobar "unless it were clearly established that the boundary line in the north would follow down the Napo River to the mouth of the Aguarico River, and ascend the Aguarico and the Lagartococha directly to the mouth of the Güepi River in the Putumayo." The mediators thereupon agreed that this stipulation would be made in the final arrangement, and Arroyo then said he would take the proposal to Tobar.

In the meeting of the Ecuadoran delegation that followed immediately on receipt of this three-hour ultimatum, it was decided that

Ecuador could not hope to obtain a better line from Peru without the assistance of the mediators, if the offer were rejected. However, when their meeting with the mediators was held at four o'clock, the Ecuadorans tried in every possible way to gain both concessions and time. The Peruvian delegates were in an adjoining room, and Tobar recalls that Aranha hustled from one room to the other with offers and counteroffers, while, outside, the delegates of the other countries awaited anxiously the call for the closing session of the conference.

Lacking any account of the talks between Aranha and the Peruvian delegation headed by Solf, we can only guess at their content. It may be assumed that Aranha told Solf that the mediation was at an end and that unless some concessions were made to Ecuador the mediators would refuse to recognize a treaty imposed by force alone, with the result that Peruvian title to the whole of the Oriente would remain in doubt. Such a "moral threat" was Aranha's only resource, and yet it was evidently of some effect.

Tobar warned Aranha that the proposal was not in accord with his instructions from Quito and that its signature would surely bring about a political overturn in Ecuador; he states, however, that he recognized that Aranha did not fear such an outcome.[37] This may have meant that Aranha did not much care, or it may have meant that Aranha had shrewdly diagnosed the situation in Ecuador, or both. There was no revolution in Ecuador as the immediate result of the Peruvian victory, probably because potential revolutionaries were quite satisfied to allow the regime of President Arroyo del Río to bear full responsibility for the position of Ecuador in 1941–42 and so burden the Liberal Party with an historic and unpopular decision.

In a last desperate move, Tobar asked Aranha to obtain from the Peruvians an agreement to allow fifteen days for the signing of the protocol if it was accepted by President Arroyo del Río. Aranha said he would do so if desired, but added ominously: " 'You may be certain that, once the conference is over, Peru will look at the agreement with a smile.' "[38] Tobar preferred not to face that Peruvian smile. Besides,

Each of the mediators urged the Ecuadoran delegation to sign the protocol, making clear in one way or another that, if it was not accepted, Ecuador could take it for granted that Peru would occupy Guayaquil. Sr. Ruiz Guiñazú, for his part, intimated that Peru had already conceded enough and that it was time for Ecuador to give away.

To one of the Ecuadoran efforts to make a change in the text, Aranha was reported to have replied: " 'The Peruvian claims are limitless; at the end of five days they will invade you.' " Questioned as to whether in that case there existed sanctions in the legal institutions of America, Aranha said that Brazil could not provide them because of the grave problems it faced; their existence depended upon the United States. Tobar does not record whether this question was asked of Welles.[39]

A glimpse of some off-stage realities of international politics in the Americas was reported to Tobar by Humberto Albornoz of the Ecuadoran delegation, who talked with an unnamed statesman, who may well have been Oswaldo Aranha but whom Tobar refers to as "X." Albornoz had asked for aid, and X inquired if X's government should have declared war on Peru. Albornoz replied that Ecuador had depended on the principles of international law and Pan Americanism. X commented that these principles "exist to solve problems. You are not a problem for America. You, with your lack of military resistance, have not made your problem an American problem." He then advised Albornoz not to leave Rio de Janeiro without a treaty.[40]

At this point, the mediators left the Ecuadorans in the Itamaraty, asking them to think over their decision. The time was short, for the mediators were already half an hour late for the closing conference session. Aranha's last words were: " 'Think over what is best for you. Decide, Dr. Tobar, and come to the session where I shall have the pleasure of announcing that Ecuador and Peru have arrived at a final agreement and that the protocol will be signed tonight.' "

The decision was Tobar's alone. He recalls that he threw himself into an armchair, transfixed by bitter thoughts of the destruction of the hopes for the greatness of Ecuador that had been cherished for a century, and by the no less bitter thoughts that, unless those hopes were renounced, Ecuador might disintegrate and even disappear as a nation through new Peruvian assaults.

My reason told me that national existence itself, liberation from the invader, and the avoidance of his threats were of greater value at this moment than the fulfillment of our dreams. History said to me, in addition, that it was not I who sacrificed those dreams, but the country itself that had broken them into pieces through many decades of inconceivable negligence and abandonment.

" 'It was the last chance.' " With these words of Aranha's ringing in his ears, Tobar decided to sign.[41]

It was not only the last chance; it was the last few minutes of the last chance, for Tobar arrived at the final session when it was well under way, and he was just in time to permit Aranha to make the announcement at the end of his final speech.

There remained a few points of difference to be arranged in the "night hours" of which Welles had once spoken. The Peruvians objected to giving to Ecuador the same navigation rights on the rivers of the Oriente as were enjoyed by Brazil and Colombia, but Welles supported the Ecuadoran position, saying that "this article had been part of the draft protocol from the beginning and could not be taken out. Thanks to the expression of opinion by Welles this fundamentally important clause was retained." [42]

The protocol was finally signed at two o'clock in the morning on January 29, 1942.[43] Solf, for Peru, is reported as saying that " 'thanks to the *friendly intervention* of the governments of Argentina, Brazil, Chile and the United States, along with the governments of Ecuador and Peru, it was possible to make an agreement of peace and friendship appropriate to sister peoples.' " For his part, Tobar emphasized the sacrifices made by Ecuador, and hoped for understanding on the part of Peru and for support by the mediators in later negotiations. Curiously enough, Tobar named Ruiz Guiñazú and Aranha in his statement as deserving "special recognition" and "gratitude" for their parts in the "promotion of the mediation," and in the "realization of the agreement." The fact that he did not mention Welles at all is significant, for it is unusual for a diplomat to refrain from giving credit to all other statesmen principally associated with a negotiation leading to a treaty of peace.[44]

At first sight, Tobar's omission of Welles's name might seem to indicate that Tobar meant to insult him and so to criticize the policy of the United States. However, Tobar had mentioned at least two occasions when Welles had insisted on changes in the protocol to the advantage of Ecuador.[45]

These references, when combined with the lack of positive criticism of Welles, and Tobar's view of the protocol as involving great sacrifices for Ecuador, suggest that Tobar had quite a different purpose in not mentioning Welles at the signing ceremony. Instead, it seems likely that, by naming the Argentine and Brazilian foreign ministers and speaking of them in ostensibly flattering terms, he was really placing upon them, and not upon Welles, the responsibility for Ecuador's having to accept a humiliating and sacrificial agreement. If this interpretation is correct, his statement may properly be regarded as an Ecuadoran tribute to Welles and to the policy of the United States for having attempted to uphold Ecuador at a time when Ecuador was defenseless against Peruvian military power.[46] It is worth noting that, on one of the rare occasions when Tobar cast aspersions on any other country than Peru, he said that the inactivity of the mediators between May 20 and July 9 "and the indecision that, unfortunately, began to be displayed—shall I say it?—by Argentina" had given encouragement to Peru.[47]

In commenting on his remarks on this occasion, Tobar states: "Had I acrimoniously declared that the protocol had been imposed on Ecuador, I would only have openly wounded the feelings of Peru and the mediators, diminished the quality of Americanism in the action, and deprived Ecuador of the glory of making a sacrifice for the good of the Continent." [48]

When Tobar left Rio de Janeiro after the Conference, Aranha told him: " 'Pull yourselves together; work hard, and have faith that injustice is not permanent.' " Tobar took this remark as a theme of a speech delivered in the extraordinary session of the Ecuadoran congress in the spring of 1942 and appealed to his compatriots to put an end to their internal disunity and give vigor to a national movement for peace and stability. "We have a frontier. Let us build within it a nation worthy of its glorious past." [49]

This attitude, based on a defense of the acceptance of the

protocol, is in sharp contrast with a very different current of thought among other Ecuadorans. In the last chapter of his book Chiriboga Ordóñez suggests that a red marble tombstone should be erected near Rio de Janeiro, with the inscription:

Here lies a country: light of America; discoverer of the Amazon, soul of honor, model of Pan Americanism. It died in the Itamaraty, comforted with all the aids known to Christianity, provided by the American Republics. In its death throes there were read to it the prayers of continental peace and of good neighborliness, and there were chanted beautiful psalms entitled: "Oh, America, Continent of Justice and of Peace."

This Ecuadoran patriot proclaims that "From the time of the birth of our sons and of our grandsons, and of all the generations born of the flesh severed by the imposition of Rio de Janeiro, we must indoctrinate our children unforgettably with the eternal watchword: REVENGE! REVENGE!" [50]

The protocol described the boundary line by naming certain points and provided that Peru would withdraw its troops from Ecuadoran territory and guarantee freedom of navigation on rivers controlled by Peru. Concerning the mediators, the protocol provided that their "activity . . . will continue until the definitive demarcation of the frontiers between Ecuador and Peru has been completed. This Protocol and its execution will be under the guaranty of the four countries." [51]

The boundary line of the protocol in general lay between the line of the *status quo* of 1936 and the most advanced positions reached by Peruvian troops in 1941. It followed the line of 1936 between the Andes and the Pacific Ocean but gave a substantial advance to Peru in the practically uninhabited central and northern sections of the Oriente, except that in the extreme northern sector, along the Güepi River, a small section east of the 1936 line was recognized as Ecuadoran. In the northern areas of the Oriente, the protocol line resulted in the withdrawal of Peruvian troops which had reached some outposts as much as one hundred miles to the west of that line at points only about one hundred miles due east of Quito.[52]

In effect, therefore, Ecuador lost no territory occupied by its civilians, nor did it "lose" direct access by river to the Marañón, since even Tobar's description of the 1936 line shows that it ran north from the Chínchipe River along the San Francisco River and demonstrates, therefore, that Ecuador did not have any civil or military establishments along the Marañón in 1936.[53] The Peruvian record in this respect was quite different, as evidenced by the existence of Iquitos and other towns. It is probable that appreciation of this situation by other American states was influential in their decisions not to give stronger support to the Ecuadorans in the later stages of the dispute.[54]

As to Ecuador's territorial "losses," Tobar estimated that on its side of the line of the *status quo* of 1936 Ecuador then possessed about one third, or 40,600 square miles, of the total Ecuadoran claims in the Oriente, which were about 120,000 square miles. Of this 40,600 square miles, Tobar estimates that Ecuador lost by the protocol only a net total of 5,392 square miles; this figure was arrived at by subtracting from Peru's gain of 7,420 square miles over the 1936 line the Ecuadoran gain of 2,028 square miles.[55]

Tobar noted that the Peruvian government had been attacked by the APRA party for not having secured all of Peru's territorial claims and said that Marshal Benavides had expressed disapproval of the protocol as not obtaining enough for Peru. As a further defense of the protocol, he remarked that Ecuador retained 40,600 square miles in the Oriente, an area "almost as large as Guatemala and Cuba, and larger than Panamá and other American states," containing mineral and petroleum deposits and good agricultural and grazing land. Peru, on the other hand, in his view, secured mainly marshy areas that would not be useful for civilized settlement for many years.[56]

Tobar was here trying to make Ecuador's residue of dreams appear as substantial as he could. He did not mention, for example, that the boundary line of the protocol was drawn so far west as to exclude navigation by launches on the Ecuadoran side of all of the rivers in the Oriente, except the Putumayo, which formed part of the northern boundary.[57]

In Peru every effort was made by the government to give the impression that Peru had won both a diplomatic and a military triumph in what was called the Zarumilla campaign. The Peruvian press, with the exception of *La Tribuna* (Lima), the APRA organ which managed to appear occasionally despite an official ban, unanimously hailed the signing of the protocol as a magnificent victory. *El Peruano* (Lima) stated editorially on February 10, 1942, that the occasion "marked a complete and transcendental triumph capable of causing all Peruvians to take pride in their nationality."

The Peruvian government's chief propaganda document was a pamphlet [58] published in Lima in 1942. It does not contain the name of an author or a publisher, but it is probable that it was prepared by the government's own office of public relations, then directed by Rául Porras Barrenechea. The pamphlet, entitled *El protocolo de Río de Janeiro ante la historia*, was evidently intended to gain support for the government by emphasizing the size and value of the territories acquired by Peru in the peace settlement. It claimed that the Peruvian government had made military preparations to defend itself against the hostile attitude of Ecuador, and in the struggle

> provoked by Ecuador, the army of Peru gloriously fulfilled its duty, putting to flight the army of the aggressor, occupying the bases that served as the starting points for the aggression, and advancing in the north and the northeast even to places more distant than those claimed by virtue of our historical rights. . . . The treaty of Río de Janeiro is one of the most honorable pages in the history of our nationhood.

There followed a quotation from *El Telégrafo* (Guayaquil) of February 8, 1942, lamenting, for Ecuador, the conclusion of the protocol " 'which consecrates the most tremendous territorial mutilation recorded in the history of America.' " The pamphlet also contained a series of five maps, which compared the line of the protocol with five earlier lines drawn in consequence of unfulfilled treaties in the period from 1830 to 1910. The line of the protocol was described as giving to Peru various areas ranging from 8,000 to 80,000 square miles more than the earlier lines. For example, the protocol line was said to have given to Peru an area of about 8,000 square miles more than the line recommended to the King of Spain by his Council of State, as well as excluding Ecuador from the Marañón, which the latter did not. In view of the smaller figures given above from Tobar, it is perhaps not surprising that this publication does not make any comparison between the 1936 *status quo* line and that of the protocol. The only reference that might be interpreted as relating to the 1936 line is the statement that "the line of the protocol is superior by 30,000 square kilometers [12,000 square miles] to the line of Peruvian possessions in any previous period of our history." There is no mention of any territory, such as the Sucumbios Triangle, that Tobar had regarded as ceded to Ecuador by Peru.[59] As one of eight main reasons why Peruvians should be "proud of the protocol," this publication listed, with some exaggeration, "the securing by Peru of Ecuador's declaration that it is not an Amazonian country."

Peruvian troops evacuated El Oro province of Ecuador on February 11, in accordance with the protocol. The protocol was ratified by Peru on February 26 and by Ecuador on the following day. In Lima the votes in both houses were unanimous. In Quito the congressional votes were 27 to 3 in the senate and 42 to 9 in the chamber of deputies. Two senators and five deputies of the Conservative Party absented themselves from the legislature at the time of the vote. Ratifications of the protocol were exchanged on March 31, 1942, at Rio de Janeiro, in the presence of President Getulio Vargas. When the news of ratification by both countries was received in Washington, Welles expressed the satisfaction of his government and said that the settlement "affords a further proof of the ability and determination of the American Republics to settle all disputes between them by pacific methods." [60]

The signature of the protocol at Rio de Janeiro was the occasion of an exchange of congratulatory telegrams reasserting the solidarity of the American states. President Roosevelt cabled to President Prado:

Once more, and in a matter which for over a century has threatened the peace of the continent, the American republics have demonstrated their determination to settle their differences through friendly consultation and mutual adjustment. This convincing application of the doctrine of the Americas cannot but hearten us all in our struggle against those who recognize only the rule of force in the relations between nations.

To President Arroyo del Río, Roosevelt stated:

The spirit of cooperation and cordial collaboration which resulted in this act is a splendid expression of the high resolve of the American republics that differences between them can and must be settled through amicable discussion and just conciliation of opposing views.[61]

In his reply, the President of Ecuador could not forbear to say that in signing the protocol Ecuador had given one more evidence of its support for harmony and peace on the continent and for hemisphere defense, since by the terms of the protocol Ecuador "had made a sacrifice of its rights to bring about a solution of the boundary controversy and so contribute to the well being of the continent." [62]

CHAPTER XII

The Protocol of Rio de Janeiro
and the Policy of the United States

THE ACCEPTANCE of the protocol ended organized fighting along the Ecuador-Peru boundary for a long period of time. Peru had mobilized some 15,000 troops, of which about 13,000 saw service on the short front in the west, while the remainder occupied widely separated points in the Oriente, notably at Rocafuerte. Ecuador had mobilized forces of a strength of about 3,000 men on all fronts. Casualties are not known with exactitude, but information from Peruvian sources indicated that about 80–100 Peruvians had been killed, while Ecuadoran losses may have been as high as 500–600 killed. Ecuador was reported to have taken five prisoners, while several hundred Ecuadorans were held by the army of Peru when fighting ended. A substantial amount of damage to property had been caused in El Oro province, both by military action and by looting and other depredations.

In Quito the response to the protocol was a mixed reaction of relief at the ending of the threat of further Peruvian advances, satisfaction that a settlement had been reached, profound disappointment over the boundary that cut the country off from access to the Amazon river system, and bitterness ar the pretenses of a so-called community of American states that could permit what Ecuadorans regarded as an imposition by force of Peru's territorial demands.[1]

In Lima the protocol was hailed as a great military and diplomatic victory. A proposal made in the Peruvian congress for the erection of a monument on the Ecuadoran frontier to symbolize peace between the two countries, was regarded by *El Comercio* (Quito), September 13, 1943, as a note of "bitter humor."

In Washington Secretary Hull said at a press conference that "this was a peaceful settlement in accordance with one of the earliest policies of the good neighbor stemming from Montevideo through all subsequent conferences for peaceful settlement of disputes. The Rio decision carries this out and makes it all the more permanent in the policies of Pan Americanism." [2]

At the Rio de Janeiro conference Welles had given to Tobar assurance of financial support from the United States for Ecuadoran economic development and currency stabilization, and also for assistance in the rehabilitation of El Oro province.[3] This aid, however, does not appear to have had any connection with the terms of the settlement of the boundary dispute; other countries, such as Bolivia, also obtained financial assistance from the United States in the course of negotiations at the conference, and Solf announced as early as March 13, 1942, that the United States government had authorized lend-lease aid "for the defense of Peru" totaling $29 million.[4]

The protocol did not refer to the question of responsibility for the outbreak of hostilities in 1941. It may be said that responsibility was shared by Ecuador and Peru, but it also may be said that the responsibility was not equally shared. Without going back beyond 1941, when each country might charge the other with actions that prevented a settlement, as in 1889 or in 1910, it appears that Ecuador was following a policy that had grown increasingly risky. With a population about a third the size of Peru's and with material resources even smaller in proportion, Ecuadoran policy in the dispute had continued to maintain claims to territory that had in fact long been occupied and settled by Peruvians. Officially sanctioned maps published in Ecuador as late as 1938 maintained the fiction that Iquitos was within the boundaries of Ecuador. The territory effectively held in 1936 by Ecuador was considerably smaller than the territory it would have possessed had the Ecuadoran government accepted in 1910 the arbitration award that his Council of State had advised the King of Spain to make. In particular, it would then have received access to the Marañón from the Santiago to the Pastaza.[5]

Quito, however, had continued to assert its traditional legal claims and had tried to gain the support of other American, and even of European, states in the dispute. These efforts were so persistent as to give rise to the observation that there are abuses of weakness, as well as those of strength.

One of the techniques of the weak is to provoke an incident with a stronger opponent in the hope that other powers may intercede and aid the weaker state to gain a relatively advantageous settlement. Peruvians were accustomed to speak of Ecuadoran "provocations," [6] and it was obvious that only Ecuador had anything to gain from the creation of a "continental pressure," which, Quito hoped, would mitigate inequalities of power by introducing considerations of equity or justice.[7]

It will be recalled that Paraguay, five years before the outbreak of the Chaco war, had tried to gain the aid of other American states by attacking Bolivian forces at Fort Vanguardia and then immediately withdrawing. The tactic resulted in attracting attention to a dangerous situation, and the settlement of that incident was arranged, but it was not successful in producing enough continental pressure on Bolivia to bring about the peaceful solution of the controversy then desired by Paraguay.

In the Marañón dispute there does not appear to be any way of determining with finality the responsibility for the incident at Brumadero or Bramador on the Zarumilla River, which was the occasion for opening hostilities on July 5, 1941. Even if there were, the Paraguayan precedent in the Chaco would not encourage the belief that, if Peruvian soldiers were then at fault, the responsibility for the conflict as a whole would fall exclusively on the government at Lima. Similarly, on July 26, when Ecuador precipitately ordered its troops to cease fire before receiving confirmation of the report from Washington that Lima had agreed to an armistice on that day, it appears that President Arroyo del Río took this action as a way both of covering up the fact that his army was already on the point of dissolution and of attempting to place Lima in an embarrassing position before the mediators.

Ecuador's responsibility for the conflict exists in the sense that its policy had permitted the dispute to drag out its weary length until a moment had been reached when all factors in the situation were to Ecuador's disadvantage. Peru was incomparably stronger militarily, and General Ureta was able and energetic. President Prado was burning with a desire to restore the honor of his family and his country. Peru had suffered an ignominious reverse in the Leticia affair, and Peruvians remembered with bitterness not only the occupation of Lima as part of their defeat by Chile in the War of the Pacific but also other defeats in a nearly unrelieved record of losses beginning with the battle of Tarquí in 1829.

In addition, the outbreak of World War II left Ecuador alone in the world, with no prospects for effective help from its friends. The League of Nations had been wrecked, and inter-American peace machinery, the absence of which had been deplored by Stimson in 1930, still had to be designed anew, on frail foundations, for each dispute. The record of the Latin American states in cooperative measures for the prevention of war was not such as to encourage Ecuador to believe that it could obtain any assistance from other countries in South America.

These considerations should not be taken as suggesting, however, that Ecuador was responsible for the employment of force in the solution of the dispute. Ecuador hoped to gain the support of other countries to induce Peru, through diplomacy, to engage in a pacific procedure of settlement that would give Ecuador an opportunity for securing a maximum of its territorial claims by an arbitration in equity. The Ecuadoran political leaders had shown disastrously unrealistic judgment in upholding unrealizable claims until a point had been reached when the power, determination, and opportunity of Peru had simultaneously joined in a combination irresistible for Ecuador, and unrestrainable by others.[8]

The responsibility for the employment of force to bring about a final settlement rests primarily on Peru. The Peruvian government massed armaments and disposed its troops along the Ecuadoran border in the early months of 1941 and made use of the Bramador incident to launch a well-planned and skilfully directed attack on Ecuador.[9] The use of tanks, artillery, and parachute troops provides a sharp contrast between this calculated military operation and the hasty, feckless improvisation of the Peruvian military effort in Leticia nine years previously.

The plans of the Peruvian government for a military campaign on the northern front were laid at least as early as January, 1941. According to an account by a former Peruvian diplomat and public official, Luís Humberto Delgado, the instructions to General Ureta were based on the claim that Ecuadoran troops were already occupying Peruvian territory in the region of the island Noblecilla–El Caucho at the mouth of the Zarumilla River. General Ureta was to remain initially on the defensive, but, if the Ecuadoran troops held their positions, the army was to drive out the Ecuadorans. If a counteroffensive were undertaken by Ecuador, Ureta was to advance toward Machala and occupy El Oro province as far as the Jubones River. This account may be given some credence, since it purports to be a summary of a document and since, except for the way hostilities commenced, these instructions were closely followed in the actual fighting.[10]

Beyond the technical military preparations of Peru for the invasion of Ecuador, Humberto Delgado emphasized that Peru "was a country accustomed to defeats." The victory over Ecuador was the "only triumph" that Peru had ever enjoyed in the course of the settlement of its boundary problems. "As a result of the military campaign with Ecuador, we were rehabilitated; we realized that Peruvians could be victorious in combat, that they could repudiate the fear of war, which was the symbol and the shame of the past." [11]

It is indicative of the state of Peruvian historical studies that Humberto Delgado, who had been a Vice-President and an Ambassador of his country, could so markedly differ from Jorge Basadre, one of Peru's most eminent historians, in his estimate of Peruvian military history. Basadre, in an essay on the wars of Peru, notes that Peru fought its neighbors nine times in the nineteenth century. Peru engaged in more conflicts than any other South American country. However, says Basadre, "Peru has been the most peaceful and generous state of South America," and its nine wars have been carried on "in a posture of self-defense." Of these nine conflicts, three were won by Peru, three were lost, and three were related to "the maintenance of Peru as a state." [12]

That the Peruvian government had calculated on the use of force to solve the ancient Marañón dispute is strongly supported by publications of other eminent Peruvians. One of these is a pamphlet by General Felipe de la Barra, the founder of the Centro de Estudios Histórico-Militares del Perú.[13] General de la Barra states that "the moment has arrived to assert that the experience of conflicts of the past, especially that with Colombia [Leticia], has demonstrated that claims derived from justice and law only have validity when they are supported by force." [14] In the Leticia conflict Peru lacked effective armament, notably aircraft, but after 1933 Peru began to procure arms, because, as had been said by President Oscar Benavides, President of Peru from 1933 to 1936, " 'the effective defense of the rights of Peru neither should or can be limited exclusively to the methods of diplomacy.' " [15] Thus, "when the Peruvian government and High Command were convinced that the traditionally peaceful and conciliatory policy of Peru was taken by the country to the north [Ecuador] as evidence of weakness, Peru began to take the necessary preparations, so that, when the boundary question became acute, there was created the Army of the North." [16]

Suggestions that the Peruvian government had decided to solve the Marañón dispute by direct methods have also been made by Alberto Ulloa:

Following the decision of President Coolidge in the Tacna-Arica question, public opinion in Peru had undergone a major change in its appreciation of international policy with regard to boundary questions. Peruvians no longer desired arbitral solutions, regarding them as always influenced by political considerations, especially when they were made by the head of a state, and that arbitrators, for these reasons or others of greater convenience and lesser responsibility, sought a compromise settlement. However, by means of direct negotiations, it was thought, there would be no obligatory compulsion that would require a country, either legally or morally, to accept an unjust decision by an external agency.[17]

In addition, the Peruvian government, convinced of "the necessity of not committing again the error made in the Leticia affair," was determined to avoid any further " 'mutilations' " of Peruvian territory.[18]

In 1941, therefore, the Peruvian government, having decided to reject arbitration, also rejected "friendly services," or any other kind of third-party assistance, in dealing with Ecuador. Furthermore, having built an effective armed force in the years after the Leticia affair,[19] it was confident that it could impose on Ecuador its solution of the boundary dispute and, in particular, could maintain its fundamental objective: "finally to remove Ecuador from the Marañón." [20]

In Washington, when Secretary Hull had "spoken firmly" to Carlos Concha, as noted above, he was aware that the Peruvian government had violated its promises on two occasions: when the armistice set by the mediators for July 26 had not been observed by Peru, despite Solf's statement that the mediators' decision would be accepted, and when Lima had agreed to withdraw its troops behind the 1936 line and had failed to do so. He was also well aware, as the head of the United States delegation to the Eighth International Conference of American States at Lima in 1938, as was Concha, of the terms of the "Declaration of American Principles," approved by the Conference on December 24, 1938, and of the following two paragraphs of the Declaration:

2. All differences of an international character should be settled by peaceful means.
3. The use of force as an instrument of national or international policy is proscribed.[21]

Another factor that affected the views of officials in Washington, although it was not mentioned in official documents, was the timing of Peru's military preparations. The point of maximum Peruvian readiness for a conflict was reached at a time during World War II, following the passage of the Lend-Lease Act in March, 1941, when the resources of the United States were being committed to the aid of the enemies of the Axis in Europe, and the United States was also preoccupied with Japanese expansion in the Far East. With Peru's predominance over Ecuador in military strength, no more favorable moment for the use of force to settle the boundary dispute had been offered to Lima since 1830. Peru's military preparedness and the political situation created by World War II crowned with laurels the tenacious, century-old Peruvian policy of "deferring treaties while its people advanced up the rivers." [22] The precise calculations made in Lima may never be known, but it may be said that, if the Peruvian government had intended to employ its power to enforce its territorial claims, it selected the most auspicious time for doing so.

When fighting first occurred in July, 1941, Welles had been asked by reporters whether "outside influences" had played a part, and he had replied that " 'very often in muddy waters fishing is good.' " [23] He meant, presumably, that Axis agents might have incited Peru to attack Ecuador. He also said, however, that it was regrettable that such an incident should occur "in view of the very critical international situation," and this remark suggested that the Peruvians were not only not averse to fishing in muddy waters, but that they were also artful anglers. The evidence, therefore, points clearly to Peru as the state primarily responsible for the use of force in the controversy. In this discussion, the term "aggression" has not been used, because it would not promote understanding. Each side accuses the other of aggression; but there were no neutral observers to view the initial military phases of the struggle. If Peru rejected "friendly services," it did not reject all modes of peaceful settlement. It would be of little use to come to the conclusion, as was done in the Walwal incident in the Italo-Ethiopian conflict, that, technically, neither side had committed aggression, so nontechnical language has been employed here in an attempt to appraise the situation.

The principal material result of the campaign of the Zarumilla and the occupation of El Oro was the consolidation by Peru of its largely peaceful penetration of the Oriente. As the Peruvians themselves claimed in *El protocolo de Río de Janeiro ante la historia,* the difference between the line of the Rio protocol and the line proposed to the King of Spain by his Council of State in 1910 was about 8,000 square miles in favor of Peru, and the gain was even less according to Tobar's figure of a net acquisition by Peru of no more than 5,392 square miles, if the protocol line were compared to that of 1936.

However, as Ecuadoran boundary experts do not cease to point out, the extent of the Peruvian advantage accorded by the protocol should not be measured alone in square miles; [24] from the Ecuadoran point of view the loss of a given amount of territory was less important than the fact that Ecuador was completely excluded from riparian rights on the Marañón-Amazon river system. Ecuador was no longer an Amazonian country, either by occupation or legal claims.

Nevertheless, the fact remains that Peru obtained little more beyond its *de facto possessions* in 1936 than the two towns of Andoas and Rocafuerte and the legal validation of its claims to the east of the line of the protocol. Why did not Peru secure greater advantages when Ecuador was defenseless? The reasons are not to be found in an attitude of moderation and restraint in Lima, for Solf's note of September 13 evinced a conqueror's intent. The conclusion seems inescapable: it was the influence of the mediators, which was decisive in first staying a Peruvian advance on Guayaquil and then inducing Prado and Solf to accept a frontier that was not much farther west than the line of the *status quo* of 1936.

The greatest tribute to the effectiveness of the mediation has been offered by Tobar. The former Ecuadoran Foreign Minister stated, on the one hand, that the protocol constituted a recognition of the results of force employed against Ecuador and that "the power of Peru prevailed over the fundamental canons of American international law, which once more were reduced to scraps of paper." Tobar admitted, on the other hand, that America did not possess military sanctions and had no opposition to offer to Peru except its advice and influence. "America, because of the existing stage of development of its legal institutions and because of the situation created by the attack of an Asiatic power, could not use force to restrain the American nation which had resorted to force to despoil its neighbor."

However, the mediation had several notable achievements to its credit, in Tobar's opinion. It had rejected the terms of the Peruvian note of September 13, and it had delivered to Lima its memorandum of October 4, which "signified that the voice of America condemned Peru's attitude as against moral law and the law of America."

Furthermore, it is evident that, without the intervention of America, the result of the conflict would have been the imposition on Ecuador of the formula of the Peruvian note of September 15 [i.e., 13] and perhaps the

retention by Peru of those parts of Ecuador occupied as a guarantee.
. . . The only effective obstacle to Peru was, without doubt, the action of
the governments which had offered their friendly services and that of the
other governments which supported and strengthened that action with
their generous help. As Foreign Minister Aranha said, the mediation
saved the life of Ecuador.[25]

In Peru, since the government and its apologists tried to depict
the whole affair as both a military triumph over Ecuador and a diplomatic triumph over the mediation, there was little inclination to
credit the mediators with any success at containing Peruvian aspirations. Alberto Ulloa argued that Peru had not only rejected the
overtures of the mediators but had even turned the mediators into
supporters of Peru:

> Despite the existence of the mediation, Peru did not bow before the
> provocations of Ecuador, but it unleashed an impressive military action
> that resulted in the occupation of parts of the province of El Oro as a re-
> prisal and as a means of obtaining security for the future. . . .
> The art of diplomacy—which Peru has fully realized on this occasion
> —consists in refusing to allow one's self to be controlled by mediations
> but to lead them in the direction one wishes them to go, in such a way
> that they first help to bring about the desired result and then they support
> it with their international prestige.[26]

In other words, the mediation that Tobar regarded as having
saved Ecuador was interpreted by Ulloa as having been first flouted
by Peru and then bent into the shape of a rubber stamp for the
validation of Peruvian claims.[27]

Another view is that the action of the mediators constitutes one
of the grounds for the Ecuadoran government's claim in 1960 that
the protocol is null and void and without legal standing, since it was
forced on Ecuador not only by Peruvian invasion but also "under
the pressure of foreign diplomats interested in presenting to the
world an American image of cordiality and mutual respect." [28]

On their own behalf the mediators were content to praise the two
countries for having come to an agreement and to express pleasure
that the mediatory action had assisted in reaching a settlement.[29]
There was, of course, good reason for this modesty. The survival of
Ecuador and the limitation of Peruvian territorial ambitions were
substantial but by no means complete successes for the mediation.

During the Rio de Janeiro conference, when the Peruvian troops were still in El Oro province poised for an attack on Guayaquil, the mediators had little room for maneuver, although even under these conditions they were able to shake the Peruvian position on one or two points. The outstanding fact, however, was that for the first time in the twentieth century an American nation, after taking the initiative in employing military force, had imposed its will on another American nation. The American community had mitigated extreme expression of that will but had felt compelled to bow before it in the extraordinary circumstances existing immediately after Pearl Harbor. In the Leticia conflict justice had prevailed and the disturbers of the peace had been repulsed. In the Chaco war, while it could be argued that the settlement had but ratified the Paraguayan victory, it was no less well established that Bolivia, the initiator of the conflict, had been defeated, so that the aggrieved party, and not the attacker, had triumphed.

In these two cases the ultimate settlements, if not the roles of mediators, could well be the source of mutual congratulations on the "success" of the "inter-American system." The results in the Chaco and at Leticia concealed the weakness of collective action because they were roughly consonant with the norms of resolutions of inter-American conferences and with the sympathies of noncombatants. But, in 1941–42, the latest achievement of the American states—consultation—was not applied; a calculated attack was not beaten off; the proposals of the mediators, particularly as set forth in their note of October 4, 1941, were flouted; and the sympathetic hopes of the American states were disappointed.[30]

In terms of the "inter-American system" as it operated in this period, the "wrong" country won the Marañón conflict, and the "system" was revealed to all as ineffectual. A Peruvian diplomat is reported to have protested in late 1941 that his country should not again, as in Leticia, be made "the victim" of the American treaty structure; it was not, but that fact demonstrated the frailty of the structure as it existed at the time.

In relation to the "system," therefore, the importance of the Marañón dispute is that, by demonstrating the inadequacy of existing American methods for preventing attacks by one country on another, it may have stimulated efforts made in 1945 toward the formation of the Organization of American States.

At the Rio de Janeiro conference the American community's principal asset in countering the military power of Peru was its capacity to withhold respectability from Peru's military victory, if Peru demanded too much. Although the leaders of Peru had successfully defied their neighbors and might have broken continental solidarity if their dignity had been outraged, they were also desirous of receiving the acceptance by the American states of their newly won territory. It was from this point of view that they had a shadow of justification for their claims to having made a contribution to inter-American solidarity at the conference. The final settlement was a compromise among the mediators, Ecuador, and Peru. Peru made a minimal compromise, since its army was in command of the terrain; but Peru did not quite secure its maximum demands because its army alone could not gain for its conquests the accolade of the other American states.

The Policy of the United States

The policy toward the dispute adopted by the United States was marked by several significant features. The United States made no use of coercion to influence the course of the conflict. There was provocation both in the intransigence of Peru and in the fact that damage was done by Peruvian bombing planes to the property of United States citizens in Ecuador. Although the suggestion was made by Quito that a United States warship be sent to southern Ecuadoran waters as a warning to Peru, there appears to have been no serious consideration given by Hull or Welles to making a show of force or to presenting any threats to Peru. Two reasons counseled restraint, either of them by itself of sufficient strength: the ten-year-old policy of nonintervention and the desire to avoid any military involvement in South America when the rest of the world was aflame. After August 1, 1941, the Peruvian army in Ecuador would almost certainly have fought any forces sent to oust them and a battle involving United States forces in El Oro province was not a commitment Washington then thought seriously of undertaking.

The absence of peremptory demands or ultimatums, however, was not the only element in this policy. There was also an absence of any attempt to appeal to public opinion in the Americas by publishing protests either against the breaking of promises by Peru or against the methods of warfare employed by Peru. Tobar pointed out that at the Panama conference in 1939 the American states had protested the bombing of cities by belligerents in Europe, but that no protests had been raised against the bombings of what he called nonmilitary towns and villages in Ecuador by the Peruvian air force. There was well-founded doubt in Washington as to the accuracy of some of the Ecuadoran reports,[31] but some air raids did take place. Even after the bombings of United Fruit Company properties, however, the United States did not protest publicly, and its private representations to Lima could hardly be described as vigorous.

When this noncensorious attitude toward Peru is compared with the freedom Washington allowed itself in condemning war measures of the Axis states in Europe and Asia, it appears that in disputes in the Western Hemisphere the United States government muted the fanfare of moral and legal indignation against invaders of foreign territory that it trumpeted when other parts of the world were involved. It is not intended here to assert that the Peruvian invasion of Ecuador was comparable to the German invasion of Poland or the Russian invasion of Finland. It is sufficient to note that, although Peruvian policy was strongly condemned in private by Secretary Hull, no criticism of Peru was given to the press by governmental spokesmen in Washington.[32] This action is understandable, since Germany and Russia were potential enemies of the United States in 1939, and in 1941 Peru was a potential ally. Indeed, on matters that Peruvians regarded as important to the defense of the hemisphere, Peruvian cooperation with the United States quickly became as complete as that of most of the other Latin American states. There may also have been in this attitude an element of defensiveness about the good neighbor policy, which had failed in this case to prevent Peru's imposition by force of its territorial demands. The public denunciation of the acts of one of the other American republics had not been part of the vocabulary of the Department of State for many years, and it was not to be indulged in until August, 1943, when Foreign Minister Segundo Storni of Argentina was blown out of office by a blast from Secretary Hull in response to Storni's request for lend-lease armaments.

An additional reason, if not a controlling one, for the failure to assail Peru publicly may well have been the feeling that such action would not have been effective. Censorship combined with defensive patriotism in Peru would have made dubiously valuable an appeal from Washington to the Peruvian people, and it is at least questionable whether the public in other Latin American countries or in the United States itself could have been aroused to any useful purpose, or even significantly diverted from its absorption with such great events as the German conquest of Yugoslavia and Greece in the spring of 1941 and, in June, the German invasion of Russia. Finally, and not necessarily cynically, it may be noted that the protests of the United States against the Soviet invasion of Finland entailed no immediate responsibility for the United States. However, had the United States gone so far as to accuse Peru, as well as the Soviet Union, of "a wanton disregard for law," it could hardly have avoided taking measures against Peru, since, in the Americas, the United States obviously possessed the ability to redress wrongs that it lacked on the shores of the Gulf of Finland. Therefore, Washington limited itself publicly to the expression of hopes that peace would be restored between Ecuador and Peru and did not express openly any indignation against the Peruvian invasion.

A third question of diplomatic method was whether the convocation of a meeting of consultation of the foreign ministers of all the American states in May or June, 1941, or in September, when Padilla raised the issue, might not have been the most effective way of trying to halt what was, even at the earlier date, recognized as Peru's preparations for settling the boundary dispute by force of arms. This question was raised at that time by Foreign Minister Alberto Guani of Uruguay, but Welles did not favor a consultative meeting in this instance, despite his previous strong support for such meetings in general terms.[33] In view of the signs of alarm in Lima that were manifest whenever this subject was raised, there remains the possibility that a meeting might have averted the conflict and brought about a peaceful settlement. However, should judgment veer in this direction, it should also be remembered that there was a real danger that Peru, given sufficient provocation, might have withdrawn from cooperation in measures for hemisphere solidarity. Considering the overt bitterness of the Peruvian reaction to the apparently innocuous offer of friendly services, the risk of an appeal to the still fragile structure of consultation, untried in an intra-American dispute, would have been great indeed.

Short of the alienation of Peru, it may be considered that Washington was unduly sensitive about creating antagonism in Lima by its participation in the mediatory effort. The impression arises, from the depth of Welles's concern on this subject, that he was genuinely surprised at the intensity of Peruvian resentment, whether or not it was feigned. There does not appear to have been in Washington any concern about resentment in Ecuador; it may have been felt that Ecuador was incapable of elevating complaints to the level of resentment, that is, of offering protests that might have policy implications, just as Aranha had told Albornoz that Ecuador was incapable of creating a problem for America. With respect to Peru, however, Welles's reaction was almost one of incredulity at the burgeoning of Peruvian ill will. One explanation for this may have been his conviction that the anti-United States feelings that had been manifest in Peru during the Leticia conflict were primarily the result of Stimson's admonitory diplomacy.[34] Probably Welles believed that he had avoided Stimson's approach, and he appeared not to have anticipated the adoption by Peruvians of the stand expressed by *El Comercio* in commenting on Padilla's support of the mediation. In Lima any move by third parties that limited Peru's freedom of action toward Ecuador was looked on as being nothing other than pro-Ecuadoran, and Peruvians did not admit the possibility that such a move might honestly be motivated by a desire to keep the peace or to prevent any lessening of the defense effort. The frontier problem was the most important thing in the world to Peru. It is doubtful that any refinement of diplomatic technique would have avoided Peruvian resentment against the United States for what Peru considered as support for Ecuadoran claims.[35]

Out of this discussion of the methods of the policy of the government of the United States the aims of its policy emerge. These aims may be summarized briefly. The Department of State desired to maintain conditions of internal stability and peace in the American countries so that the flow of raw materials for defense preparations might be uninterrupted. It wished to avoid a conflict that might give an opportunity to agents of the Axis powers to limit or reduce the contributions of the American states to the war effort of Great Britain and its allies and sympathizers. It hoped to avoid the shedding of blood—its traditional, humanitarian aim in previous intercessions in Latin American disputes. It did not really care where the boundary lines were drawn so long as a formal settlement was reached. Finally, it wished to maintain the friendship and prestige gained through its good neighbor policy and so to achieve a high degree of continental solidarity against the growing menace of the totalitarian powers. After Pearl Harbor, solidarity meant not only economic cooperation but military collaboration, in the form of bases for United States patrol planes, and political cooperation in such matters as the internment of Axis agents.

The great importance that the United States government attached to the restoration of amicable relations with Peru was made abundantly evident during a state visit by Manuel Prado, President of Peru, in May, 1942. Responding to an invitation from President Roosevelt, Prado spent fifteen days in the United States, visiting Washington, Detroit, Boston, and New York. Roosevelt personally met him at the Washington airport and gave a banquet in his honor at the White House.[36] Prado placed wreaths on the Tomb of the Unknown Soldier and on the grave of George Washington and made addresses to the House of Representatives and the Senate. In New York he received honorary degrees from Columbia University and Fordham University, and a banquet was given in his honor by the Council on Foreign Relations. In Boston he was received by Governor Leverett Saltonstall, and he visited the campus of Harvard University.[37]

President Arroyo del Río of Ecuador later visited the United States at the invitation of President Roosevelt, who met him at the Washington airport "in a cold November rain," accompanied by Vice President Henry A. Wallace, Secretary Hull, Secretary of the

Treasury Henry Morgenthau, Under Secretary Welles, and other cabinet officers. Arroyo was also tendered a state banquet at the White House and made addresses to both houses of Congress; he was given honorary degrees by Columbia and George Washington universities.[38]

These visits brought to an end a phase of the boundary dispute and a phase of United States relationships with both Ecuador and Peru. Fresh starts in new directions were made toward close co-operation during World War II.

The violence of 1941 has not recurred, but the boundary dispute goes on.[39] The stipulations of the protocol were so vague that differing interpretations of its meaning were soon made by the two governments concerning two sectors of the boundary—one near Lake Lagartococha in the far northeast and the other in the Santiago-Zamora-Chínchipe area in the southwest. Incidents still occur along the frontier, and "doctors of boundaries" still write books discussing the details of the still unquiet settlement.[40] If, as one United States Ambassador has said, there are internal advantages for the government of a strong state in having an unsettled boundary dispute with a weak neighbor, there are also advantages seen by governments of weak powers in desperately keeping open some doubts about the finality of a boundary settlement that in its broad application cannot be seriously questioned. Even Tobar, in closing his memoir, called on Ecuadorans to keep their hopes alive, and quoted Gabriel Hanotaux as saying that "the victory of the vanquished is the secret of history."

Ecuador, as the vanquished, is trying to discover history's secret. The first technique of discovery is to keep the question open, and this had been solved by Ecuador's refusal to agree to place boundary markers on a stretch of about forty-nine miles in the region of the Cenepa River, which lies between the Santiago and Zamora rivers. The protocol mistakenly refers to the "watershed" between these rivers, because it was not known at the time that the Cenepa lay between them.[41]

A second technique is to create Ecuadoran heroes in the conflict with Peru, to keep their memory green, and thus to maintain the national aspiration to become an Amazonian country. The principal national hero is Lt. Hugo Ortiz Garcés, who was killed while fighting Peruvians near Yaupi, in August, 1941. It is reported that he replied to a Peruvian demand that he yield: " 'An Ecuadoran soldier does not surrender,' and that he died, having dedicated his last moments to a benediction to his country and a farewell to his mother." [42] The slogan "Ecuador has been, is, and will be an Amazonian country" is repeated regularly by radio stations in Ecuador, was emblazoned on postage stamps issued in 1961, is currently carried on postmarks, and in 1962 decorated the bumpers of many automobiles in Quito. On the wall of the Cathedral that faces the Plaza Independencia in Quito there is a bronze plaque with the inscription: "The Discovery of the Amazon River Is One of the Glories of Quito."

A third technique is to take every opportunity to deny legal status to the protocol of Rio de Janeiro on the ground of its forcible imposition and to claim Ecuador's "right" to territory along the Marañón, at least between the Santiago and Pastaza rivers.[43] This stand was taken most forcefully by President José María Velasco Ibarra in his inaugural address of September 1, 1960, when he asserted that Ecuador no longer regarded the protocol as a valid treaty with Peru.[44] The claims of Ecuador were presented in the Assembly of the United Nations in the autumn of 1960 and hotly contested there by the representative of Peru.[45]

The Ecuadoran representative asserted that his country was "the victim of aggression, of occupation, of invasion," of "a Pearl Harbor against Pan-Americanism." Furthermore, he noted that the protocol was signed "when Peruvian troops were occupying extensive provinces of Ecuador." The Peruvian delegate stated:

Peru could not commit aggression against any country. All it did was defend itself; and of course, in repelling aggression, its forces advanced and a peace treaty had to be signed. It goes without saying that Peru did not keep an inch of territory its advance had covered. . . . It would be an affront to such great nations as the United States of America, Argentina, the United States of Brazil and Chile, to think that they would give their guarantee to a Protocol which sanctioned an act of spoliation.

He did not deny that the protocol had been signed when Peruvian troops were occupying Ecuadoran territory; he answered this charge only by saying that the protocol was ratified "after the normal frontier situation had been restored. Hence the Ecuadoran Congress ratified the Protocol without any material pressure being placed upon it."

This exchange in the General Assembly of the United Nations gave Ecuador the opportunity to make its claim of the injustice of the protocol, and Peru the chance to defend itself, before a world audience.

The United States and "the other guarantor countries" replied to Ecuadoran claims that the Protocol was "null and void" by asserting in identic notes of December 7, 1960, that the Rio de Janeiro protocol, almost entirely carried out in practice, "is a valid instrument and should be complied with." [46] Further, any dispute over the undemarcated part of the frontier should be resolved amicably with the assistance of the guaranteeing powers, in accordance with article 7 of the protocol. Finally, the mediators warned Ecuador that "no American country could today challenge the peaceful conscience of the continent."

So far, Ecuador has refused to accept this judgment, although its regimes since 1960 have retreated from the claims of nullity made by Velasco Ibarra. The present position appears to be that the Ecuadoran government assails the protocol as having been imposed by force of arms and asserts its intent to secure its modification by pacific procedures. The gap between the frontier markers persists in the Cordillera del Condor. Similarly, there is a gap in the continuity of the conferences of American states. A meeting should have been held in Quito in 1959, had the regular five-year interval been maintained, but Ecuadoran demands for inclusion in the agenda of its dispute with Peru, and a consequential Peruvian refusal to attend, have been influential in postponing the conference. Meanwhile, Ecuadorans continue to issue books and pamphlets protesting the boundary settlement.

The Peruvian defense consists, first, in denying the existence of a controversy. The most succinct statement of the Peruvian position is: "There is no boundary problem." [47] The boundary, in this view, was settled by the terms of the protocol and subsequent determinations by Col. Braz Díaz de Aguiar, a Brazilian army engineer. Second, the Peruvian claim is that "it has been fully proved that Ecuadoran troops committed aggression on July 5 and 6, 1941." [48] Finally, Lima bases its stand on the notes of December 7, 1960, sent by the mediators to the government of Ecuador. Since the notes were written in reply to an Ecuadoran declaration rejecting the protocol, their effect is to consolidate the Peruvian position. This statement of the mediatory powers also indirectly consolidates Colombia's acquisition of Amazonian status at Leticia by way of the Solomón-Lozano treaty, since the mediators assert in this note that "it is a basic principle of international law, that the unilateral will of one of the parties is not sufficient to invalidate a boundary treaty nor to liberate it from the obligations imposed." So long as the Peruvian government accepts this position of the mediators, which is to its maximum advantage vis-à-vis Ecuador, it will certainly not make any effort to question the validity of the treaty that made Colombia an Amazonian power. [49]

As a consequence of the mediators' statement, the boundary dispute continues, and means for its settlement are lacking. The mediators' note referred to the desirability of an amicable settlement in accordance with article 7 of the protocol, which states that any doubt or disagreement that may arise over the execution of the protocol, "will be resolved by the parties with the assistance of the representatives of the United States, Argentina, Brazil, and Chile, as soon as possible." The protocol was to be carried out "under the guarantee" of the above four powers. Consequently, the guarantors, and not the Organization of American States, are responsible for the execution of the protocol. Since the Peruvian government is able to keep the question from being considered by any agency of the Organization of American States, since the guarantor powers have in effect recommended that Ecuador comply with the protocol, since Ecuador has refused to accept this recommendation by not completing the demarcation of the boundary, the dispute has not been settled. It may not be settled until a time, apparently far distant, when, as one United States diplomatic representative has privately suggested, a Peruvian government becomes strong enough to be generous and an Ecuadoran government simultaneously becomes strong enough to be reasonable. [50]

PART FOUR

Solicitude in Anarchy

CHAPTER XIII

Anarchy in the Americas

DURING THE PERIOD from 1932 to 1942 the American states made a melancholy record as keepers of the peace. In no case could they claim to have prevented a war, so they could point to no success comparable to that of the League of Nations in the Greco-Bulgarian affair of 1925. They could not even offer the excuse that they had been surprised by war. The Chaco and Marañón conflicts were two of the most clearly anticipated struggles in history, and, although the first blow at Leticia was unexpected, the American states were incapable of arranging a settlement during the five months' opportunity given to them before the battle of Tarapacá by the elaborately and ostentatiously dilatory voyage of the Colombian fleet up the Amazon—the hesitation waltz of Vásquez Cobo.

If the American states could not prevent wars, neither could they bring them to an end. Ultimately, of course, a formal settlement was arranged for each conflict, although the Marañón dispute still drags on.

Diplomacy always resumes its normal course after wars are over, but diplomacy in the Western Hemisphere can hardly be credited with shortening the struggles in the Chaco, at Leticia, or along the Marañón. In the Chaco conflict in 1935 Bolivia and Paraguay resembled two unhorsed and wounded warriors, capable of nothing more than feeble gestures of defiance. Quite ingeniously, the conference was able to assist the warriors back to their camps with their dignity nearly unimpaired, but the fighting itself had not been prevented by the American states. In the Leticia dispute it was the assassination of Sánchez Cerro, and not the action of the American states, that was decisive in making it possible for Peru to withdraw from a rash commitment. In the Marañón incident the Peruvians agreed to an armistice when they were sure that Ecuador was helpless, but not in response to appeals from other nations of the continent.

Before and during these conflicts, however, the American states did not ignore their existence; on the contrary, they lavished attention upon their warring brothers. Order they would not attempt to impose, weapons they would not in common withhold. Nevertheless, occasionally with one voice and frequently with many, they urged and sometimes went so far as to beseech the combatants to cease their strife. Moreover, in many different ways they offered honorable paths to peace. Ultimately, some of these paths were entered upon by the gladiators, and then, during long months of armistice, the American states maintained their solicitude that the truce should not be broken. It was here that their attention was well rewarded. The American states found their only successful role in the last acts of a war drama; they starred in the part of transforming an armistice into a treaty of peace. They could not prevent wars, nor could they stop the fighting, but they could effect formal reconciliations and so take part in what were hailed as happy endings.

If this success in the final phase of conflicts was the main achievement of the American states, it was considerably less impressive than is sometimes claimed. Nevertheless, it was a meritorious, if limited, accomplishment. After the armistices in the Chaco and Leticia disputes there were some anxious moments when war might have been renewed, and, after the Talara truce there remained the possibility that the Peruvian army might still march on Guayaquil. It is largely to the credit of the Chaco Peace Conference and Afranio de Mello Franco that the first two armistices were not broken. Not as much credit may be given to the delegates of the principal states at the Rio de Janeiro conference for maintaining the Talara truce, but the circumstances in that case were extraordinary and the fact remains that there was no more bloodshed.

In the broadest terms, the reason for the limited accomplishment of the American states in dealing with the problem of war was that they did not constitute a social entity competent to maintain order.

In the first place, a major inadequacy was their lack of a common legal obligation of *American* origin to refrain from the use of force. The Kellogg-Briand Pact had not been ratified by Bolivia. Although it is true that all the states involved in the three conflicts were members of the League of Nations, they behaved toward each other as though they were in a primitive society, unhampered by the Covenant, and they used the mass of inter-American treaties of peaceful settlement rather as a source of excuses or charges against an opponent than as a source of legal or moral obligation. Whatever the legal status of their obligation under the Covenant, the political fact was that the sense of obligation derived from the Covenant was weak in the Americas. This may have been partly because of the physical distance from Geneva, but a more compelling reason seems to have been the pervasive desire of the American states to find an American solution for American disputes. Brazil and the United States, as nonmembers of the League, may have felt this desire most keenly, but it was shared in some degree by all the American states.

In the second place, the American states had developed no principle of social cohesion, no common consciousness sufficiently intense to enable them to work together as a whole or by commission to proscribe recourse to war. There was no concert of America in 1932, or even in 1942, and no working understanding or common fear or sense of responsibility that made politically significant the maintenance of peace. In the Americas peace was universally recognized as a good thing, but peace had not yet come to be an important consideration, at least in the case of the only American conflicts during this period.

Third, there was no single meeting place in law or in mutual sympathy for effective collaboration by the American nations for the expression of their common concern for the maintenance of peace. The Americas had never known a general territorial settlement like that achieved by the Congress of Vienna for Europe, nor was there a tradition of collaboration for peace. Secretary Stimson on more than one occasion complained about the lack of peace machinery as an obstruction to his peace efforts, but this inadequacy was not remedied until after World War II. In the natural relief and satisfaction following the Chaco peace, Spruille Braden spoke of "the practicability of the American peace machinery," and Cordell Hull expressed his pride in "our inter-American system of consultation and cooperation." However, it would be easy to overestimate the degree to which "machinery" or "system" played a part in the three settlements that have been reviewed. The American states in the 1930s were still in the "handicraft" stage of peace production. As Sir Edward Grey once had bewailed his inability to find Europe, so, as late as 1942, Tobar Donoso lamented that there was no America to help Ecuador *in extremis*. The American "peace machinery" as exemplified by the Chaco peace conference was specially designed for the Chaco problem and was never operated again. The American "system of consultation and cooperation" as established at the Buenos Aires conference and supplemented at the Lima conference was not used in the Marañón conflict. The remarks of Braden and Hull may be taken as signs of joy or examples of hortatory diplomacy but hardly as descriptions of the behavior of the American states. In each case the procedures of conciliation and mediation were improvised when the fighting was at an end and in none of them, except when the Kellogg-Briand Pact was ineffectually invoked, was the latent moral influence of the American community brought to bear through solidary action by nonbelligerents.

Finally, there was no socially sanctioned way of exercising force to keep the peace. The United States was the only American state that possessed sufficient power to prevent, without a major effort, other states from fighting, but it would not unilaterally employ its strength, and there was no agency that could give it leave.

The single feature of a social entity that the American states had was a steadfast attachment to the ideal of continental peace. Although the temper of their statesmen did not permit the governments to go beyond vain persuasion in attempts to prevent war or restore order, they professed an abiding concern for peace while war was raging, and they were indefatigable in the exploration of the resources of mediation and conciliation. It was this untiring quest for peace that entitled them to claim credit for success in the post-armistice phase of each conflict, and their experience in these protracted negotiations, combined with their recognition of the causes of their failures in earlier phases, may have contributed to their desire for finding more effective ways of cooperation for peace after 1942.

Since their mutual bond was little more than a desire for peace, the American states could be successful in bringing about peace only when, finally, the contending states desired peace but were in need of help in negotiating a treaty. In providing help the American states performed several essential functions. They could furnish an *ad hoc*, impersonal, nonpolitical organization, like the Chaco confer-ence to which the governments of Bolivia and Paraguay could shift responsibility for the terms of a treaty that was less than wholly sat-isfactory and so enable them to remain in power in spite of domestic opposition. Such a conference represented for a brief period an ideal of American solidarity and pacification for which governments might make territorial or other sacrifices with some show of moral justification. In this way the American states enabled the ex-belligerents to save face by accepting a settlement that met with the approval of the temporarily recognized representatives of this ex-pression of social cohesion. The nonbelligerent countries, and especially the United States, had an interest in performing this func-tion, for it was a face-saving technique for them as well; this was the least they could do in order to demonstrate to the world that the Americas were capable of the pacific settlement of disputes.

Another function of the American states was that of ratifying the results of the conflicts. If there was acceptance of the final treaty by representatives of an expression of a societal ideal, there would be rather less chance that the conflict would be reopened than if the terms of peace were unilaterally imposed. In the Marañón conflict, for example, it appears that the Peruvians were anxious for approval of the boundary settlement at the Rio de Janeiro conference, and for the guarantee by the mediators that was written into the proto-col. The evidence of such social approval was desired by Peru, it may be assumed, not so much to deter Ecuador from upsetting the settlement, for Ecuador was too weak for that, but rather to make it difficult for other states subsequently to come to Ecuador's assist-ance against Peru or to question the legitimacy of the settlement.

From the point of view of the government of Ecuador, the approval of the American states was needed to keep the Peruvian forces from extending their invasion of Ecuadoran territory.

The performance of these functions represented the limits of the urge toward cooperation by the American states in this period. If these accomplishments were small, they were none the less real, and they alone gave substance to the ideal of international peace in the Americas.[1]

To most of the Latin American countries the conflicts that took place in the decade under consideration were not matters of acute concern. War between sister states was to be deplored, of course, but the governments of the smaller states preferred to adopt an impartial attitude and to refrain even from attempts at mediation. This policy was due in part to the nature of the conflicts, which were not only bilateral struggles over territorial claims but were also fought out in areas remote from centers of population. The issues of the conflicts were not of continental concern, ideological causes were not involved, nor was it plausible that any of the contestants were aspiring to continental hegemony. The smaller states with limited financial resources and prestige could not hope to affect the outcome of the conflicts, and they prudently determined, on the whole, to refrain from making diplomatic enemies by pretending to interfere.

The larger states undertook the responsibility of trying to conciliate the antagonists, and in the Chaco War the interests of Argentina, Brazil, and Chile were significantly involved. However, there does not appear to have been any moment between 1932 and 1935 when there was a serious danger of war involving these major states. Argentine assistance to Paraguay was generally known, although it was kept under diplomatic cover, and the Chilean officers who fought with the Bolivians appear to have acted without their government's support or even permission. Open Argentine intervention might have occurred had the Bolivians threatened to occupy Asunción, but the course of the war was such as to make it fairly easy for the three powers to avoid becoming embroiled. A renewal of the war in 1938 might have involved one or more of the three powers, but all of them, after the disappearance of Saavedra Lamas from the scene, worked together to bring about a final settlement. This is not to say that considerations of power politics were absent from the Chaco affair; however, Argentina, Brazil, and Chile did not take advantage of the situation in order to embark on policies of conquest or to go so far as to shift significantly the balance of power among them. The three powers were content to let Bolivia and Paraguay fight it out in distant and nearly resourceless territory, and such aid as they may have given to either belligerent represented a concern for limited objectives. Although control of the Tarija oil fields was of great importance to Bolivia and Paraguay, it was not a vital matter to Argentina, Brazil, and Chile. The fields lay near the Argentine border, and the geographical situation, combined with relatively good Argentine communications, made it appear highly probable that whether or not the Paraguayans gained control of the fields, the petroleum would find both a principal market and an outlet to world commerce in Argentina.

It was a well-known and publicly expressed ambition of the Argentine government to reconstitute the eighteenth century viceroyalty of La Plata, but Argentina did not take advantage of the Chaco conflict to make any effective progress toward its realization. Power relationships, therefore, do not appear to have strongly motivated any state or group of states either to prevent war or to prolong it.

There was one possible stimulus to common action by the South American countries that arose briefly in the Chaco dispute, only to fade away quickly. There existed in some countries, including Argentina, Chile, and Peru, but not Brazil, a desire to settle South American disputes without the aid either of the United States or the League of Nations. This tendency reached its highest point in February, 1933, at the Mendoza conference between Saavedra Lamas and Cruchaga Tocornal, and in the subsequent effort of the neighboring powers to effect a Chaco peace. Saavedra Lamas, on arriving in Buenos Aires from Mendoza, said: "From now on . . . South America will possess an international personality of its own and a genuine instrument for peaceful settlement." From the point of view of the relationship between Latin America and the United States, the Mendoza conference was held at a time when the bonds of inter-American solidarity were exceedingly weak. If South America, under the leadership of Argentina, was to attain a personality of its own quite independent of the influence of the United States, this was the most favorable moment of the epoch. However, Saavedra Lamas evidently did not believe his own bold words, for he soon asked the help of the United States for the Mendoza plan that sought to effect a Chaco settlement, and shortly afterward he permanently alienated Cruchaga Tocornal and other Chileans by engaging in separate negotiations with Brazil for peace in the Chaco dispute.

This action was a second demonstration of Saavedra Lamas's incapacity to collaborate with others in the cause of peace. The first had occurred when, in November, 1932, he commenced individual negotiations with Bolivia and Paraguay, three months after he had signed the agreement of August 6 with representatives of Brazil, Chile, and Peru containing the provision that the four governments would "keep united in order to offer their adherence and their collaboration to the Commission of Neutrals . . . with the aim of preventing, in their character as limitrophe countries, war between the republics of Bolivia and Paraguay." [2]

Another man might have created in South America what Saavedra Lamas called "a new organ of pacification" that would have excluded the United States, and this might have had incalculable consequences for the political development of the Western Hemisphere. Such a task, however, was quite outside the range of the abilities of the Argentine Foreign Minister. The Mendoza plan was Saavedra Lamas's South American substitute for the work of the neutral Commission whose efforts he had obstructed; after he destroyed it, the desire to find an exclusively South American settlement was less openly expressed in Buenos Aires, and the United States became in effect one of the neighboring powers.

The absence of compelling political motives for the maintenance of peace permitted Latin American statesmen to be politically irresponsible in their peace-seeking activities. If they failed to find a way to peace, no disaster would ensue, and each government knew that this was so. There was no common need for peace, no common ruin to be faced if these wars broke out or if one country or the other were vanquished. Therefore, the statesmen who initiated peace maneuvers could afford to indulge impulses that were almost wholly unconnected with the vital interests of the states they served.

Political irresponsibility for peace together with the ineffectiveness of the League of Nations in the Americas and the absence of American institutions charged with the maintenance of peace combined to create a situation of maximum maneuver for Latin American statesmen. It was an anarchic situation so far as the methods that might be used in seeking peace were concerned, and the result of this type of anarchy was an intense and even bitter rivalry among Latin American statesmen for the role of peace-maker.

Unfortunately, this rivalry was not ennobled by the goal of peace. Instead, it was demeaned by personal ambitions and accentuated by the urge to win the Nobel Peace Prize, which had never been accorded to a Latin American statesman. It may not be an exaggeration to say that in the 1930s the winning of the Prize appeared to become an obsession on the part of a number of Latin American diplomats.

It was not necessary to be the author of a successful peace plan in order to receive the Prize, as Norman Angell, Lord Cecil, and others had demonstrated. However, the conditions prevailing in the Americas in the 1930s offered what seemed to be an unprecedented opportunity for Latin American statesmen. There was war in the Chaco and an anarchic situation that gave free rein to private enterprise for peace. Interest in the Prize had been manifested by the unsuccessful nomination of Afranio de Mello Franco in 1934 by Colombia, Cuba, Ecuador, and Peru, following the settlement of the Leticia dispute. The aspiration to receive the Prize was manifested in various other ways. The Foreign Minister of El Salvador publicly proposed in 1934 that the Chaco War be terminated by a year's armistice arranged through the Pan American Union; shortly afterward, articles appeared in the Salvadoran press stating that the Foreign Minister's candidacy for the Nobel Prize was being presented by the Atheneum of El Salvador.[3] President Rafael Leonidas Trujillo of the Dominican Republic proposed to the Nobel committee the name of President-elect Franklin D. Roosevelt as a candidate for the Peace Prize on the basis of the speeches made by Roosevelt in the electoral campaign of 1932.[4] Later, President Trujillo's own Foreign Minister nominated him for the Prize for having completed a boundary treaty with Haiti.[5]

Carlos Saavedra Lamas, who won out in this competition for reasons to be discussed later, seems to have been the only American diplomat who requested, through his Ambassador in Washington, that his own candidacy be supported by the government of the United States; others who had better manners unquestionably also had aspirations for the Prize, and some may even have allowed their desire to keep Saavedra Lamas from getting it to affect the positions they adopted in peace negotiations during the Chaco conflict.[6]

The importance of the element of personal rivalry in limiting the capacity of the major Latin American states to cooperate for peace may, of course, be exaggerated. However, the rivalry certainly existed; it was regarded by Braden and others as adversely affecting peace negotiations, and it may possibly have prolonged the Chaco War.[7]

It should be recognized that this was a rivalry that adversely affected the only feasible type of peaceful cooperation, that of unifying nonbelligerent countries in support of a plan of mediation or conciliation. The Latin American countries at no time during any of the disputes evinced a disposition to unite in the application of economic or military sanctions or even to agree on the naming of one belligerent as an aggressor. The formal assessment of blame for a conflict was a responsibility that no Latin American government wished to accept. Although in the armistice of June 12, 1935, provision was made for an international commission to determine responsibility for the Chaco War, the commission was never established and in the final treaty Bolivia and Paraguay renounced all claims deriving from war responsibilities. In the Leticia settlement Peru "sincerely deplored" the events resulting from the attack on Leticia, but this was a unilateral act, and the protocol of Rio de Janeiro ignored entirely the problem of responsibility for the Marañón conflict.

It is, of course, by no means certain that, if all the principal American states had been able to agree on what they felt was a reasonable

plan for settlement in any of the three disputes, the fighting would
have been prevented. The contending states were in deadly earnest,
and in deadly earnest they resented being chid. To Hugh Gibson
the Chaco War was a "public nuisance," and a "senseless" dispute,
but to Bolivians and Paraguayans it was the most important event in
their lives. It meant life or death to soldiers, glory or obloquy for
the nations, and success or failure in the careers of statesmen. In the
Leticia affair, President Olaya of Colombia said he would prefer to
lose the territory by war than to be "cheated out of it by any sort
of diplomatic negotiations." Time and again the compromise proposals of mediators were rejected by intransigent contestants who
insisted on the satisfaction of their legal rights. The Peruvians were,
or pretended to be, infuriated by the proposal of the mediators that
an "equitable solution" be found for the Marañón controversy. In
the face of such intransigence, mediation was a frustrating occupation.

The intransigence of the contending states was of course most
intense during the conflicts, after the governments had committed
themselves to violence, but it was also exhibited before fighting had
broken out. Perhaps the principal although by no means the only
source of this intransigence was the ferocity that characterized the
domestic politics of some of the Latin American states and the
frailty of their civic institutions. It was a standard response of Latin
American diplomats and presidents to suggestions for compromise
solutions of their disputes that their governments would immediately be ousted by revolution. Peruvian Foreign Minister Solf y
Muro told Ambassador Norweb in 1941 that "Peruvians are much
more concerned with the internal situation and with matters of
prestige and pride than are the United States and other mediatory
governments." Zavala, Foreign Minister of Peru a decade earlier, may
have been exaggerating, but he said that, if he made the suggestion that the Peruvians should withdraw from Leticia before revision of the Salomón-Lozano treaty, he would be "hanged." In another instance, President Ayala of Paraguay was probably right in
saying that his acceptance of a proposal of the Neutrals in 1932
would have meant that he would not have been able to remain in
office for twenty-four hours.[8]

Sometimes it was "the people" who would not accept a compromise, and sometimes it was said to be "the army" that would revolt. This argument of imminent revolution usually won the day, although it failed in the Marañón dispute when Tobar warned Aranha in a feeble bluff that acceptance of the so-called "Aranha line" would cause a political upheaval in Ecuador. This small risk was accepted by Aranha and the other mediators, and the government remained in office, partly because its political opponents were satisfied to let it take responsibility for the settlement for which they had no alternative policy and partly because the Ecuadoran army at that time had neither the prestige nor the power to mount a rebellion.

Apathy among the weak states, disunity and rivalry among the strong, and intransigence on the part of the disputants were the continuing causes of disorder in Latin America that the United States, the only great power in the Western Hemisphere, strove to overcome in the conflicts concerning Leticia, the Chaco, and the Marañón.

CHAPTER XIV

The Policy of the United States

Mulitilateral Collaboration Short of Force

THE PRECEDING SUMMARY of the accomplishments of the American states as a whole and some features of Latin American international politics is intended to suggest the setting in which the policy of the United States toward war in the Americas was developed from 1932 to 1942. From historical precedents, the Department of State lacked the guidance to anticipate the problems here described. Secretary Stimson, in the summer of 1932, was confronted with the specific situations of the outbreak of major fighting in the Chaco, and by the Loretanos' coup at Leticia. These were the first serious conflicts between states in South America in the twentieth century. Stimson's equipment to deal with them in a positive way consisted largely of a tradition of serious concern for peace on the part of the United States, acquaintance with the successful compromise solution of the Tacna-Arica question, a rooted attachment to legal principles such as the sanctity of treaties, and a precedent in the Manchurian affair for a stand by the United States for the nonrecognition of territorial annexation by force. However, since Stimson was sensitive to Latin American criticisms of forceful action by the United States, he was determined to refrain from landing the armed forces of the United States on Latin American soil as a result of his experience in Nicaragua, and he may well have been rendered cautious not only by inhibitions arising from the Depression but also by an unwillingness to commit the government of the United States shortly before a presidential election.

In the Chaco dispute Stimson encouraged Francis White to work through the Commission of Neutrals with which Bolivia and Paraguay continued to negotiate until the spring of 1933, and he approved the joint declaration of August 3, 1932, that applied the so-called "Stimson Doctrine" to the Americas. In the Leticia dispute it appears that Stimson had some difficulty in believing that the Peruvian government would go so far as to back up the filibusterers from Iquitos. The Chaco fighting grew out of a recognizable type of territorial dispute, but there is surprise and shock in Stimson's communications about Leticia; he seemed to think that what Peru was doing was akin to what Japan had done and that it was hardly conceivable on the part of one of the American nations. Indeed, Stimson could hardly be expected to understand the position taken by Ambassador Freyre y Santander, in the statement to Francis White that "whatever the juridical position may be, we must get down to facts and the facts are that unless the two countries can get together and discuss this matter there will be war and that we should not run the risk of a war to save a juridical principle." [1]

Stimson's action in the Leticia dispute was both more partisan and more forceful than in the Chaco War. He believed Peru had broken its obligations under the Pact of Paris; he sent his note of January 25, 1933, only to Peru; and he lent the prestige of the United States government to the plan of settlement proposed by Brazil. This was the boldest unilateral move made by the United States in any of the three disputes. Not only was it a complete failure in itself; it gave rise to long-standing resentment in Lima against the United States. It is an example of the futility, in the pre-armistice phases of these disputes, of appeals to equity and law, however well justified and however firmly supported by the prestige of the United States. It did no good to talk of the law to men who had no respect for the law, and both the principle of the sanctity of treaties and the principles of the Pact of Paris were damaged when, after being invoked in this dispute, they were defied with impunity.

Nevertheless, Stimson would not use the economic or the military power of the United States to force a settlement in Leticia even against a Peruvian action he regarded as devoid of legal or moral justification. The policy of the government of Sánchez Cerro could have been changed only by the speedy exercise of superior force; this Stimson was not prepared to apply, and he therefore was unable to prevent the imminent conflict. Stimson is described as being "annoyed by his own restraint," and he wrote in his diary: " 'I am getting quite blue over the bad way in which all Latin America is showing up. It seems as if there is nothing we could count on so far as their having any courage and independence is concerned, and yet if we try to take the lead for them, at once there is a cry against American domination and imperialism.' " [2]

The government of the United States made no effort to hide its intention to refrain from using force in any way. Francis White stated publicly that none except "moral guarantees" could be given to Bolivia or Paraguay; more importantly he told the Bolivian minister as early as January, 1932 that "of course" the United States had no intention of forcible intervention if war should break out but that its "moral support" would be used against any country that resorted to arms. Taking into consideration Bolivia's preparations for war, this was quite likely a most satisfactory statement from the Bolivian point of view. Similarly, the Department of State was unwilling to follow Minister Feely's suggestion in December, 1932, for "forcible measures" by the Commission of Neutrals, such as the appointment of a group of military observers to supervise a neutral zone.

When Cordell Hull became Secretary of State, the policy of abstention from force was continued with equal vigor. He has written that "we could not hope to point the better road to nations like Germany and Japan, unless we first showed that cooperation could work in the areas of the Monroe Doctrine," and, when he and President Roosevelt decided to "work side by side" with the League in Leticia, Hull states that the decision meant a "willingness to cooperate with other nations in the settlement of Latin American questions. Unilateral action on our part was now in the discard." The United States would not act without consulting all interested nations, since "only in this way could we work from under the deep-seated resentment engendered in Latin America by previous one-sided actions of our country." [3]

The basis of the policy of the United States toward South American conflicts in this period consisted, then, of three main elements: a lasting concern that there should be peace in America; a determination to refrain from the use of force; and a desire to avoid Latin American resentment. The chief difference between the policies of Stimson and Hull was that Hull would not undertake, unilaterally, to follow the example of Stimson's note of January 25, 1933, to Peru. He would, of course, unilaterally plead for peace on the part of all belligerents, but he would not single out one of them as responsible for a conflict, nor would the Department of State engage in single-handed enterprises of conciliation. This significant difference established as a fundamental tenet of the policy of the United States the principle of consultation with all American states in matters of mutual concern, a principle that subsequently was adopted, first in theory and then in practice, by all the American states. It was not put into service, however, in any American territorial dispute during this period.

These basic elements of policy responded to feelings and attitudes that were deeply and widely held by persons influential in public life in the United States. Without endeavoring to analyze the special ethic growing up at this time toward the other American countries, it may be suggested that it was formed in part from a half-remorseful reaction against earlier coercive policies of the United States; from impulses associated with the idea, expressed by Alfonso Reyes, that the Americas were "the last refuge of mankind"; from the simple desire for the good opinion of, and friendly relations with, the people of Latin America symbolized by the notion of the good neighbor; and from a genuine and humanitarian concern for the avoidance of bloodshed.

Former Secretary of State Dean Acheson has called the good neighbor policy "the renunciation of domination." In domestic affairs of Latin American countries the "good neighbor" followed policies of nonintervention and noninterference. In South American international relations the United States did not intervene, but it did interfere on occasion in its own style, which may be called "solicitude in anarchy."

The nature of the international anarchy in the Americas in this period has already been described. The quality and technique of the solicitude expressed by the United States in seeking peace in the Americas may be sampled if not fully plumbed by reviewing two types of action adopted by the Department of State: its exploration of the resources of multilateral methods of influence short of force; and its experimentation with unilateral measures by the United States that might promote peace without causing resentment in Latin America.

In a general sense, solicitude connotes devoted and painstaking attention; it may imply concern and worry; it frequently involves anxious inquiry as to well-being; it is often carried to a point where the object of solicitude shows signs of exasperation and a desire to be left alone. These aspects of solicitude were often exemplified in the peace-seeking relationships between the United States and Latin American countries.

In a more specific sense, the United States made a remarkably sustained effort at testing the limits of collaborative and noncoercive methods of bringing about peace in Latin America. Other countries, such as Argentina and Chile, also maintained their efforts over a period of several years in the Chaco conflict, but their record was atomistic rather than collaborative. Brazil alone among the major states rivaled the United States in the expenditure of time and energy devoted to the cooperative search for peace.

There were several types of collaboration available to the United States in trying to maintain peace in the Americas. One of these was to associate itself with the League of Nations. The United States went so far as to allow one of its army officers to serve on the League's mission in the Leticia dispute. In the Chaco conflict it placed no obstacles in the way of League action, once it was clear that its own action through the Commission of Neutrals could not possibly succeed. More positive association with the League was restrained not only by the rising tide of isolationism after 1933 but also by the pervasive desire to find an American settlement for American quarrels. When the Commission of Neutrals abandoned its efforts, it did not invite the League to undertake negotiations but turned to South America in hopes that the neighboring states might find a solution. The League's activities were tolerated, but they were not welcomed. Although Hull expressed to Geneva the hope that the League Commission might be successful in the Chaco dispute, he also informed the Argentine government that this expression of hope did not mean that he approved the Commission's plan of settlement. Later, however, Washington agreed to appoint a representative to meet with the League's proposed Neutral Supervisory Commission, which was to have been composed of "American states meeting on American soil." The Commission never met, but it is of interest to recall that one of the principal reasons for Hull's willingness to work with it was to offset the suspicion on the part of some American states that the United States might attempt to dictate the terms for the settlement of the controversy. It is also of interest that Hull was willing to go as far as this despite the raising of the question, by Foreign Minister Macedo Soares of Brazil, whether the Monroe Doctrine was to be an all-American principle or whether it would be undermined by non-American handling of American affairs. Apparently the allaying of Latin American suspicions about "dictation" by the United States was of greater importance to Hull than adherence to what might be called a Brazilian corollary to the Monroe Doctrine that would have excluded the League of Nations from interfering in American quarrels. The high point of United States collaboration with the League of Nations that was reached in the Leticia dispute was not attained again; the League's activities did not shorten the Chaco War and it played no part in the Chaco question after May, 1935, nor, of course, at any stage of the Marañón conflict.

A type of collaboration actively but vainly sought by the United States was that of joint mediation by all the American governments. Hull asserted that "the furtherance of peace should be a matter of joint moral responsibility for all of the American Republics" and that their efforts should not be limited to "any bloc or clique." However, Hull's principle was never realized in practice; he was unable even to attain that declaratory unanimity that Stimson had achieved for his nonrecognition doctrine in the Chaco War. When Hull repeatedly tried to arrange representation of all American states in the Chaco Peace Conference, he was rigidly and successfully opposed not only by Saavedra Lamas but also by other foreign ministers.

A third method of collaboration favored by the United States was also found to be impossible of realization. This was the attempt at the Buenos Aires conference in 1936 to formulate a multilateral treaty or treaties that would place legal obligations on all American states both to refrain from warfare and to cooperate in halting fighting if it should break out.

This conference did not fulfill the purpose Secretary Hull had in mind when he said that he wished to use the end of the Chaco War "as a springboard from which to reach agreement to outlaw further war between American Republics." The Latin American states were not ready to outlaw war nor to agree to the formation of anything in the nature of an American league of nations, even though the latter idea had been warmly urged by a few of them, notably Colombia and Uruguay. The acceptance of the principle of consultation by all twenty-one states in case of a threat to the peace from any source was, however, a notable achievement of this conference. Ironically enough, the United States government did not propose the application of this principle in the Marañón dispute, and consideration of the settlement of this conflict did not even appear on the agenda of the inter-American conference at Rio de Janeiro in 1942.

It was only through a fourth method of collaboration that the United States was able to achieve the strictly limited measure of success that was attained in the last phases of the Chaco and Marañón conflicts. This method, if it deserves the name, was the willingness of the United States to associate itself with one or more Latin American states in a series of *ad hoc* groups that sought avenues to peaceful settlement. These groups, except for the Chaco peace conference, had no foundation in treaties but were examples of the opportunistic use of good offices. The Department of State also worked with such groups in the prewar and wartime phases of each dispute, but the political irresponsibility of some of the Latin American members of these groups kept them from holding together or operating with mutual frankness and confidence. It was proven time and again that it was impossible to carry on effective negotiations in five or six capitals at once; it was also proven that the negotiators had not enough real concern about peace to organize their negotiations. If peace were to be made, or a settlement reached, two essential conditions had to be met; first, it was necessary for one group to monopolize the mediatory function and for that group to include all the governments that had, or could seriously claim, a significant interest in the dispute; and, second, it was necessary that the mediators meet with delegates of the disputants in one place. The final settlement in each dispute was not reached until these conditions were satisfied, following the failure of other methods, and in each dispute they were satisfied only in the post-armistice phase, after fighting had come to an end.

The Department of State was well aware of the requirements of the situation. It was quiescent when the neighboring states or the League of Nations were active in the first two phases of the Chaco problem, and it tried to discourage other states from interfering with the group that seemed at a given moment to have the best prospect for hopeful negotiations. However, after the Commission of Neutrals retired from the arena, the field was free and open to anyone who wished to enter the contest of proposers, and the limitations the Department of State had imposed on its own freedom of action rendered it helpless to exercise effective leadership in order to centralize the negotiatory function. It pleaded for continental responsibility for peace, but, self-shorn of power, it was able to do little more than encourage the successive whims of foreign ministers. The formation of the Chaco peace conference was possible only when the Latin American foreign ministers had exhausted the possibilities of freedom of enterprise in seeking peace and the belligerents had given up hope of being able to impose peace by military means. Then, and then only, were the resources of collective diplomacy exploited.

Unilateral Action Short of Resentment

At the same time that the United States was loyally supporting the various multilateral efforts for peace in these disputes, it was able to undertake some small measure of unilateral action. Having forsworn the use of force and still earnestly desirous to aid the cause of peace, what were the policy limits within which the Department chose to operate? Broadly speaking, the limit to unilateral action was set by the desire to avoid resentment, an objective that successfully competed with that of furthering peace in the Americas.

This policy objective is stated negatively because that is the way policy problems came before the Department of State. Officials were frequently asked to do something to prevent or stop a war or to hasten peace negotiations, and their principal test for acceptability of a suggestion was whether or not it would cause resentment in Latin America. This was not because of caprice nor because the Department was headed during this period by men of exceptionally thin skins. This position was taken because, unless the United States was to be completely indifferent to the course of conflict in Latin America, there was no reasonable alternative to a policy aimed at the cultivation of good will when coercion was renounced. The averting of anger against himself is the first objective of an empty-handed pacificator.

Nearly empty-handed the United States was, for it sought to bring about peace holding neither a carrot nor a stick. It was armed only with sweet reasonableness; as Peruvian Foreign Minister Zavala irritably told Ambassador Dearing, the United States was "dealing in Aristotelian logic," while he himself had to deal with "immediate practical necessities."

The government of the United States did not carry even a little stick. Renouncing the use of threats of armed force, it also cast aside all other forms or threats of coercion; it carried only an olive branch. It did not on any occasion during these disputes apply economic pressure in an attempt to change the policy of a Latin American government. It refused to accept a suggestion that it employ nonrecognition of the Paiva government in Paraguay as a form of coercion. After Stimson's note to Peru of January 25, 1933, the Department of State refrained almost entirely from the use of publicity as a form of coercion, and no further attempts were made at the "mobilization of public opinion" against one or another of the contestants. Stimson's use of publicity was no less a failure, as was the single threat of publicity made to Lima by Welles in the Marañón dispute.

Moving further down what may be called the scale of insistence, the United States also avoided the use of what it considered to be pressure, or even the appearance of pressure, against a Latin American government. Pressure is different from coercion in that it is defined subjectively; it may be intended by, or inferred from, the use of words, such as "prompt" in the mediators' first note to Peru in the Marañón affair, but it is not necessarily accompanied by any threat of a material act beyond conversation and the writing of notes. "Pressure" was a favorite word used by Latin American diplomats to describe an attitude, a phrase, or an action of the United States that they did not like, such as, for example, when the Bolivians accused the United States of exerting pressure with no more reason than that the McCoy Commission had proposed arbitration of the Chaco dispute. Francis White denied that such a proposal constituted pressure; on the other hand, White had his own understanding of this concept, for on one occasion he asked Minister Wheeler "discreetly" to try to speed negotiations "without giving the impression that this Government is pressing Paraguay too hard and hence cause resentment." Many other examples of the desire of the United States to abstain from pressure are found in the diplomatic correspondence. These examples suggest that the category of "pressure" as understood by the United States ranged downward in substance from "insistence" and in method from "importunity." The Department of State substituted "urge strongly" for "insist" in a document of the Chaco Peace Conference; and in manner and frequency it was willing to "plead" but wished not to appear to "importune."

As for material inducements, the United States had the capacity to offer them, but it refused to do so. Welles rejected Braden's suggestion that an offer of a favorable trade agreement might induce Paraguay to make peace with Bolivia. When Saavedra Lamas proposed that the United States government could support the Mendoza plan by suggesting that bankers in the United States offer aid to Bolivia if it accepted the plan, White replied that his government "does not practice economic imperialism such as is envisaged by the mention of aid from American bankers." Similarly, the Department of State did not attempt to make use of the resources of the Export-Import Bank as a means of influence in the cause of peace.

In still another sphere the United States government followed the policy of impartial denial of access to its resources. In the Leticia dispute, if it refused to allow Peruvian ships to be refitted in the Panama Canal Zone, it also put a stop to Colombia's recruiting of airplane pilots in the United States; it rejected a Colombian request to send an air mission to Bogotá, and it prevented the holding of a military review at Panama in honor of the officers of the Peruvian cruiser *Almirante Grau*. Francis White's remark that the United States was acting in "an impartial manner" in the Leticia dispute was echoed by the acts of the Roosevelt administration. Similarly, during the Chaco dispute, the United States arms embargo was enforced equally against each belligerent.

The kind of action the United States allowed itself to take, then, fell within the range of unimportunate persuasion and nonmaterial rewards. This is an area of meager influence, but, since it comprised the gamut of constructive activities by the Department of State, it was explored with diligence and ingenuity. Like the Statue of Liberty, if slightly less immobile, the United States government held up the beacon of the ideal of peace. Much more vocal, but with mildness appropriate to its shackled power, it addressed the belligerents with earnest pleas to cease their strife and called for unity among the peacemakers.

Even in the area of unimportunate persuasion, however, there were limits to the action of the United States that were set by the desire to avoid resentment. Without attempting to codify the diplomatic etiquette of the good neighbor as practiced by the United States in this period (a mode of behavior only slightly less rigid than that prescribed by manuals of protocol), it is possible to obtain an impression of the keenness and pervasiveness of the desire of the Department of State to avoid creating resentment. To what extent, for example, should the Department of State attempt to influence the negotiating personnel selected by a Latin American government? In Stimson's day, before the code was refined, the minister in La Paz was instructed to request that the Bolivian government refrain from appointing a negotiator in whom the United States had no confidence. In 1936, however, Welles would not accede to Braden's request that the Department ask President Toro of Bolivia to prevent the replacement of the Bolivian representative at the Chaco conference, because, said Welles, the Bolivian Foreign Minister would "properly resent" any attempt to go over his head to the President. The Argentine government, interestingly enough, had no such scruples; it sent a special envoy who tried unavailingly for its own reasons to do what Braden had in mind. To this same order of manners belong such decisions as the refusal to allow a United States army officer to accompany Vásquez Cobo's squadron up the Amazon; the establishment of the principle that a United States military observer on an inter-American team should not outrank his colleagues; and Ambassador Dearing's remark that he did not wish to be "unduly curious about Peru's internal affairs" when inquiring about the alleged relationship between a domestic "menace" in Peru and the attitude adopted by the Sánchez Cerro government in the Leticia dispute.

At this level of political niceties the Department of State was actually concerned with pique and embarrassment rather than resentment; its justification was that this distinction was not always made by Latin American diplomats who, to a greater degree than North American officials, were sensitive in matters affecting personal dignity, inclined to allow even minor affronts to influence their conduct of affairs of state, and not at all reluctant to exploit the policy potential of contrived resentment.

Despite this narrow circumscription of the diplomatic activity of the United States, there remained a few initiatives at Washington's disposal. The Department of State sometimes felt free to make independent suggestions for procedures of peaceful settlement in all three phases of the dispute, as in the case of Welles's useful suggestion for convening a meeting of mediators in Buenos Aires to deal with the Chaco problem. The Department was, however, much more cautious when it came to suggestions for the substantive solutions of disputes; it would not appear as the lone initiator of a proposed boundary line, and it tried in various ways to erect a screen behind which its work for peace might be effective but unperceived, or at least diplomatically unassailable. The question of the avoidance of initiatory responsibility arose in all three disputes in one form or another. In the Chaco conflict, for example, Francis

White attempted to persuade Saavedra Lamas to sponsor the August 3, 1932, declaration; Saavedra Lamas refused, although he was characteristically willing to accept credit for the idea after finding that the declaration was favorably received. Washington's desire to escape prominence was also exemplified by the convening of conferences in capitals other than Washington, and by the refusal to allow Braden to negotiate in Asunción without being accompanied by the Brazilian delegate to the Chaco conference.

The self-effacing characteristic of the policy of the United States in these disputes did not mean that the United States expected comparable modesty from other Latin American governments. Secretary Hull more than once repeated his preference for the exercise of continental responsibility for peace, but, since this was an unattainable ideal, he was not unwilling that Latin American states should try to restore peace by methods with which the United States would not permit itself to be identified. Francis White at one point suggested that Argentina, Brazil, and Chile should "tell Bolivia and Paraguay" that a temporary boundary line "will be patrolled and policed" by their "forces," as one means of strengthening a proposal by the Commission of Neutrals; such a responsibility the United States at no time offered to shoulder or to share. On many occasions the Department of State encouraged other foreign offices or groups to undertake peace initiatives and, if they seemed to be lagging, quietly urged them to move more quickly or to increase the intensity of their pressure on the disputants. In the late days of the Chaco negotiations Braden told Cantilo that "the one time a mediator had pounded the table" Paraguay had backed down; this unprecedented action had been taken by Rodrigues Alves, the representative of Brazil, and Braden proposed that Cantilo should follow this excellent example.

The one area of policy with respect to these disputes where the Department of State felt least inhibited was that of offering nonmaterial rewards. The ceremonial aspect of inter-American relations became more highly developed in this period than ever before. The United States took the initiative in offering effusive congratulations to the signers of armistices and treaties with no fear of resentment in Latin America. Braden was permitted to arrange for the "theatricals" he considered helpful in creating a favorable atmosphere before the final meeting of the Chaco conference. Presidents Prado of Peru and Arroyo del Río of Ecuador were invited to the United States following the ratification of the Protocol of Rio de Janeiro; they were received and feted by the White House.

Flattery as a diplomatic technique was frequently employed by the United States, and it was regarded by Braden as of some value. He reported that he and other mediators had been able "to circumvent Dr. Saavedra Lamas' personal peculiarities, delays and obstructions by reasoning, flattery, and other means"; and it may be recalled that Soler had recommended flattery to Francis White in dealing with the Argentine Foreign Minister.

This technique had its limitations, however. White once noted that flattery of Saavedra Lamas had been effective "doubtless because his and our final objectives were then identical; now they are different and it has been amply proven that our former methods with him no longer are successful."

The most spectacular example of United States action of this type was the support given by Secretary Hull to the candidacy of Saavedra Lamas in 1936 for the Nobel Peace Prize. It was the settled policy of the Department of State that the support of the government of the United States would not be given to the candidacy of citizens of foreign countries for this prize, and this policy had been followed in 1934 when a request had been made for United States participation in the presentation of the name of Afranio de Mello Franco to the Nobel committee.[4]

Early in 1936 Saavedra Lamas requested that Secretary Hull or President Roosevelt advance his claim for consideration before the Nobel committee,[5] and Hull complied, dubiously maintaining the established policy by stating that he was acting only in his personal capacity and not as Secretary of State of the United States.[6] Hull's own account of his part in this episode links his action to Saavedra Lamas's friendly collaboration at the Montevideo conference: "Throughout the conference I could not have asked for more cordial and understanding cooperation on all important questions than I received from Saavedra Lamas. I later urged him for the

Nobel Peace Prize, although my own candidacy had been proposed, and he received the award." [7]

Saavedra Lamas's receipt of the award was announced in November, 1936, just before the Buenos Aires conference at which he presided, at the very height of his career. Hull's attempt, as he said, to "make a friend of Saavedra Lamas" at Montevideo had apparently been successful at that time, although Hull should have been warned by the fact that Saavedra Lamas had not agreed to cooperate until Hull had told him that otherwise "it will be necessary to select the next most suitable person" for the "outstanding task" of introducing one of the two resolutions the United States government wished to have considered by the conference. Hull intended to ask Afranio de Mello Franco of Brazil if Saavedra Lamas refused his request. [8]

At the Buenos Aires conference, however, Hull recalls that Saavedra Lamas was not so friendly as he had been at Montevideo, and that he had "formulated an inflexible policy of opposition" beforehand. Hull had discussions with Saavedra Lamas that "became increasingly animated. Our last conference was heated, some sharp words were exchanged at least on my side, and we parted with no signs of complete agreement." [9]

Less than a month before this conversation, the Department of State, on November 24, issued a press release expressing gratification at the decision of the Nobel committee: "The award is a fitting recognition of Dr. Saavedra Lamas's broad and sustained service in the cause of peace, signalled by such achievements as the Argentine Anti-War Pact, ratified by the United States on June 27, 1934, and his statesmanlike conduct of the Chaco Peace Conference, which has made steady progress toward the peaceful settlement of the conflict between Bolivia and Paraguay." [10] It may have been a bit galling to officials in Washington that the speech of award by Dr. C. L. Lange on December 10, 1936, linked Saavedra Lamas to the campaign in Latin America against the former United States policy of intervention and said that Saavedra Lamas had been led by the abandonment of that policy "to take active part in the work of the Pan American Union, which had been suspected of being a screen for the imperialism of the United States." [11]

In view of the uncomplimentary reports in the possession of Department of State about the character and activities of Saavedra Lamas, it must be assumed that Hull's support for his Nobel Peace Prize candidacy was premised, not on Saavedra Lamas's obstructive record in the Chaco dispute, but rather on the hope that the award would encourage him not only to continue at the Buenos Aires conference the collaboration begun at Montevideo but also to engage in a more cooperative and less independent role in the Chaco mediation that began in the summer of 1935. Both these hopes were unfulfilled. It is unfortunate that the honor given to Saavedra Lamas should have marked him as the publicly esteemed model of the Latin American man of peace. Successful he was to uninformed observers, and spectacularly brilliant in his attainment of public position and renown. More worthy of emulation, however, and higher in the regard of his diplomatic colleagues was Mello Franco, whose quiet and perhaps decisive contribution to peace between Colombia and Peru was a solid achievement that Saavedra Lamas never closely approached.[12]

No less unfortunate was Hull's sponsorship of Saavedra Lamas, however unofficially, for it seems not unreasonable to presume that Hull's advocacy was greatly influential in Norway. If, on the most favorable assumption, Hull intended that the award of the Nobel Peace Prize should encourage the observance of higher standards of statesmanship in the Americas, it was strange that the approval of the Secretary of State of the United States should have been bestowed on a man of intrigue. If, less creditably, aid to secure the Prize were to be given in order to obtain political cooperation from Saavedra Lamas, the anticipation of such cooperation should have been more substantial than it was. Hull did not even salvage political success from this dubious enterprise. He was left in the position of having vainly rewarded recalcitrance and ill will, when he might have given aid and comfort not only to statesmen who wholeheartedly strove for peace but also to those whose political objectives were in harmony with those of the United States. Even on personal grounds Hull's effort was barren. At the termination of the Buenos Aires conference, as he simply and austerely relates: "I saw no more of Saavedra Lamas before leaving Buenos Aires. He did not extend the usual courtesy of seeing me off." [13] So ended, sourly, the most notable single example of flattery as a technique of the good neighbor policy.[14]

Responsibility and Leadership for Peace

The characteristic features of the policy of solicitude in anarchy reflected one fundamental change that took place after 1927 in the Department of State's conception of the place of the United States in the Americas. This change was a drastic modification of the bases of the prestige of the United States among its neighbors. The formerly valued element of prestige that consisted of apprehensive respect on the part of Latin American countries was replaced by a many-sided campaign to cultivate good will. This campaign did not go quite so far as Dearing had intimated in saying that the United States was leaving the Latin American countries to work out their own salvation if international conflict should occur, but it went a long way in that direction.

This campaign may be said to have begun, insofar as it related to warfare in the Americas, with the determination not to employ coercion in the Chaco dispute. In the Leticia affair further progress was made with the failure of Stimson's several pressures on Peru. It was this affair, indeed, that provided Sumner Welles with an object lesson in the creation of resentment. There were several things Stimson had done in this case that were not done again, either in the Chaco dispute or in the Marañón conflict. He had censured Peru; he used the word "aggression" in his note of January 25, 1933; he stated that Peru had violated an international treaty; he had shown partiality by sending his note only to Peru; he had warned Peru, by speaking of the denial of the benefits of the Kellogg-Briand Pact; and, finally, he had published his censorious note for all the world to see. These causes for resentment against the United States were henceforth almost entirely absent from the policy of the United States. This catalogue of pressures is not necessarily a criticism of Stimson, although it appears that Welles so regarded it. Stimson stood at a transitional point in the making of policy, and the Peruvian attitude was certainly a provocative one. He valued the maintenance of peace more than he cared about Peruvian good will; and in 1933 both the sanctity of treaties and the reputation of the Kellogg-Briand Pact were more highly valued than they were in the later 1930s.

Did the United States, the only great power in the Americas, by relinquishing its great-power attributes in dealing with international conflicts among its neighbors, place itself on the same level as other American states who also sought to keep the peace? This question can hardly fail to arise as one surveys the course of the American states in the 1930s, but the answer is in the negative. There were at least three significant characteristics possessed by the United States that continued to distinguish it from other American countries.

In the first place, the government and the officials of the United States had no selfish interests in the territorial disputes in South America. Neither in the Tacna-Arica dispute nor in any of the three conflicts here considered did the United States care about the position of the boundary lines. The fact that the Standard Oil Company of New Jersey held a concession in southeastern Bolivia did not influence the policy of the United States in the dispute. The Standard Oil Company apparently did not urge Bolivia to undertake the war, nor did it assist Bolivia during the war beyond continuing to produce oil, paying taxes, and performing such services as in the circumstances it could not avoid. Before the Marañón conflict the United States disclaimed any desire to obtain a naval base in the Galápagos Islands, and its policy was certainly not that of a power that looked for any favors from Ecuador.

The United States was disinterested in all matters save the avoidance of bloodshed and the attempt to uphold in the Americas higher standards of international conduct than were exhibited elsewhere in the world. In this feature of its policy the United States occupied a position apart from the diplomatic battle waged by the Latin Americans among themselves. It is of interest in this connection to recall that, when Francis White suggested to Pablo Max Ynsfrán that he desist from a newspaper controversy with a Bolivian diplomat in order to avoid giving the affair further significance, Ynsfrán replied that such action might be all right for the United States, "but the weak, smaller countries, just because they are weak, are not serene enough to look at things in that way."

In the second place, if the serenity of disinterestedness could be enjoyed by the United States, so could its probity. The United States government maintained in the negotiations over these disputes a higher standard of probity than that of any major Latin American country except Brazil. The United States government was loyal to the mediatory groups it joined. A United States representative engaged in no negotiations without the knowledge of his associates, and he could be depended upon by them to fulfill faithfully his agreements, written or unwritten, without subterfuges or deviations. This standard of diplomatic rectitude was not met by other countries, nor did they expect it of each other. Deviousness and deceit are usual diplomatic techniques among sovereign states that are striving for advantage. The United States was not striving for any advantage but was earnestly seeking peace without utilizing its military or economic power; it sought to maintain friendly relations with all Latin American countries, and a frank and straightforward diplomacy was an essential part of its whole endeavor to form an American society of states.

On the other hand, the Latin American statesmen, struggling for territory, for fame, or for economic gain, sought advantage with all the means at their command. The maneuvers of Saavedra Lamas were unique combinations of guile, audacity, and double-dealing, but other Latin American statesmen attempted now and then to emulate him, or by counterintrigue to foil his aspirations. The United States avoided any kind of underhanded diplomacy, even in response to Saavedra Lamas's twists and turns; in consequence, the Department of State was more than once made to appear naive and gullible by a Saavedra Lamas or a Maúrtua. This was an appearance the United States could afford to give as part of the responsibility of a great power; it was willing to put up with occasional, gleeful impudence on the part of a weak state, such as Argentina or Peru, and to refrain from treating trickery in kind.

A third factor combined with disinterestedness and probity to give the United States a unique position in the Americas; this was the inexpugnable, latent prestige of power, even though held in check. Coercion aside, the weight of the opinion of the government of the United States was greater than that of the other governments.

Small states, distant from the conflicts, might be no less disinterested and honorable than the United States; they might make equally earnest pleas for peace, but they were disregarded. The opinions expressed from Washington might be rejected, but they were not wholly disregarded.

It was the total effect of these three factors that may have given special importance to the judgment of the United States at certain crucial moments in negotiations. On at least two critical occasions, it appears that the stand of the United States may have made the difference between agreement and disagreement. When the Paraguayan government submitted to a plebiscite the final conference plan that had originated with the United States delegation, it called the plan the "Roosevelt formula" despite the desire of the Department of State that this phrase should not be used. In the final negotiations at Rio de Janeiro between Ecuador and Peru, the disputants and the mediators looked to Sumner Welles for the decisive words on the right of freedom of river navigation for Ecuador and on the definition of the northern sector of the boundary. In both cases, according to Tobar Donoso, Welles's decision was quickly and unquestioningly accepted by all concerned. Welles was not acting as an arbitrator here but as the representative of the United States; he was regarded as first among equals and was expected to provide a solution to a dispute that could not be settled by majority vote or other peaceful means.

It is clear that within the severe limitations it imposed on itself, the United States spared no effort to prevent war or to secure peace. Braden's "incorrigible optimism" and indefatigable diligence typified the persistence of the Department of State in the search for peace and exemplified the depth of its concern. The haunting question that arises at the end of this consideration of the role played by the United States in relation to these conflicts is whether or not it should have used its power to prevent or shorten them. It is probably too early to formulate a judgment on the policy of the United States, but one may seek to understand the decisions made and try to estimate the relative significance of the alternatives.

The problem was posed explicitly at an early stage in the Leticia dispute. Dr. Leo S. Rowe of the Pan American Union proposed to

Francis White on October 22, 1932, that the United States should "take the leadership" in the Leticia affair and initiate another continental declaration like that made in the Chaco. White demurred, saying that the United States was not "the policeman of South America." Rowe then stated the political issue by saying that no country except the United States would

take the leadership. Our [United States] leadership is the only one that would be respected in Peru. He thought that despite my [White's] reluctance to have us play a predominant role that it was one of the prices this country has to pay for its great power. We are the only one who can take the lead and we would be respected for doing so. We may well be criticized afterwards, but he thought we could be callous to that.

White did not reply to this challenge in policy terms other than to say he hoped "something would be worked out." [15] The previous day, when asked by Peruvian Ambassador Freyre for "suggestions," White had said that the United States "did not want to butt into this matter in any way whatsoever or to seem to take any preponderant role"; the United States desired to be "helpful" but would not do anything that would not be agreeable to both Colombia and Peru. Similarly, shortly after the invasion of Leticia, White had told Rowe that the United States was not "the sole guardian of peace in South America, and there is no reason why we should always jump in and assume such a role. Such action on our part might well be resented in other parts of South America."

White, presumably in accord with Stimson, had earlier made a similar decision concerning the Chaco dispute. It seems not unreasonable to assume that the Bolivians and Peruvians, both contemplating aggressive policies at the time, based their future courses on the conviction that the United States would not intervene. Rowe, understandably concerned about the outbreak of two international conflicts in South America in one year, may with some justification have believed that the Leticia affair presented an excellent opportunity for the United States to assert its "leadership"; Peru had no shadow of legal right in this case, its government appeared to be uncertain for some weeks as to whether it should try to take advantage of the situation, and the ability of the United States to affect the course of the fighting was unquestionably greater in Leticia than it was in the Chaco. However, the moment, or the month, was allowed to pass, when a minimum of "leadership" might have prevented war, and Lima was given every expectation that it would have no cause to fear intervention by Washington.

The issue of United States leadership, its exertion of predominant power, or the meeting of its responsibilities, as it was variously phrased, was also posed to the Department of State by Latin American diplomats. It was to be expected that the contending states would ask the United States to assert its power, as, for instance, when President Olaya said that the United States could, if it wished, settle the Leticia dispute in forty-eight hours, or when a former Colombian president expressed the hope of "intervention" by the United States. When Olaya asked for a "supreme effort" for peace by the United States, the Department of State did not respond and Edwin C. Wilson commented that this was another example of Olaya's "almost pathetic conviction" that the United States government was "omnipotent and can settle anything if it so desires." The attitude of the Department was further exemplified by White when he asked a Colombian envoy for a suggestion as to action by the United States; the reply was that the United States should tell Peru to get out of Leticia, and White could do no more than reply that he "had said this in no uncertain terms to both Freyre and Maúrtua but Peru had not gotten out." This admission of frustration and ineffectuality was a low point in United States policy; a month later a more positive stance was adopted by Stimson's invocation of the Kellogg-Briand Pact. By that time, however, Stimson's note was too weak to influence the defiant Peruvian government, although it might have been decisive had it been sent in early September, 1932.

On more than one occasion Latin American states which were not parties to conflicts suggested that the United States should take strong and independent measures. The Brazilian Ambassador suggested early in the Chaco dispute that the United States could operate more expeditiously alone than with the neutral Commission, and the Chilean delegate to the Chaco conference told Braden that the refusal of the United States to exert pressure of any kind was giving "these minor states an inflated opinion of themselves." He added that the United States should "demonstrate its authority and the fact that a strong hand of control still exists." These and similar suggestions had no influence on the Department of State, nor did requests for action in specific cases, such as Saavedra Lamas's insistence that the United States "must push Bolivia since you have the means to do it."

Within the Department of State there seems to have been no wavering; leadership would be exercised by means no stronger than those of example, exhortation, and unwearying helpfulness—in a word, solicitude.

When the critics of the Department of State spoke of leadership and responsibility, they appear to have assumed that there was a necessary relationship between the possession of power by the United States and its exercise to prevent other American states from violating treaties and shedding blood. The Department of State in effect denied that such a necessary relationship existed when its interests were not directly affected. It argued that its power was not unlimited, and it claimed that it had no duty to keep order. Moreover, it was commencing in 1932 to consider that the interests of the United States lay rather in the cultivation of friendship by the way of nonintervention and impartiality than in the upholding of international law or the maintenance of peace by the use of force. An important element in the Department's policy that was in harmony with these arguments was the contractive effect of the Great Depression on military adventures; Stimson had already discovered that Congress was unwilling to vote funds to pay for the supervision of elections in Nicaragua.

If the influence of public opinion in the United States had any important effect on the attitude of the Department of State toward Latin American conflicts, it appears to have been in this negative direction and in a very general sense. The Depression years were not a time for foreign crusading and, in any case, there was practically no popular interest in the United States about South American boundary disputes. The issues were unknown, and there were no groups of immigrants in the United States from the contending countries to make an outcry, much less exert any political influence. Furthermore, the Department of State does not appear to have been under any serious pressure from private groups or organizations to adopt a different policy. Finally, after Stimson's failure to mobilize American opinion against Peru in the Leticia case, the negotiations were carried on by the Department of State, if not in secret, at least in such a way as to avoid creating any concern or excitement on the part of the public. The tone of public statements was consistently hopeful, vague as to the precise nature of direction of developments, and empty of drama or tension. The Department proceeded as though convinced of the wisdom of Hugh Gibson's remark, referring to Argentina: "If we are to deal with this problem effectively it will have to be through some . . . mechanism which puts an end to the acute public interest in this region and allows a solution to be worked out under wholesome conditions of a bored public opinion."

The case for the assertion of leadership had no effect on the Department of State when presented in general terms, and the Department was not confronted with any specific issue of national interest that appeared to make it advisable to change its policy. There were, however, two additional points that were advanced in Latin America that were more substantial than those that have been mentioned. Even these, however, were predictions of potentialities that seemed insufficiently important to justify a policy change by the Department of State.

In the first days of the Leticia affair, Olaya told Caffery of his hope that the United States would take action to preserve the peace. "Anything else," he said, "means that every Latin American country must stay armed to the teeth in order to guard its legitimate rights." Colombia was nearly unarmed at the time; not only was it necessary to recall General Vásquez Cobo from his residence in France, but many of the most highly skilled men in Vásquez Cobo's flotilla were non-Colombians. In addition, Colombia was one of the few Latin American countries that had established a tradition of supremacy of civilian over military elements in the state. Olaya "resents . . . the fact that he is compelled to spend a great deal of money on war supplies (without question, he is anti-militarist and dislikes spending his money in that way)," and he therefore regretted that the United States had not taken measures to prevent fighting over

Leticia. In the course of the 1930s Olaya's prediction was largely fulfilled; there was a substantial rise in the armaments of several of the more important Latin American countries, including Colombia. In the case of Colombia in particular, the position of the military was greatly strengthened as a result of the Leticia affair and the concomitant expenditures on armaments, and subsequent developments in Colombia have given to the military a new role in political affairs comparable to that of army elements in many other Latin American countries. It is impossible to demonstrate conclusively that this sequence of events would not have occurred had the United States acted decisively to block Sánchez Cerro's ambitions in 1932; on the other hand, it is equally difficult to show satisfactorily that the United States remains free from any responsibility for it.[16]

In the Marañón dispute a different issue also raised a question about the exercise of the influence of the United States. It was known in Washington that the Ecuadorans were more vitally concerned with retaining access to the Marañón-Amazon system via the Santiago or Morona rivers than with any other aspect of the controversy. It was also recognized that acceptance of the Peruvian demands would constitute an imposed, rather than a negotiated peace, and therefore a bad settlement, in view of Peru's mood. Consequently, despite Tobar Donoso's signing of the protocol, it might have been anticipated that future Ecuadoran governments would have found ways to keep this issue open, as, in fact, they have done. It would perhaps be going too far to compare this controversy with that over Alsace-Lorraine in Europe, if only because of the great disparity in the strength of the contending states and because it is highly improbable that a renewal of the Marañón struggle would spark a general conflagration. Nevertheless, the affair remains unsettled, the Ecuadorans continue to refuse to accept their exclusion from the ranks of Amazonian countries—a status that they have treasured from the sixteenth century journey of Orellana—and frontier affrays occur from time to time.

On political grounds, therefore, the United States might have been justified in taking a stiffer stand against the Peruvian demands. Furthermore, the United States might have refused to allow itself to be associated so completely with the desire for an expression of continental solidarity at the Rio conference as to have agreed to assist in providing a "guarantee" of a frontier excluding Ecuador from the Marañón that was dictated by a Peruvian government, whose army had invaded Ecuador and remained in occupation of Ecuador's province of El Oro until fifteen days after the conference was ended and the protocol signed.[17] In reply to such questions, however, it might be pointed out that the United States no longer possessed great freedom of action; it was a beleaguered government that sent Sumner Welles to the Rio conference, one that could hardly fail to consider that even a formal continental solidarity, combined with Peruvian cooperation against the Axis states, was of such immediate importance as to overshadow any doubts that may have been entertained about future difficulties along the upper Amazon. These considerations also provide the political answer to those who would assert on moral grounds that the United States failed to lift its voice against the Peruvian invasion of Ecuador when it had vigorously denounced the Russian invasion of Finland. If the moral issues were comparable, the political features were quite different, and in January, 1942, the United States could not but have given greater weight to the latter. In one sense, this is another way of saying that the Peruvians chose well the time to settle the boundary dispute, just as they chose well the time, five days before the protocol was signed, to break diplomatic relations with the Axis powers. In 1938 the United States might have taken the lead to bring about consultation among all the American states. Such action might have prevented conflict; if not, it would very probably have avoided the kind of confirmation provided at the Rio de Janeiro conference for the Peruvian victory, a confirmation that is now regarded in Lima as one of Peru's most precious diplomatic possessions.

The responsibility imputed to the United States to take the long view, to guard the common good, to speak out for justice and not alone for peace was incompletely accepted by the United States in its attitude toward South American conflicts from 1932 to 1942. But this was no more than an imputed responsibility, urged from time to time by those who lacked the power themselves. Harassed first by economic stringency in 1932 and by its own involvement in war in

1941, the government of the United States reached decisions of self-effacement rather than those of assertiveness. These decisions may in part have entailed certain undesirable consequences, but intervention in the conflicts would probably have had disadvantageous, if different, effects. Resentment would certainly have been engendered on the part of some states, and conflicts might have been postponed rather than averted.

Nonintervention in affairs between Latin American states was consistent with nonintervention in their domestic politics. The policy aided in dispelling claims to the predominance of the United States in the Western Hemisphere that had begun with the Monroe Doctrine. Nonintervention in "internal or external affairs" was the policy pressed upon the United States at the Havana conference in 1928 and later, and its strict pursuance played an important, if incalculable, role in the attainment of hemispheric solidarity as manifested at the Lima conference and subsequent conferences of foreign ministers that dealt with problems of the defense of the Americas.

The role of the United States toward South American conflicts was not one of refusing to accept leadership in an interstate system in which great power leadership was the acknowledged method for establishing political norms. On the contrary, these three conflicts arose at a time of transition from great-power predominance and from a situation in which standards of conduct were enforceable by intervention or blockade to relationships in which equality of states was both demanded by the weak and recognized by the strong as in its own interest. During the transition there was a period of anarchy among the unshepherded weaker states, as is indicated by the courses of these conflicts. Was not this period also one of education in the disadvantages of anarchy, at least on the part of the smaller states of Latin America? Was their desire for an organization of American states as expressed at Chapultepec in 1945 motivated in part by the experience in the Chaco and in Leticia disputes and, more importantly and more recently, in the Ecuador-Peru conflict? If so, then it may be said that the United States did fulfill a responsibility by its policy of solicitude toward these conflicts. One of the justifications for the policy of nonintervention in internal politics was the view that only by abstention on the part of the United States would Central American peoples learn to govern themselves with a maximum of liberty and a minimum of force. This view has found justification in some countries, but it remains only a hope in others. In Latin American international relations, it may be suggested that the unfortunate consequences of anarchy, unmitigated by the exercise of benevolent power or influence by the United States, were realized so keenly that a favorable political climate was created for the establishment of cooperative institutions for the maintenance of peace. This is not to say that the formation of the Organization of American States sprang only from this source, since the desire for defense against extra-hemispheric dangers was of great importance in 1945, but it does suggest that the motives that had inspired the Uruguayan proposals for an American league of nations in the 1920s had become more widely and more deeply appreciated in Latin America by 1945. It may well have been true that the common experience of failure to keep the peace was the ineluctable prelude to the common conviction that a change in methods was necessary. Unless the United States had refrained from enforcing peace unilaterally the futility of the unorganized efforts of all twenty-one republics might not have been demonstrated. The power to prevent war existed, but its employment on the sole decision of the government of the United States would have been regarded as a breach of the principle of equality of states that had been accepted in Washington and demanded by all of Latin America. Consequently, if the employment of power to prevent war was to become collectively acceptable, the decision to employ it had to be a joint decision. But such a decision could only be attained through a system of collective security in the Americas, and the need for collective security was bitterly experienced before it became a driving motive for governmental action. It was not before some American states had been invaded by their greedy sister republics and had felt the losses, the pain, and the cost of war that they took seriously the proposals for an American league of nations that had formerly been dismissed as mere rhetoric. It was not before other American states had been defied, insulted, and ridiculed by sister republics who attacked their neighbors that they, too, responsibly sought effective ways to keep the peace.

This aim demanded organization. Common action in the disputes reviewed here was limited to a few states, and it was utterly ineffective in averting fighting. Mutual aid had developed in many technical and cultural fields, but progress in this sphere had little if any effect upon political relationships. The unifying principle of consultation was found applicable before 1945 only to issues of hemisphere defense and not to American conflicts. What has come to be called the inter-American system was a source of unity against external aggression before it became a method for preventing or limiting war in the Americas. However, the foundation for organization was built upon the urge to end both the armed strife and the failures to deal with it during the decade before World War II, and on the association of the United States with the Latin American countries as one among equals. These forces, stimulated by wartime collaboration, made possible an organization for limiting conflicts and for other types of cooperation in the postwar world.

The imperatives of such an organization, as they emerged from the 1932–42 experience, included the following. First, it was essential to depersonalize diplomacy. There should no longer exist the scope for a Saavedra Lamas to be a prima donna of pacification. Interestingly enough, even in the Americas, it has recently become rare for bilateral treaties to be identified by the names of their signers. Instead of Salomón-Lozano or Muñoz Vernaza–Suárez, for example, names for treaties are now found in cities or other places (such as the Pact of Bogotá), or in the subjects covered (such as Inter-American Mutual Assistance Treaty of 1947). This tendency is, of course, one reflection of the increasingly multilateral character of inter-American diplomacy; it may also bear a relationship, however, to an awareness of the difficulties created by familial identification with a treaty, as exemplified by Lozano Torrijos's opposition to the Leticia settlement of 1934.

In the second place, it was essential to establish legal obligations accepted by all states. Third, acceptance of the rapid arrival of neutral observers at the scene of fighting had to be agreed upon and then made technically feasible. Fourth, a large measure of publicity about the activities of the organization was required. Fifth, one central body, adequately staffed, should exercise a monopoly over peace-keeping action. And, finally, provision was necessary for the taking of appropriately severe sanctions against violators of the peace.

A direct relationship between these empirically discovered imperatives and the relevant provisions of the charter of the Organization of American States and the American Treaty of Pacific Settlement would be interesting but difficult to trace, and an effort to do so is outside the scope of this study, as is an examination of the record of the Organization. It may be noted, however, that in one way or another the charter and the treaty contain articles that, directly or indirectly, deal with all the issues discussed above, and the existence of a connection between them seems a likely hypothesis. Procedurally, therefore, the Organization of American States is equipped to cope with problems that baffled the American states in the Chaco, Leticia and Marañón disputes. Whether the procedure will be utilized depends, of course, on factors of motivation and common interest that will be variously tested.

A substantial number of disputes involving armed conflict have been effectively dealt with by the Organization in the past fifteen years, and it is apparent that in maintaining peace in the Americas the United States now enjoys far greater influence that it possessed during the years 1932–42. This apparently paradoxical development is due to the ability of the United States to use its prestige as a great power more effectively behind the shield of the Organization of American States than in the days when it refrained from unilateral coercion and there existed no collective authority either for the use of sanctions in international conflicts in the Americas or even for the swift use of such methods of peaceful settlement as teams of neutral observers. The enhancement of the capacity of the United States to fulfill responsibilities as a great power as a consequence of accepting membership in an organization that apparently limits the scope of its independent action is a notable political development. The ability to initiate action based on institutionalized obligations and procedures permits the United States to give the full weight of its support to pacific solutions to disputes, at the same time that the risk of resentment against it individually is reduced. This suggestion is made only in broad terms; and its refinement through close examination of political processes within the Organization may be of future interest both to statesmen and to scholars.

The Organization of American States is the heir of the Bolivarian intellectual and ethical tradition of peace and cooperation among American states. More recently and more specifically José Batlle y Ordóñez of Uruguay and Henry L. Stimson of the United States, among others, have urged the establishment of institutions to safeguard peace. However, during the decade 1932–42 the institutions and the tradition could have been combined effectively only when three conditions arose simultaneously: the American countries experienced notable failure to prevent international armed conflicts in their midst; the United States demonstrated firmness in its policy of nonintervention; and threats of further violence at home and unprecedented dangers from abroad made collaboration for peace and protection mutually advantageous.

Sources

Note on Sources

THE PRINCIPAL SOURCES used for the accounts of the Chaco and Leticia disputes are unpublished documents of the Department of State. These have been supplemented by publications of the governments concerned and by commentaries by Latin American statesmen and scholars.

As in the case of sources for *The Making of the Good Neighbor Policy*, the author is indebted to the Committee on the Use of Departmental Records of the Department of State for the opportunity to consult unpublished documents. The Department of State did not restrict access to materials, but quotations from and citations to documents required the approval of the Department before use could be made of them in published form.

Such approval may be obtained in two ways. One way is to take notes on documents in verbatim or paraphrased form and to submit the notes for clearance by officers of the Department. A second way is to prepare a manuscript incorporating quotations from and citations to documents and to submit the whole manuscript for clearance.

In the present study the second method for securing clearance was followed for all three disputes, and quotations from and citations to every document regarded as important were included in the manuscript. In the sections on the Chaco and Leticia disputes, officers of the Department suggested a half-dozen minor changes; these were made, and none of them significantly affected information about or interpretation of the policy of the United States.

In the case of the Marañón dispute, however, such extensive restrictions were placed on the excerpting and citing of official documents in the manuscript that it seemed preferable to base the account of the dispute on sources other than those in the files of the Department of State. The action of the Department is, of course, understandable, since the United States is one of the guarantors of the Protocol of Rio de Janeiro and since the Marañón dispute continues to smolder, at least in the sense that Ecuador maintains its protests against it, whereas the settlements in the other two conflicts now appear to have been accepted by all parties.

For the Marañón conflict, therefore, published materials form the principal cited sources. The account has benefited from acquaintance with the archival materials to 1943, and it has been supplemented by interviews with diplomats such as ex-Foreign Minister Julio Tobar Donoso, former Ambassador Mauricio Nabuco, and others, and by documents made available by foreign offices of Latin American governments.

Substantial reliance has been placed for documentation and interpretation on Tobar Donoso's *La invasión peruana y el protocol de Río.* This memoir was written not so much to present Ecuador's case to the world as to explain Tobar's signing of the protocol to the Ecuadoran people. It is nearly unique in the first half of the twentieth century among comparable publications by Latin American statesmen in its frankness, accuracy, clarity, and moderation. Wherever possible, Tobar's account of negotiations and quotations from documents have been compared with relevant data from other sources, and there appears to be good reason for giving it serious consideration. Since it is an Ecuadoran source, it would be comforting to be able to contrast it with a memoir by a Peruvian diplomat, but none has appeared so far. The outstanding Peruvian statement is found in the works by Alberto Ulloa listed in the bibliography; these, however, are less in the nature of memoirs than affirmations and justifications of the foreign policy of Peru, expounded with firmness and precision.

Diplomatic memoirs in the United States are barren as far as the Marañón dispute is concerned. Cordell Hull's memoirs do not mention it; the books by Sumner Welles and Laurence Duggan are no more informative, and it is ignored in a two-volume biography of Hull published in 1964. A few useful references were found in papers at the Franklin D. Roosevelt Memorial Library, and citations have been made with permission of the Library.

In view of the above difficulties with respect to primary sources, a study of the unofficial literature has been made; most of this is polemical, and very little of it either adds to or detracts from Tobar's record of the diplomatic relationships. If it may be said that it is less than fully satisfactory to have to depend so largely on Tobar's book, it may also be said both that an orderly account would be impossible without it and that we are fortunate that it tells a story that is internally coherent and gives evidence of being fair and dispassionate. This is not to say that Tobar's record is complete, nor that his interpretations are not open to challenge now or later. His signature of the Protocol has been denounced in Ecuador, but, so far, his account of the negotiations from April, 1941, through January, 1942, does not appear to have been seriously questioned in Quito, Lima, or elsewhere.

Public official records are scanty, although some information is available from annual reports of the Ecuadoran and Peruvian foreign offices. (See, for example, Peru, Ministerio de Relaciones Exteriores, *Memoria de Relaciones Exteriores* [Lima, Tall. Gráf. Villaneuva, 1956], for documents on the frontier incident of 1955.) Archives are not open for intensive scholarly research, although it may be occasionally possible to secure in foreign offices access of one kind or another to a few documents which can be specifically described because their existence is known. The 42 pages of documents in *Foreign Relations of the United States*, 1941, VI, are very useful, although their gaps are regrettable, notably the "attached description" in the Peruvian note of September 13, 1941, and the text of the mediators' note of October 4, 1941. However, these gaps have been filled in the present study, as indicated in Part III. No documents relevant to the Marañón dispute are printed in FR, 1942, V, or FR, 1943, V. The Hull Papers in the Library of Congress are of no use in the study of these three disputes.

Despite these limitations, it is believed that this account of the Marañón dispute includes textual excerpts or summaries from all of the principal intergovernmental notes and memoranda exchanged between the mediators and the disputants. Missing are the flavor, insights, and predilections offered by the reports of officers of the Foreign Service of the United States and of memoranda of conversations between Hull and Welles and Latin American envoys.

Missing also are interpretive histories and biographies of statesmen by Latin Americans. There are a few useful memoirs by Bolivians, Ecuadorans, and Paraguayans, but Colombian and Peruvian diplomats have left almost no personal records of their work on behalf of their countries. Benjamin Disraeli once warned: "Read no history; nothing but biography, for that is life without theory." Biography in Latin American countries is a rare art form, and diplomatic histories of the twentieth century are little more than chronologies, unillumined by any display of motivation, attitudes, and prejudices that exist in the diplomatic correspondence. "History is too important to be left to the historians," appears to be the motto of diplomats and the officials of foreign offices who jealously guard the fundamental records.

Notes on Maps

MAP I. The map for the Chaco War has been developed from the four maps at the end of *The Chaco Peace Conference: Report of the Delegation of the United States of America to the Peace Conference held at Buenos Aires July 1, 1935–January 23, 1939*, with the aid of the maps of the American Geographical Society, relevant sections of the World Aeronautical Chart, maps in David H. Zook, Jr., *The Conduct of the Chaco War* (New York, Bookman Associates, 1960), and several other sources, some of which have been useful in fixing a single *fortín*.

MAP II. The map for the Leticia dispute has been based on *The Times Atlas of the World*, Vol. V (Boston, Houghton Mifflin, 1957), with the assistance of Francisco Terán's *Geografía del Ecuador*, Herbert Boy's *Una historia con alas* (Madrid, Ed. Guadarrama, 1955), and other sources.

MAP III. This map derives from several sources, including the *Mapa geográfico del Ecuador compilado por el Instituto Geográfico Militar, 1950;* the description of the Talara Truce lines as given in *Foreign Relations, 1941*, VI, p. 234; and the "Croquis de la Frontera del Zarumilla," in Felipe de la Barra's *Tumbes, Jaén y Maynas* (Lima, Centro de Estudios Históricos Militares del Perú, 1961), p. 48.

MAP IV. The *status quo* line of 1936 is taken from Julio Tobar Donoso's

La invasión peruana y el protocolo de Río (Quito, Ed. Ecuatoriana, 1945), p. 80, and from the text given there of the Peruvian description of the *status quo,* which Tobar calls "malicious" but does not question geographically. It should be noted, however, that in the last of the end-maps in Julio Tobar Donoso and Alfredo Luna Tobar, *Derecho territorial ecuatoriano* (Quito, Ed. La Unión Católica, 1961), there is given a line called "Peruvian positions before 1936." This line is drawn south of the Marañón northeastward from the mouth of the Chínchipe in the Marañón to the Manseriche Rapids, and is north of the Marañón thereafter. There is also an incomplete line showing Ecuadoran positions before 1936, but this line does not at any point touch the Marañón; this is consistent with Tobar Donoso's statement on p. 80 of *La invasión peruana y el protocolo de Río* that there were no Ecuadoran military posts "nor other signs of possession" on any of the mouths of the northern tributaries of the Marañón. It seems probable that the Tobar Donoso–Luna Tobar line of the Peruvian positions has been drawn for propaganda purposes, and that the line as given in Map IV is a closer approximation to the actual situation in 1936. Peruvian maps since 1941 do not show the *status quo* line of 1936, presumably because the differences between it and that of the Protocol are not great, and therefore the image of the "victory" of 1941 might shrivel, and, also, because in at least two places the line of the Protocol is more favorable to Ecuador.

The line of the Peruvian note to the mediators of September 13, 1941, has been drawn from the text of the "attached description" as given in the text, pp. 293–94, and with the aid of the *Mapa geográfico del Ecuador.* There are some problems of reconciling maps (for example, Andoas on the *Mapa geográfico del Ecuador* is about 40 miles south of the position given for it by the map of the American Geographical Society, as revised, 1962, although both are drawn to the scale of 1:1,000,000), but an effort has been made to establish correct relationships, particularly as between the several lines.

The line of the Protocol of Rio de Janeiro is taken from the *Mapa geográfico del Ecuador,* as checked with Peruvian and other maps. The two "zones in dispute" listed on that map are shown (Laguna Lagartocohca near Güepi in the north, and the Cordillera del Condor area including the Cenepa River in the south), together with dotted lines in the gaps. The dotted line in the south is the proposed line skirting the source of the Cenepa River as drawn in the map contained in Felipe de la Barra's *Tumbes, Jaén y Maynas* (Lima, Centro de Estudios Históricos Militares del Perú, 1961), p. 90. The dotted line in the Laguna Lagartocohca area fills in a gap in the line of the Protocol as given in the *Mapa geográfico del Ecuador* that is not recognized as a gap in de la Barra's map. In the south, the Ecuadoran map indicates that about 125 miles in the Cordillera del Condor is not demarcated, but the map in de la Barra's book shows only about 50 miles where boundary markers have not been placed by officials of the two countries, and de la Barra claims that this gap exists precisely between two markers named, on the south, "Cunchuime Sur," and on the north, "20 de noviembre."

The line recommended by the Spanish Council of State, 1910 is taken from *El protocolo de Rio de Janeiro ante la historia* (Lima, Sanmartí y Cía.?, 1942), Map No. 5.

In addition to the above mentioned sources, there have been used geographical texts and other works listed in the section in the Bibliography on the Marañón Conflict, as well as strictly cartographical sources that include the following, some of which exist only as sheets sold as such in bookstalls:

American Geographical Society of New York. *South America*. Scale 1:1,000,000, 1939–1962, with revisions.

Banco Comercial del Perú, Perú. *Mapa Físico-Político*. Escala 1:2,500,000, 1960?.

Ecuador. *Sistema fundamental de vias de comunicación*. Escala 1:2,000,000, Ministro de Obras Públicas y Comunicaciones, Quito, 1956.

Ecuador. *País Amazónico* (El Ecuador y sus desmembraciones territoriales en su litigio con el Perú, desde el año de 1,829). Cartógrafo: Jaime Jaramillo Espinosa, Escala 1:5,000,000. (Not dated.)

Ecuador. Ministerio de Relaciones Exteriores. *El Ecuador y el Amazonas: Tradicionalmente conocido como Río de Quito o de Orellana*. Quito, 1961. 8 pp.

Mapa del Chaco Boreal. Buenos Aires, Amengual Litograph, Piedras 636, 1938.

Mapa de la República del Paraguay, destinado para uso de las instituciones de enseñanza. Escala: 1:2,000,000. Autorizada por el Instituto Geográfica Militar, Asunción, Alberto da Ponte, 1962.

Mapa geográfico del Ecuador, compilado por el Instituto geográfico militar. Escala: 1:1,000,000. Quito, 1950.

Morales y E., Juan. *Ecuador: Texto-Atlas Geográfico del Ecuador*. 116 pp., 30 maps.

Peru. Ministerio de Relaciones Exteriores. Departamento de Propaganda e Informaciones. *Peru* (Travel information and map, 1962).

La Prensa (Buenos Aires), January 28, 1942. Map of Ecuadoran and Peruvian *status quo* lines of 1936.

Ríos Valdivia, Alejandro, and L. René del Villar. *Atlas Universal: Edición especial para el Perú*. 1st ed. Chile, Zig-Zag, 1957. 43 pp. with 7 maps of Peru.

World Aeronautical Chart, Nos. 1192, 1259, 1261, 1314, 1315. Scale 1:1,000,000, Bolivia, Brazil, Paraguay. St. Louis, Mo., United States Air Force Aeronautical Chart and Information Center, 1951.

Notes and Bibliography

Abbreviations

DS U.S. Department of State unpublished documents. File numbers in the 720s deal with disputes among American states. For example, 724.3415 includes documents on the Chaco War, and 724.34119 comprises documents on the Chaco Peace Conference; 721.23 covers the Leticia affair, and 722.2315, the Marañón dispute. A citation such as 721.23/1698 means that the document in question (see footnote 31 for Chapter VI in the Leticia dispute) is the 1698th received or sent by the Department of State relating to this dispute. The number of the document may not be strictly in chronological order; in some cases a document with a single number may have attachments, such as newspaper clippings or memoranda, that are not separately numbered. Whenever possible, citations have been given to documents published in FR (see below). Documents dated through December 31, 1933, are now generally available in the National Archives; for permission to use later materials, application should be made to the Historical Office, Department of State.

FDRL Franklin D. Roosevelt Library, Hyde Park, New York. Materials in this library are generally available, but permission for direct quotation should be requested of the director.

FR *Foreign Relations of the United States,* Washington, D.C., U.S. Government Printing Office, 1 to 5 or more volumes annually, at present, through 1943. Comprehensiveness of documentation varies greatly. The Chaco dispute is given relatively full treatment, whereas that on the Marañón conflict is much more limited, and no documents on the latter are provided in the volumes for 1942 or 1943.

Notes to Text

Introduction

Full bibliographical information about the works cited will be found in the General section of the Bibliography.

1. On changes in the policy of intervention, see the author's *The Making of the Good Neighbor Policy*.

2. Instruction 137, to Panama, April 28, 1915. FR, 1915, 1147.

3. Note of April 27, 1921. FR, 1921, I, 212.   4. FR, 1934, IV, 361.

5. On this point, an editorial in *El Imparcial* (Santiago), January 18, 1937, commenting on the Buenos Aires conference, reviewed the failure of South American efforts in the previous twenty-five years to achieve more than "a disconcert of nations" and rejoiced that a "fraternal society of nations" was now being formed under the leadership, but without the tutelage, of the United States. A coolness in official relations between Argentina and Chile in 1937 might account for the editorial's judgment that the responsibility for earlier failures lay with Argentina, which "had committed the capital sin of always placing its own interests before those of other states," after it had achieved a position of predominant influence in South America. However, *El Imparcial* lived up to its name by criticizing Pedro Montt, President of Chile in 1910, for refusing a Brazilian invitation to pay a visit to Rio de Janeiro.

6. Hull, *Memoirs*, I, 309–10.

7. It is worth recalling, however, that Fred Morris Dearing, Ambassador to Peru, remarked in 1935: "To have delivered into Saavedra Lamas's hands the primary responsibility for peace in this continent proves itself more and more to have been far sighted and wise . . . it contributes as well to what seems to me to be of prime necessity in this part of the world—that is, leaving these nations free to learn how to assume and discharge responsibilities and take care of themselves." Letter to President Roosevelt, Lima, March 4, 1935. FDRL, PSF, Box 20. Carlos Saavedra Lamas was the Argentine Foreign Minister.

Part One. The Chaco War, 1928–1938

Full bibliographical information about the works cited will be found in the section of the Bibliography on the Chaco War.

I. The Failure to Prevent War

1. On physical conditions in the Chaco, see Estigarribia, *The Epic of the Chaco*, and González, *La guerra del Chaco*, where the arable forest and desert zones are described.

2. *Commission of Inquiry and Conciliation, Bolivia and Paraguay*. Report of the American Commissioner to the Secretary of State, Washington, December 15, 1929. DS, 724.3415/942. See also Cardozo, *Paraguay independiente*, who says, perhaps with unconscious humor, that the first incident in the Chaco was that at Fort Sorpresa on the Confuso River (p. 297).

3. Each side of course denounced any action by the other that improved its position in the Chaco. For example, the Paraguayans objected to the establishment in 1906 of Bolivian military posts at Guachalla and Ballivián, and the Bolivians protested the settlement at Colonia Mennonita. See Zook, *The Conduct of the Chaco War*, pp. 31, 37; and Rodas Eguino, *La guerra del Chaco*, p. 77. There is a vast juridico-historical literature on the rival claims that Zook describes as a "bog from which the unwary investigator must extricate himself lest he squander years in an unrewarding pursuit of a definitive title" (p. 37). We have taken his advice, at least for the pre-1928 period.

4. Minister Edward Francis Feely in Bolivia reported that the belief existed in that country "that Argentina would welcome the addition of Paraguay as its northernmost province, with the Bolivian petroleum deposits as a rich prize in the northwest; that Brazil is desirous of extending its boundary westward; and that Chile would view with favor the acquisition of the rich mineral district of Southwestern Bolivia." Despatch 183, from La Paz, July 18, 1931. DS, 724.3415/1332. A high Argentine official was reported as saying that Chile was "pushing Bolivia towards the Atlantic for the outlet Bolivia seeks so as to rid herself of the complication of a Bolivian exit on the Pacific." Despatch 1264, from Buenos Aires, July 8, 1931. DS, 724.3415/1291.

5. Secretary Frank B. Kellogg to American diplomatic officers in Latin America, February 28, 1929. FR, 1929, I, 698. This important instruction expressed a position essentially the same as that in the memorandum to the Secretary of State printed in *Memorandum on the Monroe Doctrine*, by J. Reuben Clark (Washington, U.S. Government Printing Office, 1930). The memorandum was dated December 17, 1928; Clark was then Undersecretary of State.

6. The term "Fort" is here used to apply to any place designated by

the Spanish word "fortín." Such places might be no more than temporary shelters for a squad of soldiers, or they might become fortified camps with trenches and breastworks of logs and sandbags. The same "forts" were given different names by Bolivians and Paraguayans as they changed hands, and the names might accompany the temporary bivouacs of squads or other detachments as they were shifted in a vaguely defined area.

7. FR, 1929, I, 694.

8. *Commission of Inquiry and Conciliation*, p. 29 (see note 2).

9. Supplementary Memorandum by the Secretary General and Counselor of the Commission (H.F. Arthur Schoenfeld and Walter Bruce Howe). Attached to *Commission of Inquiry and Conciliation* (see note 2).

10. *Ibid.*, pp. 47–48.

11. *Ibid.*, p. 103. This attitude was for a time thought by President Hernando Siles of Bolivia to represent the policy of the State Department or of President Herbert Hoover, because, as Siles said, "No Latin country would ever have permitted its representative to act without interference," as the Department of State had done in the case of General McCoy. FR, 1929, I, 925. See also FR, 1929, I, 918–20.

12. The arrival of French planes in Asunción at the beginning of 1930 was reported by the Minister in Paraguay, on January 3. Despatch 979, DS, 724.3415/984. See also FR, 1930, I, 331, 333, for references to British Vickers planes purchased by Bolivia. As early as 1925, Paraguay had commenced purchases of arms for a force of 24,000 men. See Zook, *The Conduct of the Chaco War*.

13. *Commission of Inquiry and Conciliation*, pp. 32–33 (see note 2).

14. FR, 1929, I, 911.

15. FR, 1930, I, 329. Leguía added that, if actual war broke out in the Chaco, "the prestige of the United States in Latin America, as well as in Europe, could not but suffer immeasurably" and said he would give "wholehearted support" to any move made by the United States.

16. FR, 1929, I, 907–8.

17. See, for example, the note of Minister of Foreign Affairs Gerónimo Zubizarreta, of April 20, 1931, FR, 1931, I, 715–17.

18. For a review of the background of the dispute, see Zook, *The Conduct of the Chaco War*, Chap. I.

19. The Bolivian government admitted that Paraguay's "civil possessions remain up to about meridian 60° " in the Chaco, in arguing that the removal of Paraguayan troops to the Paraguay River would not mean "disoccupation." Note by the Bolivian Minister for Foreign Affairs to the Chairman of the Commission of Neutrals, September 22, 1932. FR, 1932, V, 93. Bolivian civilian settlement in the Chaco was limited to a few places along the western Pilcomayo, and to Fort Muñoz, an important base in the southern Chaco. Telegram 53, to Asunción, December 2, 1932. FR, 1932, V, 113.

20. González, *La Guerra del Chaco*, p. 205.

21. Despatches 305 of October 10, 1931, DS, 724.3415/1402, and 271

of September 5, 1931, DS, 724.3415/1402, from Asunción. See also González, *La Guerra del Chaco*, p. 14: "In January 1931 the war was inevitable. The political leaders of Paraguay still cherished the ingenuous hope that the neutrals, our legal titles, the American spirit, 'the Department of State,' would make an armed conflict impossible in this 'traditionally pacifist part of the world.' However, some military leaders, more practical in outlook, urged the taking of concrete measures to meet the threat from Bolivia."

22. October 9, 1931. FR, 1931, I, 758.

23. October 14, 1931. FR, 1931, I, 764. The Chilean Minister of Foreign Affairs telegraphed La Paz "urging Bolivia to attend conference at Washington and to restrain troops. He stated he has now a definite reply that Bolivia has yielded." For Bolivian claims of "Paraguayan usurpation of the entire right bank of the Paraguay River" and charges that Paraguay was the "permanent aggressor," see its note to the neutrals of October 18, FR, 1931, I, 767–68. For a brief statement of the Paraguayan position, see note of April 20, 1931, FR, 1931, I, 715–17, in which reference is made to "the military advances of Bolivia in the Chaco," which have "craftily and in violation of the compacts designed to regulate the conduct of the two parties, brought about a proximity exposed to every kind of incidents."

24. FR, 1931, I, 733, June 25, 1931, and I, 736, June 27, 1931. On September 30, 1931, Feely reported that a high official had told him, in view of a recent clash in the Chaco, that "if Paraguayan aggression continued the government might be forced into open warfare both by public sentiment and because of a growing restiveness amongst younger army officers." Despatch 115, DS, 724.3415/1397. See also report by Minister Post Wheeler in Paraguay that officials there thought that reports of Bolivian threats to bomb Asunción were made to give the impression in Brazil and Chile that the situation was "too explosive to permit discussion at the present time," but that "acute pressure" both by the neutrals and other American governments caused Bolivia to decide to send representatives to Washington to discuss the nonaggression pact. Telegram 105, from Asunción, October 21, 1931. DS, 724.3415/1481.

25. July 18, 1931. FR, 1931, I, 747–48.

26. The text of the Hayes Award did not give any reason for the decision. See FR, 1878, 711. This award determined claims only as between Argentina and Paraguay to the area between the Verde, Pilcomayo, and Paraguay rivers and did not relate directly to Bolivian claims.

27. Despatches 53 of January 20, 1931, DS, 724.3415/1168, and 183 of July 18, 1931, DS, 724.3415/1332, from La Paz. Francis White wrote to Minister Feely on February 18, 1931, explaining that the Department did not give instructions to General McCoy, that it did not even know very much about the work of the Commission during its activities, and that in any case none of the neutral governments was in any way committed by the work of the Commission. Mr. White added that, in the past seven

years, the Department of State had aided in settling eight American boundary disputes and that only two of these had been settled on the basis of possession or occupation of territory. In both of these, however, as in the other cases, the solutions had appeared to be the "common sense arrangements." White assured Feely that "any conversations coming up now before the Department will be handled as a new matter without any preconceived notions being entertained regarding it in an endeavor to do justice to both parties." DS, 724.3415/1175.

28. Despatch 53 (see note 27). In the letter quoted in the same note, Francis White stated that the United States had not brought any pressure to bear on either country in the Tacna-Arica case.

29. FR, 1931, I, 766, 768. The term "American" is used here and elsewhere to refer collectively to the United States and the twenty Latin American states. Canada is also, of course, an "American country," but it has not participated, except indirectly, in the settlement of "inter-American" disputes. The term "Latin American" is used because, while not entirely satisfactory, it seems to be in most general usage in the United States, and it is perhaps the most inclusive of the general expressions, such as "Ibero-American," "Indo-American," "Hispanic-American," which have been suggested from time to time.

30. Text of the draft pact in FR, 1932, V, 8–13. For a detailed review of the drafting process see note from White to Juan José Soler, the Paraguayan delegate, July 28, 1932, FR, 1932, V, 41–6. When the pact was not accepted in Asunción, Soler apparently tried to disclaim responsibility for its terms and represented it to his government as "the White draft." White records his "intense surprise" that Soler claimed that the pact "is absolutely inacceptable." FR, 1932, V, 45. White thought that Soler had communicated with his government during the informal negotiations in order to get instructions, but this the latter had not done. See also Soler's reply of August 4 to this note, FR, 1932, V, 52–56.

31. June 1, 1932. FR, 1932, V, 16.

32. Despatch from the Minister in Paraguay (Wheeler), June 2, 1932. FR, 1932, V, 13–15.

33. The Bolivians referred to this incident as that of Fort Mariscal Santa Cruz, at Laguna Chuquisaca. Despatch 628, from La Paz, July 1, 1933. DS, 724.3415/3232. This difference in nomenclature recalls Ayala's statement that "Bolivia's custom is, when she has made an attack on a Paraguayan post, to give out a statement at La Paz wherein she calls the post by another name, claims it her own, and alleges that it has been attacked by Paraguayan troops." Telegram 95, from Asunción, August 21, 1932. FR, 1932, V, 76.

34. Memorandum of telephone conversation with the Ambassador in Argentina (Robert Woods Bliss), August 17, 1932. DS, 724.3415/2090–1/14.

35. Full text in FR, 1932, V, 169f. The declaration did not mention the Kellogg-Briand Pact, as had been done in the Manchurian case, but

it did include some of the language of the Pact, for example, "The American nations . . . are opposed to force and renounce it . . . as an instrument of national policy."

36. Memorandum by Assistant Secretary Francis White, "Bolivia-Paraguay Negotiations," August 5, 1932. DS, 724.3415/1965–1/2. The Mexican Ambassador, José Manuel Puig Casauranc, suggested the idea independently in the Commission of Neutrals on July 11.

37. FR, 1932, V, 37.

38. "Bolivia-Paraguay Negotiations" (see note 36).

39. FR, 1932, V, 37.

40. Minutes of Meeting of July 30, 1932, between Representatives of the Neutral Countries and Representatives of Countries Neighboring on Bolivia and Paraguay. FR, 1932, V, 154–56.

41. Despatch 1740. DS, 724.3415/2072. Bliss added: "Both in editorial comment and in a statement given out by Dr. Saavedra Lamas, the United States has been acclaimed for its 'magnanimous' action in turning to Argentina and other South American republics to come to the rescue of the Neutral Commission . . . for a solution of the problem with which it has been wrestling." In the margin of this despatch is the comment: "Argentina was offered the chance to take the initiative but refused for fear she couldn't pull it off. When we succeeded she then jumped in to try to take the credit. F. W.[hite]."

42. When the Governor of Buenos Aires province sent a message to Saavedra Lamas, stating that the widespread approval given to the " 'Argentine formula' " signified " 'the consolidation of South American peace,' " Saavedra Lamas expressed his " 'profound thanks' " for this appreciation of the " 'pacific policy' " of the President of Argentina. *La Prensa* (Buenos Aires), September 13, 1932.

43. See the debate in the Argentine senate reported verbatim in *La Prensa* (Buenos Aires), September 13, 1932. An amusing exchange took place when the senator accused Saavedra Lamas of never hearing those who asked him questions. He said: " 'It is not possible to have a dialogue with you,' " and Saavedra Lamas replied: " 'This time I will listen; I shall depart from my custom and hear what you have to say.' " *Ibid.* The next day, *La Prensa*, as was its custom, defended the foreign minister in an editorial that characterized the debate as "confused."

44. Memorandum by the Assistant Secretary of State (White). FR, 1932, V, 182–83. See FR, 1932, V, 245, for White's remarks concerning *La Prensa* and the reasons for suggesting that Saavedra Lamas take the initiative.

45. Memorandum of conversation, August 22, 1932. DS, 724.3415/2090–8/14.

46. *Ibid.* In this same talk, however, Finot objected to a suggestion of White's that the forthcoming Montevideo conference might draw up an arbitration treaty, on the ground that it was a "political conference." Finot added: "It is felt in Bolivia that this country [the United States] dominates the Pan American Conferences and also dominated the Amer-

ican nations in their recent declaration; that all the American nations have been lined up hostile to Bolivia, and that they would support Paraguay and not Bolivia at the Conference." White said that it was "absurd to think that the whole continent of nineteen nations would bank together against one. . . . It [the declaration of August 3] was drawn up to apply to Paraguay in the first instance but by force of circumstances it had actually applied to Bolivia and no hostility had been directed against Bolivia at all." If the Bolivians had stopped negotiations before Soler's return, and had based their action on Soler's leaving Washington, the declaration of August 3 would have applied to Paraguay rather than to Bolivia.

47. For example, the Chilean Foreign Minister told Ambassador Culbertson on August 9 that "the insistence upon the cessation of hostilities on the basis of occupations as of June 1st is merely a detail compared with the major issue of a possible war." Telegram 162, from Santiago, August 9, 1932. FR, 1932, V, 169. White, on the other hand, considered that the declaration of August 3 would be violated unless a return to the June 1 line were accepted by Bolivia, an acceptance already made by Paraguay.

48. Telegram 46 to Minister Wheeler in Asunción, November 5, 1932. FR, 1932, V, 108. In the note of the Commission of Neutrals to the Argentine Ambassador (Espil), of November 4, 1932, White, for the Neutrals, wrote of the declaration of August 3: "This deliberate declaration by nineteen American States of the policy by which each of them proposes to be governed in future can not be treated as lacking in weight or effectiveness. On the contrary, considering the serious circumstances under which it was made, it must be considered as of the most solemn character, carrying with it the faith of each signatory, and as of quite as much weight as instruments of more formal execution." FR, 1932, V, 211.

49. The first concerned a request by Saavedra Lamas for the good offices of the United States in restoring diplomatic relations between Argentina and Uruguay. After the United States had begun negotiations, the Argentine Foreign Minister brought up new conditions that he had not previously mentioned, causing Ambassador Bliss to say to him "that his attitude amounted to a flat reversal of the assurances upon which United States good offices were proffered." FR, 1932, V, 324.

50. On Hull's support for Saavedra Lamas's candidacy for the Nobel Peace Prize, see below, pp. 370–72. A Bolivian comment was that Saavedra Lamas "could have become the principal figure of South American diplomacy had he acted honorably in the Chaco conflict." Baldivia G., *La guerra con el Paraguay y la diplomacia argentina*, p. 4.

51. Memorandum of conversation by Francis White, August 11, 1932. DS, 724.3415/1920–5/14.

52. Minister Wheeler reported from Asunción on December 4, 1932, that "apparently as a result of Soler's cables . . . the feeling has grown that they [the other four Neutrals] are merely figureheads, that the

United States dictates the Commission's actions and that she is so greatly under the influence of Bolivian propaganda that she cannot be fair." FR, 1932, V, 116. For a comparable Bolivian example, see note 46.

53. Despatch 476, from the Minister in Asunción (Wheeler), July 28, 1932. DS, 724.3415/2211. It appeared that this blouse had been sold by the United States government to private firms as surplus equipment, and that, contrary to law, the buttons bearing United States Army insignia had not been removed before resale to Bolivia. The information appeared in Asunción papers, although governmental influence was exercised to prevent sensational treatment of the news.

54. Despatch 2175, from the Secretary of Embassy in Peru (Garret G. Ackerson, Jr.), September 29, 1932. DS, 724.3415/2401.

55. Telegram 14, from La Paz, April 15, 1932. FR, 1932, V, 138. This suggestion, however, is open to the interpretation that Bolivia, aware that the Neutrals would not employ sanctions in the Chaco, feared that the neighboring powers might do so and were trying in this way to play one group off against the other in such a way that no action would be taken.

56. For some of the less wealthy countries of Latin America, financial considerations occasionally influenced diplomatic negotiations. Referring to the draft nonaggression pact, Francis White noted that, on May 6, the two delegations had revised and rewritten the draft pact "and sent it to their Governments for instructions. Rather than pay a little extra and cable down the text, both Delegations sent it by mail and got their instructions back by mail. As they had to reply to that again, you can imagine that we marked time for a long period. Just as we were about to get under way again early in July, came word to the Paraguayan Delegation that a Paraguayan fort had been attacked." Letter to the Minister in Switzerland (Hugh R. Wilson), August 15, 1932. DS, 724.3415/2067A.

57. Despatch 446, from La Paz, October 10, 1932. DS, 724.3415/2512.

58. Memorandum of conversation, January 23, 1932. DS, 724.3415/-1641-4/5.

59. Wheeler reported that the Paraguayan president felt the most practicable guarantee to be reciprocal retirement of troops in the Chaco "and a setting up of a body of international police in the vacated area." Telegram 38, from Asunción, June 4, 1932. DS, 724.3415/1795.

60. Memorandum of conversation between White and the Paraguayan delegates, Juan José Soler and César Vasconcellos, June 13, 1932. DS, 724.3415/1803-5/9. Memorandum of telephone conversation, June 3, 1932. DS, 724.3415/1803-5/9. Soler told White that the Neutrals had told him "definitely that Mexico would give no guarantee whatever." Memorandum of conversation, June 13, 1932. DS, 724.3415/1803-5/9.

61. Memorandum of conversation, January 12, 1933. FR, 1933, IV, 253.

62. Memorandum of conversation regarding the Chaco Dispute, by J. Butler Wright, Montevideo, December 1933. DS, 724.3415/3425-1/2. See also telegram 60, from Montevideo, December 16, 1933, FR, 1933, IV, 376, for statement by Hull that he had taken steps to avoid any obligation on the part of the United States to "agree to sanctions" at the conference.

63. Instruction 35, August 20, 1932. FR, 1932, V, 75.

64. Memorandum of conversation, February 29, 1932. DS, 724.3415/1663–10/19.

65. Telegram 50, to Asunción, November 21, 1932. DS, 724.3415/2538A.

66. Memorandum of conversation, November 28, 1932, written by Francis White. DS, 724.3415/2683–2/11. Two years later, Secretary Hull had to admit that "the time has not yet come when efficient machinery is functioning, nor have the peace agencies created by common agreement between the American nations so far acquired sufficient prestige to prove their usefulness at this juncture." FR, 1934, IV, 115.

67. FR, 1932, V, 21. Minister Wheeler expressed the opinion that "an attack on the Government" would probably have occurred otherwise. FR, 1932, V, 23.

68. FR, 1932, V, 125. Wheeler commented: "Judging by the temper of the people generally, the press and the military party, I am of the opinion that he does not greatly exaggerate." Earlier Wheeler had noted that the "war fever had been steadily growing here and mobilization is being rapidly completed." Ayala had told him: "'If I opposed the Army further I should have no army.'" Telegram 93, August 19, 1932. FR, 1932, V, 73.

69. August 11, 1932. FR, 1932, V, 173.

70. Despatch 455, from Asunción, June 24, 1932. DS, 834.00/736.

71. Memorandum of conversation, October 21, 1932. DS, 724.3415/2414–6/13.

72. This interpretation of the outbreak of fighting in the Chaco and of Salamanca's underestimation of Paraguayan military capability is strongly supported by the testimony of Colonel Rogelio Ayala Moreira in his *Por que no ganamos la guerra del Chaco*, pp. 99, 112–13, 165.

73. Despatch 466, from La Paz, November 9, 1932. DS, 724.3415/2614. It should also be noted that on August 10, 1932, the neighboring countries, considering "that they are peculiarly well situated to estimate conditions in Bolivia and Paraguay," agreed to request the Neutrals to ask the parties to agree to a truce, in view of the neighboring countries' fear that "if Salamanca should yield further to the representations of the Commission he would be overthrown by the military and the outbreak of war would follow." FR, 1932, V, 171.

74. Memorandum of conversation, August 8, 1932. FR, 1932, V, 165.

75. Memorandum of conversation, July 7, 1932. DS, 724.3415/1815–4/14.

76. Memorandum of conversation, by Francis White, March 16, 1932. DS, 724.3415/1663–15/19. White had advised the neighbors to "go slowly" but did not regard this as "calling off" their efforts at peace.

II. The Search for Peace

1. Memorandum of conversation, April 7, 1932. DS, 724.3415/1724–5/14.

2. Memorandum of conversation between White and the Argentine Ambassador (Espil), April 12, 1932. DS, 724.3415/1723-9/14.

3. The Secretary of State to the Ambassador in Argentina (Bliss), August 13, 1932. FR, 1932, V, 180.

4. Letter to Hugh R. Wilson, Minister in Switzerland, September 19, 1932. DS, 724.3415/2322A.

5. Telegram 63, to the Ambassador in Chile (Culbertson), August 13, 1932. FR, 1932, V, 181.

6. See telegram 187, from Ambassador Culbertson in Santiago, August 25. FR, 1932, V, 187.

7. Memorandum of conversation, August 26, 1932. FR, 1932, V, 189.

8. Telegram 71, August 26, 1932, to Santiago. DS, 724.3415/2154.

9. FR, 1932, V, 80.   10. FR, 1932, V, 95-96.

11. FR, 1932, V, 99-100. Military setbacks interested La Paz in the Neutrals' plan for stopping the fighting, and the Bolivian representative in Washington "who, as one of the Neutrals said, was a 'Sleeping Beauty' for some weeks, has recently been honoring us with his visits two and even three times a day to express the eagerness of Bolivia to comply with the Neutrals' suggestion." Letter from White to Wilson, September 19, 1932. DS, 724.3415/2322A.

12. This and the previous quotation are taken from a Memorandum of the Press Conference, Friday, September 23, 1932. Department of State, Division of Current Information. DS, 724.3415/2356.

13. Telegram from the Commission of Neutrals to Asunción, September 25, 1932, FR, 1932, V, 96; and note from the Paraguayan delegate (Soler) to the Chairman of the Commission of Neutrals, September 28, 1932, FR, 1932, V, 98. The Bolivians had indicated earlier their preference for "a civil commission of neutrals." Telegram from La Paz, undated, received September 18, 1932. FR, 1932, V, 91.

14. See Map I, and memorandum of conversation between White and Soler, October 3, 1932, and note of the Bolivian Legation to the Neutrals of October 9, 1932. FR, 1932, V, 99-100, 101-2.

15. Memorandum from Soler to the Commission of Neutrals, October 6, 1932. FR, 1932, V, 100.

16. Telegram 126, October 7, 1932. FR, 1932, V, 100-1.

17. FR, 1932, V, 112-13.

18. Instructions to the ministers in Paraguay and Bolivia, December 2, 1932, and December 3, 1932. FR, 1932, V, 112-13, 114-15.

19. FR, 1932, V, 117-19. Stimson stated that this line represented "about 98 or 99 per cent of what Paraguay asked." The question here as at other times was: "Who is Paraguay?" Soler had given White the impression that he considered the offer a "fair" one by saying that "he could not say that it was not a fair proposal," although he did not think his government would be willing to accept Bolivian policing south of the line. He added that he could not say openly that he thought the proposal fair and that if White said that Soler "was in favor of the proposal, he would deny it." Memorandum of conversation between White and the Argentine Am-

bassador (Espil), December 22, 1932. DS, 724.3415/2683–8/11. At least, Soler had not said that the proposed line would be rejected by his government, and his instructions may not have been precise. However, he may have desired to avoid responsibility both in Washington and Asunción for acceptance or rejection of the proposal. This he might do because of an ambiguity; when Stimson referred to "a retirement to parallel 62° 30'," he meant only the point on the Pilcomayo at Fort Ballivián, which was almost that far west, but Ayala meant, and Soler presumably knew it, a retirement of Bolivian troops entirely west of that meridian. See FR, 1932, V, 120–21, for Wheeler's telegram 168, December 7, 1932, from Asunción. Wheeler also reported that the Neutrals' proposal "was received here at first from Soler in a spirit of incredulity. The impression prevailed that he must have misunderstood." Despatch 549, from Asunción, December 23, 1932. DS, 724.3415/2764.

20. FR, 1932, V, 118. White took a similar line, remarking in a telegram of December 23, 1932, to Wheeler, that "it seems perfectly evident that Paraguay can not drive the Bolivian forces back to Ballivián and even if she could it would be a Pyrrhic victory." DS, 724.3415/2693B. This was a mistaken judgment.

21. Telegram of Foreign Minister Justo Pastor Benítez to the Commission of Neutrals, December 17, 1932. FR, 1932, V, 129–30. Text of the Neutrals' proposal in FR, 1932, V, 126–29.

22. Telegram from Foreign Minister Franz Tamayo to the Commission of Neutrals. FR, 1932, V, 131. For Feely's comments, see telegram 138 from La Paz, December 10, 1932, FR, 1932, V, 124.

23. See Feely's telegram 132, from La Paz, December 6, 1932, in which he gives as his impression that "the acceptance of a middle line is only a remote possibility." FR, 1932, V, 119–20. White later remarked that the December 15, 1932 proposal "had not been accepted by Paraguay nor had it been categorically accepted by Bolivia." Memorandum, June 1, 1933. FR, 1933, IV, 339.

24. Wheeler reported on November 23, 1932, that Paraguayan losses were about 700 killed, 1,400 wounded, and 65 prisoners. Bolivian casualties were estimated in Asunción as about 3,000 killed, 3,500 wounded and 1,500 prisoners. Telegram 159, from Asunción. DS, 724.3415/2541.

25. FR, 1932, V, 107, 123. President Ayala told Wheeler that "he hopes very strongly that the Neutrals may find it possible to register disfavor of his [Kundt's] coming" not only because his arrival would "stiffen the Bolivian Government against any agreement for the cessation of hostilities" but "on principle, as amounting to an undesirable interposition of an European militarism in a matter whose solution should be left to the Americas." Telegram 145, from Asunción, November 4, 1932. FR, 1932, V, 107. The Neutrals apparently did not find it possible to "register disfavor" of Kundt's importation by Bolivia. The general arrived in La Paz about December 1, 1932.

26. See telegram 135, from Asunción, October 21, 1932, FR, 1932, V, 207, for Wheeler's statement that "the opinion prevails here however that the neutrals are without authority and that nothing is to be expected

from them." On December 1 Wheeler reported from Asunción that Paraguayan distrust of the Neutrals, which he first reported on July 9, 1932, had increased. "There are now in Asunción but two opinions: one is that they all, including the United States, are pro-Bolivian; the other is that the United States is the only one sincerely interested in the matter, and that she is not considering the merits of the controversy and for *amour propre* would sacrifice either party thereto in order to gain a solution, her unjust pressure being brought to bear on Paraguay in the belief that the latter is the weaker of the disputants." Apparently both Soler and Vasconcellos had told their government that, while they had previously obtained some reaction from the Neutrals favorable to Paraguay, now the only reaction they got "was controlled by Mr. White and was distinctly in favor of Bolivia." "It is, of course, common knowledge here that the President himself [Ayala] has no faith in the Commission's ability to accomplish anything." Despatch 538, December 1, 1932 (received December 27, 1932). DS, 724.3415/2702.

27. FR, 1932, V, 136.

28. An example of editorial opinion is given from the following extract from *El Orden* (Asunción): "'Before the Neutrals and Bolivia carry this through . . . the whole nation will be exterminated. In our last national stronghold our last soldiers must fall and the women and children perish with them. Let them close our ports. Let them deny us war materials and bread. We will produce both. It is time for the comedy to cease. Let us die with our honor before the criminal attitude of the Neutrals and the timid complicity of the League of Nations.'" Quoted from Minister Wheeler's telegram 175, from Asunción, December 19, 1932. DS, 724.3415/2661.

29. Telegram 177, December 21, 1932, from Asunción. DS, 724.3415/2679. Two days later, Wheeler said: "It is safe to say that there is not in Asunción a political leader of the smallest segment of public opinion who would venture to approve the acceptance of the proposal." He added that the formal submission of the proposal, after the Neutrals had learned of Paraguayan opposition, had aroused the anger of the entire cabinet, "who counted it tantamount to asking the Government to abdicate. . . . I regret to say that feeling here, from the President down, is at the moment bitter against the United States." Despatch 549, December 23, 1932, from Asunción. DS, 724.3415/2764.

30. Telegram 180, from Asunción, December 25, 1932. DS, 724.3415/2693. Wheeler said: "I am convinced that nothing can qualify Paraguay's absolute rejection of the Ballivián-Vitriones line and that she will at present consider no other suggestion from the neutrals which does not envisage the security she demands which in her opinion can be given only by the demilitarization of virtually the whole Chaco. She is convinced that it is futile to talk of lines and policing and the real peace can never be obtained so long as Bolivian armies remain in the territory."

31. Despatch 550, from Asunción, December 24, 1932. DS, 724.3415/2849.

32. Telegram 61, December 28, 1932. DS, 724.3415/2678.

33. Despatch 553, from Asunción, December 25, 1932, quoting an editorial in the issue of December 23, 1932. An editorial in *La Tribuna* (Asunción), December 22, 1932, charged that Mr. White had made errors as a member of the Commission of Neutrals but coupled the charge with assurances to the Paraguayan people that White's "errors" should not be imputed to the United States as a whole nor to the immutable spirit of justice which characterized the United States. DS, 724.3415/2851.

34. See, for example, Cooper, *American Consultation in World Affairs*, Chap. IV; Royal Institute of International Affairs, *Survey of International Relations, 1936* (London, Oxford University Press, 1937), Part VI, II; FR, vols. for 1932–35; La Foy, *The Chaco Dispute and the League of Nations*.

35. Letter of September 19, 1932. DS, 724.3415/2322A. The Argentine and Chilean intrigues were clearly uppermost in White's mind.

36. FR, 1933, IV, 262. Telegram 86, from Geneva, January 27, 1933.

37. Telegram 60, from Washington, January 30, 1933. FR, 1933, IV, 263–64. In reply, Wilson said that Drummond had remarked "that he recognized the difficulty of long distance negotiation and that it was with the hope of avoiding this difficulty that the Council Committee suggested a commission to the two capitals." Telegram 87, from Geneva, January 31, 1933. FR, 1933, IV, 264.

38. Letter to Minister Wilson in Switzerland, August 15, 1932. DS, 724.3415/2067A. White also noted that the Chilean Minister for Foreign Affairs was carrying on "certain conversations" with Bolivian Foreign Minister Zalles concerning the importation of armament through Arica. See FR, 1932, V, 156–58 and 163, on these talks. White, in a talk with the Chilean Ambassador, Emilio Edwards Bello, on September 1, 1932, expressed his "surprise" at learning from Asunción that the Chilean Minister there had asked President Ayala "whether Paraguay would not entertain the idea of transferring the negotiations from the Neutrals to the group of the neighboring countries. This is not cooperation but is destructive intrigue and I thought that if this sort of thing continued it would end up in no settlement being arrived at." DS, 724.3415/2214–1/15. Peruvian diplomats were also active at this time, having suggested to the other three neighbors that Bolivia might agree to "evacuate positions occupied since June first on the understanding that these positions will be neutralized and will not be reoccupied by Paraguay." Washington was informed that Argentina had privately accepted this suggestion and had proposed it in La Paz and Asunción, without informing the Neutrals. Circular telegram, August 18, 1932. FR, 1932, V, 184.

39. Telegram 75, from Buenos Aires, August 17, 1932. DS, 724.3415/2088.

40. Memorandum of telephone conversation between White and Bliss, August 17, 1932. DS, 724.3415/2090–1/14. Caffery reported from Bogotá that the Colombian foreign minister was incensed at Saavedra Lamas's playing against the Neutrals and had cabled his legation at Buenos Aires, stating that in his opinion "the Argentine Government's activities were

prejudicial to the interests of South American peace." Despatch 4223, August 19, 1932. DS, 724.3415/2195.

41. Memorandum of conversation, January 12, 1933. FR, 1933, IV, 252–53. For individual Argentine and Chilean proposals, see FR, 1933, IV, 246, 248. The Ambassador in Argentina (Bliss) reported that his impression of Saavedra Lamas was that he "will try to block any proposal not his own." Telegram 7, from Buenos Aires, January 12, 1933. FR, 1933; IV, 255.

42. FR, 1933, IV, 257.   43. DS, 724.3415/2824–7/16.

44. Text of the Act of Mendoza in FR, 1933, IV, 288–91.

45. Despatch 1957, from Buenos Aires, February 3, 1933. DS, 724.3415/2875. This interpretation is supported by the words of Saavedra Lamas on his return from Mendoza: "We have incorporated a new organ to Pan Americanism, and in the future, any disturbance of the peace will find us organized to fight against it in South America. The appearance of this new organ of pacification, which accentuates the individuality of this part of the continent, ought to be received with satisfaction by those other countries which, like the United States, willingly offered their collaboration in the initial acts of solidarity brought about by the conflict between Bolivia and Paraguay.

"From now on, with the agreement of Brazil and Peru and other countries, South America will possess an international personality of its own and a genuine instrument for peaceful settlement." *La Nación* (Buenos Aires), February 4, 1933.

46. Memorandum of conversation with Ambassador Espil, February 28, 1933. FR, 1933, IV, 275.

47. Despatch 2205, from Buenos Aires, August 23, 1933. DS, 724.3415/3310, and Instruction No. 2 to Buenos Aires, September 26, 1933. DS, 724.3415/3310.

48. Despatch 1987, March 8, 1933. DS, 724.3415/2964. The Ambassador commented that this request for United States pressure "is inconsistent with the attitude he [Saavedra Lamas] took during the months when his support was earnestly solicited to uphold the formulas proposed by the Neutral Commission. As reported at the time, the Minister expressed to me his aversion to bringing any sort of pressure to bear on the Governments at La Paz and Asunción."

49. Despatch 572, from Minister Wheeler in Asunción, January 29, 1933. DS, 724.3415/2895.

50. Note of March 20, 1933. FR, 1933, IV, 293. Although it was not so stated in the note, it appeared that the Peruvian government made a reservation to the effect that an armistice should be made on the basis of existing troop positions, with no withdrawal. Telegram 9, to the Minister in Paraguay (Wheeler), Washington, March 22, 1933. FR, 1933, IV, 293–94. This Peruvian position was apparently influenced by intense Bolivian diplomatic activity after the Mendoza conference and perhaps by factors related to Ambassador Dearing's report that "Peru is said to have found at last one friend in the Leticia dispute, namely: Bolivia." Telegram 78, from Lima, February 14, 1933. DS, 724.3415/2822.

51. Note of March 23, 1933. FR, 1933, IV, 295.

52. The Secretary of State to the Minister in Paraguay (Wheeler), telegram 10, March 27, 1933. FR, 1933, IV, 296. In addition, Bolivia continued to maintain that any arbitration must be limited to a small part of the eastern Chaco.

53. Telegram 25, from La Paz, March 30, 1933. FR, 1933, IV, 297.

54. Telegram 7, March 30, 1933. FR, 1933, IV, 297. In his report on this incident, Minister Feely remarked that he had reminded the Undersecretary of Foreign Affairs "of several instances in which information received from the Minister in Washington was subsequently found to be without foundation in fact." Despatch 580, from La Paz, April 4, 1933. DS, 724.3415/3013.

55. Telegram 8, to La Paz, April 6, 1933, and telegram 11, to Asunción, April 6, 1933. FR, 1933, IV, 299–300.

56. Memorandum of conversation, April 27, 1933. FR, 1933, IV, 313. The Counselor of the American Embassy in Chile reported that an adviser in the Chilean foreign office said he was "discouraged at what he characterized as the negative attitude taken by Washington and . . . felt doubtful in view of the attitude of the United States whether they would be successful in influencing Bolivia." Despatch 1439, from Santiago, April 26, 1933. DS, 724.3415/3071.

57. Telegram 37, from La Paz, April 23, 1933. FR, 1933, IV, 312.

58. Memorandum of conversation, April 27, 1933. FR, 1933, IV, 314–15. In his memorandum, Foreign Minister Cruchaga said that, "if the present occasion is lost, the war in the Chaco would continue and the responsibility for having raised the final objection to conciliatory plans would rest on Bolivia." On this point, White told the Paraguayan Minister in Washington, who had said Bolivia was responsible for the continuation of the war, that "there were many times during the course of the negotiations in the last four years when immediate blame could be imputed to either one or the other." Memorandum of conversation, May 6, 1933. FR, 1933, IV, 317. Compare White: "We are dealing with two of the most difficult of a rather difficult lot of countries and immediate results can not always be obtained." Letter to the Minister in Switzerland (Wilson), August 15, 1932. DS, 724.3415/2067A.

59. Text of note in FR, 1933, IV, 316.

60. Memorandum of conversation between Francis White and the Chilean Chargé, May 19, 1933. DS, 724.3415/3143. On learning that Bolivia had not sent replies to the last Argentine and Chilean notes, White called the Bolivian Minister (Finot) and told him that neither country was willing to take further action about the Chaco dispute until it received more friendly replies from Bolivia. White said he "did not want to try to influence the action Bolivia would take," but that some indication that Bolivia still desired cooperation from Argentina and Chile "might be all that was necessary to get things going." DS, 724.3415/3143. The Bolivian government replied on May 23, to the Argentine and Chilean notes, so courteously that no open break resulted, and without such warmth that negotiations on the Mendoza plan were reopened. FR, 1933, IV, 334.

61. FR, 1933, IV, 318–19. The representatives of Argentina and Chile

in Washington sent word that they could not meet with the Neutrals on the day this invitation was sent as their governments "were provoked by the last Bolivian note." FR, 1933, IV, 318. The Bolivian note was that of May 5.

62. Telegram 58, from Rio de Janeiro. FR, 1933, IV, 338. The previous chronology is taken from FR, 1933, IV, 323–28.

63. FR, 1933, IV, 363–64.

64. Despatch 1561, from Santiago, October 25, 1933. DS, 724.3415/3378. Chargé Norweb in Santiago reported in this despatch that "Cruchaga has repeatedly reproached the Argentine Ambassador in Santiago for this 'act of treason' on the part of his Chief [Saavedra Lamas]."

65. Despatch 158, from Santiago, July 28, 1934. DS, 724.3415/3086.

66. Telegram 45, May 26, 1933. FR, 1933, IV, 336. White told Ambassador Espil: "I realized that Argentina had never wanted to cooperate with the Neutral Commission. . . . As long as Argentina continues the policy of not supporting effectively other peace moves, it continues the uncertainty as to what her action and desires are, and makes it possible for one of the contesting parties to try to play off one group against the other. . . . I personally knew nothing which would justify my feeling that Argentina was backing the League." Memorandum of conversation, May 23, 1933. FR, 1933, IV, 332–33.

67. June 9, 1933. FR, 1933, IV, 340–41.

68. Letter from Francis White to the Minister in Uruguay (Wright), Washington, June 30, 1933. DS, 724.3415/3221A.

69. Despatch 4182, from Rio de Janeiro, July 29, 1933. FR, 1933, IV, 350.

70. Memorandum of conversation, October 4, 1933. FR, 1933, IV, 362. Caffery stated in his typically laconic fashion that he "explained the reasons why" to Finot, but he did not put the reasons down in his memorandum.

71. Despatch 41, from Asunción, April 3, 1934. DS, 724.3415/3647.

72. Telegram 220, from Geneva, September 1, 1934. FR, 1934, IV, 76.

73. March 6, 1934. FR, 1934, IV, 64.

74. Instruction 5, to Buenos Aires, January 5, 1934. FR, 1934, IV, 38–39.

75. Telegram 17, from Buenos Aires, January 17, 1934. FR, 1934, IV, 45.

76. Telegram 46, to Rio de Janeiro, May 16, 1934. DS, 724.3415/3673.

77. Department of State, Division of Current Information, No. 114. Memorandum of a special press conference, May 18, 1934. DS, 724.3415/3736. See also President Roosevelt's Press Conference No. 123, May 18, 1934, Vol. 3, pp. 355–57. FDRL.

78. Note of June 1, 1934. FR, 1934, IV, 290–91.

79. The Secretary of State to the Bolivian Minister (Finot), June 13, 1934. FR, 1934, IV, 291–92.

80. Telegram 33, from Asunción, August 1, 1934. FR, 1934, IV, 296–97.

81. FR, 1934, IV, 296. Minister Nicholson in Asunción reported on July 28 that "Havas Agency despatches from Washington were published in Asunción this morning in which it was stated that munitions valued at over three million dollars, including five planes, were to be shipped to

Bolivia, while material valued at about two million dollars was not to be allowed to leave the United States. . . . Havas, as it often does, has again published inaccurate and misleading information prejudicial to the interests of the United States." Despatch 95. DS, 724.3415/3999.

82. Minister Des Portes reported from La Paz that "the general tone is that the United States is an altruistic, foolish idealist, who made a grand but ineffective gesture." Despatch 117, July 10, 1934. DS, 724.3415/3937. Rumors reaching the Minister were that arms were on the way from Italy and Czechoslovakia to Bolivia; others might come from Japan, while Chile would continue to permit their transit through Arica.

83. Despatch 17, January 15, 1934. DS, 834.00 General Conditions/79. Shortly after the war began, an article in the Communist paper, *International Press Correspondence* (Moscow), August 18, 1932, by A. L. Maggi, charged that one of the purposes of Bolivia was to establish good relations with the United States "by securing the Gran Chaco oil for the Standard Oil Company." Despatch 681, from Riga, August 31, 1932. DS, 724.3415/2273.

84. Despatch 71, from Asunción, June 8, 1934. DS, 724.3415/3871. The Long charges loosed attacks on Standard Oil and on the United States government not only in Asunción but also in the press of other American capitals. *El Diario* (Asunción), June 24, 1934, suggested that the Roosevelt administration was not strong enough to control Standard Oil and that proof was to be found in the exceptions made to the application of the prohibition on sales of arms in the United States.

85. Despatch 106, from Asunción, August 23, 1934. DS, 724.3415/4095. Nicholson added that government officials had assured him that "they do not allow their suspicions of the Standard Oil to affect their attitude toward the Government and people of the United States."

86. Senator Long may not have desired the identification, but he was on the side of the Marxist interpreters of the Chaco conflict. See, for example, Colle, *El drama del Paraguay*, p. 105. This is the frequent fate of United States citizens who attack their government on grounds that it has been unduly influenced by "monopolists" or "greedy corporations."

87. Telegram 29, to Asunción, August 1, 1934. FR, 1934, IV, 298.

88. Despatch 222, from Asunción, May 4, 1935. DS, 724.3415/4891.

89. Earlier Ambassador Weddell had reported that the British member of the League of Nations Commission, General A. B. Robertson, had told him that "while in Bolivia the Commission had carefully investigated the persistent rumors that American oil interests were helping Bolivia to carry on the war and that they were all convinced that this gossip was without foundation; the General added that in his opinion the Standard Oil Company had been very badly treated by the Bolivian Government." Despatch 185, from Buenos Aires, February 23, 1934. DS, 724.3415/3587.

90. Despatch 338, from Buenos Aires, July 6, 1934. DS, 724.3415/3923. At about this time, Secretary Hull was asked at a press conference about Chaco peace efforts. He said they were progressing slowly and there were "a great many wheels within wheels. In view of this situation, it would be futile to attempt to give a clear picture of the present position." Memorandum of the Press Conference, July 11, 1934, No. 161. DS, 724.3415/

3942. The Secretary added that the United States was acting as a "peace loving nation" in the situation.

91. Telegram 64, to Rio de Janeiro, July 14, 1934. FR, 1934, IV, 144-45.

92. July 16, 1934. FR, 1934, IV, 145-46.

93. Telegram 12, to La Paz, July 20, 1934. FR, 1934, IV, 152-53.

94. Telegram 66, to Buenos Aires, July 17, 1934, FR, 1934, IV, 147; telegram 101, from Buenos Aires, July 19, 1934, FR, 1934, IV, 150-51.

95. Telegram 68, to Buenos Aires, July 20, 1934. FR, 1934, IV, 153-54. In this telegram Ambassador Weddell was asked whether Saavedra Lamas had approached the Chilean government. Weddell reported that the Foreign Minister had said in response to an inquiry that the Chilean Ambassador had asked for information; "that he had informed the Ambassador that 'exploratory conversations' had been negotiated by him with the two Governments at war; that a natural modesty had restrained him [Saavedra Lamas] from discussing the matter with Chile when there was a chance of a second rebuff by one or the other of the combatants; that of course it had always been his idea promptly to inform the Chilean Government as soon as something like an understanding had been reached." Telegram 103, from Buenos Aires, July 23, 1934. FR, 1934, IV, 155-56.

96. An official of the Chilean foreign office told Counselor of Embassy Robert McGregor Scotten that "Chile was deeply offended that Saavedra Lamas had not consulted Chile in regard to this plan. He alluded to the pact of March 6, 1932, and stated that in his opinion the Argentine Government was not living up to this Pact [the Mendoza Pact]. . . . He inferred that Saavedra Lamas had acted in bad faith stating that the latter, when questioned recently by the Chilean Ambassador in Buenos Aires regarding the alleged formula, had replied that he had submitted no formula whatsoever. . . . The Chilean Foreign Office was at that time in possession of the text of the formula which it had received through Bolivian sources." Despatch 158, from Santiago, July 28, 1934. DS, 724.3415/3986.

97. Telegram 96, to Rio de Janeiro, August 4, 1934. FR, 1934, IV, 164-66.

98. Telegram 175, from Rio de Janeiro, August 16, 1934, FR, 1934, IV, 171-72; telegram 176, from Rio de Janeiro, August 17, 1934, FR, 1934, IV, 173.

99. Gilbert reported from Geneva: "It is . . . accepted here that the Argentine representative is speaking for the United States in respect of the status of the Buenos Aires negotiation and thus reflects the attitude of the three negotiators in regard thereto and as a natural consequence that action by the League is acquiesced in or even approved by the United States and Brazil. It would thus appear that the League will proceed at once with this matter unless some direct action intervenes. . . . I wish nevertheless to make entirely clear that Cantilo has at no time stated specifically that he spoke for the United States but that this has been a natural inference from the general tenor of his statements." Telegram 245, September 18, 1934. DS, 724.3415/4146, and telegram 218, from Rio de Janeiro, September 13, 1934, FR, 1934, IV, 200.

100. Telegram 157, from Buenos Aires, September 13, 1934. FR, 1934,

IV, 199–200. Saavedra Lamas also told the Brazilian and United States ambassadors that "nothing should be communicated which would damage either country before the League although he said Argentina's position before that body is 'very delicate.' He said that this would leave to the League to determine whether 'the good offices' of the mediating countries should now come to an end and in that case the League to accept the responsibility for success or failure in further negotiations."

101. Telegram 224, from Rio de Janeiro, September 15, 1934. FR, 1934, IV, 207–8.

102. Telegram 109, to Buenos Aires, September 14, 1934. FR, 1934, IV, 203–4.

103. Telegram 250, from Geneva, September 20, 1934. DS, 724.3415/4150.

104. Telegram 262, September 22, 1934. DS, 724.3415/4173.

105. Telegram 170, from Buenos Aires, September 30, 1934. FR, 1934, IV, 91–92.

106. Telegram 94, from Santiago, September 26, 1934. FR, 1934, IV, 84.

107. Telegram 162, to Rio de Janeiro, October 29, 1934. FR, 1934, IV, 231–32.

108. Telegram 322, from Rio de Janeiro, November 22, 1934. DS, 724. 3415/4362.

109. Despatch 897, from Montevideo, December 29, 1934. DS, 724.3415/4481.

110. Telegram 94, to Geneva, September 20, 1934. FR, 1934, IV, 80.

111. Department of State, Division of Current Information. Memorandum of the Press Conference, September 28, 1934. DS, 724.3415/4232. The Secretary generously added that "what appears to have happened is that there has been a large number of movements designed to promote peace in the Chaco. These movements . . . frequently dove-tail and merge into each other and as one movement develops and goes forward, a new one appears, conditions, meanwhile, undergoing a change but everybody concerned is endeavoring, to the best of his ability, and without bias or jealousy, to effect a peaceful settlement."

112. Telegram 255, from Rio de Janeiro, October 1, 1934. FR, 1934, IV, 93–95.

113. Telegram 143, to Rio de Janeiro, October 2, 1934. FR, 1934, IV, 97–98.

114. Telegram 162, to Rio de Janeiro, October 29, 1934. FR, 1934, IV, 231–32.

115. Letter from the Secretary of State to the President, November 28, 1934. DS, 724.3415/4373. These views are summarized in telegram 176, to Rio de Janeiro, December 1, 1934, FR, 1934, IV, 114–16.

116. Memorandum for the Secretary of State, Warm Springs, Ga., December 3, 1934. DS, 724.3415/4390–1/2. Also, with Hull letter of November 28, 1934 in FDRL, OF338-C.

117. FR, 1934, IV, 117–21. It appeared that the first inclination of the Brazilian Foreign Minister had been to refrain from participating in any way in the League Committee and Commission but that the emphasis

given by Washington to the changed circumstances since September, particularly the approval by other Latin American states of the League report, had brought about a modification of opinion in Rio de Janeiro. Memorandum of conversation between the Assistant Secretary of State (Welles) and the Brazilian Ambassador (Aranha), November 30, 1934. DS, 724.3415/4389.

118. Telegram 128, to Geneva, December 11, 1934. FR, 1934, IV, 129.

119. Telegram 396, from Geneva, December 21, 1934. FR, 1934, IV, 134–35.

120. Memorandum for the Undersecretary of State (Phillips), January 7, 1935. DS, 724.3415/4492.

121. Memorandum, January 17, 1935. Changes were made in this memorandum by the President in his own handwriting. DS, 724.3415/4601.

122. Memorandum, February 28, 1935. DS, 724.3415/4523.

123. This situation was, of course, variously viewed. Cardozo considered that "the bureaucracy of Geneva demonstrated a notably hostile attitude toward Paraguay." Cardozo, *Paraguay independiente*, p. 351. Manley O. Hudson rejoiced that for the first time in history "a number of States joined together in discriminatory action against a belligerent which failed to meet the conditions of the collective system of dealing with international disputes. These departures make a very decided progress in the effort to proscribe war upon which our generation has embarked." Hudson, *Munitions Industry: The Chaco Arms Embargo*, p. 1. One aspect of the sanctions was that the Advisory Committee on Opium and Other Dangerous Drugs of the League of Nations, supported the lifting of the arms embargo on Bolivia alone by recommending to Member states the withholding from Paraguay of morphine and other drugs useful in treating soldiers wounded in combat. Interview with Herbert S. May, of the Secretariat of the League of Nations, spring, 1935. This was one of the most extreme actions ever taken by the League Secretariat against a Member state. Another aspect so far as Paraguay was concerned, was that "the application of sanctions against the attacked nation [Paraguay] and the exculpation of the aggressor definitively discredited the League of Nations in America, and the dispute, therefore, had to be returned to America." Julio César Chaves, *Compendio de historia paraguaya*, p. 230.

124. See, among other papers, *La Prensa* (Buenos Aires), March 2, 1935.

125. Memorandum of conversation, March 7, 1935. DS, 724.3415/4718.

126. Despatch 96, from Buenos Aires, December 7, 1935. DS, 724.34119/321. Braden added that Nieto had told him of his negotiations in La Paz in February, 1935, "among other things saying that he first became very friendly with the heads of the Banco Central, gradually built up a group around that organization, and through them he eventually caused the overthrow of the Minister of Foreign Relations who was opposed to any peace moves."

127. Memorandum of conversation with E. C. Wilson, January 15, 1935. DS, 724.3415/4495.

128. Telegram 217, from Rio de Janeiro, September 13, 1934. DS, 724.3415/4116.

129. Telegram 126, to Rio de Janeiro, September 14, 1934. DS, 724.3415/4116.

130. Telegram 143, to Rio de Janeiro, October 2, 1934. FR, 1934, IV, 97–98.

131. Secretary Hull reported to President Roosevelt: "While it would unquestionably be desirable that all inter-American disputes be adjusted by purely American peace agencies, the time has not yet come when the necessary machinery is functioning, nor have the peace agencies created by common agreement between the American nations so far acquired sufficient prestige to prove their usefulness at this juncture." Letter, November 28, 1934. DS, 724.3415/4373.

132. Text of statement in FR, 1935, IV, 21–22.

133. Telegram 62, from Rio de Janeiro, March 18, 1935. FR, 1935, IV, 19. These maneuvers apparently caused something like exasperation in Geneva: "There seems to be a feeling on the part of certain European powers that the limitrophe states [the ABCP group] have again given evidence of a definitely obstructionist policy toward the League's handling of the Chaco dispute and that this time their tactics should be frankly recognized as such and should no longer be allowed to impede the integral application of the Covenant." Telegram 97, from Geneva, March 22, 1935. DS, 724.3415/4664.

134. Telegram 158, from Geneva, May 6, 1935. DS, 724.3415/4839. Gilbert added: "As a part of the general adjustment for the League's 'relinquishment' of the Chaco matter is seen the possibility of Paraguay's return to the League."

135. For material on these arrangements, see FR, 1934, IV, 32–135 and FR, 1935, V, 7–91.

136. Text in *The Chaco Peace Conference*, pp. 49–52.

137. The Bolivian debate over acceptance of the protocol was of course intense. The clearest statement of the problem is in Saavedra, *El Chaco y la conferencia de paz de Buenos Aires*. Saavedra laments what he considers the gullibility of Tomás M. Elío, the Bolivian delegate in Buenos Aires. Saavedra Lamas, he asserts, assured the Bolivians that they would not be "swindled" out of an arbitration of the claims in the Chaco, but, in fact, he "hypnotized" Elío with "dithyrambic phrases" and in fact eliminated the possibility of an arbitration in law as a means for concluding the conflict (pp. 116–30). The Bolivian decision to accept an armistice was of course a difficult one, and the literature on the decision, both concurrent and reflective, is voluminous. See, for example, Rodríguez, *Autopsía de una guerra;* Toro Ruilova, *Mi actuación en la guerra del Chaco;* Vergara Vicuña, *La guerra del Chaco.*

138. Braden, "A Résumé of the Rôle Played by Arbitration in the Chaco Dispute," *The Arbitration Journal*, II, 387–95.

III. The Nature of the Conflict

1. White remarked to the Chilean Ambassador, Miguel Cruchaga Tocornal, that, "if the zone of the Hayes Award were included in the arbitration . . . this would take in all the territory right down to Asunción. He said that that was his understanding also. I then remarked that should Bolivia win the arbitration Paraguay would virtually disappear as a nation, to which he again assented." Memorandum of conversation, February 19, 1932. DS, 724.3415/1663–5/19.

2. See the appeal on June 5, 1932, by President José P. Guggiari of Paraguay that Argentina and Brazil "jointly take possession of the Chaco and impose an arbitration upon both Paraguay and Bolivia." FR, 1932, V, 141.

3. Despatch 315, February 15, 1932, from La Paz. DS, 724.3415/1666. Minister Feely concluded that "it may easily be seen that public opinion in Bolivia at the present moment is not at all in favor of arbitration of the Chaco dispute either by the United States, or, presumably, by any other nation." The Department of State had received "very disquieting reports that Bolivia is in fact preparing for an attack against Paraguay in the Chaco"; these were confirmed by Minister Feely, who noted that in April, 1932, Bolivia had some 7,000 men in or near the Chaco, "the largest concentration of troops since the mobilization of 1928." Telegram 7, to La Paz, March 31, 1932, DS, 724.3415/1684A, and despatch 344, from La Paz, April 5, 1932, DS, 724.3415/1736.

4. See telegram 53, December 2, 1932, from the Secretary of State to Minister Wheeler in Asunción. FR, 1932, V, 112–13.

5. Memorandum of conversation between Mr. White and Ambassador Espil, August 8, 1932. FR, 1932, V, 165. More formally, White added that, while the United States "did not want to take an intransigent position . . . we should do nothing which would impair or invalidate the doctrine of August 3." Chile, although less strongly than Argentina, also supported the Bolivian position. FR, 1932, V, 169.

6. FR, 1932, V, 162. Compare Feely, who stated that, in July, 1932, "after the attack at Lake Chuquisaca, it was the President [Salamanca] who ordered the Bolivian advance by way of reprisal that resulted in the capture by Bolivian forces of Forts Boquerón, Toledo and Corrales, and thus precipitated open hostilities. At that time, the Chief of the General Staff, General Osorio, protested against a Bolivian advance on the ground that the positions could not be held." Despatch 466, November 9, 1932. DS, 724.3415/2614.

7. Letter to the Secretary of State, Buenos Aires, February 26, 1934. DS, 724.3415/3616.

8. Text of address in *El Diario* (Asunción), August 16, 1934. Ayala went on to say that some "noble philanthropists" abroad were surprised "that Paraguay should prefer to sacrifice its youth and its wealth, rather than cede to Bolivia some thousands of square kilometers of swamps."

. . . Happily for humanity, the world is ruled by moral interests rather than by the criterion of utility. The blood spilled by a people from time to time is fruitful, not because of its material results, but because it exalts the virtues which form the moral personality of a nation. . . . When a nation loses the respect of others, and its faith in itself, it suffers civic death, which is more horrible than defeat and annihilation."

9. Telegrams 166, December 4, 1932, and 169, December 9, 1932, from Minister Wheeler in Asunción. FR, 1932, V, 116, 122. In general, on military aspects of the conflict, see Zook, *The Conduct of the Chaco War*, *passim*.

10. Despatch 466, November 9, 1932. DS, 724.3415/2614.

11. Telegram 130, from La Paz, December 6, 1932. DS, 724.3415/2595.

12. Telegram 104, from La Paz, October 15, 1932. FR, 1932, V, 103. Feely followed up this suggestion with the statement that "the only part of the recent proposals that Bolivia has really accepted or is likely to accept without reservation is that regarding a military commission and I believe that the Neutral Commission should give serious consideration to the immediate appointment of such a commission with full powers to establish and supervise the proposed neutral zone." Telegram 130, from La Paz, December 6, 1932. DS, 724.3415/2595. There seems to have been no response to either of these suggestions from the Department of State.

13. Telegram 52, from Buenos Aires, July 8, 1932. DS, 724.3415/1814. In despatch 1708, reporting more fully on this talk, Ambassador Bliss reported Ayala as saying that he understood that the United States might hesitate to act alone "because of the tendency in some South American countries, especially Argentina, to look upon the United States as domineering and imperialistic," but he thought that the result in the Tacna-Arica case had been most happy for all concerned. Ayala had apparently talked with Saavedra Lamas who felt that "Argentina was the one Power to intervene in the controversy," but Ayala preferred to have the United States and Brazil participate in any "strong recommendation." July 8, 1932. DS, 724.3415/1834.

14. Despatch 572, from Feely in La Paz, March 25, 1933. DS, 724.3415/2998. Feely added that the Bolivian determination was "without regard to the negotiations now in progress," which were those on the Mendoza formula. Feely also reported that the Bolivian reply, rejecting the Mendoza formula, "was received with applause in La Paz as representing a consensus of Bolivian hopes and aspirations . . . and the outcome of the controversy with Chile as to free transit of arms via Arica hailed as a great victory for Bolivian diplomacy." Despatch 578, from La Paz, April 3, 1933. DS, 724.3415/3012.

15. Telegram 7, to Asunción, February 27, 1933. FR, 1933, IV, 274. White told Finot that "it would be most anomalous, to say the least, for us to try for so many months to prevent fighting and now, when fighting has broken out, to take measures to facilitate the entry of arms into one of the countries." Memorandum of conversation, February 13, 1933. DS, 724.3415/2900–5/7.

16. Telegram 25, from Asunción, February 21, 1933. FR, 1933, IV, 272.

17. Telegram 7 (see note 15). FR, 1933, IV, 274. The ambāssador in Chile (Culbertson) explained that: "We may assume that Ramírez' inexcusable action was resorted to in an effort to explain the failure of his strenuous efforts to block the transit of arms to Bolivia." Telegram 36, from Santiago, February 28, 1933. DS, 724.3415/2908.

18. Telegram 5, from Asunción, January 8, 1933. FR, 1933, IV, 244.

19. Despatch 623, from La Paz, June 14, 1933. DS, 724.3415/3199. In this despatch, Feely noted that Bolivians tended to blame Argentina and Chile for the breakdown of the ABCP negotiations, and stated as his view that "an impartial study of the negotiations for a peaceful settlement that have taken place since the outbreak of hostilities, however, cannot but lead to the conclusion that Bolivia has spared no effort to prolong the diplomatic discussion in the hope of obtaining a stronger position by the force of arms. One of the reasons for the Bolivian Government's preference that the negotiations continue under the auspices of American entities is that the latter have not the power to apply sanctions, while the League has such an attribute." Bolivia brought the case to the attention of the League in May, on the basis that Paraguay had declared war and that sanctions should therefore be applied to Paraguay.

20. Letter from Francis White to the Minister in Switzerland (Wilson), Washington, February 2, 1933. FR, 1933, IV, 265–66. *El Diario* (La Paz), November 18, 1932, charged that Argentine officers were aiding the Paraguayan army and that Argentine guns were turned against the Bolivians in the Chaco. White stated that "Argentina is correctly recognized in Bolivia as being an out-and-out supporter of Paraguay." Letter to the Minister in Switzerland (Wilson), November 5, 1932. FR, 1932, V, 245.

21. Telegram 103, from Asunción, August 30, 1932. DS, 724.3415/2187. See also Rivarola, *Memorias diplomáticas,* Vol. II, Chap. 7, for an account of Rivarola's success in securing loans for Paraguay from the Argentine government.

22. Letter of September 20, 1932. DS, 724.3415/2322B.

23. Telegram 115, from Buenos Aires, May 18, 1938. FR, 1938, V, 123.

24. Telegram 142, from Buenos Aires, June 4, 1938. FR, 1938, V, 134.

25. Despatch 232, from Asunción, May 17, 1935. DS, 724.3415/4922.

26. Despatch 245, from Asunción, June 11, 1935. DS, 724.3415/5031.

27. Telegrams 112, from Asunción, December 11, and 97, from La Paz, December 12, 1933. FR, 1933, IV, 371–72. The number of troops captured was reported as "over 5,000" by La Paz, and "18,000" by Asunción.

28. Despatch 680, from La Paz. DS, 724.3415/3325. He added: "The Indians from the Altiplano, of which the rank and file of the Army is largely made up, cannot resist the intense heat of the Chaco, and soon fall victims to tuberculosis, dysentery, or beri-beri."

29. See Map I. A strictly military account of the war from the Paraguayan point of view is given by the Paraguayan Commander-in-

Chief, Marshal Estigarribia, in his *The Epic of the Chaco*. For a Bolivian account, see Rodríguez, *Autopsía de una guerra*.

30. Letter from La Paz, March 14, 1933. DS, 714.1515/1359–1/2.

31. Despatch 600, from La Paz, May 9, 1933. DS, 724.3415/3125. Feely had protested in May, following a raid on Puerto Pinasco in which American-owned property had been damaged. Feely stated in this despatch that General Kundt's "personal reputation, if not his life, is dependent upon a military decision, or at least an important military victory." Later, he reported that Kundt "will brook no interference, even from the President." Despatch 647, from La Paz, July 25, 1933. DS, 724.3415/3258. It should be noted that in 1927 United States planes had bombed the village of Ocotal in Nicaragua, during the campaign against General A. C. Sandino.

32. Larden, "Blind Man's Buff in the Chaco," *The Journal of the Royal Artillery*, LXI (April, 1934), 32–48.

33. Despatch 647, from La Paz, July 25, 1933. DS, 724.3415/3258.

34. Despatch 687, from La Paz, September 23, 1933. DS, 724.3415/3349. "The reader might better understand the vicious tenacity of the Chaco struggle if the author had made him realize that Bolivia and Paraguay had lost all their other boundary disputes." Roland D. Hussey, review of Harris Gaylord Warren, *Paraguay: An Informal History*, in *American Historical Review*, October, 1949, p. 178.

35. Despatch 628, from La Paz, July 1, 1933. DS, 724.3415/3232. The political opposition in Bolivia accused Salamanca of precipitating the war by these declarations, since it was argued that Paraguay began preparing for war when Salamanca was elected. Despatch 586, from La Paz, April 8, 1933. DS, 724.3415/3038.

36. Despatch 619, from La Paz, June 7, 1933, citing an article by Saavedra in *La República* (La Paz). DS, 724.3415/3189.

37. Article in *El Diario* (La Paz), May 14, 1933, cited in despatch 606, from La Paz, May 16, 1933. DS, 724.3415/3144.

38. Feely reported that this information had come to him from "a reliable source." Despatch 655, from La Paz, July 31, 1933. DS, 724.3415/3270.

39. Memorandum of Conversations regarding the Chaco Dispute, by J. Butler Wright. Montevideo, undated, probably written during the Montevideo conference. DS, 724.3415/3425–1/2.

40. One of Wright's informants said: "In Paraguay every available man was at the front; schools, universities, colleges, and other institutions of learning, social welfare, etc., were completely deprived of the services of the professors, doctors and other officers and other individuals who customarily pursued these occupations." DS, 724.3415/3425–1/2 (see note 39).

41. DS, 724.3415/3425–1/2 (see note 39). This development was thought to have been demonstrated by the apparent violation of the armistice arranged during the Montevideo conference.

42. Despatch 41, from La Paz, February 20, 1934. DS, 724.3415/3577.

43. Despatches 84 and 117, from La Paz, May 23, 1934, and July 10, 1934. DS, 724.3415/3777, and DS, 724.3415/3937, respectively. Paraguay protested the participation of Chilean officers, and Chile enacted legislation prohibiting the enlistment of Chileans in armies of foreign countries in September. Despatch 113, from Asunción, September 8, 1934. DS, 724.3415/3170, and FR, 1934, IV, 300–20.

44. Despatch 548, from La Paz, February 28, 1933. DS, 724.3415/2939.

45. Memorandum of conversation by E. C. Wilson, January 21, 1935. The Australian referred to above stated that, in addition to the Russians, there were also some Germans, Canadians and English officers with the Paraguayan forces. DS, 724.3415/4513.

46. Despatch 121, from Asunción, September 29, 1934. DS, 724.3415/4263.

47. Telegram 6, from Asunción, February 2, 1935. DS, 724.3415/4526. In this despatch, President Ayala was quoted as expressing concern lest the United States government should believe "that Argentina had given Paraguay material assistance in the conflict. He declared emphatically that such was not the case whereas Uruguay had pursued a much more friendly policy."

48. Despatch 164, from Asunción, February 19, 1935. DS, 724.3415/4613.

49. Despatch 180, March 5, 1935. DS, 724.3415/4677.

50. Despatch 217, from Asunción, April 26, 1935. DS, 724.3415/4860.

51. Despatch 245, from Asunción, June 11, 1935. DS, 724.3415/5031. However, as Cardozo points out, the distance of the Paraguayan forces from their bases, the difficult economic situation, and the general war-weariness in Paraguay prevented the Paraguayans from increasing their effort sufficiently "to carry the war to Bolivia and impose the peace that patriotism might have desired." Cardozo, *Paraguay independiente*, p. 357.

52. Despatch 190, from Asunción, March 18, 1935. DS, 724.3415/4738. This view was echoed by President Ayala who said that Paraguay could not relinquish the territory it held and added that "the Chaco boundary is now established." Telegram 61, from Asunción, September 8, 1935. DS, 724.3415/5088.

53. There are many books by Bolivians containing material relevant to the reasons for Bolivia's defeat. See, for example, Díaz Arguedas, *Como fué derrocado el hombre símbolo: (Salamanca)*; Díaz Machicao, *Historia de Bolivia: Salamanca, la guerra del Chaco, Tejada Sorzano, 1931–1936*, Vol. 3; Rodas Eguino, *La guerra del Chaco: Interpretación de política internacional americana*; Rodríguez, *Autopsia de una guerra*; Salamanca, *Archivo: Documentos para una historia de la guerra del Chaco*; Toro Ruilova, *Mi actuación en la guerra del Chaco*; Urioste, *La encrucijada*; Vergara Vicuña, *La guerra del Chaco*.

54. FR, 1934, IV, 225.

55. Francis Paul Walters, *A History of the League of Nations* (New York, Oxford University Press, 1952), II, 526.

56. For example, Warren, *Paraguay: An Informal History*, p. 314; and

Hubert Herring, *A History of Latin America*, 1st ed. (New York; Knopf, 1961), p. 678.

IV. The Chaco Peace Conference—Frustration

1. *The Chaco Peace Conference*, p. 7. This volume contains a formal account of the negotiations at the conference and a collection of documents, including texts of the protocol of June 12, 1935, conference proposals for settlement, and the final treaty of July 21, 1938. There are also four maps.

2. Braden remarked that "the mediation undertaken in this Conference differs from all other mediations," since the conference not only negotiated but had certain duties such as fixing the lines of separation of the armies and supervising them. Despatch 280, from Buenos Aires, September 24, 1936. DS, 724.34119/639.

3. Telegram 77, to Buenos Aires, June 18, 1935. FR, 1935, IV, 81–82. For Gibson's telegram 84, June 16, see FR, 1935, IV, 78–79.

4. Gibson noted that "the Uruguayan delegate is merely an echo of the Argentine Minister of Foreign Affairs." Telegram 120, from Buenos Aires, July 6, 1935. FR, 1935, IV, 95.

5. See, for example, Gibson's report that Saavedra Lamas might propose that the United States provide financial aid for "rehabilitation of the belligerent countries," in telegram 135, from Buenos Aires, July 16, 1935. FR, 1935, IV, 100. Gibson said that such a proposal would probably be based "on the assumption that a large part of the money received by both countries would find its way to Argentina in the form of the refunding by Paraguay of Argentine advances (Saavedra Lamas has repeatedly stated that Bolivia will have to pay a large sum in reparation to Paraguay)." On learning of this suggestion, the Department of State immediately instructed Gibson that "it would be well for the matter to be quashed emphatically at the outset." Telegram 104, to Buenos Aires, July 18, 1935. FR, 1935, IV, 100.

6. Rivarola, *Memorias diplomáticas*, II, 230. For details, see *ibid.*, III, 82f, 100f, and 165f.

7. *Ibid.*, III, 100, 168.

8. *Ibid.*, III, 107. This claim was mentioned in a letter of April 12, 1934, from Rivarola to President Ayala.

9. *Ibid.*, III, pp. 100–1.

10. Memorandum of conversation, November 15, 1934. DS, 724.3415/4337–1/2.

11. Gibson noted that Pedro Manini Ríos, the special Uruguayan delegate, seemed to take little interest in the conference, and left Uruguayan representation to the Uruguayan ambassador to Argentina. He said that the position of the Peruvian and Uruguayan diplomatic representatives, "coupled with their lack of force and ability makes them tend to be subservient to Saavedra Lamas. Typical of their timidity it may be mentioned that Peruvian Ambassador absented himself from seventh plenary meeting

on the ground that he could not be present at so delicate a discussion as that on setting up a tribunal to deal with the question of responsibility." Telegram 156, from Buenos Aires, July 29, 1935. FR, 1935, IV, 108.

12. Gibson said of Saavedra Lamas that "there is no doubt that he formulates and directs Argentine foreign policy which President Justo leaves strictly to him." Telegram 279, from Buenos Aires, November 15, 1935. FR, 1935, IV, 180.

13. Telegram 156, from Buenos Aires, July 29, 1935. FR, 1935, IV, 106–7.

14. Telegram 170, from Rio de Janeiro, July 6, 1935, and telegram 121, to Rio de Janeiro, July 8, 1935. DS, 724.34119/20. This view was also taken by Gibson, who wrote: "No matter how skillfully the matter were handled through the President [Justo] there would be keen resentment in the Argentine Foreign Office and any non-Argentine Secretary General brought in would be faced with sabotage." He did not share Macedo Soares's fear that the Bolivians would seriously protest Podestá Costa's appointment. Telegram 121, from Buenos Aires, July 7, 1935. DS, 724.34119/25.

15. Telegram 120, from Buenos Aires, July 6, 1935. FR, 1935, IV, 95.

16. Telegram 156, from Buenos Aires, July 29, 1935. FR, 1935, IV, 107. Gibson ended this telegram by stating: "When we come to real work the chairman's mischievous activities will be an unavoidable hazard but if there is to be a period of 6 weeks or more of deliberate delay, it would be well to avoid unnecessary risks by a recess. Experience has shown that under present circumstances practically all our time and effort are devoted to straightening out the tangles created by the chairman." That these views on Saavedra Lamas were not held only by North Americans was indicated by Gibson's report that Miguel Cruchaga Tocornal, the Chilean Foreign Minister, was leaving on July 3, "convinced that his presence here was not only productive of no good but that there was definite resentment on the part of Saavedra Lamas of any constructive ideas which he or anybody else might advance." FR, 1935, IV, 92. Telegram 112, from Buenos Aires, July 2, 1935.

17. Telegram 156, from Buenos Aires, July 29, 1935. FR, 1935, IV, 105–6. In a supplementary despatch, Gibson said that Saavedra Lamas usually conducted himself in public in "an exceedingly adroit and able manner" but "occasionally allows himself to get into what is practically an hysterical condition. . . . Should he be in such a state at one of the Conference meetings he is capable of disrupting the Conference." Despatch 18, from Buenos Aires, July 23, 1935. DS, 724.34119/90.

18. His alleged remark on this occasion is a frequently repeated slur on Bolivian army officers: " 'This is the only encirclement in which you have been successful.' " Díaz Arguedas, *Como fué derrocado el hombre símbolo: (Salamanca)*, p. 178.

19. It was reported that Salamanca's last words were: " 'The Buenos Aires Protocol has killed me—the Chaco is lost.' " Despatch 393, from La Paz, July 20, 1935. DS, 724.3415/5063.

20. There is of course an extensive literature on this extraordinary

overthrow of a government responsible for a great military victory. See, for example, Artaza, *Ayala, Estigarribia y el Partido Liberal;* Prieto, *Eusebio Ayala, presidente de la victoria;* Stefanich, *Capítulos de la revolución paraguaya;* Angel F. Ríos, *La defensa del Chaco: Verdades y mentiras de una victoria.*

21. Since Estigarribia's death in an airplane accident in September, 1940, Paraguay has been ruled by opponents of the Liberal Party. Anti-Liberal historians have carried on an intense campaign to obliterate in Paraguay any recollection or impression that the Liberal Party and its leaders, such as Eusebio Ayala, should be given any credit or remembered with any sympathy as men who saved the Chaco for Paraguay and, possibly, Paraguay for the Paraguayans. Estigarribia remains a hero, and his mementos are preserved in the military museum in Asunción as administered by the present government. Ayala and his immediate predecessors as Liberals and as those responsible for the preparations for the defense of Paraguay and for the conduct of the war, are vilified and denigrated by apologists for succeeding regimes. The intensity of party politics in Paraguay is intimated by the fact that at present it is estimated that not much less than one third of all Paraguayans are exiles, mainly in Argentina, and that a large portion of these are at least nominally adherents of the Liberal Party. From a historiographer's point of view the situation is piquant. For ten years before the Chaco War and for a year after its termination the Paraguayan government was administered by members of the Liberal Party. However, the peace is called a surrender of the rightful possessions of Paraguay (Ramírez, *La paz del Chaco,* p. 279); and it is alleged that the preparation for the Chaco War was utterly inadequate and that Paraguay was saved only by the heroism of its soldiers (see González, *Preparación del Paraguay para la guerra del Chaco).* For a moderate statement of the defense of the Liberal Party and its leaders, see Ríos, *La defensa del Chaco: Verdades y mentiras de una victoria.* For a more lyrical view of the Liberal Party's accomplishments, see Artaza, *Ayala, Estigarribia y el Partido Liberal.*

22. Despatch 179, from Asunción, March 5, 1935. DS, 724.3415/4676.

23. Telegram 194, from Buenos Aires, September 2, 1935. FR, 1935, IV, 131.

24. Telegram 232, from Buenos Aires, October 5, 1935. FR, 1935, IV, 155.

25. Telegram 234, from Buenos Aires, October 8, 1935. FR, 1935, IV, 158.

26. Telegram 136, to Buenos Aires, October 7, 1935. FR, 1935, IV, 156–57.

27. Telegram 244, from Buenos Aires, October 12, 1935. FR, 1935, IV, 160–61. Compare Rivarola, *Memorias diplomáticas,* II, 212: Saavedra Lamas "is without question intelligent and thoughtful, but his intellectual vanity makes him vacillating and insufficiently courageous to assume great responsibilities and to insist upon his proposals to the end: *he has a horrible fear of failure."* (Italics added by author.)

28. FR, 1935, IV, 175ff.

29. Telegram 234, from Buenos Aires, October 8, 1935. FR, 1935, IV, 158.

30. Despatch 29, from Asunción, November 29, 1935. DS, 724.34119/310. Ayala also told Howard that "the present line is so far from the Paraguayan base it is unlikely that it could be permanently held against Bolivia if the conflict should be renewed."

31. Despatch 96, from Buenos Aires, December 7, 1935. DS, 724.34119/321. According to this despatch, Braden said the same thing to Ambassador Nieto Del Río of Chile on November 28. The reference to the Italo-Ethiopian conflict evoked a marginal "?" by an unknown hand in the Department of State, but there seems to be no reason for doubting Braden's sincerity in making the remark.

32. The "permanent" character of the Conference was stipulated by Article I of the protocol of June 12: "the Peace Conference cannot relinquish its functions as long as the arbitral *compromis* is not definitively agreed upon."

33. Telegram 283, from Buenos Aires, November 23, 1935. FR, 1935, IV, 183, 184.

34. Telegram 295, from Buenos Aires, December 12, 1935. FR, 1935, IV, 190.

35. Telegram 28, from Rio de Janeiro, January 21, 1936. DS, 724.34119/337.

36. Despatch 198, from Buenos Aires, June 23, 1936. FR, 1936, V, 53.

37. Telegram 159, from Buenos Aires, August 12, 1936. FR, 1936, V, 58. See also, telegram 193, from Buenos Aires, September 13, 1936, FR, 1936, V, 64.

38. Despatch 202, from Asunción, June 25, 1936. DS, 724.34119/518.

39. Telegram 159, from Buenos Aires, August 12, 1936. FR, 1936, V, 58. Later, when some progress seemed to have been reached on one occasion, Braden sceptically stated: "Because of Ramírez' frequent repudiation of his verbal agreements, I still question whether the Paraguayans will readily concede to the Conference such an effective control and supervision of their police forces as to prevent any incident occurring along the Villa Montes road." Telegram 197, from Buenos Aires, September 27, 1936. FR, 1936, V, 66. With such a diplomatic record, Ramírez' memoirs should be approached with all the caution they deserve. However, see his charges that Braden's speech of May 24, 1938 (see p. 143) was not in accordance with the good neighbor policy of the United States. Ramírez, *La paz del Chaco*, pp. 127f.

40. Memorandum dated December 10, 1935, "Summary of Chaco Mediation Efforts and of the Work of the Buenos Aires Peace Conference: April to November, 1935." DS, 724.34119/311-1/2.

41. Despatch 255, from Buenos Aires, September 4, 1936. DS, 724.34119/606. A little later Braden expressed the fear that in neither of the ex-belligerents was public opinion in a frame of mind to accept a compromise solution in the Chaco and that the newspaper press was not helping to educate them toward approval of an equitable agreement.

Despatch 260, from Buenos Aires, September 11, 1936. DS, 724.34119/611.

42. Telegram 2, from Asunción, January 9, 1934. DS, 724.3415/3477. The Paraguayan minister in Washington, however, told Welles that "no outlet to the River Paraguay for Bolivia would be agreed to by the Paraguayan Government." He added that "Bahía Negra was of no value whatever to Bolivia as an outlet inasmuch as ocean going vessels could only reach that point approximately three times during the year and then only for a brief period." Memorandum of conversation, March 2, 1934. DS, 724.3415/3608.

43. Telegram 39, from Asunción, August 27, 1934. FR, 1934, IV, 186.

44. Telegram 200, from Buenos Aires, September 28, 1936; telegram 128, to Buenos Aires, September 29, 1936. DS, 724.34119/621. See also telegram 240, from Buenos Aires, October 27, 1936, FR, 1936, V, 72, telegram 148, to Buenos Aires, October 28, 1936, FR, 1936, V, 73.

45. Despatch 332, from Buenos Aires, December 24, 1936. Memorandum by Braden, December 23. DS, 724.34119/721. Braden indicated that this conversation had not been resumed.

46. Despatch 318, from Buenos Aires, November 13, 1936. DS, 724.34119/704.

47. *Ibid.*

48. Despatch 519, from Buenos Aires, September 30, 1937. DS, 724.34119/1057.

49. Despatch 174, from La Paz, March 19, 1937. DS, 824.6363 St2/82.

50. Despatch 332, from Buenos Aires, December 24, 1936. DS, 724.34119/721.

51. Memorandum of conversation, March 11, 1935. DS, 724.3415/4719.

52. Despatch 406, from Buenos Aires, April 20, 1937. FR, 1937, V, 4–9.

53. Instruction, May 7, 1937. FR, 1937, V, 10.

54. Despatch 415, from Buenos Aires, April 30, 1937. DS, 724.34119/853.

55. An account of the meeting on April 23 with Roca and the discussion at the April 29 dinner is given in a long memorandum drafted by Nieto del Río and approved by Braden and Rodrigues Alves. FR, 1937, V, 10–18, transmitted with despatch 420, from Buenos Aires, May 7, 1937. The English translation was transmitted by Braden; its style is of a quaintness that was certainly not Braden's own.

56. Braden quoted Major John A. Weeks, Military Observer for the United States in the Chaco, as reporting that "if the Conference fails he considers that there is an 80% probability that war will be renewed within a year and thereafter this percentage will increase rapidly." FR, 1937, V, 14. In a memorandum to Braden, Weeks stated that: "The Bolivians believe that they are in a much better tactical position than the Paraguayans and that it would be a simple matter to move in from the north and south (Parapetí River and Pilcomayo River areas), secure and hold the area for some 50 miles or more to the east of the Boyuibe–Villa Montes road. (This is my opinion.)" Despatch 422, from Buenos Aires, May 10, 1937. DS, 724.34119/869.

57. FR, 1937, V, 18–19.

58. Memorandum of conversation between the Under Secretary of State and the Argentine Ambassador, July 27, 1937. DS, 711.00 Statement July 16, 1937/67.

59. Despatch 474, from Buenos Aires, August 4, 1937. FR, 1937, V, 20.

60. *Ibid.*

61. FR, 1937, V, 23. Incidentally, Braden noted that the reading of this statement "brought out the fact that my Uruguayan and Peruvian colleagues apparently have not been presenting to their governments a true picture of the sad course of this Conference, and they made it clear to me that were my statement to appear in the minutes they would be subject to criticism by their governments. I therefore agreed that it should not appear in the minutes but threatened to read it in should there be any further cancellation of meetings and procrastination. This mild piece of blackmail will, I hope, have a salutary effect." FR, 1937, V, 21.

62. Telegram 127, from Buenos Aires, August 10, 1937. FR, 1937, V, 25.

63. Despatch 251, from La Paz, June 14, 1937. DS, 724.34119/908.

64. Despatch 479, from Buenos Aires, August 25, 1937. DS, 724.34119/1000.

65. *Ibid.* While Zubizarreta and other refugees were allowed to return by an amnesty in September, Ayala and Estigarribia were excluded from the amnesty.

66. Telegram 73, to Buenos Aires, August 18, 1937. DS, 724.34119/978.

67. Despatch 479, from Buenos Aires, August 25, 1937. DS, 724.34119/1000.

68. Despatch 509, from Buenos Aires, September 23, 1937. DS, 724.34119/1043.

69. Despatch 464, from Buenos Aires, July 22, 1937. DS, 724.34119/949.

70. Over three years previously, Ambassador Bliss had reported that Saavedra Lamas had frequently said that "the logical outlet for the eastern and southern portions of Bolivia is by means of the Argentine railways and the Pilcomayo River." Despatch 1957, from Buenos Aires, February 3, 1933. DS, 724.3415/2875.

71. Despatch 509, from Buenos Aires, September 23, 1937. DS, 724.34119/1043; and letter from the Under Secretary of State (Welles) to Braden, Washington, October 13, 1937. DS, 724.34119/1043.

72. Despatch 540, from Buenos Aires, October 21, 1937. DS, 724.34119/1087-1/2.

73. Despatch 608, from Buenos Aires, January 10, 1938. DS, 724.34119/1174.

74. Despatch 606, from Buenos Aires, January 7, 1938. DS, 724.34119/1172.

75. Memorandum to the Under Secretary of State (Welles), October 30, 1937, summarizing a part of despatch 541, from Buenos Aires, October 21, 1937. DS, 724.34119/1095.

76. Despatch 609, from Buenos Aires, January 10, 1938, and memorandum of January 26, 1938. DS, 724.34119/1175.

77. Despatch 615, from Buenos Aires, January 18, 1938. DS, 724.34119/

1184. Braden's impression was that the other mediators were mainly interested in saving face for themselves and their governments.

78. Telegram 4, from Buenos Aires, January 20, 1938. DS, 724.34119/1181.

79. Letter from Welles to Braden, February 1, 1938. DS, 724.34119/1183.

80. Despatch 634, from Buenos Aires, February 8, 1938. DS, 724.34119/1219; and telegram 11, from Buenos Aires, February 3, 1938. DS, 724.34119/1199.

81. Despatch 144, from La Paz, February 9, 1938. DS, 724.34119/1216.

82. Despatch 636, from Buenos Aires, February 11, 1938. DS, 724.34119/1221.

83. Telegram 29, from Buenos Aires, February 18, 1938. FR, 1938, V, 89–90.

84. Telegram 15, from Buenos Aires, February 10, 1938. DS, 724.34119/1209.

85. Despatch 636, from Buenos Aires, February 11, 1938. DS, 724.34119/1221.

86. Telegram 21, from Buenos Aires, February 13, 1938. DS, 724.34119/1211.

87. Telegram 40, from Buenos Aires, February 24, 1938. FR, 1938, V, 91.

88. Telegram 57, from Buenos Aires, March 15, 1938. FR, 1938, V, 95. Later, Braden stated that "Saavedra's machinations will become unimportant once his prognostications have been proven false. It is pertinent to observe, however, that he continues to be so dangerous an element that Alvarado has twice told my colleagues and me it would be up to us to convince Dr. Cantilo, on his arrival, of the nefariousness of the former Argentine Minister for Foreign Affairs." Despatch 661, from Buenos Aires, March 22, 1938. DS, 724.34119/1274. Manuel P. Alvarado was Acting Minister for Foreign Affairs.

V. The Chaco Peace Conference—Fulfillment

1. Telegram 21, from Buenos Aires, February 13, 1938. DS, 724.34119/1211. Braden meant that either an agreement would be reached on a boundary or the conference could decide that agreement was impossible and try to arrange an arbitration.

2. Despatch 637, from Buenos Aires, February 15, 1938, and telegram 26, to Buenos Aires, February 28, 1938. DS, 724.34119/1226.

3. Telegram 49, from Buenos Aires, March 8, 1938. FR, 1938, V, 92.

4. Telegram 56, from Buenos Aires, March 14, 1938. FR, 1938, V, 94.

5. Telegram 51, from Buenos Aires, March 9, 1938; draft telegram, March 10, 1938; note from Welles to Laurence Duggan, Chief, Division of Latin American Affairs, March 11, 1938. DS, 724.34119/1250.

6. Telegram 58, from Buenos Aires, March 17, 1938. FR, 1938, V, 96.

7. Despatch 661, from Buenos Aires, March 22, 1938. DS, 724.34119/ 1274.

8. Telegram 69, from Buenos Aires, March 25, 1938, and telegram 38, to Buenos Aires, March 26, 1938. FR, 1938, V, 100.

9. Despatch 668, from Buenos Aires, April 4, 1938. DS, 724.34119/1294.

10. Letter from the Under Secretary of State (Welles) to Braden, Washington, October 6, 1937, and memorandum from the office of the legal adviser, September 22, 1937. DS, 724.34119/1009.

11. Despatch 464, from Buenos Aires, July 22, 1937. DS, 724.34119/949.

12. Telegram 14, from La Paz, April 12, 1938. FR, 1938, V, 107–8.

13. Telegram 93, from Buenos Aires, April 19, 1938, FR, 1938, V, 110, citing telegram 18, from La Paz, April 14, 1938; and interview with Spruille Braden, March 18, 1963. With regard to informal diplomacy, Braden recalls that on one occasion, during a talk with Saavedra Lamas and Zubizarreta, he overturned a coffee table to successfully divert attention from what he regarded as an embarrassing *démarche* by the Paraguayan diplomat.

14. FR, 1938, V, 110. Braden recalls that at this time he regarded himself as being very nearly in the position of Ortiz' "ambassador" as well as Roosevelt's, with respect to the conference.

15. Telegram 66, from Buenos Aires, March 24, 1938. FR, 1938, V, 99.

16. Telegrams 113 and 115, from Buenos Aires, both dated May 18, 1938. FR, 1938, V, 122, 123.

17. *The Chaco Peace Conference*, pp. 138–42. It should be noted that the very action Braden asserted was in accord with the Good Neighbor policy, was claimed to violate that policy by the Paraguayan delegate to the Chaco conference under the Franco regime. See Ramírez, *La paz del Chaco*, p. 127.

18. Telegram 126, from Buenos Aires, May 26, 1938. DS, 724.34119/ 1365. While the immediate press reaction was favorable, and so had maximum effect on the occasion of the arrival of the foreign ministers, a subsequent attack was made on Braden, as a result of this speech, in the form of a syndicated editorial appearing in about twenty Argentine newspapers in early June. It described his attitude as "rather antipathetic . . . in trying to impose by coercion a peaceful formula on Paraguay, a method opposed by Argentina, which insisted that the formula be presented only as a suggestion." The editorial gave further currency to reports that Braden had financial interests in mining companies in Bolivia, and Braden therefore read into the minutes of the conference a declaration that he had never owned stock in Standard Oil Company of New Jersey nor had any investment "directly or indirectly in Bolivia." Despatch 696, from Buenos Aires, June 14, 1938. DS, 724.34119/1420.

19. Telegram 115, from Buenos Aires, May 18, 1938, and telegram 62, to Buenos Aires, May 20, 1938. FR, 1938, V, 123–25. Braden's references in the speech to informing the public of America as to reasons for failure of the conference plan were mildly expressed as a result of the Department's suggestion that credit or blame should not be assigned for failure, but that "any views regarding statements to be made in

the event of a failure of the negotiations might better be expressed to representatives of one or both of the parties verbally rather than included in a public address."

20. Telegrams of May 25, 1938. FR, 1938, V, 126–28.

21. Telegram 74, to Buenos Aires, June 6, FR, 1938, V, 136; and telegram 117, from Buenos Aires, May 20, 1938, FR, 1938, V, 124–25. The consideration was £200,000.

22. Telegram 137, from Buenos Aires, June 2, 1938. FR, 1938, V, 131–32. The six kilometers in question was Braden's estimate of the distance between Puerto Caballo and the mouth of the Otuquis to the north.

23. Telegram 139, from Buenos Aires, June 3, 1938. FR, 1938, V, 132–33. Minister Findley B. Howard reported that a Paraguayan had told him that the Liberal Party was "holding Dr. Zubizarreta in reserve for future political contingencies because as long as he does not cede on any of Paraguay's pretensions he is one man upon whom the army and the country generally could patriotically unite. . . . I tried to suggest that this was a very shortsighted and in the long run unpatriotic point of view and might lead to a renewal of the conflict with Bolivia. He depreciated this possibility but, as many others have done, expressed the opinion that such a war was preferable to a revolution within the country." Despatch 614, from Asunción, May 26, 1938. DS, 724.34119/1379.

24. Telegram 129, from Buenos Aires, May 27, 1938. DS, 724.34119/1370. Báez later told Braden that these remarks were occasioned by the speech in question, "but he now esteemed me as entirely fair in my dealings." Telegram 159, from Buenos Aires, June 15, 1938. DS, 724.34119/1410.

25. Telegram 140, from Buenos Aires, June 3, 1938. FR, 1938, V, 134.

26. Telegram 74, to Buenos Aires, June 6, 1938. FR, 1938, V, 136.

27. Telegram 147, from Buenos Aires, June 7, 1938. FR, 1938, V, 139.

28. Telegrams 151 and 154, from Buenos Aires, June 10 and June 13, 1938. FR, 1938, V, 141, 143.

29. Telegram 164, from Buenos Aires, June 24, 1938. FR, 1938, V, 145–46. Nine days previously the entire Paraguayan delegation, including Zubizarreta and Báez, had signed a recommendation to the government in Asunción "that the counter-proposal should reject any river front for Bolivia but should otherwise accept the conference line." Telegram 159, from Buenos Aires, June 15, 1938. DS, 724.34119/1410. This suggests that, at worst, Zubizarreta was only the most intransigent of Paraguayan civilians and also that the firm Argentine attitude, plus Braden's speech, may have been of some effect. Minister Howard reported that he judged that "the Government will not enter any agreement which it feels might cause its overthrow. Practically speaking, this means that any agreement must have the almost solid support of the army." Because of the internal political situation, however, and the position of Zubizarreta as "a defender of Paraguayan interests in the Chaco," it was not likely that the government "would dare accept any agreement which Dr. Zubizarreta refused to approve." Despatch 629, from Asunción, June 23, 1938. DS, 724.34119/1437. Howard added that for months he had tried to persuade Paraguayans

of "the advisability of a campaign of education designed to inculcate a more conciliatory spirit and prepare the public mind for the acceptance of such an agreement as it might be possible to secure, which would, of course, embrace something less than the maximum Paraguayan pretensions to the Chaco."

30. Telegram 164, from Buenos Aires, June 24, 1938, FR, 1938, V, 146; and telegram 159, from Buenos Aires, June 15, 1938, DS, 724.34119/1410.

31. Telegram 166, from Buenos Aires, June 25, 1938. FR, 1938, V, 147.

32. Telegram 167, from Buenos Aires, June 26, 1938. FR, 1938, V, 149. According to this telegram, Finot, for Bolivia, said he thought he could get this proposal accepted "with alterations in the west and north, for instance, D'Orbigny."

33. Telegram 82, to Buenos Aires, June 27, 1938. DS, 724.34119/1425. Similar action was taken by the governments of Argentina, Chile, and Brazil about June 28, and on June 29 the minister told Welles that instructions had been sent to Diez de Medina in Buenos Aires authorizing him to withhold publication if he thought it desirable. This amounted to "an instruction to desist from publication," since it was Finot and not the Foreign Minister who was insisting on publication. Memorandum of conversation between the Under Secretary of State (Welles) and the Minister of Bolivia (Luís Fernando Guachalla), June 29, 1938. DS, 724.34119/1452.

34. Despatch 256, from La Paz, June 29, 1938. DS, 724.34119/1490. Prendergast also observed that the Bolivians believed, "with what would appear to be a good deal of justification, that at all events it is not they who have impeded the progress of the peace negotiations, and the local press continues to flay Paraguay for what it regards as a most intransigent attitude."

35. Telegram 168, from Buenos Aires, June 26, 1938. FR, 1938, V, 150–51. Zubizarreta said that he "would not be an obstacle to signature of such an agreement but would simply resign." Telegram 169, from Buenos Aires, June 27, 1938. DS, 724.34119/1427.

36. Telegram 170, from Buenos Aires, June 28, 1938. FR, 1938, V, 152.

37. This arrangement has given rise to some controversy, since the armistice agreement of June 12, 1935, provided for a "juridical arbitration." See La Foy, *The Chaco Dispute and the League of Nations*, pp. 131–32, who notes that the arbitration *ex aequo et bono* was quite different from the provisions of the armistice, and Ramírez, *La paz del Chaco*, p. 276, who asserts that the arbitration *ex aequo et bono* was disadvantageous and should not have been accepted by Paraguay in 1938.

38. Telegram 172, from Buenos Aires, June 29, 1938, FR, 1938, V, 153–55; and telegram 164, from Buenos Aires, June 24, 1938, FR, 1938, V, 145–46.

39. Telegram 86, to Buenos Aires, June 30, 1938. FR, 1938, V, 155–56. Braden reported later that, although the Braden-Cardozo suggestion was not proposed by President Roosevelt, "in Paraguay the leaders found useful the prestige of the President's name as an additional evidence of the Treaty's excellence," during the pre-plebiscite campaign. He quoted

from a speech by Dr. Luis A. Argaña, Acting Foreign Minister, in which it was said that on June 30, "under the high auspices of the President of the United States of America, Mr. Roosevelt, the Peace Conference presented the saving formula." Despatch 781, from Buenos Aires, October 4, 1938. DS, 724.34119/1651.

40. Despatch 65, from Bogotá, April 17, 1939. DS, 724.34119/1776. This despatch was written as a commentary on the draft report of the Chaco conference.

41. Cardozo, *Paraguay independiente*, pp. 378–79. On other aspects of the proceedings of the Chaco conference, see *ibid.*, pp. 380ff.

42. Despatch 257, from La Paz, July 4, 1938. DS, 724.34119/1470. Prendergast obtained this information from an individual who had personally talked with President Busch.

43. Telegram 178, from Buenos Aires, July 1, 1938. FR, 1938, V, 157–58.

44. Telegram 182, from Buenos Aires, July 4, 1938. FR, 1938, V, 159–60. Finot was known for his use of the resources of domineering techniques in diplomacy; a Paraguayan is reported to have told the story that on one occasion General Frank R. McCoy said of Finot: "'When I hear him thunder, I tremble for the safety of my own country.'" Despatch 401, from Asunción, June 12, 1937. DS, 724.34119/910. The "Finotesque manner" was a diplomatic byword at this time.

45. Telegram 180, from Buenos Aires, July 2, 1938. FR, 1938, V, 158–59. This action may have been taken out of irritation at Zubizarreta's attempt to repudiate the Braden-Cardozo formula. Telegram 178, from Buenos Aires, July 1, 1938. FR, 1938, V, 157–58.

46. Telegram 182, from Buenos Aires, July 4, 1938. FR, 1938, V, 159–60.

47. Braden cabled that on July 2 Cardozo said he was authorized by Asunción to accept the Braden-Cardozo formula, which had been accepted by Diez de Medina on the morning of July 1 and then repudiated by him and by Finot the same afternoon. "Thus, if the Paraguayan acceptance of today and Bolivian acceptance of yesterday had coincided, the peace would have been made but due to the Bolivian about-face we must get them back in line." Telegram 180, from Buenos Aires, July 2, 1938. FR, 1938, V, 158.

48. Text in *The Chaco Peace Conference*, pp. 148–51.

49. Telegram 182, from Buenos Aires, July 4, 1938. FR, 1938, V, 160. The triangle was the Brazilian cession to Bolivia along the Paraguay River above the limit of navigation.

50. Telegram 146, from Buenos Aires, June 7, 1938, and telegram 75, in reply, June 9. FR, 1938, V, 137–38. Hull added: "Experience indicates that it would not be possible to keep the terms of such an agreement secret for any length of time."

51. There is in the FDRL a memorandum, unsigned, with no letterhead, dated June 1, 1939, with an attached note to President Roosevelt from Basil O'Connor stating: "Be sure to read *before* you see General Estigarribia." (The General was to see the President on that day.) The memorandum asserts that Estigarribia had been assured in Buenos Aires

by Braden and Welles "in the presence of foreign ambassadors" that he would be given assistance to build a highway from Asunción to the Brazilian border. It is stated that Estigarribia "assured his own people that these things would be done . . . and he was authorized to conclude the Chaco Settlement in the light of those assurances." Further: "It should be borne in mind that the Chaco Peace was arrived at directly as the result of the efforts of General Estigarribia and he, in turn, was authorized to conclude that Peace by his military supporters in reliance upon the performance of the program of the public works hereinabove indicated." It is likely that this document was prepared in the Paraguayan legation and that it stretched the truth; for example, Welles was not in Buenos Aires at the time when Estigarribia was a member of the Paraguayan delegation to the Chaco Peace Conference. It would be interesting to know how this document got to O'Connor and why he considered it so important that Roosevelt should read it. Cardozo notes that Estigarribia had returned from Washington via the west coast of South America, where he had learned about new preparations by Bolivia for carrying on hostilities. He adds that, with regard to the final peace plan, "the opinion of Estigarribia was decisive." Cardozo, *Paraguay independiente*, pp. 381, 383.

52. Telegram 209, from Buenos Aires, July 21, 1938. DS. 724.34119/1493.

53. Despatch 280, from La Paz, July 25, 1938. DS, 724.34119/1525.

54. Despatches 635 and 644, from Asunción, July 14, July 27, 1938. DS, 724.34119/1496 and /1532. To a suggestion that all mediatory countries declare at least a half holiday on the occasion, Braden reported he had "expressed doubt that this could be done in the United States giving as excuse President Roosevelt is on the high seas. If you think of something to do please advise me." Telegram 204, from Buenos Aires, July 18, 1938. FR, 1938, V, 172.

55. The opposition groups in Paraguay, the Colorado party and the supporters of ex-President Franco, published manifestos after August 10, declaring that the ratification of the treaty by plebiscite was unconstitutional. This alleged defect, however, was removed by approval, by both houses of congress, of the treaty on February 8, 1939. Despatch 750, from Buenos Aires, August 26, 1938. DS, 724.34119/1603 and despatch 794, from Asunción, February 16, 1939. DS, 724.34119/1771.

56. Text of speech in *El País* (Asunción), February 10, 1939.

57. Memorandum of conversation with Ambassador Espil, August 8, 1932. FR, 1932, V, 166.

58. Despatch 663, from La Paz, August 10, 1933. DS, 824.032/116. Feely commented that the Bolivians knew that "to have accepted such a proposal would have been a direct repudiation of the declaration of the nineteen American nations of August 3, 1932, which proclaimed the doctrine that territory captured by force would not be recognized. . . . The President's reference to it here is intended no doubt for home consumption, as an argument to prove that Bolivia was not responsible for the failure of the negotiations of that time."

59. Despatch 879, from Montevideo, December 15, 1934. DS, 724.3415/4456. Later, the minister reported that "the representatives of the upland countries of South America in Montevideo" believed that the Chaco settlement would raise grave problems "such as the interpretation of the doctrine of non-recognition of territory acquired by force of arms, which may have serious repercussion throughout South America." Despatch 1072, from Montevideo, April 16, 1935. DS, 724.3415/4819. Compare the comment: "America does not yet dare to fix responsibilities," Pastor Benítez, *Bajo el signo de marte*, p. 14.

60. Despatch 152, from Asunción, January 26, 1935. DS, 724.3415/4539.

61. Despatch 276, from La Paz, March 6, 1935. DS, 724.3415/4651. This circular was published in *Ultima Hora* (La Paz), March 5.

62. *The Chaco Peace Conference*, pp. 41–42.

63. *Ibid.*, pp. 160, 41, 42.

64. The Spanish is: *Homenaje al valor y heroísmo de dos pueblos hermanos que por error e injusticia de los hombres se agredieron.* There is another plaque on the tank stating that this is a "Light Tank, Mk. E. Mf. by Vickers-Armstrongs, Ltd., Elswick Works, Newcastle-on-Tyne, Nov. 1932. 324841 319122."

Part Two. The Leticia Dispute

Full bibliographical information about the works cited will be found in the section of the Bibliography about the Leticia Dispute.

VI. Background and Outbreak

1. League of Nations, Treaty Series (No. 1726), Vol. 74, p. 9.

2. Quoted in Francisco Andrade S., "Límites entre Colombia y Ecuador," *Boletín de Historia y Antigüedades* (Bogotá), XLVII (March-April, 1961), 201–19, at p. 217. On this subject see also: Cabeza de Vaca, *La posición del Ecuador en el conflicto colombo-peruano*; López, *Los tratados de límites y la paz internacional americana*; Muñoz Vernaza, *Exposición sobre el tratado de límites de 1916 entre el Ecuador y Colombia y análisis jurídico del Tratado de límites de 1922 entre Colombia y el Perú*; Pérez Serrano, *El tercero en la discordia*. Pérez Serrano considers that Colombia, by the Salomón-Lozano treaty, "gave us to Peru, tied hand and foot" (p. 123). Muñoz Vernaza defends the 1916 treaty as a good one for both parties—"the only thing lacking was the good faith of the government of Colombia" (p. 58). For a defense of the Colombian position, see Rivas, *Historia diplomática de Colombia*, p. 666. Alberto Ulloa asserts that "Colombia not only kept the terms of the treaty from Ecuador, but deceived Ecuador as to its nature by repeatedly affirming that Ecuador's rights were not affected." Ulloa, *Posición internacional del Perú*, p. 174. The Colombian Senator and Ambassador Carlos Uribe Echeverri is reported to have condemned the conduct of his country in

this affair by saying that it "might be juridically acceptable, but it was not in good faith (*no es moralmente leal*)." Pérez Serrano, *El tercero en la discordia*, pp. 141–42. Also quoted in Cavelier, *La política internacional de Colombia*, III, 153.

3. Telegram 36, to Lima, October 8, 1923. FR, 1923, I, 352.

4. Telegram 47, to Lima, December 4, 1923. FR, 1923, I, 353.

5. Despatch 657, to Bogotá, March 28, 1924. FR, 1924, I, 295.

6. Telegram 3, to Rio de Janeiro, January 19, 1925. FR, 1925, I, 437–38.

7. For details of the negotiations, see FR, 1925, I, 436–63.

8. Despatch 2134, from Lima, September 19, 1932. DS, 721.23/135.

9. Instruction 385, to Lima, October 18, 1932. DS, 721.23/135.

10. Telegram 8, to Lima, February 28, 1925. FR, 1925, I, 453–54. In this telegram, Hughes noted that Peruvian Foreign Minister, Alberto Salomón Osorio, had stated that "it would be contrary to the Peruvian constitution to recommend to Congress the approval of the treaty" and proceeded briefly to dispute Salomón's interpretation of his country's constitution, a rather unusual action for the foreign minister of one sovereign state in dealing with his counterpart in another sovereign state.

11. Text of the agreement is in FR, 1925, I, 461–63. Brazil also agreed to "establish in perpetuity in favor of Colombia freedom of navigation on the Amazon and other rivers common to both countries."

12. Telegram 1, to Lima, January 6, 1927. FR, 1927, I, 332–33.

13. Telegram 55, from Lima, November 12, 1927, and telegram 44, to Lima, November 15, 1927. FR, 1927, I, 341–43.

14. The large majority did not, however, reflect the intensity of the minority's emotions. See, for example, the views of Senator Julio C. Araña of Loreto, set forth in Evaristo San Cristoval, *Páginas internacionales: Antecedentes diplomáticas del tratado Salomón-Lozano;* and Ugarteche, *Documentos que acusan: El tratado Salomón-Lozano;* Valcarcel, *Crítica del tratado Salomón-Lozano.*

15. Antonio Miró Quesada, Civilista and editor of *El Comercio*, was regarded by Fred Morris Dearing, United States Ambassador in Lima, as "the real author of the Leticia dispute. . . . His motive was primarily to destroy the work of Leguía, whom he hated, and I may mention that he hated our Government too, particularly because Leguía was friendly to us." Letter to President Franklin D. Roosevelt, May 27, 1935. FRDL, PSF Box 20.

16. Telegram 131, from Lima, September 2, 1932. FR, 1932, V, 270. Dearing's description of the filibusterers as Apristas (members of APRA, a political party founded by Victor Raul Haya de la Torre), was apparently based on the President's assertion. The United States had no consul at Iquitos and was forced to rely on Colombian and Peruvian reports, occasional information from the British consul there, and infrequent United States travelers for on-the-spot coverage. The Embassy in Lima reported that "the people in Lima likely to have freshest information are the 7th Day Adventists." Despatch 2075, September 6, 1932. DS, 721.23/69.

17. Telegram 141, from Lima, September 5, 1932. DS, 721.23/20. Polo

said that the Leticia attack was a movement that "was really revolutionary" and "was for the purpose of cloaking a serious uprising in Lima and elsewhere in the country."

18. Dearing reported that "a trustworthy American source informs the Embassy that for several months it has been publicly known in Iquitos that Leticia would be forcibly seized." Despatch 2091, from Lima, September 8, 1932. DS, 721.23/72. Later, Dearing reported that the Colombian Minister in Lima, Fabio Lozano y Lozano, son of the signer of the treaty, claimed to have information that an agent of Sánchez Cerro had been sent to Iquitos on August 9 to provoke the Leticia incident, both to open the way to revision of the treaty and to give a justification to the government for further repression of the APRA Party. This latter reason was being asserted in Peru by APRA Party members. Despatch 2157, from Lima, September 25, 1932. DS, 721.23/199. From Bogotá came word that Brazilian authorities at Tabatinga reported that Leticia had been seized by two hundred civilians and fifty soldiers from the garrison at Chimbote. Despatch 4312, from Bogotá, September 5, 1932. DS, 721.23/47. This report was supported by a letter from a French resident of Iquitos to his minister in Lima. Despatch 2172, from Lima, September 28, 1932. DS, 721.23/240.

19. On the question of military preparedness, see p. 444, note 51.

20. Telegram 54, to Lima, September 13, 1932. DS, 721.23/52.

21. Despatch 2129, from Lima, September 17, 1932. DS, 721.23/134. Dearing reported that he got no definite answer from Zavala, as might have been expected.

22. Despatch 2139, from Lima, September 20, 1932. DS, 721.23/172.

23. Telegram 183, from Lima, September 21, 1932. DS, 721.23/108.

24. Despatch 4511, from Bogotá, October 5, 1932. DS, 721.23/262.

25. Several telegrams from Caffery, especially Telegram 57, from Bogotá, September 4, 1932. DS, 721.23/11.

26. Telegram 135, from Lima, September 4, 1932. DS, 721.23/15.

27. See, for example, Colombia, Consulate General, *International Opinion and the Leticia Controversy;* Colombia, Legación, España, *Un gran triunfo de Colombia;* Colombia, Legacíon, Mexico, *Información sobre el actual conflicto entre Colombia y el Perú.*

28. Despatch 2232, from Lima, October 16, 1932. DS, 823.032/147.

29. Despatch 4785, from Bogotá, November 25, 1932. DS, 721.23/550. The alternative to Lima's backing of the Junta Patriótica in Iquitos " 'would have been a revolt against the Government' " in Loreto, according to this source. At the time, Dearing cabled that the "Government's position is dangerous. Siding with Loreto means war. Abandonment of Leticia against public feeling may cause government's fall unless it is strong enough to suppress ensuing resentment." Telegram 146, from Lima, September 7, 1932. DS, 721.23/30.

30. This letter was republished in *El Espectador* (Bogotá) on April 22, 1933. These statements are largely borne out by disinterested sources. See FR, 1933, IV, 401–3, for corroborative statement by Assistant Secretary of State Francis White in a talk with the Peruvian Ambassador,

January 13, 1933. White commented that, if some arrangement had been made by Colombia with Vigil, "it would have been much better." On excessive port charges at Leticia, see Memorandum of conversation, March 2, 1933. DS, 721.23/1413. "Loretanos feel that with Colombians at Leticia Colombia can at any time block traffic on the Amazon and bottle up and isolate Iquitos."

31. Report from Manaos, by the United States Military Attaché in Brazil, April 12, 1933. DS, 721.23/1698. Major William Sackville, the Attaché, had visited Leticia at the end of March and had talked with Colombians and Peruvians.

32. Quoted in *El Espectador* (Bogotá), April 22, 1933.

33. Telegram 134, from Lima, September 3, 1932. FR, 1932, V, 272–75. The report of the sending of the "América" was naively thought by Dearing at the time to be part of a cooperative action by Peru and Colombia to " 'join armed forces to capture' " the captors of Leticia.

VII. Fighting and Mediation

1. Telegram 73, to Rio de Janeiro, September 7, 1932. DS, 721.23/32A.
2. Telegram 50, to Lima, September 3, 1932. FR, 1932, V, 271.
3. Telegram 134, from Lima, September 3, 1932. FR, 1932, V, 272–73.
4. Telegram 57, from Bogotá, September 4, 1932. DS, 721.23/11.
5. The expression is Dearing's, reporting his first talk with Sánchez Cerro. Despatch 2074, September 5, 1932. DS, 721.23/51.
6. Telegram 35, to Bogotá, September 7, 1932. DS, 721.23/12.
7. Memorandum of conversation, September 7, 1932. DS, 721.23/75. The memorandum was written by Edwin C. Wilson, Chief, Division of Latin American Affairs.
8. Telegram 192, from Lima, September 28, 1932, and Telegram 62, to Lima, October 1, 1932. The Navy Department concurred in the instruction. DS, 721.23/149, and despatch 2174, from Lima, September 28, 1932. DS, 721.23/242. See also despatches 2225 and 2234, from Lima, October 14 and 15, 1932. DS, 721.23/306 and 721.23/333. The second of these includes a report on his activities by the chief of the Naval Mission, which is described in a Department of State memorandum as "very lame." Edwin C. Wilson later advised the head of the Naval Mission that he understood that the Mission "was to assist in improving technical methods and training and that they were not to engage in drawing up offensive plans against particular countries, and this would be especially so in a period in which the countries were actually preparing to go to war." Memorandum of conversation, March 24, 1933. DS, 721.23/1507.
9. Telegram 149, from Lima, September 7, 1932. DS, 721.23/31.
10. Telegram 151, from Lima, September 8, 1932. DS, 721.23/39. Dearing stated he was "not completely convinced" the government would fall in this case. Despatch 2088, from Lima, September 8, 1932. DS, 721.23/71.
11. Telegram 65, from Bogotá, September 8, 1932. DS, 721.23/37.

12. Memorandum of conversation, September 9, 1932. FR, 1932, V, 276.

13. Memorandum by E. C. Wilson to the Secretary of State, September 12, 1932. DS, 721.23/77.

14. Memorandum of conversation, September 13, 1932. DS, 721.23/97. The memorandum was written by Francis White. On the declaration of August 3, 1932, see p. 28. For a similar expression of the Department's views, see the instruction to Dearing, September 15, 1932, FR, 1932, V, 277–78.

15. Memorandum of telephone conversation, September 13, 1932. DS, 721.23/96.

16. Memorandum of conversation, September 21, 1932. DS, 721.23/152. In this same vein, see Telegram 39, to Bogotá, September 17, 1932, FR, 1932, V, 279–80.

17. Despatch 2147, from Lima, September 22, 1932. DS, 721.23/177.

18. Telegram 169, from Lima, September 16, 1932. DS, 721.23/79. The pressure referred to here was the action of Hughes in 1925. An additional justificatory argument used by some Peruvians at this time was that the Leticia affair was like that of Fiume.

19. See the letter by Alberto Ulloa, a Peruvian international lawyer, in *El Comercio* (Lima), September 26, 1932. Ulloa noted that Peru had not denounced the treaty, but he said: "There is no people in the world which would fail to take advantage of an occurrence which revealed a situation which concerned it, not, of course, to violate a juridical instrument, but in order to demonstrate its inconvenience, and secure its modification."

20. Dearing reported a talk with the Ecuadoran minister in Lima, Augusto Aguirre Aparicio, who said that Lozano Torrijos had played on Leguía's vanity through flattery and had persuaded him that he would make a great contribution "to the Americanista ideal if he signed the treaty." Aguirre's view was that the Peruvian congress that ratified the treaty was "undoubtedly hostile, but that the more devoted Leguía supporters therein felt they must ratify the treaty in order to uphold the Leguía regime and because they trusted him and believed in his sincerity in supporting the Americanista ideal." Despatch 2146, from Lima, September 22, 1932. DS, 721.23/176. For the official, more restrained statement of this position, see the note of February 20, 1933, from the Peruvian Foreign Minister to the Secretary of State. FR, 1933, IV, 486.

21. *La Realidad Nacional* (Paris), 1931, quoted in Alayza y Paz Soldán, *Mi país: Algo de la Amazonia Peruana*, p. 77.

22. *Ibid.*, p. 76.

23. Ulloa, *Posición internacional del Perú*, pp. 157, 160, note 233. Ulloa asserts that Salomón opposed the treaty that he had signed but was constrained to complete it by the will of Leguía, which in turn was strongly influenced by "the pressure of the government of the United States." *Ibid.*, p. 169. On this point, see also Ugarteche, *Documentos que acusan: el Tratado Salomón-Lozano*, pp. 32–33, and "La cuestión de Leticia," *Boletín de la Sociedad Geográfica de Lima*, LI, 87–242. The Colombian signer of the treaty quotes Sánchez Cerro as saying that

Leguía had " 'sold the fertile land of the Putumayo' " to Colombia and thus planted the seed of the Leticia affair. Lozano Torrijos, *El tratado Lozano-Salomón*, p. 387.

24. Editorial, February 2, 1933.

25. Despatch 2170, from Lima, September 27, 1932. DS, 721.23/238. See also *La Crónica* (Lima), January 17, 1933, for the suggestion that the United States government may have aided Leguía to obtain a loan in the United States in order to get the treaty through and establish friendly relations with Colombia. Such an argument ignored the fact that the United States–Colombian treaty of 1922, settling the Panama question, antedated by three years Hughes's alleged pressure in 1925.

26. Despatch 4438, from Bogotá, September 23, 1932. DS, 721.23/144.

27. Despatch 2174, from Lima, September 28, 1932. DS, 721.23/242, and Telegram 197, from Lima, September 30, 1932. DS, 721.23/183.

28. Telegram 63, to Lima, October 3, 1932. DS, 721.23/183. This cable was sent before the receipt of Dearing's despatch 2174, but it answered his question. In that despatch, Dearing commented that "Sanchez Cerro is a gambler, is at home in the midst of military activity and greatly prefers the dangerous life and lots of action to any course which calls for thought and patience." In connection with "military life" in Peru, it may be noted that Dearing reported the following rumors going around Lima: "In the South it is said that the Fourth Military Division, based on Cuzco and Puno, favors the retention of Leticia, whereas the Third Division, based on Arequipa, stands for the fulfillment of the provisions of the Salomón-Lozano Treaty." Despatch 2152, from Lima, September 25, 1932. DS, 721.23/197.

29. Memorandum of conversation, October 3, 1932. DS, 721.23/245. The note of September 30 is called by Ulloa "one of the immortal pages of the diplomatic history of Peru." Ulloa, *Posición internacional del Peru*, p. 190.

30. Memorandum of conversation, October 5, 1932. DS, 721.23/291.

31. Memorandum of conversation, October 14, 1932. FR, 1932, V, 283–84.

32. Memorandum of conversation, October 10, 1932. DS, 721.23/298. In this same talk, Freyre tested White with the argument that Leticia was comparable to Fiume, but White, forewarned by Dearing, was ready with the statement of the Italian Chargé in Lima who had pointed out that there had been no comparable treaty in the Fiume case; the Chargé had said that, if this line were persisted in by the Peruvian government, he would have to make a correction in the press.

33. Memorandum of conversation, October 21, 1932. DS, 721.23/370. In discussing the Colombian attitude, Freyre remarked that "the essence of statecraft is not to be too rigid," and White commented that, before Colombia could be expected to "show some flexibility," the demands of the Loretanos would have to be reduced.

34. Memorandum of conversation, October 22, 1932. DS, 721.23/371.

35. Despatch 722, from Quito, October 25, 1932. DS, 721.23/386.

36. Memorandum of conversation, October 29, 1932. DS, 721.23/407.

Concerning the origin of the treaty of 1922, Maúrtua said that, during the ten-year period when Lozano Torrijos was Colombian Minister in Lima, he had formed a close relationship with Leguía and had negotiated the treaty with him "the terms of which were not even known by the Minister of Foreign Affairs, Mr. Salomón, until he was called in to sign it." Maúrtua and Salomón were both opposed to the treaty, and Maúrtua said that he "was put in the very anomalous position of conniving with the Minister of Foreign Affairs who had signed the treaty to find a way by which it could be modified. Mr. Maúrtua admitted that he had stirred up the Brazilian opposition to the treaty and had helped in drafting the Brazilian protest" to Peru, which had been the occasion of Secretary Hughes's making arrangements that resulted in the protocol of March 4, 1925. Secretary Hughes's success, however, was Maúrtua's failure, since the protocol made possible the treaty's ratification.

37. Memoranda of conversations, October 27, 1932, and November 10, 1932. FR, 1932, V, 285.

38. Memorandum of conversation, October 31, 1932. FR, 1932, V, 286–90. Illustrative of White's attitude was this remark: "I told him that personally it was pretty hard to ask President Olaya to take a position contrary to the firm convictions and public feeling in Colombia in order to save the Peruvian authorities from carrying out their obvious duty."

39. Details of the proposal and of Stimson's argument for it are in Telegram 49, to Bogotá, November 16, 1932. FR, 1932, V, 295–97.

40. Despatch 4757, from Bogotá, November 19, 1932. FR, 1932, V, 297–98.

41. Despatch 4703, from Bogotá, November 7, 1932. DS, 721.23/496. In Despatch 4757 (see note 40), Caffery said that " 'Dr. Olaya is not open to reason on these matters and it is better to let matters remain as they are and say nothing at all in this connection.' "

42. Despatch 4805, from Bogotá, November 28, 1932. DS, 721.23/558.

43. Despatch 4813, from Bogotá, November 29, 1932. DS, 721.23/540.

44. Memorandum of conversation, December 14, 1932. DS, 721.23/634.

45. Memorandum of telephone conversation with Mr. George Rublee, November 28, 1932. DS, 721.23/572.

46. Despatch 4399, from Bogotá, September 17, 1932. DS, 721.23/113.

47. FR, 1932, V, 302–4. Especially telegram 167, from Panama, December 8, 1932. The legation in Bogotá considered that this was one of several instances in which Cruchaga had "fancied himself as an arbiter . . . he was extremely anxious to figure prominently in any international controversy in Latin America in which he could get added prestige from the publicity received." Despatch 4923, December 19, 1932. DS, 721.23/628.

48. Telegram 130, from Rio de Janeiro, December 30, 1932. FR, 1932, V, 313.

49. Telegram 100, to Rio de Janeiro, December 30, 1932. FR, 1932, V, 314.

50. FR, 1932, V, 306–15, at p. 310. Maúrtua's first talk with White was on December 20. Maúrtua later submitted a memorandum, but it was disregarded because attention had shifted to the Brazilian formula. When

White told Freyre about "l'affaire Maúrtua," Freyre "said he appreciated the difficulties; that I [White] was not the first one who had found Maúrtua a very difficult man to deal with." Memorandum of conversation, January 4, 1933. DS, 721.23/699.

51. Memorandum of conversation, December 22, 1932. DS, 721.23/640. In this connection it may be noted that Colombia was so far from having an army at this time, that Vásquez Cobo, the general who led the expedition up the Amazon, was domiciled in France and that many of the men in the expedition were not Colombians but foreign adventurers. Colombia had not one amphibian plane, the type necessary for operations near Leticia because of the absence of airfields, and the pilots of those that were acquired after the incident were nearly all German nationals. Peru's position in and around Leticia was stronger than Colombia's, principally because of the substantial population in and near Iquitos. Dearing estimated that the "Peruvian defense in Loreto consists of about 2000 armed men with four antiquated Krupp guns, nine airplanes, and two old gunboats armored with galvanized iron and armed with 37-millimeter guns. The 2000 men are mostly volunteers but are sprinkled with ex-service men and are officered by regular officers and non-coms who have been sent to Loreto by air. Efforts are being made to transport 3-inch mountain guns from Lima to Iquitos by airplane. The Krupp guns, which are 1895 3-inch field pieces, mounted on wheels, are stationed on shore, two at Leticia and two at Tarapacá." Despatch 2474, from Lima, December 30, 1932. DS, 721.23/664. There were two cruisers in the Peruvian navy. One of these had been damaged in a mutiny in 1931. The other was not sent to the Amazon; Dearing reported in the despatch above that "this delay is in line with the lack of military preparedness in general, not from a desire to avoid sending a warship through Brazilian waters. Peru has believed there would be no war and has done very little to prepare for it. Colombia is forcing the situation. Interior politics is to blame for much of the Peruvian delay, as the officials hesitate to take any action which might injure their own political fortunes." Dearing added: "It is possible that instructions from Lima to Loreto may precipitate war in spite of the fact that the overwhelming majority of Peruvian opinion heartily wishes to avoid war and is thoroughly frightened and surprised at the failure of the Colombians to back down." This possibility became nearer a reality on January 3, when Dearing reported that the Constituent Assembly rejected the Brazilian proposal and voted confidence in the government's position that Peru should resist Colombian attempts to retake Leticia. Dearing stated that troop movements had begun and the Minister of War had left that day for Iquitos. Telegram 2, from Lima, January 3, 1933. DS, 721.23/651.

52. Memorandum of conversation, December 21, 1932. DS, 721.23/637.

53. FR, 1933, IV, 400. Acting Secretary of State William R. Castle, Jr., instructed Dearing to stress with Peruvian officials that "the support of the invaders of Leticia by armed Peruvian forces is contrary to the obligations of the Peruvian Government under the Kellogg Pact and that

Peru should welcome means now offered for extricating herself from her untenable position." FR, 1933, IV, 400.

54. Telegram 13, from Lima, January 12, 1933. FR, 1933, IV, 401. Dearing's source was the Brazilian minister in Lima. Dearing reported that Manzanilla, "infuriated by our note, has approached Dean of Diplomatic Corps trying to make an incident out of the way the note was presented." However, the Dean, the Papal Nuncio, "recognizes it as trivial and merely an exhibition of temperament." Telegram 15, from Lima, January 12, 1933. DS, 721.23/717. Manzanilla's charges, according to the Nuncio, were that Dearing had "come alone to the first reception he had given for the purpose of presenting the members of the Diplomatic Corps to his wife, that I had not been suitably dressed, and that I had insisted upon his reading immediately the note." Dearing's explanation was that his wife had not attended because the Embassy was in mourning following the death of former President Coolidge, that he had worn a dark gray suit, and that he had with some misgivings given the note to Manzanilla at the reception, saying that it was important, but had not asked him to read it immediately. Despatch 2517, from Lima, January 12, 1933. DS, 721.23/799. The incident was no more than a minor flurry, but the Foreign Minister's anger at the United States "pressure" seems to have been real.

55. Note of January 14, 1933. FR, 1933, IV, 404–5.

56. See FR, 1933, IV, 409–11, for text of the Peruvian note of January 16, to Brazil, and FR, 1933, IV, 413, for telegram 21, from Bogotá, January 21, 1933. The text of the Brazilian offer of January 13, is given in FR, 1933, IV, 408–9.

57. The proposal of December 30 provided that Brazil would return Leticia to Colombia if Colombia agreed to undertake negotiations in Rio de Janeiro to settle the dispute. This proposal Colombia accepted. However, the January 13 proposal to Peru did not provide for the return of Leticia to Colombia, and, in addition, it stated that Colombia and Peru would meet in Rio de Janeiro for the purpose "of considering the Salomón-Lozano Treaty," with the implication that that treaty might be replaced by another "territorial statute."

58. Commenting on this effort of Mello Franco to employ the *fait accompli* as a mediatory technique, Second Secretary Allan Dawson in Bogotá stated: "It seems probable that the Brazilian Foreign Minister, having been successful in securing acceptance by Colombia of the substance of the formula originally presented by him and having met with failure in his efforts with Peru, thought that it might be possible to take advantage of the more conciliatory temper of the Colombian Government by presenting to the Peruvian Government a formula somewhat more favorable to it than that accepted by Colombia with the incorrect assurance that Colombia had accepted the modified formula; Dr. Mello Franco apparently realized that if Peru accepted the modified formula, Colombia would be placed in a position where it would be very difficult for it not to accept it also. Without definite knowledge of the public temper here

it would seem safe to rely on the Colombian Government's earnest desire for peace to cause it to make concessions. If Dr. Mello Franco's maneuver succeeded, his prestige, as the guiding genius of the settlement of a delicate international question, would be greatly enhanced; otherwise, if the Brazilian negotiations failed, as they seemed about to do, his prestige would naturally suffer." Despatch 5102, from Bogotá, January 26, 1933. DS, 721.23/947.

59. Despatch 2532, from Lima, January 16, 1933. Received January 26. DS, 721.23/884.

60. Memorandum of conversation, November 16, 1932. DS, 721.23/492. In the course of this talk, which apparently became heated on more than one occasion, despite White's cool account, White said that once Maúrtua "flew off and said that the United States would never be able to get the countries of America to join in any declaration against Peru, as happened in the case of Bolivia and Paraguay." White replied that he would reserve a discussion of that until the point should come up. White also told Maúrtua: "I had no patience with an argument based on the premise that the people of a country [Peru] had risen up and could not be controlled. In that event the Government was not a government at all and it did not control its territory unless it denounced the action of its people and called on them to evacuate the foreign territory."

61. Text attached to memorandum of conversation between White and Lozano Torrijos and Guzmán, December 16, 1932. DS, 721.23/635.

62. Memorandum of conversation with Lozano Torrijos, December 21, 1932. DS, 721.23/638. At this interview, White told Lozano of Maúrtua's plan (p. 195) and said he "thought it had great promise and that it offered a far better chance of a satisfactory solution than procedure along the lines we had just been discussing." It is clear that White's hopes had been seriously raised by what he thought was a straightforward move by Maúrtua; his strong endorsement of the plan added to his embarrassment when he learned he had been tricked. It is possible that this episode, as well as the Colombian refusal to accept the jurisdiction of the permanent commission in Washington, may have influenced Jacobo Varela Acevedo to take the unusual step of going over White's head to Secretary Stimson to ask if he would "personally take the matter up with Mr. White and see what could be done." Memorandum by the Secretary of State, January 5, 1933. FR, 1933, IV, 385–86. Varela was the Uruguayan member of the commission.

63. Telegram 10, from Bogotá, January 9, 1933. DS, 721.23/686. This "ultimatum" was said by Dearing to have been "somewhat unsatisfactorily disavowed" by Sánchez Cerro and Manzanilla to the Brazilian Minister in Lima. Telegram 12, from Lima, January 11, 1933. DS, 721.23/708.

64. FR, 1933, IV, 418–19.

65. FR, 1933, IV, 421–22. Memorandum by the Assistant Secretary of State (White), and Comment thereon by the Secretary of State. White's memorandum contains discussion arising from questions asked by some of the ambassadors. Stimson commented: "While the foregoing accords with my recollection as to the ultimate facts stated and agreed upon, the mat-

ter was presented much less abruptly and forcibly than would appear from this. First of all the facts as presented in the Colombian-Peruvian correspondence was [*sic*] brought out gradually and discussed by question and answer in reference to the obligations of the Kellogg Pact, and then the conclusions were gradually summed up with the apparent concurrence of every one present, even the Japanese Ambassador made no dissent and several times nodded his head. The British Ambassador seemed to have considerable antecedent acquaintance with the situation." When asked at his press conference on January 25 why he had asked these five ambassadors to confer with him, Stimson replied that "he consulted the representatives of the same powers which he consulted a few years ago regarding the Kellogg Pact. Furthermore, the representatives of those five countries represent the powers who have been most prominent in regard to the Kellogg Treaty. Furthermore, they were easier to reach at the moment than were the others." Memorandum of the press conference, Wednesday, January 25, 1933. No. 20. DS, 721.23/988.

66. Text in FR, 1933, IV, 423–28. Asked by a correspondent at his press conference "if there was any question at all as to the Secretary's having invoked the Kellogg Pact in his recent note to Peru," Stimson replied that "if the correspondent would tell him just what he meant by invoking the Kellogg Pact he would be glad to answer that question . . . he did not know just what was meant by the words 'invoking the Pact.'" He said that Colombia had sent a note to the Department, and "he would say in this case, as his interpretation, that Colombia had invoked the Pact and had asked us to take the same action which she requested of the other nations." Memorandum of the press conference, Thursday, January 26, 1933, No. 21. DS, 721.23/987.

67. FR, 1933, IV, 429–30. Gilbert reported that he had sent word to Drummond of the gist of Stimson's note to Peru during the session at which the above cables were discussed. It is not clear whether Drummond informed the Council members of the note at that time. Later, on the same day, Drummond asked that the note be formally communicated to him so he could circulate it, and this was immediately authorized by the Department of State. FR, 1933, IV, 429–31.

68. *El Comercio* (Lima), on January 5, carried an article stating that the Colombian expedition was like the tower of Babel, made up of soldiers of many nationalities. There were, however, some foreigners also in the service of Peru. It was reported that a French military adviser was assisting the Peruvian army command and that an Englishman with the rank of colonel was superintending military transport on the main trail down the eastern slope of the Andes. Despatch 2751, from Lima, April 7, 1933. DS, 721.23/1586. Persistent rumors that Japanese engineers were laying mines in the Amazon near Leticia were not proved. These and other rumors came from Colombian sources and may have been part of a campaign to enlist sympathy in the United States. The Ambassador in Japan, Joseph Grew, later reported that the embassy had been told that the Colombian minister in Tokyo "was alleging in Tokyo diplomatic circles that by frightening the United States, through the American Ambassador at

Tokyo, with threats of Japanese colonization in Colombia in return for Japan's support for Colombia in the Leticia dispute, he had succeeded in enlisting the aid of the United States in forcing acceptance of the settlement of the dispute upon Peru." Grew noted that the Colombian minister had said nothing to him on this subject, and that the allegations, if they had been made, were "obviously unfounded." Despatch 951, from Tokyo, September 5, 1934. DS, 721.23/2379. The minister may have been merely trying to enhance his reputation, but the incident demonstrates that the notion of exploiting the potentialities of existing United States–Japanese relations was not unfamiliar in Latin American diplomatic circles. Note may be made in this connection of an article in *El Perú Ilustrado* (Lima) of March 29, 1933, stating that " 'in view of the similar conflicts arising in Manchuria and in Leticia, which have been treated with the same intransigence by the League of Nations and by the United States, Peru and Japan feel the need of uniting themselves and inaugurating a healthy and frank cooperation. The presence of the Japanese in Manchuria, like the presence of Peruvians in Leticia, does not arise from capricious motives but from a serious economic necessity. . . . Peruvians and Japanese, let us work together for the triumph of our just aspirations.' " Quoted in Despatch 2727, from Lima, March 31, 1933. DS, 721.23/1551.

69. FR, 1933, IV, 434–37.

70. Note of January 30, 1933. FR, 1933, IV, 439.

71. Note of January 31, 1933. FR, 1933, IV, 440.

72. This request was sent to twelve Latin American countries. FR, 1933, IV, 441.

73. FR, 1933, IV, 451, n. 89.

74. Telegram 30, from Santiago, February 10, 1933. FR, 1933, IV, 471–72. Culbertson added: "Obviously the point is more clever than it is sound."

75. Letter from Francis White to the Counselor of American Embassy in England (Ray Atherton), February 4, 1933. DS, 721.23/998.

76. *Aide mémoire* by the Department of State to the French Embassy, February 9, 1933. DS, 721.23/1208.

77. Memorandum by the Chief of the Division of Latin American Affairs (Edwin C. Wilson), January 27, 1933. FR, 1933, IV, 431–33.

78. Telegram 25, to London, February 1, 1933. FR, 1933, IV, 441–43. White and Stimson were seriously concerned about the British plan. White cabled Dearing: "Department has been very much disturbed by this proposal as it indicates a disposition on the part of the British to further the Peruvian aim to force at least an arbitration regarding sovereignty over Leticia and the British Government appears to be taking no action on the request of Colombia that it call Peru's attention to her obligations under the Kellogg Pact." Telegram 23, to Lima, February 1, 1933. DS, 721.23/936. It does not appear, however, that London was motivated by any desire other than to make what it regarded as a more practical move toward peace than had so far been offered. The British minister in Lima, said Dearing, had the "feeling that since the arbitration would unquestionably assign the territory to Colombia, Colombia could afford to

agree beforehand to an arbitration, and Peru would be able to save her face, get out of the situation and remove the difficuly of Loreto." Despatch 2579, from Lima, February 3, 1933. DS, 721.23/1123. Manzanilla apparently gave the minister the impression that the British plan would be acceptable to Peru, but Dearing thought that Manzanilla had hoodwinked the minister, as a means of confusing the situation and so gaining time in the struggle to get the treaty revised. He also thought Lima did not want to "build bridges" or "save its face"; it desired to use any and all methods to hold on to Leticia.

79. Telegram 21, from London, February 3, 1933. FR, IV, 448–49. In his message to the Chargé in Washington, for delivery to Stimson, Sir John said: "The juridical arguments set forth in the note from the United States Government, have throughout been present to our minds. Our primary object however was to prevent a conflict and believing that Peru only needs a bridge over which to retreat, we consider that such an avenue of escape can be provided with less danger to the sanctity of treaties than would be involved in an armed conflict between the two countries." Despatch 643, from London, February 3, 1933. DS, 721.23/1121. The acidity of this appeal to realism was diluted by the Foreign Minister's decision to drop his proposal.

80. Despatch 2579, from Lima, February 3, 1933. DS, 721.23/1123. These various notes are referred to above, pp. 204–5.

81. Telegram 51, from Lima, January 31, 1933. DS, 721.23/935. In his despatch supplementing this cable, Dearing said that "unless we can make use of a real and compelling restraint in some form or another . . . we must abandon any hope of bringing about any change for the better" in Sánchez Cerro's attitude; however, he did not suggest that such restraint be exercised. Despatch 2569, from Lima, January 31, 1933. DS, 721.23/1094.

82. Telegram 68, from Lima, February 6, 1933. FR, 1933, IV, 457–58.

83. Telegram 41, from Lima, January 26, 1933. DS, 721.23/853.

84. Telegram 9, from Bogotá, January 9, 1933. FR, 1933, IV, 398. It is probable that the decision to go up the Putumayo to Tarapacá was made as early as Vásquez Cobo's stop at Manaos. The German-born chief pilot of the SCADTA airlines in Colombia reports that he took part in talks resulting in the dissuasion of Vásquez Cobo from sailing directly for Leticia. See Boy, *Una historia con alas*, pp. 200f. From Boy's account, it would appear that control of the air over the Putumayo both at Tarapacá and later at Güepi was of major importance in Colombia's military victories over Peruvian troops. On the fight at Güepi, see the account by J. Lozano y Lozano, *La patria y yo*.

85. Telegram 12, from Bogotá, January 10, 1933. DS, 721.23/691. García Calderón was said to have told Mello Franco that the vote of confidence in the government of Peru, passed by the Constituent Assembly on January 3, had been based on his mistaken report that the Mello Franco formula contained the provision that Leticia would be returned to Peru if negotiations should fail. Despatch 5020, from Bogotá, January 11, 1933. DS, 721.23/774.

86. Telegram 5, from Lima, January 10, 1933. DS, 721.23/692.

87. Telegram 18, from Lima, January 13, 1933. DS, 721.23/730.

88. Despatch 2540, from Lima, January 20, 1933. DS, 721.23/889. The text of the note of January 16 is in FR, 1933, IV, 409–11. This note is a good example of the able fashion in which Manzanilla exploited the resources of diplomacy for purposes of delay.

89. Telegram 18, to Rio de Janeiro, January 30, 1933. FR, 1933, IV, 439–40.

90. Telegram 25, to Rio de Janeiro, February 10, 1933. FR, 1933, IV, 469–70. This proposal had been sent to Rio on February 6.

91. Memorandum of telephone conversation between White and Chargé Walter Thurston in Rio de Janeiro, February 6, 1933, FR, 1933, IV, 453–55; telegram 27, from Bogotá, February 6, 1933, FR, 1933, IV, 456; telegram 18, to Bogotá, February 6, 1933, FR, 1933, IV, 460; telegram 28, from Bogotá, February 7, 1933, FR, 1933, IV, 463.

92. Telegram 28 from Bogotá, February 7, 1933, FR, 1933, IV, 463. Caffery added that he "must emphasize" his telegram of January 9 (see note 84), warning that the patience of Colombian opinion was nearly exhausted.

93. Telegram 29, from Bogotá, February 9, 1933. FR, 1933, IV, 469. The Santos referred to was Eduardo Santos, Colombian representative at the League of Nations, and, as director of *El Tiempo*, the leading Liberal newspaper in Colombia, a powerful influence on Colombian public opinion. Caffery advised: "The Department will readily understand that it would be very serious for President Olaya to have *El Tiempo* turn against him at this juncture." Despatch 5163, from Bogotá, February 9, 1933. DS, 721.23/1162.

94. Telegram 25, to Rio de Janeiro, February 10, 1933, 11 A.M. FR, 1933, IV, 469.

95. Text of telegram 19, from Rio de Janeiro, February 10, 1933, received 2:10 P.M., in FR, 1933, IV, 470–71.

96. Telegram 26, to Rio de Janeiro, February 10, 1933, 6 P.M. FR, 1933, IV, 472–73. Washington's position was entirely clear since it was also stated that "until the new Brazilian proposal is straightened out in the sense of the above this Government will make no representations in support thereof."

97. Telegram 29, to Rio de Janeiro, February 11, 1933. FR, 1933, IV, 473–74.

98. Telegram 23, from Rio de Janeiro, February 13, 1933. FR, 1933, IV, 475. The other main point at issue was the use of the term "compensation" in referring to Colombia's agreement to enter negotiations immediately. Mello Franco took the unassailable position that in Portuguese *compensação* did not have the same meaning as *compensation* in English, so that Colombia should not be concerned about appearing to be willing to negotiate in return for Peru's agreement to surrender Leticia to Brazil. Mello Franco, having sent copies of his note of February 10 to the other American states, did not feel he could later change it at Stimson's behest.

99. Telegrams 37 and 38, from Bogotá, February 14 and 15, 1933. FR,

1933, IV, 477, 478. The Colombian version of the encounter is given in the telegram from Foreign Minister Roberto Urdaneta Arbeláez to Secretary Stimson, FR, 1933, IV, 476, February 14, 1933. This version was substantially corroborated by the reports of Major William Sackville, United States Military Attaché in Brazil, who visited the Leticia area later. Memorandum by H. Freeman Matthews, May 6, 1933, DS, 721.23/1697 and report by Major Sackville, April 12, 1933, DS, 721.23/1697, from Manaos. Major Sackville stated: "The capture was accomplished without apparent opposition, as no Peruvians could be found." The Peruvian side of the case, reported by Dearing, was that "Colombian vessels had fired from Brazilian waters upon Peruvian troops in Tarapacá and had retired to Brazilian waters after the engagement." Telegram 82, from Lima, February 15, 1933. FR, 1933, IV, 478–79.

100. Despatch 5455, from Bogotá, April 8, 1933. DS, 721.23/1602.

101. Despatch 3193, from Lima, December 16, 1933. DS, 721.23/2070. The disease was known as Putumayo fever. Dearing's figures were obtained from "a trustworthy source in Iquitos."

102. Memorandum of conversation with George Rublee, February 15, 1933. DS, 721.23/1333.

103. Telegram 29, to Bogotá, February 17, 1933. FR, 1933, IV, 482.

104. Telegram 35, to Rio de Janeiro, February 17, 1933, and telegrams 27 and 28, from Rio de Janeiro, February 18 and 20, 1933. FR, 1933, IV, 482, 484–85. Major Sackville was instructed that the Department's purpose in sending him to the "area of hostilities is to get accurate and impartial information regarding the situation there."

VIII. Pacification

1. Memorandum to Francis White, February 14, 1933. DS, 721.23/1198.

2. Memorandum of conversation between H. F. Matthews and Pomponio Guzmán, special representative of Colombia, March 3, 1933. DS, 721.23/1396. Guzmán argued that, since the United States had in effect said that Peru had violated the Pact, and that, "if the violator of the Pact was to be treated equally with victim of her aggression, in other words, if the Department were to be 'neutral' he didn't see what advantage was to be gained from observation of the obligations of the Pact," or how the violator would be deprived of the "benefits" of the Pact. Matthews's reply was that "there was nothing which we could do about such munitions passing through the Canal."

3. Despatch 884, from Quito, February 13, 1933. DS, 721.23/1235. Dr. Guerrero's assertion was incorrect, since the Sánchez Cerro regime had strongly resented the appeals of the United States concerning Leticia. Even before Stimson's note of January 25, Dearing had proposed, through a mutual friend, a talk with one of Sánchez Cerro's close associates; the latter had replied that "the feeling in the Government against our Government and this Embassy is so strong that he did not think a talk would be of any use. . . . He stated that our country was considered to have

taken the Colombian side." Despatch 2550, from Lima, January 24, 1933. DS, 721.23/979.

4. Telegram 39, from Bogotá, February 15, 1933. FR, 1933, IV, 479.

5. Telegrams 90 and 91, from Lima, February 19, 1933. FR, 1933, IV, 550–51. Dearing stated that the publication on February 18 of news that the United States had accepted Colombia's request to assume charge of Colombian interests in Peru "lends a sinister significance to mob's attack." See also Woolsey, *The Destruction of the Colombian Legation at Lima, Peru, February 18, 1933: A Disgrace to History*. Woolsey, a prominent international lawyer, asserted that the evidence "points to the implication of Peruvian authorities in the outrageous assault" (p. 40).

6. FR, 1933, IV, 551. The reasons given by Dearing for this suggestion were the "Government's failure or disinclination to give protection last night, the large number of Americans here, the Government's direct enmity to us, its threat to force foreign companies to contribute to war funds, and the general uncertainties."

7. Telegram 36, to Lima, February 20, 1933. FR, 1933, IV, 552.

8. Despatch 2637, from Lima, February 22, 1933. DS, 721.23/1358.

9. Note of February 20, 1933. FR, 1933, IV, 485–88.

10. Note of February 25, 1933. FR, 1933, IV, 492. The text of the Council's plan is in telegram 124, from Geneva, February 23, 1933, FR, 1933, IV, 490.

11. Telegram 82, from Lima, February 15, 1933. FR, 1933, IV, 478–79. Dearing added that on February 14, they "again present Peruvian thesis in all its wrongness." Dearing considered that the Miró Quesada family's influence was anti-United States as well as anti-Leguía, and he frequently referred to its behind-the-scenes activities. See, for example, despatches 2500, 2508, 2529, 2533, 2577; January 7, 11, 16, 16, and February 3, 1933. DS, 721.23/744, 721.23/794, 721.23/826, 721.23/885, and 721.23/1096.

12. Quoted in despatch 2755, from Lima, April 7, 1933. DS, 721.23/1587.

13. Text in telegram 112, from Lima, March 9, 1933. DS, 721.23/1382. The cable from Dearing commented: "Embassy believes Society's message will be beneficial for the protection of American interests."

14. Despatch 2673, from Lima, March 5, 1933. DS, 721.23/1406, and telegram 110, March 7, 1933, DS, 721.23/1362. The Embassy apparently considered that the transmission of such a message, particularly when its inspiration was known, could do no harm, and it might ease somewhat the relationship between the Peruvian government and the business firms, who were under some pressure to make loans or contributions to promote Peruvian war preparations or to aid the government in other ways.

15. Henry L. Stimson and McGeorge Bundy, *On Active Service in Peace and War* (New York, Harper, 1947), pp. 292–93, and New York *Times*, January 17, 1933.

16. A communication to the Department from the All-American Anti-Imperialist League on November 30, 1932, may be quoted in part as representative of perhaps the leading sector of opinion opposed to the Department's policy. "WHEREAS, these wars between Bolivia and Paraguay

and between Colombia and Peru are directly instigated by American and British Imperialism through their native puppet governments in rivalry of these imperialist powers for domination and exploitation of South America as an attempt to find a way out of the crisis at the expense of the toiling masses. BE IT THEREFORE RESOLVED, that we protest most vehemently against these bloody imperialist wars, that we declare our solidarity with the mass demonstration against war in Bolivia, that we declare our solidarity with the refusal of Paraguay soldiers to shoot down Bolivian soldiers and with the *Anti-War Congress* in South America, that we denounce the sale of the S.S. Bridgeport to Colombia by American imperialism and the supplying of United States military instructors to the Bolivian army, that we demand cessation of the shipment of munitions from the United States to the warring countries." The characteristic misrepresentations of this document demonstrated the source of its political inspiration, and it had of course no influence in Washington. A resolution in almost identical terms was also received on November 27 from the Latin American Affairs Committee of the National Student League. DS, 810.43 Anti-Imperialistic League/118.

17. Despatch 5150, from Bogotá, February 6, 1933. DS, 721.23/1239.

18. Quoted in editorial in *Mundo Al Día* (Bogotá), April 17, 1933, citied in despatch 5478, from Bogotá, April 18, 1933. DS, 721.23/1636. Caffery commented: "This editorial is typical of the change of attitude in Colombia toward the United States which has been evident for some time, and particularly since the Leticia incident."

19. FR, 1933, IV, 493, February 27, 1933. Text of the proposal in FR, 1933, IV, 490–91. This position was firmly upheld by White in a talk with Freyre on March 3. He said that "the League proposal was made without consultation with us. . . . We were asked to support it and as we found the proposal a fair one we had cabled our support thereof to both Peru and Colombia, This was a matter which the League was handling and which we came into only incidentally at their request to support their proposal because we thought it offered an honorable way out." Freyre asked that, if the League should change its plan, the Department "would recommend to both countries the acceptance thereof." White did not fall into this trap; he said he could not tell Freyre "that we would be in favor of a change in the League plan which he might then cable to Geneva and might be understood as our advocating a change in the plan. I said that that was not the case at all but that any solution acceptable to both Peru and Colombia would be welcomed by us. . . . For the moment I saw no prospect better than acceptance of the present League proposal." Memorandum of conversation, March 3, 1933. DS, 721.23/1419.

20. Telegram 88, to Geneva, March 15, 1933, and telegram 154, from Geneva, March 18, 1933. FR, 1933, IV, 499. This was the same arrangement as had been made for Wilson's participation in the work of the Advisory Committee established to deal with the Manchurian question; telegram 86, to Geneva, March 11, 1933, FR, Japan, 1931–1941, I, 117–18. On the League's activity in general see the account in Russell M. Cooper,

American Consultation in World Affairs (New York, Macmillan, 1934), Chap. VI; and League of Nations, Council, *The Verdict of the League: Colombia and Peru at Leticia.* For a Colombian attack on the "naive cosmopolitan bureaucracy" of Geneva, see Villegas, *De Ginebra a Río de Janeiro.*

21. Telegram 156, from Geneva, March 22 1933. FR, 1933, IV, 509.

22. *Ibid.;* see also FR, 1933, III, 231–34, for discussion of arms embargoes in connection with the Leticia and Manchurian questions; *Aide mémoire* to the British Embassy, March 11, 1933; telegram 85, to Geneva, March 11, 1933.

23. Quoted in despatch 5427, from Bogotá, March 30, 1933. DS, 721.23/1538.

24. Telegrams 92 and 95, from Lima, February 20 and 21, 1933. FR, 1933, IV, 551, 554. Dearing reported: "*Comercio* estimates 100,000 participants, which is possibly an exaggeration. People seemingly took occasion as a holiday. Enthusiasm shown due chiefly to fostering by the Government and *Comercio's* campaign and can be regarded as spontaneous only to a moderate degree. Nevertheless Government for the moment has a certain moral advantage and mandate making its task easier."

25. Despatch 2671, from Lima, March 3, 1933. DS, 721.23/1390.

26. Despatches 5298, 5300, 5311, from Bogotá, March 3, 7, 1933. DS, 721.23/1399.

27. Despatch 5257, from Bogotá, February 24, 1933. DS, 721.23/1375.

28. Memorandum of talk with Pomponio Guzmán, in telegram 26, to Bogotá, February 15, 1933. FR, 1933, IV, 479–80.

29. Telegram 40, from Bogotá, February 16, 1933. FR, 1933, IV, 480–81.

30. Despatches 5322, 5361, from Bogotá, March 8, 17, 1933. DS, 721.23/1473, 1466. Caffery said, however: "I admit that if the Peruvians attack Colombian boats on the Putumayo River the Colombian forces certainly have the right of defending themselves." Both Stimson and Caffery made it clear that the decision was one for Colombia to make for itself.

31. New York *Times*, March 27, 28, 29, 31, April 18, 1933, and telegram 185, from Geneva, May 22, 1933, FR, 1933, IV, 536.

32. Text of this plan in telegram 167, from Geneva, April 7, 1933, FR, 1933, IV, 513–15. Sean Lester, the representative of Eire, was chairman of the Advisory Committee.

33. This view was also taken by William C. Burdett, First Secretary of Embassy in Lima, who commented: "The Lester suggestion seems to be merely another astute move of Manzanilla to cloud the real issue and to emerge creditably from a wrong position." Despatch 2766, from Lima, April 14, 1933. DS, 721.23/1605. The Department of State declared that it had "reason to believe that instead of the British urging the Peruvians to accept the earlier formula [Lester modifications], Peru prevailed upon the British to urge Colombian acceptance thereof. . . . The British Minister at Lima appears to be greatly influenced by the Peruvian Foreign Minister: in fact, the British Minister at Bogotá recently informed Mr. Caffery in strict confidence that the British Minister at Lima QUOTE had gone so

far as to say (in effect) in a report to the British Foreign Office that the 1922 Treaty was really not completely binding on Peru because it had been imposed on Peru by force by the United States END QUOTE. (The charge is of course utterly without foundation.)" Telegram 86, to London, May 2, 1933. DS, 721.23/1644.

34. Despatch 5496, from Bogotá, April 25, 1933. DS, 721.23/1674. Urdaneta asked Caffery if he thought the British had received a promise of some concession in Peru; Caffery said he did not believe that was the case but suggested to the Department that the British attitude might have resulted from "considerations connected with Anglo-Irish relations." (Sean Lester was the representative of the Irish Free State on the Council.) Later, Colombian "suspicions regarding the attitude of the British Government during the latter stages of the negotiations for a settlement of the Leticia incident" were reported to be responsible for Colombian opposition at Geneva to the appointment of a British member of the Leticia commission; Colombia also objected to the appointment of an Italian member. Despatch 5602, from Bogotá, May 26, 1933. FR, 1933, IV, 538–39.

35. Telegram 40, to Bogotá, April 8, 1933. FR, 1933, IV, 515–16.

36. Telegram 44, from Bogotá, April 11, 1933; received 11:25 P.M., April 11. FR, 1933, IV, 516–17. Olaya had emphasized that "no government here can possibly enter into any agreement that does not provide first for the recovery of Leticia (as March 18th recommendations did)." Caffery added that Lima had asked Argentina to sponsor the Lester plan. Olaya's position was that he would be happy to end hostilities. "However," wrote Caffery, "it is clear that he will not do so unless he can do so with honor and by 'honor' he means the restoration of Leticia to Colombian sovereignty. He feels very strongly on this point. He . . . would prefer losing the territory by war than to be cheated out of it by any sort of diplomatic negotiations. When he made the remark, he had in mind the recent Lester modifications. I do not believe that his extreme indignation at the Lester proposals is justified, but the fact is that the indignation exists." Despatch 5465, from Bogotá, April 11, 1933. DS, 721.23/1593.

37. Memorandum of conversation, April 13, 1933. FR, 1933, IV, 518–19.

38. This account of Manzanilla's plans is based on a memorandum supplied to Dearing. Despatch 2790, from Lima, April 27, 1933. DS, 721.23/1676.

39. Despatch 2790, from Lima, April 27, 1933. DS, 721.23/1676. Dearing reported that he had made no comment when this suggestion was made to him.

40. Telegram 46, from Bogotá, April 21, 1933. FR, 1933, IV, 520–21. This cable gives the full text of the Colombian response.

41. Telegrams 80 and 96, to London and Geneva, April 27, 1933. FR, 1933, IV, 521.

42. Telegram 42, to Bogotá, May 3, 1933. FR, 1933, IV, 522.

43. Telegram 96, from London, May 3, 1933. FR, 1933, IV, 523–24.

This position was similar to that expressed by Sir John Simon in presenting the first British suggestion, before Tarapacá. Craigie's remark about "purely academic and legal viewpoints" was apparently directed both at Colombian and United States policy.

44. Report by Caffery, despatch 5465, from Bogotá, April 11, 1933. DS, 721.23/1593. The Peruvian forces were also meeting difficulties. Soldiers accustomed to mountain conditions fell victims of disease in the Amazonian lowlands. The obstacles to supplying Puerto Arturo by land from Leticia were so great that military men in Lima were reported to be advising a withdrawal from the Putumayo port. Because of the shortage of planes and the absence of road communications with Iquitos, it was not possible to send more than "a few dozen men per day from the mountains to Loreto." Report by Burdett from Lima, despatch 2766, April 14, 1933. DS, 721.23/1605.

45. Report by the U.S. Military Attaché in Colombia, April 24, 1933. DS, 721.23/1788. Olaya had visited Vásquez Cobo at La Esperanza; it seems probable that the decision that the General should not visit Bogotá was made principally for reasons of internal politics.

46. Telegram 99, to Geneva, May 9, 1933, and note 69. FR, 1933, IV, 525. Also letter from the Secretary of War to the Secretary of State, May 2, 1933. DS, 721.23/1691.

47. Letter from the Secretary of State to the Secretary of the Navy, January 20, 1933. FR, 1933, IV, 412–13. Also, telegram 18, to Lima, January 19, 1933. DS, 721.23/860.

48. Telegram 99, to Geneva, May 9, 1933. FR, 1933, IV, 525. Olaya told Caffery that he was satisfied with the Department's handling of the *Grau's* transit of the Canal. Despatch 5537, from Bogotá, May 6, 1933. DS, 721.23/1701.

49. On May 3, a new move had been made in London, with the presentation to Santos of the "Craigie formula," changing the Lester modifications slightly in the direction desired by Bogotá but failing to provide specifically for the return of Leticia to Colombia. Urdaneta told Caffery that the formula "implied that Colombia should put its case in the hands of the League, in other words in those of the British Foreign Office, and Colombia trusted neither of them." Despatches 5538, 5539, from Bogotá, May 6, 1933. DS, 721.23/1702.

50. Memorandum by Edwin C. Wilson of talk with George Rublee, May 5, 1933. FR, 1933, IV, 524. Wilson and Rublee agreed that there was nothing useful the United States could do at the moment.

51. The assassin, Abelardo Hurtado de Leiva, appears to have acted from political motives unconnected with the Leticia dispute. Alfonso Reyes commented that the assassination was an act that many Peruvians considered as a "national execution." Reyes, *La conferencia colombo-peruana para el arreglo del incidente de Leticia*, p. 1. See also, however, Miró Quesada Laos, *Sánchez Cerro y su tiempo*, for a sympathetic defense of the dictator and for praise of his determination to continue the struggle over Leticia for "the honor of the nation" (p. 286). The restraint of the United States government in dealing with Peru is suggested by the follow-

ing judgment of one of its senior officials: "The Sánchez Cerro regime is thoroughly unscrupulous and its brutal massacre of its own citizens after the Trujillo uprising of last year has shown its complete want of humanity. It has undoubtedly victimized foreigners and foreign interests as far as it felt that it could with impunity, and Americans being the most important foreign element have suffered accordingly." Memorandum, April 21, 1933. DS, 823.00/960.

52. Despatch 2724, from Lima, March 27, 1933. DS, 721.23/1529.

53. This fact invites speculation about the possible influence on Sánchez Cerro's policy of an acrimonious debate with Vásquez Cobo some years previously during which the discussion got so heated that, when Sánchez Cerro reached into a back pocket to get a calling card, Vásquez Cobo thought he was reaching for a pistol. Memorandum of conversation between Francis White and Freyre, January 13, 1933. FR, 1933, IV, 401–3. This memorandum also contains a bit of diplomatic gossip about bad feeling between Maúrtua and Olaya. The above story gave some color to a rumor reported from Rio de Janeiro that Sánchez Cerro had talked about flying to Leticia to challenge Vásquez Cobo to a duel. Memorandum of telephone conversation between White and Morgan, January 7, 1933. DS, 721.23/724.

54. Telegram 178, from Geneva, May 10, 1933. FR, 1933, IV, 525–27. The Peruvian government protested to the Netherlands because drydocking had been refused; the Dutch apparently followed a policy similar to that of the United States.

55. Text of the proposal in FR, 1933, IV, 526–27.

56. Telegrams 45 and 59, to Bogotá, Lima, May 11, 1933. FR, 1933, IV, 527–28.

57. Telegrams 141, from Lima, and 61, to Lima, May 12 and 13, 1933. FR, 1933, IV, 529–30.

58. Telegram 180, from Geneva, May 13, 1933. FR, 1933, IV, 530–31. This telegram summarized a discussion in the Advisory Committee about policies of League members on the treatment of the Peruvian warships. Sir Eric Drummond said that "in his opinion Peru was playing for time until the squadron could arrive in the Upper Amazon; that giving of facilities to the warships was playing Peru's game; that withholding of facilities and delaying the arrival of the Peruvian fleet was the best support possible for the Committee's proposals of settlement." The British government was apparently reluctant to refuse facilities for fear of creating a precedent that might be used against its own vessels in future. It had sent instructions to Trinidad to refuse facilities to the ships, but the instructions had not arrived in time.

59. Despatch 5564, from Bogotá, May 12, 1933. DS, 721.23/1733. López's acceptance was sent with the approval of Olaya, although López did not go with governmental authority to negotiate.

60. Despatch 2848, from Lima, May 26, 1933. DS, 721.23/1803. These views could not have been expected to be held by Sánchez Cerro, whose disregard for public opinion abroad had been commented on by Dearing and had been manifest in his policy.

61. Telegram to Olaya, May 21, 1933, quoted in telegram 56, from Bogotá, May 22, 1933. DS, 721.23/1762.

62. The formula found to save Peruvian face was that Lima would be "confidentially apprised" of the "confidential letter from the President of the Council" to Bogotá. This subterfuge was probably of value to Benavides in holding off his political opponents, since the latter would not know that he was aware that Colombian troops would reoccupy Leticia under the aegis of the League. Telegram 178, from Geneva, May 10, 1933. FR, 1933, IV, 526.

63. Telegrams 185 and 187, from Geneva, May 22, 25, 1933. FR, 1933, IV, 535–38.

64. Despatch 2905, from Lima, July 7, 1933. FR, 1933, IV, 545.

65. Letter from the Secretary of State to the President, May 27, 1933. DS, 721.23/1784.

66. Despatch 2839, from Lima, May 22, 1933. DS, 721.23/1793. *El Comercio* was quoted as referring editorially to " 'the good impression caused by the termination of the conflict of Leticia according to diplomatic means which preserve the national dignity and guarantee a respect for the legitimate interests of Peru.' " Despatch 2866, from Lima, June 9, 1933. DS, 721.23/1844.

67. Despatch 5608, from Bogotá, May 27, 1933. DS, 721.23/1795.

68. Despatch 5815, from Bogotá, August 28, 1933. DS, 721.23/1956; and despatch 5462 from Bogotá, April 11, 1933. DS, 721.23/1590.

69. Despatch 53, from Bogotá, December 21, 1933. DS, 721.23/2076.

70. Memorandum of conversation, December 22, 1933. DS, 721.23/2085.

71. Memorandum of conversation, January 25, 1934. DS, 721.23/2102.

72. Telegram 16, from Rio de Janeiro, January 29, 1934. FR, 1934, IV, 321.

73. Telegram 27, from Rio de Janeiro, February 16, 1934. FR, 1934, IV, 323. The insertion of "prompt?" was made in the Department of State because of a garble in the code.

74. Despatch 107, from Bogotá, February 19, 1934. DS, 721.23/2131. The organization came to be known as the Export-Import Bank.

75. Despatch 109, from Bogotá, February 19, 1934. DS, 721.23/2133. Dawson commented that there were a considerable number of foreign technicians employed by Colombia in the area and that, apart from "military and attached personnel and Indians practically untouched by civilized influence," there were almost no Colombian civilians. "In the entire trip between Tarapacá and Caucayá (over 700 kilometers) not a single settlement was visible on the Colombian bank of the Putumayo." He considered that Colombian confidence in victory, if fighting should start again, was unjustified; their past success had been based on German pilots flying American-made planes, and on French artillerymen, and on the fact that the Peruvians they had previously defeated were less well trained and less steady than the regular troops which by this time had replaced them near Leticia.

76. Letter from Bogotá, February 20, and reply to Bogota, March 26, 1934. DS, 721.23/2145.

77. Despatch 108, from Bogotá, February 19, 1934. FR, 1934, IV, 323–24. The minister added that "all of the members of the Commission are of the opinion that immediately after Colombia has again assumed administration of Leticia an attack by Peruvian forces, either regular or irregular, is inevitable." The three commission members did not wish to remain in Leticia after June, although they thought that the term of the commission should be extended as the only way of keeping peace if the Rio talks failed.

78. Telegram 230, from Geneva, March 14, 1934. FR, 1934, IV, 325–27.
79. Telegram 135, to Geneva, March 17, 1934. FR, 1934, IV, 328.
80. Memorandum of conversation, March 19, 1934. DS, 721.23/2161.
81. Telegram 11, from Bogotá, March 19, 1934. DS, 721.23/2143. The reports from Peru at this time told also of haste in rearmament, partly encouraged by fear of arms embargoes such as that applied in the Chaco war. Peruvian arms purchases were said to be stimulated by President Benavides: "Apparently, he will concede much to the armed forces in order to insure the quiet internal conditions necessary to the resurgence of the nation." Despatch 3319, from Lima, March 19, 1934. DS, 721.23/2157.

82. Telegram 14, from Bogotá, March 22, 1934. DS, 721.23/2151. Earlier the foreign minister had hinted that Colombia would welcome it if the United States, in case war broke out, should declare that fighting would not be permitted in a zone on either side of the Panama Canal wide enough to include parts of the Colombian coastline. Despatch 137, from Bogotá, March 20, 1934. DS, 721.23/2156. Whitehouse transmitted at this time a memorandum from the foreign ministry, asserting that Peru was obtaining arms and technical assistance from Japan; these things had not at first appeared important, stated the memorandum, "but their repetition creates the impression of systematic activities which form part of a plan which, if developed, could profoundly disturb the normal life of this part of the continent." Despatch 136, from Bogotá, March 20, 1934. DS, 721.23/2154. Several despatches from Peru had reported rumors, but no confirmation, of Japanese arms sales to Peru. The Japanese consul in Bogotá officially denied, in a statement in *El País* (Bogotá), May 4, 1933, reports that two Japanese aviators were killed in the service of Peru and that Japan was furnishing arms and credits to Peru; he tried in general to discredit propaganda in Colombia that Japan was aiding Peru in various ways.

83. Telegram 232, from Geneva, March 29, 1934. FR, 1934, IV, 330–31. Among the points mentioned were a request to the League from Peru that the term of administration by the Leticia commission should be extended, and a protest by Peru against the commission's relinquishing Leticia to Colombian control, as an action that "would destroy the very basis of the Geneva Agreement, since the latter would have had no object if Peru had been disposed to hand over the territory of Leticia to Colombia."

84. Telegram 32, to Rio de Janeiro, April 4, 1934. FR, 1934, IV, 332–33.

85. Telegram 57, from Rio de Janeiro, April 5, 1934. FR, 1934, IV, 336–37.

86. Telegram 56, from Rio de Janeiro, April 5, 1934. FR, 1934, IV, 335.

87. This incident seems to have been typical of Maúrtua. Alfonso Reyes, who was in Rio de Janeiro at the time, remarked that Maúrtua was "a dangerous negotiator because of his excessive distrust of his adversary, his collaborators and himself." Reyes states that other members of the Peruvian delegation complained to Lima that Maúrtua "always gave three different versions of each point discussed—one to other Peruvian delegates, another to the Colombians, and a third to the government of Peru." Benavides finally sent Jorge Prado to Rio to bring order into the negotiations. Reyes, *La conferencia colombo-peruana para el arreglo del incidente de Leticia.*

88. Telegram 35, to Rio de Janeiro, April 6, 1934. FR, 1934, IV, 339. It appeared that Mello Franco had a reaction to Maúrtua's communications no less cautious than Francis White had earlier learned to cultivate.

89. *Ibid.*

90. Telegram 63, from Lima, May 8, 1934. DS, 721.23/2266.

91. Despatch 3343, from Lima, April 5, 1934. DS, 721.23/2195. Dearing's judgment, however, was that "neither the Loretanos nor the Peruvians at large desire to go to war." This view was supported by another high Peruvian official, who, however, pointed out that the government was being urged to maintain Sánchez Cerro's policy toward Leticia by some of the men who were responsible for the original incident. Despatch 3370, from Lima, April 17, 1934. DS, 721.23/2234. It was reported that "enthusiasm over the Sánchez Cerro policies is not translated into any desire to serve with the colors. The Government has prohibited the departure from Peru of young men of draft age, a step which has prevented an exodus of the young men of the better families of Lima." Despatch 2604, from Lima, February 10, 1933. DS, 721.23/1182.

92. Despatch 3370, from Lima, April 17, 1934. DS, 721.23/2234. Benavides spoke of the necessity to find an honorable solution at Rio. To his remark that Peru had offered Colombia at Rio "extensive territory in exchange" for Leticia, Dearing suggested that the territory in question would hardly compensate Colombia for its "doorway on the Amazon." This territory was the so-called Sucumbios triangle on the upper Putumayo, which Colombia had recognized as Peruvian in 1922 but which Peru had not been able to occupy as its own, pending the outcome of its territorial dispute with Ecuador.

93. Letter to the Secretary of War, July 7, 1933. DS, 721.23/1879. The Department did not, however, consider that the War Department should accede to a request by the Peruvian Chargé in Panama that a review of U.S. troops should be held for the officers of the *Almirante Grau.* Edwin C. Wilson noted that he had called the United States Legation in Panama to say "that we felt strongly that in view of the present status of Peruvian-Colombian relations it would be most inappropriate . . . to accede to the request." Note, attached to telegram 101, from Panama, August 1, 1933. DS, 721.23/1922. Although the review had already been announced

in the Panamanian press on August 2, the military authorities in Panama were able to call it off. They delicately arranged, instead, that a regiment of U.S. infantry marched past the Peruvian legation on its way to training maneuvers. Despatch 1607, from Panama, August 9, 1933. DS, 721.23/1936.

94. Memorandum of conversation by Edwin C. Wilson, April 6, 1934. FR, 1934, IV, 377–78. The law referred to was the United States neutrality statute, which was not in effect since there had been no declaration of war by Colombia or Peru, and no declaration of neutrality by the United States.

95. Press release, April 11, 1934. FR, 1934, IV, 381.

96. Instruction 46, to Bogotá, May 4, 1934, FR, 1934, IV, 387–88. The possibility that such pilots would themselves engage in hostilities for Colombia against Peru was explicitly recognized in this instruction, but the Department had done all it could under existing legislation. When reporting the Department's action in stopping the recruiting of combat flyers, Dearing said that President Benavides "expressed incredulity and was not to be appeased." Benavides was angry about a report that Colombia had offered a prize of $1,000 "to any American aviator for every Peruvian plane brought down and said he wondered whether he should not engage some American aviators himself and offer them a higher price for every Colombian plane brought down. He wondered what would happen if Americans should find themselves fighting each other!" Despatch 3373, from Lima, April 19, 1934. FR, 1934, IV, 384–86.

97. FR, 1934, IV, 384.

98. Telegram 31, to Lima, April 11, 1934. FR, 1934, IV, 380–81. That the officials at the Panama Canal held views differing from those expressed by the Department of State is suggested in the communication transmitted to Secretary Hull by Secretary of War George H. Dern. Letter of May 14, 1934. FR, 1934, IV, 388–89.

99. Despatch 3351, from Lima, April 11, 1934. DS, 721.23/2216.

100. Telegram 63, from Lima, May 8, 1934, DS, 721.23/2266, and despatch 3403, from Lima, May 10, 1934, DS, 721.23/2320. This explanation by Dearing may be compared with Secretary Hull's offer to Freyre of "a simple remark here or there," which has been mentioned earlier.

101. Gordon Ireland, *Boundaries, Possessions, and Conflicts in South America* (Cambridge, Mass., Harvard University Press, 1938), p. 204.

102. Despatch 3359, from Lima, April 12, 1934. DS, 721.23/2217.

103. Despatch 166, from Bogotá, August 2, 1935. DS, 721.23/2486.

104. Despatch 3429, from Lima, May 21, 1934. DS, 721.23/2335. See also Ulloa, who refers to "the defects of our military establishment" and states that President Benavides was aware that, "unfortunately, our country was not materially prepared for a war in the extraordinary conditions presented by the Amazonian terrain." Ulloa, *Posición internacional del Perú*, pp. 194, 196.

105. Memorandum of November 12, 1932. FR, 1932, V, 293.

106. Despatch 2360, from Lima, November 18, 1932. FR, 1932, V, 364–65.

107. Telegrams 18 and 40, to Bogotá and Lima, May 17, 1934. FR, 1934, IV, 356–57.
108. Despatch 3446, from Lima, June 3, 1934. DS, 721.23/2351.
109. Text in FR, 1934, IV, 361–69.
110. Telegrams from Washington, May 21, 1934, DS, 721.23/2319, and despatch 3429, from Lima, May 21, 1934, DS, 721.23/2335.
111. Despatch 3446, from Lima, June 3, 1934. DS, 721.23/2351. Dearing noted that Benavides accepted the congratulations of the diplomatic corps by saying that they were "merely a recognition of the justice and the rectitude of the Peruvian policy. The President's statement does not represent the facts . . . the record will show that Sánchez Cerro meant to have what he wanted or to wage war, and nothing President Benavides can say will ever alter this fact."
112. Telegram 46, from Bogotá, June 19, 1934. FR, 1934, IV, 369.
113. Despatch 481, from Bogotá, December 29, 1934. DS, 721.23/2421. It was "freely stated" in Bogotá that President López had offered diplomatic posts to Conservatives "in the hope that some of them might abstain from voting and allow the pact to pass. However, the Conservative Party shows unexpected signs of solidarity." Chargé Samuel W. Washington reported that among important factors in the situation were "Gómez' personal hatred of Olaya and Urdaneta . . . and the maneuvers of the Conservatives to increase their power over the Government. They may allow the Pact to pass after they have secured some concessions from the Liberals, but as yet they show no sign of being influenced by considerations of internationalism." Telegram 103, from Bogotá, December 12, 1934. FR, 1934, IV, 370–71. Lozano's opposition was understandable on the basis that he "is a fanatic on the subject of the Colombian-Peruvian boundary treaty which he regards as his life work." Memorandum, Department of State, June 14, 1933. DS, 721.23/1852.
114. Telegram 126, from Lima, December 13, 1934. FR, 1934, IV, 372. Chargé Washington reported that Olaya and Luis Cano thought that "inquiries from individual American nations and more especially from the appropriate committee of the League of Nations as to the present status" of the protocol might result in "a change in attitude on the part of those opposed." Telegram 106, from Bogotá, December 14, 1934. FR, 1934, IV, 373.
115. Telegram 71, to Bogotá, December 15, 1934. FR, 1934, IV, 374.
116. Despatch 481, from Bogotá, December 29, 1934. DS, 721.23/2421.
117. Telegram 114, from Bogotá, December 29, 1934. FR, 1934, IV, 376. Chargé Washington added that the "alleged forceful intervention of Brazil and the United States at the request of the President of Peru was the subject of criticism in the public session of the House of Representatives yesterday."
118. Telegram 3, from Bogotá, January 3, 1935. FR, 1935, IV, 199.
119. Telegram 6, from Bogotá, January 8, 1935. FR, 1935, IV, 200–1. The Chargé commented, in a telegram on January 11, that "the principal cause of the difficulties with the pact here has been and is the failure of

President López to assume any responsibilities of leadership in securing ratification." Telegram 7, from Bogotá. FR, 1935, IV, 201–2.

120. Memorandum of conversations, January 24, 25, 1935, FR, 1935, IV, 205–8; and memorandum by Edwin C. Wilson, January 24, 1935, FR, 1935, IV, 206. Wilson recalled the message of December 15, and noted that "there was some criticism expressed in the Colombian Congress by opposition senators" concerning messages sent by foreign countries; he thought that no action was desirable at this time, since Colombian officials were doing everything they could.

121. Telegram 12, to Bogotá, February 6, 1935. FR, 1935, IV, 211.

122. Telegram 13, from Bogotá, January 24, 1935. FR, 1935, IV, 206–7.

123. Telegram 15, from Lima, February 7, 1935. FR, 1935, IV, 212. Lozano's pride was understandably great, for the treaty had made of Colombia an "Amazonian power," although it seems unfortunate that he should have carried his concern about highly improbable changes in the treaty to the point of opposing the ratification of the Rio agreement. In his book on the treaty, Lozano notes that he had been accused in Peru of "excessive egotism" and declares: "I defend my personal work because it belongs to Colombia, to America and to the universal and eternal cause of justice." F. Lozano Torrijos, *El tratado Lozano-Salomón*, p. 8. The book may have been published at this time as part of Lozano's campaign against any change in the treaty.

124. Memorandum of conversation between Edwin C. Wilson and the Peruvian Ambassador, February 11, 1935. FR, 1935, IV, 213–14. Wilson said he thought this attitude "was admirable and most encouraging in its understanding of the real difficulties which had beset the Colombian Government in its sincere effort to obtain ratification of the protocol within the stipulated period, and that it would be an example to the rest of the world." The Ambassador said he had reported to Lima that the Department believed the Colombian government "had been sincere in its effort to obtain ratification of the protocol and was not merely maneuvering for an advantage, and he believed that this view of the Department had been of influence in the decision reached by the Peruvian Government."

125. Despatch 351, from Bogotá, November 2, 1935. DS, 721.23/2515.

Part Three. The Marañón Conflict

Full bibliographical information about the works cited will be found in the section of the Bibliography on the Marañón Conflict.

IX. Origins

1. Minister William C. Fox reported that the President of Ecuador had told him that he had first learned in 1900 that the "arbitration award was certain to be against Ecuador" and that, although he did not oppose

arbitration in general, Ecuador "never could submit to a decision by the King of Spain under all the circumstances." FR, 1910, 491. Telegram from Quito, July 27, 1910. See also Gordon Ireland, *Boundaries, Possessions and Conflicts in South America* (Cambridge, Mass., Harvard University Press, 1938), pp. 221–27. Twenty-six years later, Dr. Homero Viteri Lafronte, Ecuadoran Minister to Peru, told Ambassador Dearing that "such feeling as existed in his country in opposition to arbitration was due to sad experience and it was necessary for him to show that element that the unsuccessful arbitration by the King of Spain was quite a different thing from what may be expected in the Republic of the United States; it being his belief that the advisers to the king in the monarchy were corrupt and subject to mercenary considerations, while this is out of the question with the Government in Washington." Despatch 4622, from Lima, June 30, 1936. FR, 1936, V, 115. Julio Tobar Donoso, Ecuadoran Foreign Minister in 1941, considered that the Ecuadoran government was in error in rejecting the presumed award; it should have remained quiet, since it is highly probable that the Peruvian government would have rejected the proposed award. Interview, August 27, 1962.

2. Text of note, delivered in Quito on May 18, and in Lima on May 23, 1910. FR, 1910, 450. There was a delay of a week in presentation in Lima due to uncertainty about formalities, which caused Acting Secretary of State Huntington Wilson to cable to Minister Leslie Combs: "The one splendid and all-important fact is the joint offer of mediation by the three Governments . . . In these happy circumstances any unnecessary quibbles would be folly." Telegram, May 18, 1910. FR, 1910, 454.

3. Telegram, August 10, 1910. FR, 1910, 495.

4. Memorandum by Laurence Duggan, December 21, 1936. FR, 1936, V, 123.

5. Telegram 50, to Bogotá, November 16, 1932. FR, 1932, V, 361–62.

6. Full text in FR, 1932, V, 292–4.

7. Despatch 2360, from Lima, November 18, 1932. FR, 1932, V, 363–64. Dearing added: "Both Colombia and Peru have hitherto treated Ecuadorian claims lightly and took the position that as Ecuador was a weak country its pretensions need not be considered seriously."

8. See FR, 1933, IV, 561ff., especially memorandum by Francis White, January 19, 1933, pp. 565–67.

9. Washington was warned as early as 1933 that Peru had been alarmed by the Ecuadoran desire to be represented at the Leticia peace conference; Ambassador Dearing reported that Peru's "heavy credits for national defense and the purchases of armaments and naval vessels is really directed against Ecuador rather than against Colombia." Despatch 2877, from Lima, June 18, 1933. DS, 722.2315/743. Earlier, Dearing had noted that "Peru is arming as never before. . . . It would consequently seem merely foresight to bring Ecuador into any conference looking toward the demarcation of boundary lines in the northwest Amazon region." Despatch 2875, from Lima, June 16, 1933. DS, 721.23/1872.

10. Letter of January 31, 1934. FR, 1934, IV, 461.

11. Text in FR, 1936, V, 116–17.

12. It should be noted that Ecuador and Peru differed on the nature of the controversy between them. Ecuador held that the problem involved the determination whether certain areas were Ecuadoran or Peruvian and that, therefore, the controversy was territorial in nature. Peru maintained that there was no question as to Peruvian rights to the areas in question and that the only controversy was over the precise location of the boundary between those areas and Ecuadoran territory.

13. Tobar Donoso, *La invasión peruana y el protocolo de Río* (referred to hereinafter as Tobar), p. 80, map at that page, and text of the Peruvian description of the line, pp. 80–82. This book, the memoirs of Tobar Donoso, is relied upon heavily in the following pages. Among memoirs by Latin American diplomats its accuracy and objectivity are outstanding. It should be noted, however, that it was written after he had spent some eight days in prison, and as a defense against efforts to censure him following the overturn of the Arroyo del Río regime in 1944. Furthermore, it should be noted that bitter attacks have been made upon his conduct of foreign affairs, particularly at the Rio de Janeiro conference, by certain Ecuadoran writers. See, for example, Villacres Moscoso, *La responsabilidad de la diplomacia ecuatoriana en la demarcación fronteriza;* and Romero Terán, *Los traidores al Ecuador;* Santamaría, *La tragedia internacional del Ecuador y sus responsables.*

14. See FR, 1936, V, 106–26; FR, 1937, V, 46–56; FR, 1938, V, 217–45, for details of negotiations.

15. Memorandum of conversation, June 10, 1937. FR, 1937, V, 49–52.

16. Despatch 881, from Quito, August 26, 1937. FR, 1937, V, 54–55. This statement did not bring about any immediate change in the position of the United States government.

17. Memorandum, January 28, 1938. FR, 1938, V, 217–18.

18. Memorandum of conversation, February 8, 1938. FR, 1938, V, 219–22. Welles told Ambassador Colón Eloy Alfaro of Ecuador of this conversation, saying that "it was always a matter of particular pleasure to the officials of this Government to be of service to the other governments of this continent in facilitating the satisfactory and peaceful solution of difficulties which existed between them, and that . . . the Ambassador knew that during these past eighteen months I had given a great deal of time and thought to this problem, always within the limitations of the course of procedure that this Government had laid down for itself." Memorandum, February 9, 1938. FR, 1938, V, 223.

19. Memorandum of conversation, March 25, 1938. FR, 1938, V, 224. Welles asked Freyre to tell Concha of "my very deep appreciation of his message and of my great gratification that the way now seemed to be prepared for a friendly solution, through arbitration, of the long-standing dispute."

20. Telegrams of June 4, 1938, to Lima and Quito. FR, 1938, V, 225.

21. Text, dated August 31, 1938. FR, 1938, V, 226.

22. See response of Secretary Hull to a telegram from Tobar Donoso, September 3, 1938. FR, 1938, V, 227.

23. Telegram 65, from Lima, September 29, 1938. FR, 1938, V, 228.

24. Circular telegram October 13, 1938. FR, 1938, V, 234–35.

25. Concha told Chargé Louis G. Dreyfus, Jr., that he believed that "Ecuador is trying to take unfair advantage of the existing situation and called Ecuador's appeal to the Chaco mediators both 'extortion' and a form of 'blackmail,' apologizing for the use of these strong words." Telegram 69, from Lima, October 14, 1938. FR, 1938, V, 235.

26. Telegram 117, from Santiago, October 14, 1938. FR, 1938, V, 238. A principal consideration behind this move was explained as "the fear that the participating countries sought to set themselves up as a permanent group to take cognizance of all the problems which could arise, a circumstance at variance with the traditional policy of Chile and favorable to the formation of opposing blocs, with attendant dangers to the harmonious development of Pan Americanism."

27. Telegram, October 17, 1938. FR, 1938, V, 240.

28. Telegram 121 to Rio de Janeiro, October 17, 1938. FR, 1938, V, 242.

X. Hostilities

1. Telegram 74, from Lima, December 27, 1938. FR, 1938, V, 244. See also Tobar, pp. 85–87.

2. Text in *Report of the Delegation of the United States of America to the Eighth International Conference of American States, Lima, Peru, December 9–27, 1938.* (Washington, U.S. Government Printing Office, 1941), pp. 190–91.

3. See, for example, Alvarado, *El protocolo de Río de Janeiro: Lo que garantizaron las potencias garantes,* Chap. XIV.

4. FR, 1939, V, 145–47.   5. Tobar, p. 115.

6. *Ibid.,* p. 137.   7. *Ibid.,* p. 140, January 3, 1941.

8. Memorandum of conversation, February 28, 1941. FR, 1941, VI, 216–18.

9. See, for example, the report quoted by Tobar, pp. 144–45, from Antonio Quevedo, Ecuadoran Minister in Lima, February 4, 1941, that Victor Raúl Haya de la Torre had told the Minister of Peruvian preparations and had even said that military action against Ecuador could be anticipated by February 22, 1941.

10. Text in Tobar, pp. 152–53, and FR, 1941, VI, 219.

11. Text of the Peruvian note in Tobar, pp. 153–54, and FR, 1941, VI, 220–21.

12. The Peruvian reply merely stated that Lima did not regard the Ecuadoran rejoinder as satisfactory and that it therefore maintained its protest against the first declaration. Text in *El Comercio* (Lima), April 21, 1941.

13. Tobar, pp. 165–66; and FR, 1941, VI, 221–22.

14. Text in Cabeza de Vaca, *Aspectos históricos y jurídicos de la cuestión limítrofe: Las negociaciones en Washington y los desenvolvimientos posteriores,* pp. 117–18. Also in FR, 1941, VI, 223–25.

15. FR, 1932, V, 168–69.

16. These articles have been collected and published by Ulloa in *Perú y Ecuador: Ultima etapa del problema de límites, 1941–42*. On this point, see p. 36. See also in text, pp. 274–75, Peruvian note of May 23.

17. See FR, 1941, VI, 226–27.

18. Details on this exchange are given in Tobar, pp. 170–71, footnote 1; text of the United States note of May 20 in FR, 1941, VI, 228–29.

19. Department of State, Press Release, No. 245, May 16, 1941. FR, 1941, VI, 225. The aid to Ecuador may have been connected with the agreement between Ecuador and the United States of December 12, 1940, for the sending of a United States naval and military aviation commission to advise on Ecuadoran defense. See Whitney H. Shepardson and William O. Scroggs, *The United States in World Affairs, 1940* (New York, Harper, 1941), p. 367.

20. See also *La Noche* (Lima) of May 16, 1941, for the text of an interview given by Roberto Mac-Lean y Estenós, a member of congress from Tacna, who charged that the initiative in the proposed mediation came from the United States and not from Argentina and asserted that the United States did not understand either Peruvian history or Peruvian rights to the disputed territory.

21. Ulloa, *Perú y Ecuador*, p. 36.

22. Text in Cabeza de Vaca, *Aspectos históricos y jurídicos de la cuestión limítrofe*, pp. 122–23, and FR, 1941, VI, 230–31. The Ecuadoran position expressed in response to this note is contained in Ecuador, Ministerio de Relaciones Exteriores, *Exposición del ministro de relaciones exteriores del Ecuador a las cancillerías de América*.

23. Summary statement, authorized by Historical Office, Department of State, July 31, 1963.

24. Tobar, p. 174. Enrique Ruiz Guiñazú had by this time become Foreign Minister of Argentina; his later role in the dispute suggests that he would not have taken the lead in the mediation in the first place, and it is possible that the influential Peruvian Ambassador, Marshal Oscar Benavides, ex-President of Peru, was successful in slowing the mediatory action.

25. *Ibid.*, pp. 175–76.

26. *Ibid.*, pp. 174–75. A different account is given by Chiriboga Ordóñez, in *Sepultureros de la patria*, p. 199. He states that some Ecuadoran women were washing clothes in the Zarumilla River when Peruvian soldiers opened fire on them; the fire was returned by Ecuadoran soldiers who ran to the defense of the laundresses.

27. Telegram 167, to Lima, July 8, 1941. FR, 1941, VI, 231–32.

28. A summary of these messages was given by Welles at a press conference on July 9, 1941; text in FR, 1941, VI, 232–33.

29. See Tobar, pp. 178ff. and 186.

30. Ambassador Claude Bowers reported that, since the Argentine and Brazilian ambassadors in Santiago had told the foreign office that Chile would be added to the three mediators, it appeared that the United States was responsible for excluding Chile. Acting Secretary Welles replied im-

mediately that the United States would "view with deepest pleasure" the association with Chile as a mediator but that the ultimate decision would rest with Ecuador and Peru. Bowers wrote to Welles, reporting that Foreign Minister Juan Bautista Rossetti had asked him to inform Washington "that in the case of any trouble such as this involving American nations on the Pacific, Chile expects to be consulted and to take a part." Bowers expressed sympathy with Rossetti's view and added: "It does seem an amazing thing that in a quarrel between two nations on the Pacific Chile should have been left out." Copy of letter of July 7, 1941, from Santiago. FDRL, OF 303 (Bowers).

31. Address, New York City, February 4, 1937. Department of State, press release, February 2, 1937. Contrasting the anticipated future with the Chaco dispute, Welles noted that in the latter "there was no continental understanding of the purposes of consultation, there was no rallying of the forces of continental public opinion, and there was no agreement such as that which we now possess for obligatory consultation between us all whenever peace is jeopardized."

32. Text in Cabeza de Vaca, *Aspectos históricos y jurídicos de la cuestión limítrofe*, pp. 129–30.

33. Tobar, p. 228.

34. Partial text of Peruvian reply to Ruiz Guiñazú's note is given in Cabeza de Vaca, *Aspectos históricos y jurídicos de la cuestión limítrofe*, pp. 137–38. See also, Tobar, pp. 222–25, quoting despatches in various Latin American newspapers on Solf's statement.

35. See Tobar, p. 207, for text of Viteri Lafronte's cable, No. 140, July 26, 1941; it arrived in Quito at 5:15 P.M., July 26.

36. *Ibid.*, pp. 198, 221. Tobar later compared the defeat to that suffered by France in 1940. It should be recognized that other Ecuadorans took a different view of Tobar's position on this point. Chiriboga claims that Alfaro, in Washington, either intentionally or naively, "deceived" the Ecuadoran army with the report of the "armistice" of July 26, and the army then retreated. Chiriboga Ordóñez, *Sepultureros de la patria*, pp. 204–5. However, Chiriboga was a bitter opponent of the Liberal Party, headed by President Arroyo del Río, and Tobar's account of the rapid acceptance of the armistice is effectively supported by evidence from non-Ecuadoran sources.

37. Tobar, p. 221.   38. *Ibid.*, p. 213.

39. The decree was annulled by Ecuador following strong pressure from the United States, Argentina and Brazil. *Ibid.*, p. 213.

40. *Ibid.*, p. 212.

41. *Report of the Delegate of the United States of America to the Meeting of the Foreign Ministers of the American Republics, Panamá, September 23–October 3, 1939*, Resolution on the "Humanization of War." Appendix 12, p. 57.

42. Tobar, pp. 216–17.

43. Texts of the slightly different messages in Department of State *Bulletin*, V, 1941, p. 93.

44. See Tobar, pp. 271ff.

45. Memoranda of conversations, August 14 and September 22, 1941, quoted in William L. Langer and S. Everett Gleason, *The Undeclared War, 1940–1941* (New York, Harper, 1953), pp. 616–17.

46. See *Ecuador: Nociones históricas—geografía física y antrópica*. This is a textbook in geography, containing on its title-page the statement that it includes a geographical atlas "considered to be an official text by decree no. 101 of the government of Ecuador, July 30, 1937."

47. Tobar, pp. 275–76, quoting the text of an observer's report made "at the end of August," [1941].

48. *Ibid.*, pp. 272–73, quoting the text of the observer's report dated August 27, 1941.

49. *El Comercio* (Lima) of August 1, 1941, stated that Puerto Bolivar had been "taken by assault by the division of parachutists."

50. Tobar, pp. 267–68.   51. *Ibid.*, pp. 280–81.

52. Text in *ibid.*, pp. 282–83.

53. New York *Times*, September 29, 1941. This bit of diplomatic finesse may be viewed in broader terms, as, for example, in Ozzie G. Simmons, "Lo 'criollo' en el marco de la cultura de la Costa Peruana," *Ciencias Sociales*, VI (April 1955), 87–98.

54. FR, 1941, VI, 233–34. Tobar, p. 287, gives a summary of this document.

55. Original text in Spanish, made available to the author by the foreign office of a Latin American government. For this line, see Map IV.

56. New York *Times*, September 16 and 18, 1941. Tenguel is in Guayas province, about twenty miles north of Machala, one of the northernmost towns subsequently held by the Peruvian army.

57. New York *Times*, September 18, 1941. The affair dropped from view after this statement, and it is not known whether the Department of State responded. No reference is made to the incident in FR, 1941, VI or VII; the Department may well have decided that Prado was no more willing to accept protests in this case than on the invasion of Ecuador itself.

58. *Message from the President of the United States Transmitting Papers Relating to the War in South America and Attempts to Bring about a Peace* (Washington, Government Printing Office, 1882), p. 296. The Minister in Peru (Christiancy) to the Secretary of State (Evarts), Lima, December 23, 1879.

59. An insight into this relationship is provided by an editorial in *Chan Chan*, a clandestine newspaper published in Trujillo by the Aprista Party, September 27, 1941, which charged that *El Comercio* (Lima) and other papers were attempting to present Prado as the "genius who planned the war," while Ureta and the army were given only second place. *Chan Chan* called on the Peruvian people to "identify themselves fully with the Army of the North, and with General Eloy Ureta."

60. See, for example, Tobar, pp. 310–11.

61. Text in *ibid.*, pp. 311–13; not printed in FR.   62. *Ibid.*, p. 315.

63. *Ibid.*, p. 316. In FR, 1941, VI, the note of October 4, 1941, is not published, so that the erroneous impression is given that the Peruvian note of September 13 (without its attachment) received no reply.

XI. Truce and Treaty

1. Text in Tobar, pp. 306–8, and in FR, 1941, VI, 234. See Map III.
2. Tobar, pp. 321–22, and FR, 1941, VI, 239, 240.
3. Tobar, pp. 320ff., and FR, 1941, VI, 241–42.
4. The Peruvian toughness at this time has aroused even Ecuadoran admiration: "*Por hidalguía* we must recognize in our enemy [Peru] the arrogance with which it humiliated the three great mediatory powers, without even giving them an answer to their famous memorandum of October 4." Palacios Bravo, *La invasión peruana y el protocolo de Río de Janeiro,* p. 18.
5. Telegram 691. The Ambassador in Peru (Norweb) to the Secretary of State, Lima, December 15, 1941. FR, 1941, VI, 247.
6. Tobar, pp. 330ff.   7. *Ibid.*, p. 337, and FR, 1941, VI, 250.
8. The Ambassador in Peru (Norweb) to the Secretary of State, Lima, December 23, 1941. FR, 1941, VI, 251–52. Peru, however, did not secure this basis for "a good case," since there was neither a definitive settlement nor a withdrawal of its troops from Ecuadoran territory in the west before the conference of Rio de Janeiro.
9. Peruvian Foreign Minister Solf y Muro suggested to Norweb that "this is not the time to complicate the international situation by raising the boundary question at the conference," and he hoped the mediators would so inform Ecuador; and it was clearly understood in Washington that Solf was "worried that the Ecuadoran boundary question might be raised" at Rio de Janeiro and that the Peruvian Ambassador in Colombia was insisting that the dispute with Ecuador "should under no circumstances even be referred to in the forthcoming consultative conference." FR, 1941, VI, 124, 126, 129.
10. FR, 1941, VI, 252–53.
11. The Brazilian proposal is described in Tobar, pp. 356–58; that of Argentina is quoted in *ibid.*, pp. 358–60. The Department of State adhered to the terms of the note of the mediators of December 23, 1941, above.
12. Tobar, pp. 356–60.
13. Tobar Donoso and Luna Tobar, *Derecho territorial ecuatoriano,* p. 210. The precise terms of the line proposed by Aranha are here given as: " 'Status quo line of 1936 from the Pacific Coast to Andoas (mouth of the Bobonaza River in the Pastaza River); confluence of the rivers Conambó and Pintoyacu; mouth of the Cononaco in the Curaray River; following the Curaray, downriver to Bellavista; mouth of the Yasuní River in the Napo River; down the Napo and to the confluence of the Lagartococha and the Aguarico Rivers; and the whole course of the Lagartococha to the watershed between the Napo and the Putumayo rivers.' " Tobar reports these quotations as from his instruction of March

2, 1942 to all Ecuadoran legations, on the protocol of Rio de Janeiro.

14. *Ibid.*, p. 211, for point-by-point description of the Argentine proposal.

15. *Ibid.*, p. 212.   16. Tobar, p. 368.

17. This is the opinion both of Tobar, and of Mauricio Nabuco, chief administrative officer of the Brazilian foreign office in 1942. Interviews, July 12, 1962, and July 27, 1962, respectively.

18. Interview, July 30, 1962, with Mauricio Nabuco, Brazilian Ambassador to the United States, 1946. Aranha departed from these established principles on this occasion, in Nabuco's opinion, because Aranha, acting opportunistically, was primarily concerned with gaining the unanimity of the American states in breaking relations with the Axis powers, rather than with the durability of a settlement between Ecuador and Peru. There was in this view a great moment for Brazilian leadership in South American affairs that was not seized by Aranha, because of momentary concern with the world, rather than the South American, scene.

19. This statement is not made without consideration of some of the attacks that have been made on Tobar, by Chiriboga Ordóñez and others. See, for example, Villacres Moscoso, *La responsabilidad de la diplomacia ecuatoriana en la demarcación fronteriza*, where Tobar and other members of the Ecuadoran delegation at Rio de Janeiro are called "traitors to the fatherland" (p. 61). Villacres Moscoso says that Peru attacked at a time of internal disaster in Ecuador. Peru knew of the "ignominious dictatorship that burdened the backs of the Ecuadoran people; it was aware of the political struggles that had weakened the nation's unity; it was informed that the army had been prevented from preparing for the defense of Ecuador" (p. 11). This pamphlet and others, however, do not come to grips with the choices facing Ecuador at Rio de Janeiro and so do not offer a serious refutation of Tobar's decision. There seems to be no Peruvian account of the conference negotiations that has been made public.

20. Tobar, p. 350. One hope apparently was that a condemnation against "aggression by Peru on Ecuador" would be expressed as well as that anticipated against Japanese "aggression" at Pearl Harbor. Muñoz, *La campaña internacional de 1941*, pp. 185–86.

21. Tobar, p. 360.

22. This "Report" is Annex 4 to the general report of the military observers appointed by the mediators to observe, on the Ecuadoran side, the course of events on the western front following the cessation of hostilities arranged for July 26, 1941. The report and annexes consist of 56 pages, mimeographed; they have not been published and were made available to the author in the original mimeographed form by Julio Tobar Donoso in Quito, August, 1962, without restriction as to their use. The "Report" was given to Minister Boaz Long in Ecuador at the end of August, 1941, and transmitted by him shortly afterward to the Department of State. Text in Spanish; translation by the author. Notes 22–28 refer to the general report of the military observers.

23. Report (see note 22), pp. 26–27.

24. *Ibid.*, p. 27. The report was signed by Col. J. B., Pate, U.S.A., Tt.

Coronel S.C. Albuquerque Lima, Brazil, and Tt. Navío, J. P. Ibarborde, Argentina.

25. This document is dated at Zorritos, Peru, August 27, 1941, and is signed by Col. U. G. Ent., U.S.A., Mayor C. Toranzo Montero, Argentina, and Tt. Coronel H. Filgueiras, Brazil.

26. *Ibid.,* pp. 30–33.

27. *Ibid.,* pp. 33–36. The meeting was held at the request of representatives in Quito of the mediatory powers, on September 25, 1941. The report of the interview was signed by Col. H. Thompson, U.S.A., Tt. Coronel S. Lima, Brazil, and Tt. Navío J. P. Ibarborde, Argentina. Present at the interview was Comandante Superior Coronel Alberto Carlos Romero Arroyo.

28. *Ibid.,* pp. 36–37.

29. Tobar, p. 368.   30. *Ibid.,* p. 372.

31. Jaramillo Alvarado, *La nación quiteña: Perfil biográfico de una cultura,* p. 163; and Yepes, *La controversia fronteriza entre el Ecuador y el Perú,* pp. 28–29. More recently it is asserted that Welles said to Ecuadoran delegates at the Rio conference: " 'Either Ecuador agrees to accept a definitive agreement, or the mediators will immediately withdraw, with the equally immediate result that the Peruvian army will continue its aggression.' " Alvarado, *El protocolo de Río de Janeiro: Lo que garantizaron las potencias garantes,* p. 38. The source of this alleged quotation is not given; the words are almost certainly not those that Welles would have used. The importance of this quotation is not its dubious authenticity, but its publication by the Casa de la Cultura Ecuatoriana. For a Peruvian lawyer's response to Yepes, see García Rendón, *El protocolo de paz, amistad y límites entre Perú y Ecuador de 1942 ante el derecho internacional,* especially pp. 34ff.

32. Tobar, p. 374.

33. *Ibid.,* pp. 389–91, text of telegram 30, from Quito to Tobar, January 20, 1942. See also Alvarado Garaicoa, *Sinopsis del derecho territorial ecuatoriano,* who states that this Ecuadoran boundary proposal was rejected by Peru "despite its having been greeted with satisfaction by the mediators" (p. 265).

34. Tobar Donoso and Luna Tobar, *Derecho territorial ecuatoriano,* p. 215.

35. Tobar, pp. 402–3. He noted that it would have been rash of him to have made his protest at the solemn closing session of the Conference since that might have provoked an uproar and harmed the interests of Ecuador. The delegation protested without success; Tobar recounts that many of the other foreign ministers and delegates "did not wish even to hear anything about the Ecuadoran-Peruvian problem, the most American of those which could have been presented to the Conference." Tobar, p. 403.

36. *Ibid.,* p. 404. This account of the interview is quoted by Tobar as from a written report by Arroyo.

37. *Ibid.,* p. 407, note 1. Tobar added with remarkable frankness that

he had cabled Quito on January 18 suggesting that President Arroyo del Río urge United States Minister Boaz Long to cable Welles that unless the boundary dispute were settled on the basis of the December 23 proposal of the mediators, there was a danger that public order in Ecuador would be subverted. Long and the Brazilian Minister in Quito sent a joint cable to Welles and Aranha on January 26, but it related the possibility of a revolution in Ecuador only to any settlement that would not provide for the immediate retirement of Peruvian forces, and so was unsatisfactory to Tobar. *Ibid.*, pp. 407–8.

38. *Ibid.*, p. 408.   39. *Ibid.*, pp. 408–9.

40. *Ibid.*, p. 504. Compare Herbert Nicholas, "UN Peace Forces and the Changing Globe," *International Organization*, XVII, No. 2 (Spring, 1963). "Since the UN can assist only those who, at any rate initially, can themselves resist . . ." (p. 322).

41. Tobar, pp. 409–11. Other Ecuadorans, lacking responsibility at the time, have expressed different views. Pio Jaramillo Alvarado states that not even "total occupation of Ecuador by the Peruvian army could have justified the signature of this Protocol" (in his *La nación quiteña*, p. 157). For a view giving major responsibility to President Arroyo del Río, see Santamaría, *La tragedia internacional de Ecuador y sus responsables*, pp. 36ff.

42. Tobar, p. 411.

43. Mauricio Nabuco recalls that he had told Sumner Welles that Welles should not support any "little Munichs" in America. Nabuco therefore refused an invitation to attend the signing of the protocol; his office in the Itamaraty Palace was next to the room in which the protocol was signed, and Tobar came out, after the signature, with tears running down his face. Interview, July 30, 1962.

44. Tobar, p. 412. At one of the final meetings of the Chaco peace conference, the chief Peruvian delegate failed to mention his own deputy, who had also signed the treaty of peace, when distributing credits to the negotiators. Spruille Braden then arranged for the conference chairman to praise the work of the deputy at a later session. Despatch 713, from Buenos Aires, July 25, 1938. DS, 724.34119/7521.

45. On the question of freedom of navigation of the rivers in the Oriente, including the Marañón-Amazon, Tobar states that Solf tried at the last minute to refuse such freedom to Ecuador. However, "it was just at that point that Mr. Welles interposed his great prestige, with the result that the Peruvian foreign minister refrained from insisting on his negative attitude." Tobar, p. 478. For the other occasion, see p. 313.

46. Juan B. Rossetti, the Chilean Foreign Minister, was not mentioned by Tobar, but this may be explained by Chile's recent joining of the mediatory group.

47. Tobar, p. 499.

48. *Ibid.*, p. 414. The idea of gaining prestige for Ecuador by laying a sacrifice on the altar of Pan Americanism was by no means shared by all Ecuadorans. Chiriboga Ordóñez called on his countrymen to "Remember

1941," "Remember the Zarumilla," and declared passionately: "There will be no peace in America for centuries and centuries, while the Peruvian usurper dominates the left bank of the Amazon and the right bank of the Tumbes; while the farce of continental diplomacy continues sponsoring and protecting the war of aggression carried by Peru into our inheritance of the Amazon, Loja and El Oro" (in his *Sepultureros de la patria*, p. 241).

49. Tobar, pp. 416–17.

50. Chiriboga Ordóñez, *Sepultureros de la patria*, pp. 241, 248. The Itamaraty is the Brazilian foreign office building in Rio de Janeiro.

51. Text of the protocol in *Documents on American Foreign Relations, 1941– 942* (Boston, World Peace Foundation, 1942), pp. 433–35, and in U.S. Department of State, *Bulletin*, VI (1942), 195.

52. This information is based principally on maps in Tobar. Since the precise extent of penetration of Peruvian troops is not known, and since Tobar was defending himself against charges that he had given up more territory than was necessary, this information should be evaluated with some caution. In general, it appears, to be fairly accurate. See Map IV, and notes, pp. 394–96.

53. Report of the military observers (see p. 471, n. 22), interview with the Minister of Defense, September 29, 1941, p. 36–37. While men and freight could be moved by road and river from Lima to Iquitos in five days in 1941, the Ecuadorans could not supply their troops in the Oriente except by shipments through the Panama Canal, and up the Amazon. Wright, "A Study of the Conflict between the Republics of Peru and Ecuador," *Geographical Journal*, XCVIII, 272.

54. Aranha is reported to have said to Tobar at Rio de Janeiro: " 'What acts of possession have your people made in 100 years in the territories you are claiming . . . where are the roads opened, or important cities like Iquitos that you have built?' " When Tobar had no good answer, Aranha said Ecuador would have to accept the offered line, and using sign language, Aranha asked: " 'Which would you prefer that they [Peruvians] should cut—the tip of your little finger or your throat?' " Santamaría, *La tragedia internacional del Ecuador y sus responsables*, p. 42.

55. Tobar, p. 462. The Peruvian gains were in the Tarquí-Rocafuerte and Huachi–González Suárez–Tarquí areas; those of Ecuador were in the Yaupi-Morona, San Miguel–Putumayo (Sucumbios), and Aguarico-Güepi areas.

56. *Ibid.*, pp. 463–64.

57. Preston E. James, *Latin America*, Rev. ed. (New York, Odyssey, 1950), p. 125.

58. See also the official communiqué commenting on the protocol and making the most of the gains achieved by Peru, published in *El Comercio* (Lima), February 7, 1942. For praise of the protocol by one of Peru's most ardent patriots, see the article by Roberto Mac-Lean y Estenós in *El Comercio*, June 7, 1942, in which the statement is made that "Peru has

remained faithful to its glorious traditions of honor, of nobility, and of good neighborliness."

59. The Sucumbios Triangle had been recognized by Colombia as Peruvian territory in the Salomón-Lozano treaty of 1922, but Peru had not been able to occupy it because of intervening Ecuadoran territory. It was not mentioned in the protocol, but since it lay to the west of the boundary line, it was regarded as Ecuadoran.

60. Department of State Press release No. 82, February 28, 1942.

61. Telegrams of January 31, 1942.

62. Text of telegram, dated February 2, 1942.

XII. The Protocol of Rio de Janeiro and the Policy of the United States

1. See, for example, *El Comercio* (Quito), February 5, 1942, "Pan Americanism Is Humbug, as Great a Humbug as the League of Nations," by Sra. Hipatía Cárdenas de Bustamente, and other Ecuadoran newspapers of about this time. In an editorial on January 21, 1942, *El Comercio* asked whether, for the first time in America, "the right of the strong over the weak was going to be consecrated."

2. Department of State, Press release No. 43, January 30, 1942. In his memoirs, Hull says nothing about this conflict. Welles's statement to the press that the United States government was satisfied with the settlement, which "affords a further proof of the ability and determination of the American Republics to settle all disputes between them by pacific methods," ignored the Peruvian invasion and occupation of Ecuador. Department of State, Press release No. 82, February 28, 1942. President Roosevelt cabled President Arroyo del Río on January 31 that "the willingness of Ecuador and Peru to reach a harmonious understanding is particularly gratifying at a time when the danger to their liberties demands that the American republics demonstrate to the world their unanimous determination to devote themselves to the preservation of those ideals of liberty and equity upon which their political institutions are founded." FDRL, OF 563 (Ecuador). The words crossed out on this copy of the draft cable were not sent; they were presumably eliminated by someone who thought them inappropriate to describe the nature of the "harmonious understanding" embodied in the protocol.

3. This promise was kept. President Roosevelt authorized the sum of $500,000 to the Coordinator of Inter-American Affairs for rehabilitation of the province of El Oro since, " 'as a result of the Ecuador-Peru boundary dispute, the farms and homes of most of the inhabitants of the Ecuadoran province of El Oro have been destroyed and their possessions lost.' " FDRL, 79 Authorization—Treasury—Numbered Letters—42–142, memorandum for the President from Harold Smith, Director, Bureau of the Budget, and OF 4512 (Coordinator of Inter-American Affairs).

4. *El Peruano* (Lima), March 14, 1942.

5. See Flores, *History of the Boundary Dispute between Ecuador and Peru*, and *El protocolo de Río de Janeiro ante la Historia.*

6. Peru, Dirección de Informaciones, *La defensa de la peruanidad de Tumbes, Jaén y Mainas por el Presidente Prado.* Ecuador, it was claimed, "had no other recourse than that of deliberate provocation with the unfounded hope of bringing about a mediation of friendly countries to keep the peace of America. This was a profound mistake. No one could believe that Peru had the slightest intention of attacking Ecuador" (p. 121). This position was also taken by Belaunde, who accused Ecuador of "planned frontier incidents" that would provoke mediation by friendly countries, and of exaggerated demands that, combined with "external influences" might induce Peru, which was "always generous," to make maximum concessions (in his *La vida internacional del Perú, Tomo I, Relaciones con el Ecuador: La constitución inicial del Perú ante el derecho internacional,* pp. viii–ix).

7. See, for example, P. B. *El litigio peru-ecuatoriano ante los principios jurídicos americanos.* This semi-official Peruvian publication charged that Ecuador, since 1938, had followed a policy of "dictator Enríquez's boundary incidents" and claimed that the existence of such a policy had been admitted by an ex-president of Ecuador. See Peru, Bureau of the Press of Ministry of Foreign Affairs of Peru, *Ecuadorean Ex-President Velasco Ibarra passes Judgement on the Aggressive Policy of Ecuador,* p. 7. This publication contains the alleged text of a letter by Velasco Ibarra to President Arroyo del Río of Ecuador, printed in *La Crítica* (Santiago de Chile), August 2, 1941. Ecuadorans have, of course, disputed the authenticity of this letter, and it has been claimed there are at least three known texts. Julio H. Santamaría in introduction to Marín, *Ecuador la gran mutilada,* p. xxxi.

8. "What have we done in a century of independent existence to take possession, in fact, of these territories that are ours by right? Our diplomats have, perhaps, talked and written as much as those of Peru, but as for highways and colonists, which constitute real and effective possession, we have not done even the hundredth part of the work of the Peruvians." Quevedo, *Texto de historia patria,* p. 147.

9. It is difficult not to agree with a Colombian commentator who stated that in 1941–42 "the opportunity was taken advantage of marvellously by Peru." Andrade S., "Límites entre Colombia y Ecuador," *Boletín de Historia y Antigüedades,* XLVII, 217.

10. Humberto Delgado, *Las guerras del Peru: Campaña del Ecuador,* I, 73–76. The document in question is entitled: "Plan de Maniobra para la campaña." Tobar claims a little too much, perhaps, in asserting that Humberto Delgado here provides "irrefutable and definitive proof of aggression" by Peru. Tobar, p. 237. Humberto Delgado states that the objective of the army of the north was "to put an end, once and for all, to the frequent aggressions of Ecuadoran forces against our frontier posts, principally in the region of the Zarumilla River" (I, 76). Humberto Delgado does not link this campaign plan to that in the Oriente. This

account, however, gives a basis for the presumption that in 1941 Lima planned to invade Ecuador in order to force acceptance of its definition of the boundary between the two countries.

11. Humberto Delgado, *Las guerras del Peru: Campaña del Ecuador*, 1, 166. Other boundary conflicts had been both "exhausting and humiliating."

12. Basadre, *La promesa de la vida peruana*, pp. 135ff.

13. Barra, *Tumbes, Jaén y Maynas*.

14. *Ibid.*, p. 36. See also Vallejo, *Datos para la historia: El conflicto Perú-Colombiano. Charlas militares*, Vol. 1. Coronel Vallejo criticized the Peruvian government in the Leticia conflict for having tried to conceal the fact that Peruvian forces had been defeated by the Colombians and to avoid publicity about scandals in the purchase of military equipment. He demanded that Peruvians should be informed about the causes of the failure of their armed forces to offer adequate resistance to the Colombians at Leticia and called for measures to improve morale in the Peruvian army. Morale was improved, and so was equipment and organization, by reforms instituted by President Benavides, beginning in 1934. See, for example, Chang Laos, *El Perú y sus hombres a través de la República*, p. 143.

15. Barra, *Tumbes, Jaén y Maynas*, p. 37.

16. *Ibid.*, pp. 37-38. It should be noted that there is another Peruvian position on this point. Ambassador Emilio Romero, accusing Ecuador of attacking an unsuspecting Peru in 1941, states: "The news of the Ecuadoran attack fell like a bomb on Lima." However, he combines this false statement with one so ridiculous that his whole analysis is manifestly absurd: "If the garrison of police at the frontier had not sacrificed itself heroically in the first Ecuadoran assault, our military forces would not have been able to organize quickly in the rear in order to contain the Ecuadoran charge. The honor of the Peruvian fatherland was saved, in the first instance, by the Peruvian police, and then by our army." Romero, *Por el norte: Ecuador*, p. 154.

17. Ulloa, *Perú y Ecuador*, pp. 114-15. See also Mac-Lean y Estenós, *El litigio limítrofe peruano-ecuatoriano*, who noted that "Peru has had a bitter experience of arbitrations in its boundary questions" (p. 29).

18. Ulloa, *Posición internacional del Perú*, pp. 131, 148.

19. Prado publicly gave tribute to Benavides "for having endowed the Peruvian army with materials indispensable to modern warfare." New York *Times*, August 8, 1941.

20. Ulloa, *Perú y Ecuador*, p. 86.

21. *Report of the Delegation of the United States of America to the Eighth International Conference of American States, Lima, Peru, December 9-27, 1938* (Washington, D.C., U.S. Government Printing Office, 1941), Appendix 120, pp. 190-91. Similar "proscriptions" embodied in resolutions, declarations, and other acts of inter-American conferences could be cited at great length, as is frequently done in Ecuadoran publications on the Marañón dispute.

22. Lozano Torrijos, *El tratado Lozano-Salomón* (México, D.F., Ed. Cultura, 1934), p. 17.

23. New York *Times*, July 8, 1941.

24. See Viteri Lafronte, *El Ecuador y su salida propia al Marañón*. The standard figure of Ecuadoran territorial "losses" cited by detractors of the protocol is 200,000 square kilometers.

25. Tobar, pp. 498–503.

26. Ulloa, *Perú y Ecuador*, pp. 70, 71. These quotations are from an article in *La Prensa* (Lima), February 8, 1942. It is not improbable that the views expressed in these articles were those of high officials in the Peruvian government; in any case the book is deserving of study as an expression of defiant Peruvian nationalism in this period of its most bellicose and successful expression. It may be noted that Ulloa said of the first mediators' note of May 8, 1941, that "it reminds one of the documents that the totalitarian states employ in their Balkan diplomacy." *Ibid.*, p. 26, article from *La Prensa*, May 17, 1941.

27. Belaunde states that the action of the mediatory states "was practically paralyzed before the unassailable barrier of the juridical position of Peru; those states were limited to aiding the re-establishment of peace" (in his *La vida internacional del Perú*, I, viii). See also the jubilant summary of Peruvian policy in *El Comercio* (Lima), February 7, 1942.

28. Tobar and Luna Tobar, *Derecho territorial ecuatoriano*, p. 240. See also Ecuador, Ministerio de Relaciones Exteriores, *El protocolo de Río de Janeiro de 1942 es nulo*, and other semi-official and official publications since 1960. It is curious to find support for the claim of nullity of the protocol in a book jointly authored by Tobar Donoso, even though the claim is made only in the portion explicitly stated to be by Alfredo Luna Tobar. It should also be noted, however, that Tobar Donoso is stated to have signed, apparently in 1960, a declaration by the Supreme Court of Justice of Ecuador to the effect that the protocol was void because imposed by force by Peru. See, for text, *Un protocolo viciado de nulidad.* Tobar was at the time a member of the Supreme Court.

29. The mediators' patience may well have been taxed by such expressions as that by *El Comercio* (Lima) in an editorial on August 14, 1941, which went so far as to declare that "the fact is that Peru and Ecuador were at peace until the offer of 'friendly services' was made and that the warlike conflict which resulted between them was the consequence of the mediation."

30. This statement is made on the basis of Hull's strictures to Concha, already mentioned; in view of the initiative by Padilla to bring the dispute before all the American states, which could only have been disadvantageous to Peru, and in light of the fact that when the Brazilian government chose to announce an honors list in early October, 1941, several Ecuadorans were named, but not a single Peruvian. Later President Getulio Vargas personally decorated President Arroyo del Río of Ecuador and his Foreign Minister, Julio Tobar Donoso, with the highest Brazilian award, the National Order of the Southern Cross. New York *Times,*

October 21, 1941. This measure of ceremonial selectivity was not the result of absent-mindedness; it was arranged by Mauricio Nabuco.

31. Tobar records with embarrassment that in the early days of July, 1941, Benjamin Welles, a newspaper correspondent and son of Sumner Welles, went to Arenillas, not far from the battle zone along the Zarumilla River. He was in the area for two or three days and saw no signs of fighting whatever, but he stated that Ecuadoran reporters who were with him had sent stories to their papers of entirely nonexistent engagements. Tobar commented that he feared that Benjamin Welles had told his father of this experience and that it might have affected the Undersecretary's attitude toward all news of Ecuadoran origin. Tobar, pp. 189–90.

32. President Roosevelt assailed the Russian invasion of Finland as " 'a wanton disregard for law,' " and he expressed sympathy for the sufferings of the Finns. Press conference reported in New York *Herald Tribune* and New York *Times*, December 2 and 3, 1939, and telegram to the Ambassador in the Soviet Union, December 1, 1939. FR, The Soviet Union, 1933–1939, 799–800. No such sympathy was accorded the people of El Oro province in Ecuador. Compare the unavailing effort of the Ecuadoran government to secure an all-American protest to the Soviet Union against the " 'invasion and occupation of Finland.' " All the American states except Chile agreed, but the protest was not made because of this abstention. It seems reasonable to assume that the Ecuadoran initiative was taken in the hope of putting the American republics on record as opposing "the invasion of weaker nations," in the expectation that Ecuador might before long be the victim of an invasion by Peru. See, FR, 1939, V, 128–40, for relevant correspondence.

33. See text of his speech of February 4, 1937 (see above p. 468, note 31).

34. In Welles's own words, Stimson's effort "to play a helpful part in composing the sharp controversy" over Leticia "was considerably weakened by an attitude which could more properly be adopted by a schoolteacher admonishing his pupils." *The Time for Decision* (New York, Harper, 1944), p. 191.

35. Afterwards, Carlos Concha could afford to be generous. He reported that in 1938 "the archives of our Foreign Office contain evidence that the Department of State did not use any diplomatic means whatever that could be objected to as an act of pressure in order to bring about the success of its suggestions." Further, the United States did not exert "pressure" in connection with the offer of friendly services in May, 1941: "Diplomatic records . . . proved that such a hypothesis lacked serious basis and that the initiative of friendly services . . . did not have North American origins." "Sumner Welles and the Good Neighbor Policy," *Turismo*, October 19, 1943.

36. Roosevelt called Prado " 'a really delightful fellow—the first civilian President of Peru for ten or fifteen years, a professor at the University of Lima, which antedates Harvard by nearly a hundred years.' " Roosevelt presumably meant the University of San Marcos, but his own ignorance of Latin America was matched in this case by his editors. This quotation

is from a letter to Mackenzie King, Hyde Park, May 18, 1942, given in *F. D. R. His Personal Letters, 1928–1945*, edited by Elliott Roosevelt, assisted by Joseph P. Lash (N.Y., Duell, Sloan and Pearce, 1950), p. 1320.

37. An account of the visit is given in a publication entitled: *El Excelentísimo Sr. Dr. Dn. Manuel Prado, Presidente del Perú: Reseña de su visita a los Estados Unidos, del 6 al 21 de mayo de 1942*. This publication, in Spanish, was apparently published in the United States by the International Business Machines Corporation on June 21, 1942. The preface is signed by Thos. J. Watson. There are many illustrations, accompanying a day-by-day story of the visit. An introduction gives the career of President Prado. This account contains one notable omission: there is no reference whatever to the settlement of the boundary dispute with Ecuador or to the protocol of Rio de Janeiro, although the participation of President Prado in "an armed conflict with Ecuador" in 1910 is mentioned. The introduction ends with the statement that President Prado's policies had brought internal peace and prosperity to Peru. "He has also taken a decisive part in the strengthening of the unity of the American nations. His efforts symbolize the ideal of the policy of the good neighbor." On his way home, Prado made an address to the Venezuelan congress, which was the first time in the history of Venezuela that the head of a foreign state had been declared a guest of honor and received by the congress. Venezuela, Congreso Nacional, *Sesión solemne celebrada el 25 mayo 1942 en honor del excelentísimo Sr. Dr. Manuel Prado*. See also "Visit of the President of Peru to Washington," *Bulletin of the Pan American Union*, July, 1942, pp. 373–79, and the editorial in the New York *Times*, May 8, 1942, that asserted that Prado "is a loyal champion of Pan-Americanism in its noblest sense." Prado was not given a degree at Harvard University, in accordance, it appears, with a standing policy of that institution. The existence of such a policy would seem to be substantiated by an earlier incident. In 1939 John Tazewell Jones wrote from São Paulo to President Roosevelt, requesting that he use his influence with Harvard University to arrange for an honorary degree from the University for General Candido Rondon of the Brazilian army. Sumner Welles did not approve of such action, and Stephen Early was said to have replied for Roosevelt to the effect that "Harvard has been approached before *re* similar requests and this effort has borne no tangible results. They were asked to confer a degree on some outstanding Brazilian or Argentine or some other distinguished citizen of another American Republic. [Early] says under these circumstances, the President does not feel warranted in taking action suggested." Memorandum, STATE, The Undersecretary of, May 12, 1939. FDRL, OF 11 (Brazil), Box 1.

38. "The President of Ecuador in Washington," *Bulletin of the Pan American Union*, January 1943, pp. 17–22. Like Prado, Arroyo visited war plants in several cities. See also *Carlos A. Arroyo del Río, apóstol del panamericanismo: Reseña de la histórica visita de confraternidad realizada a través de seis naciones de América, del 16 de noviembre al 16 de*

diciembre de 1942, with a preface by Thos. J. Watson. This is apparently the companion volume to that issued in honor of President Prado of Peru; apparently both were printed in the United States, by the International Business Machines Corporation. Both volumes lack a table of contents and an index; both are unpaged, so that precise citations are difficult. Both are profusely illustrated, sometimes with identical pictures, such as St. Patrick's Cathedral in New York City, and occasionally both have identical texts, such as the descriptions of the history of Columbia University. The principal textual material consists of speeches by the presidents and their hosts, which provide useful examples of the diplomatic idiom of contemporary inter-American relations. The description of Arroyo del Río as the "Apostle of Pan-Americanism" has not echoed happily in Ecuador. See, for example, Linke, *Ecuador: Country of Contrasts*, p. 30.

39. See Sociedad Bolivariana del Ecuador, *La Revisión del Protocolo de Río*. The Society does not favor war as a means of revision but hopes to present a petition to the United Nations. The argument for revision is based on charges of Peruvian aggression and on threats made at Rio de Janeiro that the mediation would be terminated if Ecuador rejected the protocol.

40. For the latest incident, see New York *Times*, April 20, 1964. An earlier charge by Ecuador that Peru was massing troops along the southwestern boundary was presented to the Council of the Organization of American States, but it was referred by the Organization to the representatives of the "guarantor states," and the tension, brought on by an incident at Yaupi, was pacifically resolved. *Annals of the Organization of American States*, VII, No. 4 (1955), 290–92. For a representative book see Tobar Donoso and Luna Tobar, *Derecho territorial ecuatoriano*. This is a textbook for a course in the Catholic University of Ecuador, and, so long as Ecuador does not have riparian rights on the Marañón, Ecuadoran texts like this one will be asserting their country's right to be an Amazonian nation, denouncing the protocol, and demanding justice in the name of Pan American principles.

41. The argument over the watershed (*divortium aquarum*, as the term is given in the protocol, article VIII, B.1), continues and is complex. The Peruvians regret the phrase in the protocol but assert that there is no question as to the intention of the signatories; the Ecuadorans make the most of this error and refuse to agree to the placement of boundary markers. See Viteri Lafronte, *El Ecuador y su salida propia al Marañón*, pp. 83ff.

42. "Homage to the National Hero, Lt. Hugo Ortiz Garcés on the 17th Anniversary of His Death," *El Comercio* (Quito), August 3, 1958. See also *ibid.*, August 4, 1958, for an account of the formation of a committee to erect a monument to Captain Edmundo Chiriboga, "a hero from Riobamba, who fell in 1941, defending Ecuadoran integrity."

43. See, for example, the full-page advertisement by the Ecuadoran government in New York *Times*, January 10, 1962. See also, among

others, the debate between Ambassador Homero Viteri Lafronte, for Ecuador, and Peruvian Chargé Marco García Arrese, in Viteri Lafronte, *El Ecuador y su salida propia al Marañón.*

44. See Ecuador, Ministerio de Relaciones Exteriores, *El Protocolo de Río de Janeiro de 1942 es nulo.* See also New York *Times,* September 2, 1960.

45. *El Ecuador exhibe ante el mundo la justicia de su causa: Octubre de 1960.* This pamphlet contains texts of statements by the Ecuadoran Foreign Minister, Dr. José R. Chiriboga Villagómez, and the Peruvian representative to the United Nations, Dr. Victor Andrés Belaunde, delivered in the General Assembly of the United Nations, September 29, 1960. For English text, see United Nations, General Assembly, *Official Records,* September 29, 1960, pp. 242–46, 259–60.

46. Text of note by the government of the United States and those of Argentina, Brazil, and Chile, in New York *Times,* December 19, 1960.

47. Full-page advertisement by the government of Peru in the New York *Times,* January 5, 1956.

48. Barra, *Tumbes, Jaén y Maynas,* p. 50.

49. This is of interest not only because of Alberto Ulloa's hopes that the Salomón-Lozano Treaty might be changed to Peru's advantage but because, in 1940, it seemed likely that the Leticia question was the most dangerous issue among American states. See Whitaker, *Inter-American Affairs, 1942.*

50. Conversation, July, 1962. Peruvian generosity would presumably not have to go further than giving Ecuador a "position" on the Marañón at the mouth of the Santiago or Zamora; Ecuador's reasonableness would involve the relinquishment of the claims to Iquitos and other areas included, for example, in the maps on its special series of postage stamps issued on February 27, 1961. Such a settlement has actually been proposed by an Ecuadoran diplomat. See Quevedo, *Sobre la política externa ecuatoriana en la post-guerra,* p. 70.

Part Four. Solicitude in Anarchy

Full bibliographical information about the works cited will be found in the General section of the Bibliography.

XIII. Anarchy in the Americas

1. There are some interesting similarities between the American states in this period and what E. E. Evans-Pritchard calls the "ordered anarchy" of the Nuer people in the Southern Sudan. Fortes and Evans-Pritchard, *African Political Systems.*

2. FR, 1932, V, 169.

3. See *El Premio Nobel de la Paz y el Dr. Miguel Angel Araujo, ministro de relaciones exteriores.*

4. Letter of January 12, 1933, from President Trujillo to the Nobel Committee in *Listín Diario* (Santo Domingo), February 8, 1933.

5. República Dominicana, Secretaría de Estado de Relaciones Exteriores, *Candidatura de su Excelencia el Generalísimo Doctor Rafael L. Trujillo Molina . . . para el Premio Nobel de la Paz.*

6. The existence of this personal rivalry did not go unrecognized at the time. *El Liberal* (Asunción) on April 13, 1935, expressed the opinion that the war in the Chaco would have come to an end earlier if foreign ministers had given more attention to the real problems of peace than to minor quarrels about the identity of the individuals receiving credit for peace initiatives. It was reported from Rio de Janeiro that a Latin American diplomat had expressed the view that "there were ulterior motives behind the exaggerated anxiety with which certain Ministers for Foreign Affairs were attempting to obtain peace in the Chaco, such as promotion of their own political future, Nobel prizes, etc." Despatch 640, from Rio de Janeiro, April 17, 1935. DS, 724.3415/4817. Julio A. Noble, a journalist and former member of the Argentine Congress, wrote in 1940 that the Nobel Peace Prize "had for three years impeded the pacification of the Chaco, by arousing the rivalry of the chancellors of the A.B.C. powers who were acting as peacemakers." *Argentina Libre* (Buenos Aires), September 12, 1940.

7. Dearing wrote to Roosevelt on March 4, 1935: "The Chilean Ambassador here tells me the causes of the feeling between Alessandri [President of Chile] and Saavedra Lamas is the fact that Chile gave her vote for Mello Franco for the Nobel Peace Prize which Saavedra Lamas covets for himself; that thus Saavedra Lamas waits the moment when he can settle the Chaco dispute as a personal performance. In short, human vanity." See also Dearing's letter to Roosevelt of May 27, 1935. FDRL, PSF, Box 20.

8. Compare the remark of the Foreign Minister of Ecuador in 1937 that he would probably "be stoned by his own people" if he made a concession in the Marañón dispute.

XIV. The Policy of the United States

1. Memorandum of conversation between the Assistant Secretary of State and the Peruvian Ambassador, October 31, 1932. FR, 1932, V, 288.

2. Stimson and Bundy, *On Active Service in Peace and War*, p. 185 and diary entry of November 11, 1932.

3. Hull, *Memoirs*, I, 309, 311.

4. Hugh Gibson had said of Mello Franco in the Leticia affair that "it was largely on account of his patience, tact and resourcefulness that any agreement was concluded." Despatch 277, from Rio de Janeiro, June 1, 1934. FR, 1934, IV, 361. On this point, see the less fulsome comments by Alfonso Reyes, in *La conferencia colombo-peruana para el arreglo del incidente de Leticia* (México, D.F., Imp. Barrie, 1947).

5. This request was preceded by effusive praise for the good neighbor

policy by Saavedra Lamas in an interview on January 23, 1936, just three days before his request to Hull was made. Text attached to letter from Welles to Roosevelt, January 27, 1936. FDRL, PSF, Box 1.

6. Braden reported the Saavedra Lamas request but noted that he stated his belief that "it is counter to our policy directly to propose anyone and that we have declined to do so in meritorious analogous cases when such action on our part has been requested (having in mind Mello Franco candidacy last year)." Telegram 11, from Buenos Aires, January 27, 1936. DS, 093.57 N 66/277.

7. Hull, *Memoirs*, I, 329. Hull's other reference is: "In 1936, I championed the candidacy of Dr. Saavedra Lamas, the Argentine Foreign Minister. This was successful." *Ibid.*, II, 1724. In 1937, Saavedra Lamas proposed Hull's name. Hull received the prize in 1945.

8. *Ibid.*, I, 322, 328–29. Hull noted that after his reference to another person "Saavedra Lamas was becoming more cordial, more interested" (p. 329).

9. *Ibid.*, I, 499.

10. The Argentine Anti-War Pact, initiated by Saavedra Lamas, was signed by Hull at Montevideo as a kind of bargain. "I believed that, if we could make a friend of Saavedra Lamas at Montevideo and at the same time get him to sign the Kellogg Pact we could well sign his Anti-War Pact." *Ibid.*, I, 322. This Anti-War Pact was never utilized in the solution of any conflict.

11. English text in Despatch 337, from Oslo, December 16, 1936. DS, 093.57 N 66/300.

12. Mello Franco was also a candidate in 1936, but the then Foreign Minister of Brazil, José Carlos de Macedo Soares, had had himself nominated by Brazil for the Prize. In the view of at least one well-informed Brazilian diplomat, Mauricio Nabuco, this evidence of indecision in Rio de Janeiro was a significant factor in the selection of Saavedra Lamas, since there appeared to be in Oslo a sentiment that it was time for a "non-European Latin" to receive the Prize, and there was certainly no doubt as to the Argentine claimant. Conversation, August, 1962. If Mello Franco, however, were to be preferred to Saavedra Lames as a Nobel candidate, there would still be dissenting voices. Olaya remarked on the "mendacious position" of Mello Franco in January, 1933, when he had misrepresented the Colombian stand to the Peruvians in the hope of "pushing" a settlement. (See above, Chap. VII, notes 57 and 58). Olaya added: "Dr. Mello Franco seemed to fancy himself as a modern Machiavelli and was not to be trusted. He said that fortunately the presence of both Colombian and Peruvian representatives at the Rio de Janeiro Conference would make it more difficult for Dr. Mello Franco to befog the issue than was the case in any long distance negotiations but that it nevertheless behooved the Colombian delegates to be on their guard and he was so warning them." The Chargé in Colombia, Allan Dawson, added: "From my own personal acquaintance with Dr. Mello Franco I am convinced that one of the major factors in his personality is inordinate personal vanity. It seems possible that he aspires to go down in history as a counterpart of

his illustrious predecessors, Baron do Rio Branco and Dr. Lauro Müller. A similar tendency may be observed in other South American Foreign Ministers now holding office such as Señor Cruchaga . . . and, judging from newspaper reports, Dr. Saavedra Lamas." Despatch 5868, from Bogotá, September 26, 1933. DS, 721.23/1991.

13. Hull, *Memoirs*, I, 499.

14. There were other possible candidates in 1936. Roosevelt, in the same year, wrote of the Prize, that "no one deserves it more than Cordell and he should have had it this year instead of Saavedra Lamas." Memorandum for the Acting Secretary of State (R. Walton Moore), December 28, 1936, FDRL, PSF, Box 24. For Sumner Welles's account of ill will between Hull and Saavedra Lamas, see his *Seven Decisions That Shaped History*, pp. 104–5. Welles seems to have had a higher regard for Saavedra Lamas than for Hull, of whom he has written: "The truth is that Mr. Hull was devoid not only of any knowledge of Latin American history, but also of the language and culture of our American neighbors." *Ibid.*, p. 119. Welles called Lamas "one of the ablest statesmen produced in the Western Hemisphere in our generation . . . astute, forceful, tireless, and intolerant . . . eloquent, brilliant, and dictatorial." Welles, *The Time for Decision*, p. 207.

15. These and other quotations have been cited in texts of Parts I-III.

16. Sentiments similar to Olaya's were expressed later in Ecuador by *El Telégrafo* (Guayaquil), July 31, 1941, which declared that the principles of the good neighbor policy had been deceptions, "as has been also the belief that the United States would guard inter-American concord and protect the weak countries of the continent," which would now have to arm themselves. The statement on Olaya's anti-militarism is by Caffery (Despatch 4703, November 7, 1932. DS, 721.23/496).

17. It should be noted that this is an interpretation of the situation that is not accepted by Peruvian official circles. The Peruvian Ambassador in Washington, Fernando Berckmeyer, has stated that "Peru's role in this dispute was limited exclusively to defensive action of her territory, as was confirmed when in January of 1942 the Rio protocol was signed between the two countries and Peru was awarded these territories. This merely confirmed her historical and legal rights in this area, with the full concurrence and approval of all the American nations, including the United States." Letter to the editor of the New York *Times,* August 7, 1956. See New York *Times,* August 14, 1956, for reply of T. Alvarado Garaicoa, Ambassador of Ecuador.

Bibliography

THIS BIBLIOGRAPHY is not intended to be exhaustive on any of the three conflicts here discussed. The principal criterion for selection is relevance to problems of the foreign policy of the United States. For example, military histories have been listed only when they included material touching on diplomatic questions. The works on the Marañón, however, are more numerous than on the Chaco or Leticia, because accounts of the former cannot now be written from official records of any of the foreign offices concerned, while those of the United States are accessible on the other two. The books cited have been consulted, for the most part, in the Casa de la Cultura Ecuatoriana (Quito), the Columbus Memorial Library of the Pan American Union; the Hispanic Foundation of the Library of Congress; or the New York Public Library.

General

Clark, J. Reuben. *Memorandum on the Monroe Doctrine*. Washington, U.S. Government Printing Office, 1930.

Cooper, Russell M. *American Consultation in World Affairs*. New York, Macmillan, 1934.

Duggan, Laurence. *The Americas*. New York, Holt, 1949.

Fortes, M., and E. E. Evans-Pritchard. *African Political Systems*. London, Oxford University Press, 1940.

Fox, Annette Baker. *The Power of Small States*. Chicago, University of Chicago Press, 1959.

Herring, Hubert. *A History of Latin America*. 1st ed. New York, Knopf, 1961.

Hull, Cordell. *The Memoirs of Cordell Hull*. New York, Macmillan, 1948. 2 vols.

Ireland, Gordon. *Boundaries, Possessions, and Conflicts in South America*. Cambridge, Mass., Harvard University Press, 1938.

James, Preston E. *Latin America*. Rev. ed. New York, Odyssey Press, 1950.

Langer, William L., and S. Everett Gleason. *The Undeclared War, 1940–1941*. New York, Harper, 1953.

El Premio Nobel de la Paz y el Dr. Miguel Angel Araujo, Ministro de Relaciones Exteriores. San Salvador, Imp. Nacional, 1934.

Report of the Delegation of the United States of America to the Eighth International Conference of American States, Lima, Peru, December 9–27, 1938. Washington, U.S. Government Printing Office, 1941.

Report of the Delegate of the United States of America to the Meeting of the Foreign Ministers of the American Republics, Panamá, September 23–October 3, 1939. Washington, U.S. Government Printing Office, 1940.

República Dominicana. Secretaría de Estado de Relaciones Exteriores. *Candidatura de su Excelencia el Generalísimo Doctor Rafael L. Trujillo Molina . . . para el Premio Nobel de la Paz . . .* Santo Domingo, La Nación, 1935.

Roosevelt, Elliott, ed., assisted by Joseph P. Lash. *F. D. R. His Personal Letters, 1928–1945.* New York, Duell, Sloan and Pearce, 1950.

Royal Institute of International Affairs. *Survey of International Relations, 1936.* London, Oxford University Press, 1937.

Shepardson, Whitney H., and William O. Scroggs. *The United States in World Affairs, 1940.* New York, Harper, 1941.

Simmons, Ozzie G. "Lo 'criollo' en el marco de la cultura de la Costa Peruana," *Ciencias Sociales,* VI (April, 1955), 87–98.

Stimson, Henry L., and McGeorge Bundy. *On Active Service in Peace and War.* New York, Harper, 1947.

Walters, Francis Paul. *A History of the League of Nations.* New York, Oxford University Press, 1952. 2 vols.

Welles, Sumner. *Where Are We Heading?* New York, Harper, 1946.
—— *The Time for Decision.* New York, Harper, 1944.
—— *Seven Decisions That Shaped History.* New York, Harper, 1950.

Whitaker, Arthur P. *Inter-American Affairs, 1942.* New York, Columbia University Press, 1943.
—— *The Western Hemisphere Idea: Its Rise and Decline.* Ithaca, N.Y., Cornell University Press, 1954.

Wood, Bryce. *The Making of the Good Neighbor Policy.* New York, Columbia University Press, 1961.

The Chaco War

Scholars in the United States have given little attention to the Chaco conflict. The only book-length study, and a very useful one, is that by David H. Zook, Jr. Margaret La Foy's dissertation is confined to the ineffectual action by the League of Nations. Otherwise, a chapter in Russell M. Cooper's volume nearly completes the list, and at least one of the general texts on Latin American history ignores the conflict entirely.

Of works by Bolivians, Ayala Moreira's *Por que no ganamos la guerra del Chaco* is notable for its frankness and analysis of hard questions, and Saavedra's denunciation of the acceptance of what he called Saavedra

Lamas's deception of the Bolivian delegation in June, 1935, illuminates the diplomatic situation at the time. For formal history, Cardozo's *Paraguay independiente* illustrates one Paraguayan view of the war. However, because of party strife in Paraguay, and especially the interdiction of political activity by the Liberal Party, and the exile of its leaders, strange exercises in historiography have been indulged in by individuals associated with the present regime.

It cannot, of course, be denied that the war was won when Eusebio Ayala, a Liberal, was president of Paraguay. It can, however, be denied that Ayala and his Liberal predecessors adequately prepared the country for the conflict, and the volumes by González attempt to make this case. The case for the Liberals is presented in the study by Ríos. The principal diplomatic memoir is that by Rivarola, which is particularly significant for the light it gives on Argentine assistance to Paraguay. The Ramírez and Stefanich works are more partisan and less substantial than that of Rivarola.

Argaña, Luis A. *El tratado de paz, amistad y límites con la república de Bolivia, del 21 de julio de 1938.* Asunción, Imp. Nacional, 1938.

Argentina. Ministerio de Relaciones Exteriores y Culto. *La conferencia de paz del Chaco, Buenos Aires, 1935–1939 (Compilación de documentos).* Buenos Aires, Frigerio, 1939.

—— *La neutralidad argentina en el conflicto boliviano-paraguayo.* Buenos Aires, Peuser, 1933.

—— *La política argentina en la guerra del Chaco.* Buenos Aires, Kraft, 1937, 2 vols.

Artaza, Policarpo. *Ayala, Estigarribia y el Partido Liberal.* Buenos Aires, Ed. Ayacucho, 1946.

Ayala Moreira, Rogelio. *Por que no ganamos la guerra del Chaco.* La Paz, Tall. Gráf. Bolivianos, 1959.

Baldivia G., José María. *La guerra con el Paraguay y la diplomacia argentina.* La Paz, Imp. Eléctrica, 1934.

Baldrich, Alfonso. *El problema del petróleo y la guerra del Chaco.* Buenos Aires, Ed. de la "Revista Americana de Buenos Aires," 1934.

Braden, Spruille. "A Résumé of the Rôle Played by Arbitration in the Chaco Dispute," *The Arbitration Journal,* II (October, 1938), 387–95.

Cardozo, Efraim. *Paraguay independiente.* Vol. 21 of Antonio Ballesteros y Beretta, *Historia de América y los pueblos americanos.* Barcelona, Salvat, 1949.

The Chaco Peace Conference, Report of the Delegation of the United States of America to the Peace Conference Held at Buenos Aires, July 1, 1935–January 23, 1939. Washington, U.S. Government Printing Office, 1940.

Chaves, Julio César. *Compendio de historia paraguaya.* 3d ed. Buenos Aires, Tall. Gráf. Lumen, 1962.

Colle, Elio M. A. *El drama del Paraguay.* Buenos Aires, Ed. Claridad, 1936.

Bibliography 489

Cooper, Russell M. *American Consultation in World Affairs.* New York, Macmillan, 1934.

Díaz Arguedas, Julio. *Como fué derrocado el hombre símbolo: Salamanca.* La Paz, 1957.

Díaz Machicao, Porfirio. *Historia de Bolivia: Salamanca, la guerra del Chaco, Tejada Sorzano, 1931–1936.* La Paz, Gisbert, 1955. Vol. 3.

—— *Historia de Bolivia: Toro, Busch, Quintanilla, 1936–1940.* La Paz, Ed. Juventud, 1957.

Estigarribia, José Felix. *The Epic of the Chaco: Marshal Estigarribia's Memoirs of the Chaco War, 1932–1935,* ed. by Pablo Max Ynsfrán. Austin, University of Texas Press, 1950.

Finot, Enrique. *The Chaco Question: An Exposition for the College Students of America.* Washington, D.C., Bolivian Legation, 1934.

—— *The Chaco War and the United States.* New York, L. & S. Printing Co., 1934.

González, Antonio E. *La guerra del Chaco.* São Paulo, Tip. Cupolo, 1941.

—— *Preparación del Paraguay para la guerra del Chaco.* Asunción, Ed. El Gráfico, 1957. 2 vols.

Hudson, Manley O. *Munitions Industry: The Chaco Arms Embargo.* U.S. Senate, 74th Congress, 2d Session, Senate, Committee Print No. 9. Washington, D.C., U.S. Government Printing Office, 1936.

Hussey, Roland D. "[Review of] Harris Gaylord Warren, *Paraguay: An Informal History,*" *American Historical Review,* LV (October, 1949), 178.

Ireland, Gordon. *Boundaries, Possessions and Conflicts in South America.* Cambridge, Mass., Harvard University Press, 1938.

La Foy, Margaret. *The Chaco Dispute and the League of Nations.* Bryn Mawr, Pa., 1941.

Laconich, Marco Antonio. *El Paraguay mutilado.* Montevideo, Ed. Paraguay, 1939.

Larden, G. H. N. "Blindman's-Buff in the Chaco," *Journal of the Royal Artillery,* LXI (April, 1934), 32–48.

Macias, Silvio. *La guerra del Chaco.* Asunción, Ed. La Tribuna, 1942?.

Marchant, Alexander. *Boundaries of the Latin American Republics, an Annotated List of Documents, 1493–1943.* Washington, D.C., U.S. Dept. of State, Office of the Geographer, 1944.

Marof, Tristán (pseud. of Gustavo Adolfo Navarro). *La tragedia del altiplano.* Buenos Aires, Ed. Claridad, 1934.

Ortiz Pacheco, Nicolas. *La justicia contra el machete.* Replica al libro "Bajo el signo de marte," del Canciller Paraguayo Justo Pastor Benítez. La Paz, Ed. Renacimiento, 1935.

Ostria Gutierrez, Alberto. *La doctrina del no-reconocimiento de la conquista en América.* Rio de Janeiro, Borsoi, 1938.

—— *Una obra y un destino: La política internacional de Bolivia después de la guerra del Chaco.* 2d ed. Buenos Aires, Imp. López, 1953.

—— *The Tragedy of Bolivia: A People Crucified.* N.Y., Devin-Adair, 1938.

Paraguay—Bolivia: Aspectos de la guerra del Chaco. Asunción, Imp. Militar, 1934.

Pastor Benítez, Justo. *Bajo el signo de marte: Crónicas de la guerra del Chaco.* Montevideo, Imp. Uruguaya, 1934.

—— *Estigarribia, el soldado del Chaco.* 2d ed. Buenos Aires, Ed. Nizza, 1958.

El Premio Nobel de la Paz y el Dr. Miguel Angel Araujo, Ministro de Relaciones Exteriores. San Salvador, Imp. Nacional, 1934.

Prieto, Justo. *Eusebio Ayala, presidente de la victoria.* Buenos Aires, Ed. Ayacucho, 1950.

Raine, Philip. *Paraguay.* New Brunswick, N.J., Scarecrow Press, 1956.

Ramírez, J. Isidro. *La paz del Chaco: La defensa de la línea de hitos y el comité de tres.* Buenos Aires, Imp. Ferrari, 1942.

Ríos, Angel F. *La defensa del Chaco: Verdades y mentiras de una victoria.* Buenos Aires, Ed. Ayacucho, 1950.

Rivarola, Vicente. *Memorias diplomáticas.* Buenos Aires, Ed. Ayacucho, 1952–57. 3 vols.

Rodas Eguino, Justo. *La guerra del Chaco: Interpretación de política internacional americana.* Buenos Aires, Bernalíe, 1938.

Rodríguez, Angel. *Autopsía de una guerra (Campaña del Chaco).* Santiago de Chile, Ercilla, 1940.

Saavedra, Bautista. *El Chaco y la conferencia de paz de Buenos Aires.* Santiago de Chile, Nascimento, 1939.

Saavedra Lamas, Carlos. *Por la paz de las Américas.* Buenos Aires, Gleizer, 1937.

Salamanca, Daniel. *Archivo: Documentos para una historia de la guerra del Chaco.* Vol. I. Prefacio y notas de Eduardo Arze Quiroga. La Paz, Ed. Don Bosco, 1960.

Salmón Baldivieso, Luis. *El Paraguay provincia argentina.* La Paz, Imp. Artística-Ayacucho, 1935.

Stefanich, Juan. *Capítulos de la revolución paraguaya.* Buenos Aires, El Mundo Nuevo, 1946.

Terán Gómez, Luis. *Bolivia frente a los pueblos del Plata.* La Paz, Imp. Arnó Hnos., 1936.

Tolten, Hans. *Enchanting Wilderness.* London, Selwyn & Blount, 1936.

Toro Ruilova, David. *Mi actuación en la guerra del Chaco (La retirada de Picuiba).* La Paz, Ed. Renacimiento, 1941.

Tovar Villa, Raul. *Campaña del Chaco: El General Hans Kundt.* La Paz, Ed. Don Bosco, 1961.

Ulloa y Sotomayor, Alberto. *Habla un maestro de derecho internacional: "El Paraguay ha sido el agresor. . . ."* Lima, Edición de la Legación de Bolivia en el Perú, 1930?.

Urioste, Ovidio. *La encrucijada: estudio histórico, político, sociológico, y militar de la guerra del Chaco.* Cochabamba, Ed. Canelas, 1942?.

—— *Mi historia anecdótica de Bolivia.* Sucre, América, 1948?.

Vergara Vicuña, Aquiles. *La guerra del Chaco.* La Paz, Lit. e Imp. Unidas, 1940–44. 7 vols.

Warren, Harris Gaylord. *Paraguay: An Informal History.* Norman, Okla., University of Oklahoma Press, 1949.
—— "Political Aspects of the Paraguayan Revolution, 1936–1940," *Hispanic American Historical Review*, XXX (February, 1950), 2–25.
Wewege-Smith, T. *War Planes and Women.* London, Hutchinson, 1938.
Zook, David H., Jr. *The Conduct of the Chaco War.* New York, Bookman Associates, 1960.

Leticia

For this study, the most important of the books listed below are the following: the work by Chocano, a significant defense by a Peruvian of the Salomón-Lozano treaty; the collection of documents and other materials by Lozano Torrijos; the apologia for the treaty of 1916 between Ecuador and Colombia by Muñoz Vernaza; the highly personal memoir of the Rio de Janeiro conference of 1934 by Alfonso Reyes; and the very formal statements of the Peruvian position by Alberto Ulloa. Regrettably, the long work by Raimundo Rivas deals mainly with the period before 1915 and has little light to shed on the treaties of 1916 and 1922, which are important for the Leticia affair; the Colombian position is more adequately stated by Cavelier. Other works listed may, of course, be useful for other purposes.

Alayza y Paz Soldán, Luis. *Mi País: Algo de la Amazonía Peruana.* Lima, Lib. Gil, 1960.
Ballon Landa, Alberto. *El sentido humano de nuestra defensa en la contienda con Colombia.* Lima, Imp. Escuela de la Guardia Civil y Policía, 1933.
Barros, Jayme de. *Ocho años de política exterior del Brasil.* Rio de Janeiro, D.N.P., 1938.
Boy, Herbert. *Una historia con alas.* Madrid, Ed. Guadarrama, 1955.
Cabeza de Vaca, Manuel. *La posición del Ecuador en el conflicto colombo-peruano.* Quito, Tall. Gráf. Nacionales, 1934.
Cano, Luis. *Semblanzas y editoriales.* Bogotá, Ed. Minerva, 1936.
Casas, Gaspar de las. *Un scandale diplomatique: Le traité Salomón-Lozano.* Paris, Bellenand, 1933.
Cavelier, Germán. *La política internacional de Colombia.* Vol. 3: 1903–1959. 2d ed. Bogotá, Ed. Iqueima, 1960.
Chocano, José Santos. *El escándalo de Leticia ante las conferencias de Río de Janeiro.* Santiago de Chile, Tall. Gráf. de "La Nación," 1933.
Colombia. Consulate General. *International Opinion and the Leticia Controversy.* Washington, D.C., Colombian Legation, 1933.
Colombia. Legación, España. *La obra de Colombia en su territorio amazónico.* Madrid, Ernesto Giménez, 1932.
—— *Un gran triunfo de Colombia. Documentos publicados por la legación de Colombia en España.* Madrid, Imp. Juan Pueyo, 1933.

492   Bibliography

Colombia. Legación, México. *Información sobre el actual conflicto entre Colombia y el Perú*. México, D.F., 1932.

Colombia. Oficina de Longitudes y Fronteras. *Arreglo de límites entre la república de Colombia y la república del Perú*. Bogotá, Ed. de la Lit. Colombia, 194(

—— *Arreglo de límites entre la república de Colombia y la república del Ecuador*. Bogotá, Ed. de la Lit. Colombia, 1941.

Colombia. Ministerio de Relaciones Exteriores. *El conflicto de Leticia*. 2d ed. Bogotá, Imp. Nacional, 1934.

Corrêa da Costa, Sérgio. *A diplomacia brasileira na questão de Leticia*. Preface by Afranio de Mello Franco. Rio de Janeiro, Imp. Nacional, 1942.

"La cuestión de Leticia," *Boletín de la Sociedad Geográfica de Lima*, LI (1934), 87–242.

Documentos sobre el protocolo de Río de Janeiro. Bogotá, Imp. Nacional, 1934.

Ferrell, Robert. *Frank B. Kellogg—Henry L. Stimson*. New York, Cooper Square, 1963.

Gálvez, Juan Ignacio. *Conflictos internacionales: El Perú contra Colombia, Ecuador y Chile*. Santiago de Chile, Soc. Imp. y Lit. Universo, 1919.

League of Nations. Council. *The Verdict of the League: Colombia and Peru at Leticia*. Notes and Introduction by Manley O. Hudson. Boston, World Peace Foundation, 1933.

López, Jacinto. *Los tratados de límites y la paz internacional americana: El tratado secreto de 1922 entre Colombia y el Perú*. New York, 1932.

López, Nicolás F. *Estudios internacionales sobre el conflicto colombo-peruana*. Quito, Tall. Gráf. Nacionales, 1934.

Lozano Torrijos, Fabio. *El tratado Lozano-Salomón*. México. D.F., Ed. Cultura, 1934.

Lozano y Lozano, Fabio. *El punto de vista colombiano en la cuestión de Leticia*. México, D.F., A. Mijares y Hno., 1933.

Lozano y Lozano, Juan. *La patria y yo*. Bogotá, Colección Antologías de "Sabado," 1933.

Malta, Aguilera. *Leticia*. Panamá, Benedette, 1932.

Martínez Landínez, Jorge. *Historia militar de Colombia*. Vol. I. Bogotá, Ed. Iqueima, 1956.

Miró Quesada Laos, Carlos. *Sánchez Cerro y su tiempo*. Buenos Aires, Ateneo, 1947.

Muñoz Vernaza, Alberto. *Exposición sobre el tratado de límites de 1916 entre el Ecuador y Colombia y análisis jurídico del tratado de límites de 1922 entre Colombia y el Perú*. Quito, Tall. Tip. de *El Comercio*, 1928.

Pérez Ayala, José Manuel. *Colombia en el Amazonas*. Barcelona, Imp. NACSA, 1933.

Pérez Serrano, Jorge. *El tercero en la discordia*. Quito, Imp. Universidad Central, 1936.

Reyes, Alfonso. *La conferencia colombo-peruana para Río de Janeiro*,

25 de octubre de 1933 a 24 de mayo de 1934, el arreglo del incidente de Leticia. México, D.F., Imp. Barrie, 1947.

Rivas, Raimundo. *Historia diplomática de Colombia, 1810–1934.* Bogotá, Imp. Nacional, 1961.

San Cristoval, Evaristo. *Páginas internacionales: Antecedentes diplomáticas del tratado Salomón-Lozano.* 2d ed. Lima, Gil, 1932.

Ugarteche, Pedro. *Documentos que acusan: El tratado Salomón-Lozano.* Lima, Lit. Tip. Estanco del Tabaco, 1933.

Ulloa, Alberto. *Posición internacional del Perú.* Lima, Imp. Torres Aguirre, 1941.

Uribe, Antonio José. *Colombia: Las cuestiones de límites y de libre navegación fluvial.* Bogotá, Ed. Minerva, 1931.

Uribe Gaviría, Carlos. *La verdad sobre la guerra.* Bogotá, Ed. Cromos, 1935–36. 2 vols.

Valcarcel, Carlos A. *Crítica del tratado Salomón-Lozano.* Lima, Imp. Lux, 1931.

Vallejo, José A. *Datos para la historia: El conflicto Perú-colombiano. Charlas militares.* Vol. I. Lima, 1934.

Valverde, Carlos A. *Por la paz de América: El tratado de límites Salomón-Lozano entre el Perú y Colombia: La actitud del Ecuador.* Lima, Tall. La Prensa, 1928.

Vasconez, Pablo Alfonso. *La cuestión tetruple.* Quito, Ed. Artes Gráficas, 1933.

Villegas, Silvio. *De Ginebra a Río de Janeiro.* Bogotá, Ed. Santafé, 1934?.

Woolsey, L. H. *The Destruction of the Colombian Legation at Lima, Peru, February 18, 1933: A Disgrace to History.* Washington, Legation of Colombia, 1933.

Marañón

The best account in English of the antecedents of the Marañón conflict is the volume by David H. Zook, Jr., which includes translations of the texts of eleven documents from the treaty of 1822 to the Protocol of 1942. Of Ecuadoran publications, those of Julio Tobar Donoso and of Manuel Cabeza de Vaca are the most useful for scholarly purposes. On the Peruvian side, the works of Alberto Ulloa and Felipe de la Barra's *Tumbes, Jaén y Maynas* are the most significant. Polemical works are numerous, notably those by Ecuadorans who attack not only Peru but also the United States, the "inter-American system," and the responsible Ecuadoran officials in 1941–42.

Peruvians have been reticent; the "problem" is minimized, and, since the result of the conflict was nearly unanimously accepted as a victory in Peru, no partisan advantage could be gained by attacking anyone for not having secured even more territory. General Ureta has retired, and Prado is in exile. The mood in Peru is, therefore, one of quietude, since the settlement rests on a formally completed treaty, reaffirmed by powerful guarantors, and, in addition, evident and increasing Peruvian military superiority over Ecuador. These factors inhibit literary efforts either by diplomats or historians in Peru, and it may well be a fairly long time before de la Barra's semi-official statement is supplemented.

Alomía, Antonio. *La defensa del oriente ecuatoriano.* Quito, Tall. Gráf. Nacionales, 1936.

Alvarado, Rafael. *Demarcación de fronteras.* Quito, Tall. Gráf. de Educación, 1942.

—— *La elocuencia de las cifras en el problema territorial ecuatoriano-peruano.* Quito, Tall. Gráf. de Educación, 1941.

—— *Memorandum sobre el problema fronterizo entre el Ecuador y el Perú en el sector Lagartococha-Güepi.* Quito, Imp. de la Universidad, 1948.

—— *El protocolo de Río de Janeiro: Lo que garantizaron las potencias garantes.* Quito, Casa de la Cultura Ecuatoriana, 1961.

Alvarado Garaicoa, Teodoro. *La demarcación territorial ecuatoriana a través de cédulas reales, protocolos y tratados.* Guayaquil, Imp. Casa de la Cultura Ecuatoriana, 1939.

—— *Sinopsis del derecho territorial ecuatoriano.* Guayaquil, Ed. Cervantes, 1952.

Andrade S., Francisco. "Límites entre Colombia y Ecuador," *Boletín de Historia y Antigüedades* (Bogotá), XLVII (March–April, 1961), 201–19.

Arroyo del Río, Carlos A. *Bajo el imperio del odio: Las sanciones en el Ecuador.* 1st Part, Vol. I. Bogotá, Ed. El Gráfico, 1946.

—— *En plena vorágine: Etapa trágico-cómica.* Bogotá, Ed. El Gráfico, 1948.

Barra, Felipe de la. *Historiografía general y militar peruana y archivos: Introducción al catálogo del archivo histórico militar del Perú.* Lima, Tall. Gráf. Diet, 1962.

—— *Tumbes, Jaén y Maynas: Estudio integral de la controversia limítrofe peruano-ecuatoriana hasta el pacto de Río de Janeiro y su renuencia por el país del norte, con sinopsis histórica de las operaciones militares en 1941 y conteniendo tres mapas.* Lima, Centro de Estudios Históricos Militares del Perú, 1961.

Basadre, Jorge. *La promesa de la vida peruana.* Lima, Mejía Baca, 1958.

Belaunde, Víctor Andrés. Speech in General Debate, United Nations, General Assembly, 15th Session, *Official Records,* 878th Plenary Meeting, Sept. 29, 1960, pp. 244–46, 260.

—— *La vida internacional del Perú: Tomo I, Relaciones con el Ecuador: La constitución inicial del Perú ante el derecho internacional.* Lima, Imp. Torres Aguirre, 1942.

Bowman, Isaiah, "The Ecuador-Peru Boundary Dispute," *Foreign Affairs,* XX (July, 1942), 757–61.

Bravomalo R., Vicente G. *Crisanto Díaz.* Quito, Casa de la Cultura Ecuatoriana, 1944.

Cabeza de Vaca, Manuel. *Aspectos históricos y jurídicos de la cuestión limítrofe: Las negociaciones en Washington y los desenvolvimientos posteriores.* Quito, Tall. Gráf. Nacionales, 1956.

Cano, Washington. *Historia de los límites del Perú.* Lima, Ed. Colegio Militar Leoncio Prado, 1962.

Carlos A. Arroyo del Río, apóstol del panamericanismo: Reseña de la histórica visita de confraternidad realizada a través de seis naciones de América, del 16 de noviembre al 16 de diciembre de 1942. Preface by Thos. J. Watson. New York?, International Business Machines Corp., 1943.

Cavero-Egusquiza, Ricardo. *La amazonía peruana.* Lima, Imp. Torres Aguirre, 1941.

Chang Laos, Consuelo. *El Perú y sus hombres a través de la república.* Lima, 1960?.

Chico Peñaherrera, Rafael. *El principio de la intangibilidad de los tratados y el protocolo de Río de Janeiro.* Cuenca, Casa de la Cultura Ecuatoriana, Núcleo de Azuay, 1960.

Chiriboga Ordóñez, Leonardo. *¿Pudo el Ecuador ser agresor en 1941? Verdades para la historia de Sud-América.* Quito, La Prensa Católica, 1952.

—— *Sepultureros de la patria: Enjuiciamiento de las responsabilidades.* Quito, 1945.

Chiriboga Villagómez, José R. Speech in General Debate, United Nations, General Assembly, 15th Session, *Official Records,* 878th Plenary Meeting, Sept. 29, 1960, pp. 238–44, 259–60.

Comité Ejecutivo Nacional pro Monumento a las Campañas de 1941. *Exposición.* Lima, 1945.

Concha Enríquez, Pedro. *Sanción 1941–1942: Trágica etapa gubernamental ecuatoriana.* Quito, Imp. Fernández, 1945.

Cravioto, Adrian. *La paz de América: Ecuador y su derecho.* Quito, Imp. del Ministerio de Gobierno, 1941.

Crespo Ordóñez, Roberto. *El descubrimiento del Amazonas y los derechos territoriales del Ecuador.* Cuenca, Núcleo del Azuay de la Casa de la Cultura Ecuatoriana, 1961.

Cuestión de límites entre el Perú y el Ecuador: Reseña histórica desde 1910. Lima, Ed. Lumen, 1936.

Dictámenes de insignes internacionalistas: Cabe el enjuiciamiento del Dr. Julio Tobar Donoso, por haber suscrito el Protocolo de Río de Janeiro. Quito, Empresa Editora "El Comercio," 1944.

Ecuador. Corte Suprema de Justicia. *Manifiesto.* Quito, 1960.

Ecuador. Ministerio de Relaciones Exteriores. *Dictámenes jurídicos acerca del problema ecuatoriano-peruano dados por ilustres internacionalistas americanos.* Quito, Ed. del Departamento de Prensa y Publicaciones, Imp. del Ministerio de Gobierno, 1942. 2 vols.

—— *Exposición del ministro de relaciones exteriores del Ecuador a las cancillerías de América: Problema territorial ecuatoriano-peruano.* 2d ed. Quito, July, 1941.

—— *Informe del Ministro de Relaciones Exteriores a la Nación, 1941–1942.* Quito Tall. Gráf. de Educación, 1942.

—— *Informe a la nación: Junio de 1951.* Quito, Tall. Gráf. Minerva, 1951.

—— *Las negociaciones ecuatoriano-peruanas en Washington Sept. 1936–July 1937.* Quito, Imp. Ministerio de Gobierno, 1937.

496 *Bibliography*

—— *Problema territorial ecuatoriano-peruano: Exposición del ministerio de relaciones exteriores del Ecuador a las cancillerías de América.* 2d ed. Quito, Imp. del Ministerio de Gobierno, 1941.

—— *El protocolo de Río de Janeiro de 1942 es nulo—de acuerdo con el sistema jurídico interamericano y con el derecho internacional.* Quito, Casa de la Cultura Ecuatoriana, 1960.

Ecuador: Nociones históricas—geografía física y antrópica. Guayaquil, Cartografía del Prof. J. Morales y Eloy, 1938.

El Ecuador exhibe ante el mundo la justicia de su causa: Octubre de 1960. Quito, Casa de la Cultura Ecuatoriana, 1960.

Ecuadorean Ex-President Velasco Ibarra Passes Judgement on the Aggressive Policy of Ecuador. Lima, Bureau of the Press of de [*sic*] Ministry of Foreign Affairs of Peru, 1941.

Efrén Reyes, Oscar. *Breve historia general del Ecuador.* Quito, Tall. Gráf. de Ed. Fray Jodoco Ricke, 1960. 3 vols.

Eguiguren, Luis Antonio. *Apuntes sobre la cuestión internacional entre el Perú y Ecuador. Part I, Maynas.* Lima, Imp. Torres Aguirre, 1941.

—— *Notes on the Territorial Question between Peru and Ecuador. Part II, Invincible Jaén.* Lima, Imp. Torres Aguirre, 1943.

El Excelentísimo Sr. Dr. Dn. Manuel Prado, Presidente del Perú, Reseña de su visita a los Estados Unidos, del 6 al 21 de mayo de 1942. Preface by Thos. J. Watson. New York?, International Business Machines Corp., 1942.

Exposition of the Minister of Foreign Affairs of Perú, Dr. Alfredo Solf y Muro, to the Governments of America. Lima, Bureau of the Press, Ministry of Foreign Affairs, 1941.

Exposición del Señor Ministro de Relaciones Exteriores ante el H. Congreso Nacional (Sept. 15, 1960). Versión taquigráfica. Quito, Tall. Graf., Nacionales, 1960.

Flores, Pastoriza. *The History of the Boundary Dispute between Ecuador and Peru.* New York, 1921.

Gallardo Nieto, Galvarino. *La conferencia de Río de Janeiro de 1942.* Santiago, Chile, Imp. Nascimento, 1942.

Gallegos B., Luis Gerardo. *Defendiendo a la patria.* Riobamba, Ed. Siembra, 1945.

García Arrese, Marco. "El Marañón Peruano," Casa de la Cultura Ecuatoriana, *Revista,* No. 12 (January–December, 1952), pp. 22–40.

García Rendón, Godofredo. *El protocolo de paz, amistad y límites entre Perú y Ecuador de 1942 ante el derecho internacional.* Lima, 1963.

García Velasco, Rafael. "El arbitraje de límites entre el Ecuador y Perú ante el rey de España," Universidad Central del Ecuador, *Anales,* 87:342 (March 18, 1958), 111–47.

Herring, Hubert. *A History of Latin America.* New York, Knopf, 1963.

Humberto Delgado, Luis. *Las guerras del Perú: Campaña del Ecuador—grandeza y miseria de la victoria.* Vol. I. Lima, Imp. Torres Aguirre, 1944.

Instituto Ecuatoriano de Estudios del Amazonas. *Manifiesto que el Instituto Ecuatoriano de Estudios del Amazonas dirige a las naciones de*

América: Hácia la efectiva solidaridad de América. Quito, Tall. Gráf. de Educación, 1941.
Jaramillo Alvarado, Pio. *Ecuador, nación amazónica.* Quito, Ed. Vicente Rocafuerte, 1940.
—— *Estudios históricos.* Quito, Casa de la Cultura Ecuatoriana, 1960.
—— *La guerra de conquista en América.* Guayaquil, Ed. Jouvin, 1941.
—— *La nación quiteña: Perfil biográfico de una cultura.* Quito, Casa de la Cultura Ecuatoriana, 1958.
—— *Los tratados con Colombia.* Quito, Imp. de la Universidad Central, 1925.
Jiménez Molinares, Gabriel, and Cenón Muñoz. *Los manumisos contra sus libertadores. (Cuestión colombo-peruana).* Cartagena, Imp. Departamental, 1934.
Linke, Lilo. *Ecuador: Country of Contrasts.* 3d ed. New York, Oxford, 1960.
El litigio territorial entre el Ecuador y el Perú. El protocolo de Río de Janeiro, su origen y sus consecuencias. Polémica entre los embajadores del Ecuador y del Perú [Antonio Parra Velasco, Ecuador; Eduardo Garland, Perú]. Caracas, Ancora, 1953.
Loaiza, Lautaro V. *Interpretación lógica del protocolo de Río de Janeiro: Penetraciones peruanas que la contrarían.* Quito, Imp. del Ministerio de Gobierno, 1942.
López, Nicolás F. *Estudios internacionales sobre el conflicto colombo-peruano.* Quito, Tall. Gráf. Nacionales, 1934.
López Rodríguez, Demetrio. *Los castillos de la frontera.* Quito, Ed. Fray Jodoco Ricke, 1954.
Mac-Lean y Estenós, Roberto. *El litigio limítrofe peruano-ecuatoriano.* Publicación autorizada por la Cámara de Diputados, a pedido de su Comisión Diplomática. Lima, Cía. de Impresiones y Publicidad, 1941.
Marín, Rufino. *Ecuador la gran mutilada.* Quito, Ed. Universitaria, 1959.
—— *Las tres bombas de tiempo en América.* 2d ed. Quito, Ed. Universitaria, 1959.
Martínez Acosta, Galo. *Ecuador: país amazónico.* Quito, Imp. Inst. Nac. Mejía, 1961.
Miró Quesada Laos, Carlos. *Ficción y realidad del Ecuador y otras cinco conferencias.* Lima, Tip. Peruana, 1942.
Muller, Richard. *The Frontier Problem between Ecuador and Peru and the Official Map of Peru of 1826.* Guayaquil, Ed. Jouvin, 1937.
Muñoz, Julio H. *La campaña internacional de 1941.* Quito, Ed. Ecuatoriana, 1945.
Owens, R. J. *Peru.* New York, Oxford, 1963.
P. B., R. (probably Raul Porras Barrenechea). *El litigio peru-ecuatoriano ante los principios jurídicos americanos.* Lima, 1942.
Palacios Bravo, M. M. *La invasión peruana y el protocolo de Río de Janeiro.* Cuenca, Casa de la Cultura Ecuatoriana, Núcleo de Azuay, 1946.
Pareja Paz Soldán, José. *Geografía del Perú.* Lima, Lib. Bil, 1937.
Patch, Richard W. "Bolivia: The Restrained Revolution," American

498 *Bibliography*

Academy of Political and Social Science, *Annals*, CCCXXXIV (March 1961), 123-33.

Pérez Concha, Jorge. *Ensayo histórico-crítico de las relaciones diplomáticas del Ecuador con los estados limítrofes.* Quito, Casa de la Cultura Ecuatoriana, 1958-61. 2 vols.

—— *El protocolo de Río de Janeiro y los problemas derivados de su ejecución.* Guayas, Casa de la Cultura Ecuatoriana, Núcleo de Guayas, 1954.

Peru. Bureau of the Press of de [*sic*] Ministry of Foreign Affairs of Peru. *Ecuadorean Ex-President Velasco Ibarra, Passes Judgement on the Aggressive Policy of Ecuador. Letter Addressed to President Arroyo del Río.* Lima, 1941.

—— Dirección de Informaciones. *La defensa de la peruanidad de Tumbes, Jaén y Mainas por el Presidente Prado.* Lima, Oficina de informaciones, 1941.

—— Ministerio de Relaciones Exteriores. *Cuestión de límites entre el Perú y el Ecuador. Exposición del Ministro de Relaciones Exteriores del Perú, Dr. Alfredo Solf y Muro, a las cancillerías de América.* Lima, 1941.

—— Ministerio de Relaciones Exteriores. *Memoria de Relaciones Exteriores, 28 de julio de 1955-28 de julio de 1956.* Lima, Tall. Gráf. Villanueva, 1956.

—— Presidente, 1939. *Mensaje presentado al Congreso, 1945.* Lima, 1945.

Pino Ycaza, Gabriel. *Derecho territorial ecuatoriano, 1493-1830.* Guayaquil, Imp. de la Universidad, 1946.

Porras Barrenechea, Raul. *Historia de los límites del Peru.* 2d ed. Lima, Lib. y Ed. Rosay, 1930. (See also P. B., R., and *El protocolo de Río de Janeiro ante la historia.*)

"The President of Ecuador in Washington," *Bulletin of the Pan American Union*, January 1943, pp. 17-22.

El protocolo de Río de Janeiro ante la historia. Lima, Sanmartí y Cía.?, 1942. [Probably compiled by the Propaganda Section, Ministry of Foreign Affairs, Raul Porras Barrenechea, director.]

Un protocolo viciado de nulidad. Editado por "Unión Interamericana de periodistas para la XI Conferencia de Quito." Quito, 1960.

Puente, Rafael A. *La mala fe peruana y los responsables del desastre de Zarumilla.* Quito, Ed. Espejo, 1961.

Quevedo, Antonio. *Sobre la política externa ecuatoriana en la postguerra.* (Speech in Central University, March 23, 1944.) Quito, Imp. de la Universidad, 1945.

Quevedo, Belisario. *Texto de historia patria.* Quito, Casa de la Cultura Ecuatoriana, 1959.

Reyes, Oscar E., and Francisco Terán. *Historia y geografía del Oriente ecuatoriano.* Quito, Tall. Gráf. de Educación, 1939.

Rodríguez S., L. A. *La agresión peruana: La campaña del Zarumilla documentada.* 2d ed. Quito, Ed. Fray Jodoco Ricke, 1955.

Romero, Emilio. *Por el norte: Ecuador.* Lima, Juan Mejía Baca & P. L. Villanueva, 1955.

Romero Terán, Domingo. *Los traidores al Ecuador.* Quito, Tall. Gráf. del Servicio de Suministros, 1952.

San Cristoval, Evaristo. *Bibliografía: La controversia limítrofe entre el Perú y el Ecuador.* Lima, Gil, 1937. Vol. I.

Santamaría, Julio H. *La tragedia internacional del Ecuador y sus responsables.* Quito, Imp. Mercantil, 1945.

Silva, Rafael Euclides. *Derecho territorial ecuatoriano.* Guayaquil, Universidad de Guayaquil, 1962.

Sociedad Bolivariana del Ecuador. *La revisión del protocolo de Río.* Quito, Imp. Colegio Técnico "Don Bosco," 1949.

Terán, Francisco. *Geografía del Ecuador.* 5th ed. Quito, 1959.

Tobar Donoso, Julio. *La invasión peruana y el protocolo de Río.* Quito, Ed. Ecuatoriana, 1945. (Referred to in the notes as Tobar.)

Tobar Donoso, Julio, and Alfredo Luna Tobar. *Derecho territorial ecuatoriano.* Quito, Ed. La Unión Católica, 1961.

Tudela, Francisco. *The Controversy between Peru and Ecuador.* Lima, Imp. Torres Aguirre, 1941. (Also published in Spanish.)

Ulloa, Alberto. *Perú y Ecuador: Ultima etapa del problema de límites, (1941–42). (Escritos publicados en "La Prensa" de Lima).* Lima, Imp. Torres Aguirre, 1942.

—— *El Perú y el mundo.* Lima, Ed. Relieves Americanos, 1943.

—— *Posición Internacional del Perú.* Lima, Imp. Torres Aguirre, 1941.

Vallejo, José A. *Datos para la historia: El conflicto perú-colombiano. Charlas militares.* Vol. I. Lima, 1934.

Venezuela. Congreso Nacional. *Sesión solemne celebrada el 25 de mayo 1942 en honor del excelentísimo Sr. Dr. Manuel Prado.* Caracas, Tip. Americana, 1942.

Villacres Moscoso, Jorge W. *La responsabilidad de la diplomacia ecuatoriana en la demarcación fronteriza.* Guayaquil, Imp. de la Universidad, 1945.

"Visit of the President of Peru to Washington," *Bulletin of the Pan American Union,* July, 1942, pp. 373–79.

Viteri Lafronte, Homero. *El Ecuador y su salida propia al Marañón.* Quito, Casa de la Cultura Ecuatoriana, 1952.

Whitaker, Arthur P., ed. *Inter-American Affairs 1942, An Annual Survey, No. 2.* N.Y., Columbia University Press, 1943.

Wright, L. A. "A Study of the Conflict between the Republics of Peru and Ecuador," *Geographical Journal,* XCVIII (December, 1941), 253–72.

Yepes, Jesus M. *La controversia fronteriza entre el Ecuador y el Perú.* Quito, Casa de la Cultura Ecuatoriana, 1960.

—— *I. El Ecuador: país amazónico; II. La nulidad absoluta del protocolo de Río de Janeiro y el panamericanismo.* Quito, Tall. Gráf. de Educación, 1961.

Zook, David H., Jr., *Zarumilla-Marañón: The Ecuador-Peru Dispute.* New York, Bookman Associates, 1964.

Index